W9-CBA-863

Hypertrophic Cardiomyopathy

Cardiomyopathy Update

Cardiomyopathy Update 2

Hypertrophic Cardiomyopathy

Editors:
Hironori Toshima, M.D. and Barry J. Maron, M.D.
Associate Editor:
Yoshinori Koga, M.D.

UNIVERSITY OF TOKYO PRESS

Published in association with the Japan Research Promotion
Society for Cardiovascular Diseases

In Cooperation with International Society and Federation of Cardiology

Published by University of Tokyo Press

ISBN 0-86008-436-1
ISBN 4-13-068130-3

Printed in Japan

Production of this book was supported by the promotion fund of the Japan Keirin Association.

Contents

Foreword

Preface

INTRODUCTION

Hypertrophic Cardiomyopathy : Historical Perspective, Nomenclature, and Definition ······ 3
B.J. Maron

PATHOLOGY

Gross Morphology and Light Microscopic Features of Hypertrophic Cardiomyopathy ······ 15
E.G.J. Olsen

Light and Electron Microscopic Features of Hypertrophic Cardiomyopathy ······ 27
V.J. Ferrans

Intramural Coronary Artery Disease in Hypertrophic Cardiomyopathy ······ 47
H. Fujiwara and C. Kawai

The Value of Endomyocardial Biopsy in Diagnosing Hypertrophic Cardiomyopathy ······ 59
M. Sekiguchi, S. Nunoda, and M. Hiroe

BASIC MECHANISMS FOR CARDIAC HYPERTROPHY

α_1-Adrenergic-Stimulated Hypertrophy in Neonatal Rat Heart Muscle Cells ······ 73
P.C. Simpson

Molecular Biological Aspects of Cardiac Hypertrophy ······ 97
Y. Yazaki, H. Tsuchimochi, I. Komuro, U. Kurabayashi, and F. Takaku

Physiologic and Pathologic Hypertrophy Produced by Chronic Norepinephrine Infusion ······ 113
M.M. Laks and W.J. Raum

SYMPATHETIC FUNCTION IN HYPERTROPHIC CARDIOMYOPATHY

Norepinephrine Kinetics in Hypertrophic Cardiomyopathy ······ 129
A.S. Maisel, M. Wright, K.D. Wilner, and M.G. Ziegler

Increased Cardiovascular Responses to Epinephrine and Norepinephrine in Patients with Hypertrophic Cardiomyopathy ··· 141
H. Toshima and Y. Koga

Autonomic Nervous Function in Hypertrophic Cardiomyopathy ··· 155
Y. Sugishita, K. Iida, and K. Yukisada

HEREDITY AND ENVIRONMENTAL FACTORS

Patterns of Inheritance and Progression of Left Ventricular Hypertrophy in Hypertrophic Cardiomyopathy ··· 171
B.J. Maron

HLA and Hypertrophic Cardiomyopathy ··· 187
A. Matsumori and C. Kawai

Genetic and Environmental Factors in Hypertrophic Cardiomyopathy ··· 193
M. Yamaguchi, K. Matsuyama, Y. Koga, M. Tsuruta, S. Matsuo, and H. Toshima

A Possible Role of Systemic Hypertension in the Pathogenesis of Hypertrophic Cardiomyopathy ··· 203
Y. Koga and H. Toshima

PATHOPHYSIOLOGICAL AND CLINICAL ASPECTS

Myocardial Ischemia in Hypertrophic Cardiomyopathy ··· 219
R.O. Cannon, III

Regional Myocardial Blood Flow and Metabolism at Rest and during Exercise in Hypertrophic Cardiomyopathy ··· 237
M. Grover-McKay, H.R. Schelbert, J.K. Perloff, and J. Krivokapich

Exercise Performance in Hypertrophic Cardiomyopathy ··· 251
B. Lösse and F. Loogen

Color Flow Mapping in Hypertrophic Cardiomyopathy ··· 271
S. Nagata, K. Miyatake, and Y. Nimura

Various Patterns of Left Ventricular Hypertrophy in Hypertrophic Cardiomyopathy ··· 283
H. Rakowski, Z. Sasson, P. Liu, and E.D. Wigle

Two Forms of Apical Hypertrophic Cardiomyopathy : Japanese and Western Forms ··· 293
Y. Koga, M. Nohara, Y. Miyazaki, and H. Toshima

INTRAVENTRICULAR PRESSURE GRADIENT

The Evidence for True Obstruction to Left Ventricular Outflow in Obstructive Hypertrophic Cardiomyopathy (Muscular or Hypertrophic Subaortic Stenosis) ··· 311
E.D. Wigle, B.P. Kimball, Z Sasson, and H. Rakowski

The Influence of the Brock Bias on Our Current Understanding of Hypertrophic Cardiomyopathy ······ 327
J.M. Criley, R.J. Siegel, and P.C.D. Pelikan

MANAGEMENT OF HYPERTROPHIC CARDIOMYOPATHY

The Management of Hypertrophic Cardiomyopathy Based on Symptoms, Natural History, and Prognosis ······ 335
J. F. Goodwin

Medical Treatment of Hypertrophic Cardiomyopathy : Influence on Outflow Obstruction and Filling Pressure ······ 343
R. Hopf and M. Kaltenbach

Diastolic Properties in Hypertrophic Cardiomyopathy and Its Modulation with Pharmacotherapy ······ 361
Y. Hirota

Medical Management of Supraventricular and Ventricular Arrhythmias in Patients with Hypertrophic Cardiomyopathy ······ 373
W. J. McKenna and M. P. Frenneaux

Keyword Index ······ 389

Foreword

Cardiomyopathies are defined as heart muscle diseases of unknown cause. Clinically they may become manifest as congestive heart failure, arrhythmias, conduction disturbances, embolic phenomena or sudden death. It is often difficult to determine the exact nature or mechanism of the disease process. In another group of diseases, referred to as specific heart muscle diseases, interaction between a general disease process and concomitant cardiac involvement is well recognized although the actual mechanisms are still ill understood.

An immense amount of scientific and clinical activity is being undertaken throughout the world, and contributory factors to pathogenetic mechanisms are slowly emerging, among which viruses, immunological idiosyncrasy and electrolytic imbalance may be cited. The role that alcohol may play is also being defined.

This annual monograph series, *Cardiomyopathy Update*, will cover all aspects of heart muscle diseases. Special care will be taken to include both clinical and basic research as well as day-to-day clinical cardiology. Topics, volume editors and authors will be selected by the series editors in close collaboration with the scientific committee and editorial board.

Publication of this series was proposed by Dr. Hiroto Yoshioka, Chairman of the Board of Trustees of the Japan Research Promotion Society for Cardiovascular Diseases, during the first International Symposium on Cardiomyopathy (ISCM), which was held in Tokyo in December 1984. We are greatly indebted to the society for its support, and to the International Society and Federation of Cardiology (ISFC) for its cooperation in effective scientific communication.

The series editors hope that these publications will provide a wealth of information not only from research but also from clinical work.

Morie Sekiguchi
Eckhardt G. J. Olsen

Preface

Numerous investigations during the last 30 years have led to a dramatic evolution in our understanding of hypertrophic cardiomyopathy since the first descriptions of this disease by Dr. Donald Teare and also Sir Russel Brock in 1958. However, hypertrophic cardiomyopathy has often been the subject of controversy, and the many different perceptions of the disease held by individual investigators are evidenced by the fact that about 75 different names or terms have been used to describe this clinical entity. In the early 1960s, investigators, primarily in North America and Europe, defined the clinical features of the disease and focused on functional obstruction to left ventricular outflow.

The advent of echocardiography in the 1970s enhanced our understanding of the broad clinical and pathologic spectrum of hypertrophic cardiomyopathy. Apical hypertrophic cardiomyopathy was subsequently reported from Japan by Sakamoto *et al.* and Yamaguchi *et al.*, as a morphologic variant of the disease in which hypertrophy is confined to the apical portion of the left ventricle.

Based on the observations of the past 30 years, it is now evident that hypertrophic cardiomyopathy is a condition of extreme diversity with regard to modes of development and disease progression, as well as patterns of left ventricular hypertrophy. While hypertrophic cardiomyopathy is often genetically transmitted, the basic underlying mechanism or pathogenesis for the left ventricular hypertrophy characteristic of this disease has not yet been elucidated. Therefore, we must confess in this regard that, as the proverb states, we are like blind men who touch only a part of an elephant and try to imagine what the whole animal is like.

The first volume of the *Cardiomyopathy Update Series* focused on the pathogenesis of myocarditis and dilated cardiomyopathy. The second and present volume is a state-of-the-art overview of hypertrophic cardiomyopathy. The editors have attempted to shed light on recent advances in molecular biological approaches to cardiac hypertrophy, as well as the genetic and environmental aspects of this complex and intriguing disease.

We wish to express our gratitude to Dr. Yoshinori Koga, the indefatigable Associate Editor, and to Ms. Etsuko Hamao and her associates at the University of Tokyo Press for their superb cooperation and dedication.

Kurume and Bethesda
August 1988

Hironori Toshima, M.D.
Barry J. Maron, M.D.

Preface

INTRODUCTION

Hypertrophic Cardiomyopathy: Historical Perspective, Nomenclature, and Definition

Barry J. Maron

Cardiology Branch, National Heart, Lung, and Blood Institute, National Institutes of Health, Bethesda, Maryland, U.S.A.

HISTORICAL PERSPECTIVE

Hypertrophic cardiomyopathy is a primary myocardial disease which is often genetically transmitted and is characterized by a diverse clinical, morphologic, and functional expression.[1–12] The disease is relatively uncommon and, while precise prevalence statistics are not readily available, the best estimate of its occurrence is probably about 0.1–0.2% of the general population.[13–15]

There is some uncertainty as to who should be credited with the first description of hypertrophic cardiomyopathy. French and German authors in the late 1800s and early 1900s described a total of four older patients with cardiac disease and gross anatomic findings at autopsy, which in retrospect may have represented early examples of hypertrophic cardiomyopathy.[16–19] These reports of Liouville,[16] Hallopeau,[17] and Schmincke[18] described hearts characterized by striking left ventricular hypertrophy; this hypertrophy appeared to the authors to be responsible for obstruction to left ventricular ejection. Also, the patients reported by Bernheim in 1910,[19] in whom a hypertrophied ventricular septum was described as bulging into the right ventricular cavity resulting in apparent impedance to right ventricular function, may have had hypertrophic cardiomyopathy. While in retrospect these papers contained important observations, none had any real impact on our future understanding of hypertrophic cardiomyopathy.

In 1952, Davies[20] described a patient having marked left ventricular hypertrophy and diffuse subaortic stenosis with a family history of sudden death. However, it was not until 1958 that the first systematic and unequivocal anatomic description of hypertrophic cardiomyopathy was published by Dr. Donald Teare in the British Heart Journal.[21] It was that paper which ultimately stimulated widespread interest in this "new" disease among cardiologists, pathologists, and surgeons.

Teare described a condition characterized by an asymmetric pattern of left ventricular hypertrophy and nondilated ventricular cavities. His novel observations were derived as part of his duties as Chief Coroner of the City of London and were based on the postmortem examinations of eight patients, seven of whom had died suddenly. The striking ventricular septal hypertrophy present in these patients was thought to represent a benign tumor or "hamartoma." A bizarre arrangement of muscle bundles and substantial variation in the size of cardiac muscle cells were described as prominent histologic features of both the septum and anterior free wall. Hence, in his report Teare documented several of the most important gross and histologic markers of hypertrophic cardiomyopathy as well as the occurrence of sudden death in this disease.

Published just three months before Teare's paper was the surgical description by Sir Russell Brock of a 63-year-old woman thought to have valvular aortic stenosis prior to surgery.[22] At operation, however, the aortic valve was normal and no mechanical or anatomic obstruction to left ventricular outflow could be identified. The patient died after operation, and a hypertrophied nondilated left ventricle was described at autopsy. These findings led Brock to conclude that his patient had experienced "functional" obstruction to left ventricular outflow that was due to the subaortic muscular hypertrophy which was thought itself to be secondary to the patient's systemic hypertension. Therefore, it seems justified to consider Brock's report as the first description of the functional (i.e., physiologic) nature of hypertrophic cardiomyopathy.

NOMENCLATURE

Numerous investigations into the nature of hypertrophic cardiomyopathy since the late 1950s[23] have led to a dramatic evolution of our understanding of the clinical and pathophysiologic spectrum of this disease. In the process, over 75 different names have been utilized in the literature to describe this clinical entity or subgroups of patients with the disease (Table 1). The multiplicity of descriptive terms given to hypertrophic cardiomyopathy has contributed to (and at the same time also reflected) the confusion that has periodically surrounded the disease during the past 30 years.

Initially, in the early 1960s, several centers in North America and Western Europe that were involved in the pioneering efforts at characterizing hypertrophic cardiomyopathy[24–33] understandably developed names for this newly discovered clinical entity based on those aspects of the disease that were most impressive to the individual investigator. Indeed, the confusion surrounding the nomenclature of hypertrophic cardiomyopathy seems largely related to the enormous clinical, functional, and morphologic diversity characteristic of this disease and the fact that only a few selected referral centers evaluate large numbers of patients with this particular condition. Hence, many investigators of hypertrophic cardiomyopathy have based their perceptions of the disease on a relatively small number of patients that may not be representative of the overall disease spectrum.

Table 1 shows that many names given to hypertrophic cardiomyopathy reflect only particular aspects of its diverse clinicopathologic expression, e.g., hemodynamic state, morphologic appearance, and familial predisposition. For example, in the 1960s the majority of names emphasized dynamic obstruction to left ventricular outflow.[22–28,30,31,33] Thus, while the terms idiopathic hypertrophic subaortic stenosis or IHSS (from the United States), hypertrophic obstructive cardiomyopathy or HOCM (from the United Kingdom), and muscular subaortic stenosis (from Canada) became widely used, they are, in fact, somewhat misleading as descriptive terms for the disease. This became evident in the 1970s when the application of echocardiography to the diagnosis of hypertrophic cardiomyopathy showed that the vast majority (about 75%) of those patients with this disease who are referred for evaluation to a major center actually have little or no evidence of obstruction to left ventricular outflow under basal conditions,[1,10,11] measured either at cardiac catheterization or estimated with echocardiography (by the timing, magnitude, and duration of systolic anterior motion of the mitral valve).

Indeed, the evolution of diagnostic echocardiography itself contributed to the complexity of the nomenclature surrounding hypertrophic cardiomyopathy.[34–37] For example, the facility with which echocardiography permits noninvasive identification of the asymmetric pattern of left ventricular hypertrophy, characteristic of hypertrophic cardiomyopathy, stimulated some investigators to name the overall disease entity after its gross anatomic marker, i.e., asymmetric septal hypertrophy (or the acronym ASH).[35,36]

TABLE 1. Terms Used to Describe Hypertrophic Cardiomyopathy

Acquired aortic subvalvular stenosis	Hypertrophic subaortic stenosis
Apical asymmetric septal hypertrophy	Idiopathic hypertrophic cardiomyopathy
Apical hypertrophic cardiomyopathy	Idiopathic hypertrophic obstructive cardiomyopathy
Apical hypertrophic nonobstructive cardiomyopathy	Idiopathic hypertrophic subaortic stenosis
Apical hypertrophy	Idiopathic hypertrophic subvalvular stenosis
Asymmetric left ventricular hypertrophy	Idiopathic muscular hypertrophic subaortic stenosis
Asymmetric septal hypertrophy	Idiopathic muscular stenosis of the left ventricle
Asymmetrical apical hypertrophy	Idiopathic myocardial hypertrophy
Asymmetrical hypertrophic cardiomyopathy	Idiopathic ventricular septal hypertrophy
Asymmetrical hypertrophy of the heart	Irregular hypertrophic cardiomyopathy
Brock's disease	Left ventricular muscular stenosis
Diffuse muscular subaortic stenosis	Low subvalvular aortic stenosis
Diffuse subvalvular aortic stenosis	Mid-ventricular hypertrophic cardiomyopathy
Dynamic hypertrophic subaortic stenosis	Mid-ventricular hypertrophic obstructive cardiomyopathy
Dynamic muscular subaortic stenosis	Mid-ventricular obstruction
Familial hypertrophic subaortic stenosis	Muscular aortic stenosis
Familial muscular subaortic stenosis	Muscular hypertrophic stenosis of the left ventricle
Familial myocardial disease	Muscular stenosis of the left ventricle
Functional aortic stenosis	Muscular subaortic stenosis
Functional aortic subvalvar stenosis	Muscular subvalvular aortic stenosis
Functional hypertrophic subaortic stenosis	Nondilated cardiomyopathy
Functional obstructive cardiomyopathy	Nonobstructive hypertrophic cardiomyopathy
Functional obstruction of the left ventricle	Obstructive cardiomyopathy
Functional obstructive subvalvular aortic stenosis	Obstructive hypertrophic aortic stenosis
Functional subaortic stenosis	Obstructive hypertrophic cardiomyopathy
Hereditary cardiovascular dysplasia	Obstructive hypertrophic myocardiopathy
Hypertrophic apical cardiomyopathy	Obstructive myocardiopathy
HYPERTROPHIC CARDIOMYOPATHY	Pseudoaortic stenosis
Hypertrophic constrictive cardiomyopathy	Stenosing hypertrophy of the left ventricle
Hypertrophic disease	Stenosis of the ejection chamber of left ventricle
Hypertrophic hyperkinetic cardiomyopathy	Subaortic hypertrophic obstructive cardiomyopathy
Hypertrophic infundibular aortic stenosis	Subaortic hypertrophic stenosis
Hypertrophic nonobstructive apical cardiomyopathy	Subaortic idiopathic stenosis
Hypertrophic nonobstructive cardiomyopathy	Subaortic muscular stenosis
Hypertrophic nonobstructive cardiomyopathy with giant negative T waves	Subvalvular aortic stenosis
	Subvalvular aortic stenosis of the muscular type
Hypertrophic obstructive cardiomyopathy	Teare's disease
Hypertrophic obstructive cardiomyopathy of left ventricle	Typical hypertrophic obstructive caridomyopathy
Hypertrophic restrictive cardiomyopathy	
Hypertrophic stenosing cardiomyopathy	

However, because patients with cardiac diseases other than hypertrophic cardiomyopathy may not uncommonly show asymmetric ventricular hypertrophy, naming hypertrophic cardiomyopathy after a finding which is not pathognomonic for the disease proved to be confusing. Finally, the explosion of interest in hypertrophic cardiomyopathy in Japan,[38–52] which followed the description of a morphologic variant with hypertrophy localized primarily in the region of the left ventricular apex,[38–40] contributed further to the proliferation of names used to describe patients within this disease spectrum.

DEFINITION

At the present time, we cannot be absolutely certain whether hypertrophic cardiomyopathy is a single, etiologically distinct disease with substantial clinical and morphologic variability, or whether it actually constitutes a number of separate disease entities with similar clinical and hemodynamic expression.[1,3,7,11] However, to regard each of the variations of this diverse clinical entity as a separate disease would create an unworkable puzzle (Fig. 1). Hence, with our current state of knowledge, it seems most appropriate to consider all patients who appear to fall within the disease spectrum of hypertrophic cardiomyopathy as a single group.

With these considerations in mind, formulation of a basic and workable definition for hypertrophic cardiomyopathy that draws all its diverse elements together is critical. The best such definition presently available is an anatomic one, relying on the single most consistent and characteristic feature of the disease: a hypertrophied and nondilated left ventricle in the absence of another cardiac or systemic disease that itself could produce left ventricular hypertrophy of the magnitude present in that patient.[53] Hence hypertrophic cardiomyopathy is most simply described as a disease in which there is unexplained left ventricular hypertrophy (usually asymmetric in distribution) in the absence of ventricular cavity dilatation. In practical terms, hypertrophy is defined as a maximal left ventricular wall thickness of $\geq$15 mm on echocardiogram in adult patients, although occasional patients with this disease (and without ventricular dilatation) may show a maximum wall thickness of only 13–14 mm.[9,54] This definition of hypertrophic cardiomyopathy is independent of whether or not obstruction to left ventricular outflow and its concomitant echocardiographic features (i.e., marked mitral systolic anterior motion, premature partial aortic valve closure, or increased left ventricular outflow tract flow velocity) are present.[55–59]

While this is a critically useful definition which applies to the vast majority of instances, it is also important to be aware of its exceptions. For example, not uncommonly patients suspected of having hypertrophic cardiomyopathy may also have more common congenital or acquired cardiac diseases such as systemic hypertension or valvular aortic stenosis.[37,60–62] In this circumstance it is often uncertain as to whether a particular patient has the coexistence of two separate disease entities, i.e., a primary myocardial disease characterized by left ventricular hypertrophy (hypertrophic cardiomyopathy) as well as a more common cardiac disease (such as hypertension), or whether hypertrophic cardiomyopathy is absent and the left ventricular hypertrophy is solely related to the acquired or congenital cardiac lesion which is present.[37,60–62] Distinguishing between these two possibilities is often difficult. However, the presence of either severe systolic anterior motion of the mitral valve (sufficient to produce left ventricular outflow tract obstruction) or particularly marked left ventricular hypertrophy (wall

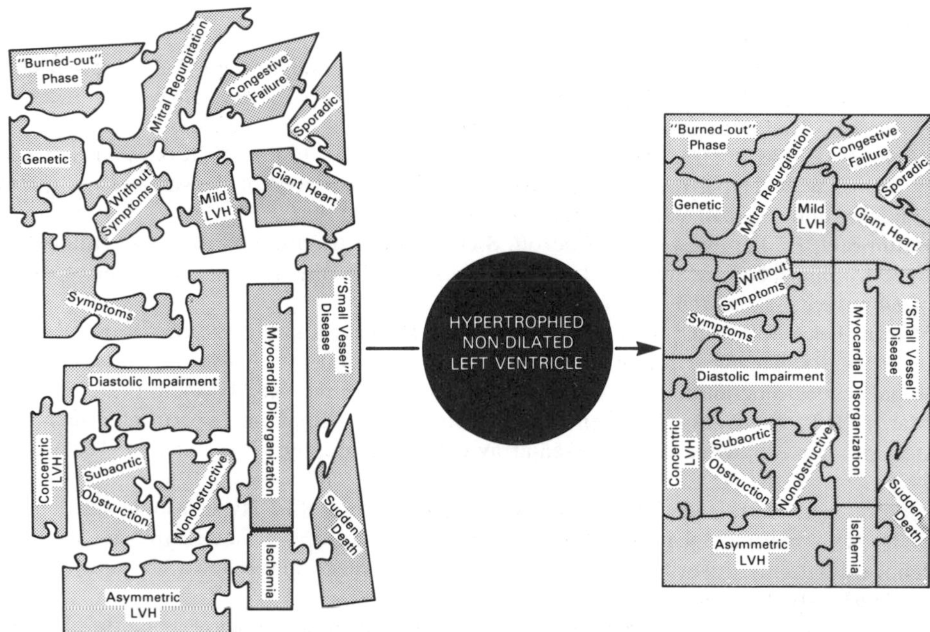

Fig. 1. Diagrammatic representation of the basic morphologic definition of hypertrophic cardiomyopathy (shown in dark circle), as it unifies the clinical and morphologic diversity characteristic of the disease spectrum.

thickness 20–25 mm),[63–66] or documentation of hypertrophic cardiomyopathy in a relative are findings which strongly support the presence of primary hypertrophic cardiomyopathy.[7,11,12] In addition, certain modifications of lifestyle such as chronic athletic conditioning involving isotonic and/or isometric training may produce relatively mild increases in left ventricular wall thickness which can mimic the appearance of the heart in some patients with nonobstructive hypertrophic cardiomyopathy.[54]

Also, because left ventricular wall thickening is not always a static and fixed feature of hypertrophic cardiomyopathy, some individuals with the disease may not fulfill the morphologic definition stipulated here at all times during their lives. For example, occasionally patients with hypertrophic cardiomyopathy may evolve from a clinical state typical of hypertrophic cardiomyopathy, in which the left ventricle is nondilated and thickened, to an atypical "end-stage" form characterized by left ventricular cavity dilatation and wall thinning (as well as severe congestive symptoms and functional limitation).[67] When examined in the latter stages of their clinical course, such patients do not have a hypertrophied and nondilated left ventricle and therefore would not conform to the basic anatomic definition of hypertrophic cardiomyopathy. Also, many patients with hypertrophic cardiomyopathy may not show morphologic (i.e., echocardiographic) evidence of left ventricular hypertrophy early in life.[68] While such patients have a genetic predisposition to develop the phenotypic expression of hypertrophic cardiomyopathy, the appearance of left ventricular wall thickening may be deferred until adolescence. Hence, at certain critical stages of life, it is possible to be affected by hypertrophic cardiomyopathy but not have evidence of increased left ventricular mass.

REFERENCES

1. Maron, B.J., Bonow, R.O., Cannon, R.O., Leon, M.B., and Epstein, S.E. Hypertrophic cardiomyopathy. Interrelations of clinical manifestations, pathophysiology, and therapy. *N. Engl. J. Med.* **316**: 780–789, 844–852, 1987.
2. Wigle, E.D., Sasson, Z., Henderson, M.A., Ruddy, T.D., Fulop, J., Rakowski, H., and Williams, W.G. Hypertrophic cardiomyopathy. The importance of the site and the extent of hypertrophy. A review. *Prog. Cardiovasc. Dis.* **28**: 1–83, 1985.
3. Braunwald, E., Lambrew, C.T., Rockoff, S.D., Ross, J. Jr., and Morrow, A.G. Idiopathic hypertrophic subaortic stenosis. I. A description of the disease based upon an analysis of 64 patients. *Circulation* **30**: 3–217, 1964.
4. Maron, B.J., Gottdiener, J.S., and Epstein, S.E. Patterns and significance of distribution of left ventricular hypertrophy in hypertrophic cardiomyopathy. A wide angle, two-dimensional echocardiographic study of 125 patients. *Am. J. Cardiol.* **48**: 418–428, 1981.
5. Martin, R.P., Rakowski, H., French J., and Popp, R.L. Idiopathic hypertrophic subaortic stenosis viewed by wide-angle, phased-array echocardiography. *Circulation* **59**: 1206–1217, 1979.
6. Maron, B.J., Gottdiener, J.S., Bonow R.O., and Epstein, S.E. Hypertrophic cardiomyopathy with unusual locations of left ventricular hypertrophy undetectable by M-mode echocardiography. Identification by wide-angle two-dimensional echocardiography. *Circulation* **63**: 409–418, 1981.
7. Ciró E., Nichols, P.F., and Maron, B.J. Heterogeneous morphologic expression of genetically transmitted hypertrophic cardiomyopathy. Two-dimensional echocardiographic analysis. *Circulation* **67**: 1227–1233, 1983.
8. Shapiro, L.M. and McKenna, W.J. Distribution of left ventricular hypertrophy in hypertrophic cardiomyopathy: A two-dimensional echocardiographic study. *J. Am. Coll. Cardiol.* **2**: 437–444, 1983.
9. Spirito, P., Maron, B.J., Bonow, R.O., and Epstein, S.E. Severe functional limitation in patients with hypertrophic cardiomyopathy and only mild localized left ventricular hypertrophy. *J. Am. Coll. Cardiol.* **8**: 537–544, 1986.
10. Maron, B.J. and Epstein, S.E. Clinical significance and therapeutic implications of the left ventricular outflow tract pressure gradient in hypertrophic cardiomyopathy. *Am. J. Cardiol.* **58**: 1093–1096, 1986.
11. Maron, B.J., Nichols, P.F., Pickle, L.W., Wesley, Y.E., and Mulvihill, J.J. Patterns of inheritance in hypertrophic cardiomyopathy. Assessment by M-mode and two-dimensional echocardiography. *Am. J. Cardiol.* **53**: 1087–1094, 1984.
12. Van Dorp, W.G., Ten Cate, F.J., Vletter, W.B., Dohmen, H., and Roelandt, J. Familial prevalence of asymmetric septal hypertrophy. *Eur. J. Cardiol.* **4**: 349–357, 1976.
13. Bjarnason, I. and Hallgrimsson, J. Hypertrophic cardiomyopathy. An autopsy study of the years 1966–78. *Icelandic Med. J.* **66**: 205–209, 1980.
14. Hada, Y., Sakamoto, T., Amano, K., Yamaguchi, T., Takenaka, K., Takahashi, H., Takikawa, R., Hasegawa, I., Takahashi, T., Suzuki, J.-I., Sugimoto, T., and Saito, K.-I. Prevalence of hypertrophic cardiomyopathy in a population of adult Japanese workers as detected by echocardiographic screening. *Am. J. Cardiol.* **59**: 183–184, 1987.
15. Svetoni, N., Casini, M., Spargi, T., Bellantonio, M., Simoni, F., Marciano, A., and Lanzetta, T. Asymptomatic hypertrophic cardiomyopathy in sport. *Int. J. Sports Cardiol.* **3**: 51–56, 1986.
16. Liouville, H. Rétrécissement cardiaque sous aortique. *Gazette Med. Paris* **24**: 161–163, 1869.
17. Hallopeau, M. Rétrécissement ventriculo-aortique. *Gazette Med. Paris* **24**: 683–684, 1869.
18. Schmincke, A. Ueber linkseitige muskulöse. Conusstenosen. *Dtsch. Med. Wochenschr.* **33**: 2082–2083, 1907.
19. Bernheim, P.I. De L'asystolie veineuse dans l'hypertrophie du coeur gauche par stenose

concomitante du ventricule droit. *Rev. Med.* **30**: 785–801, 1910.

20. Davies, L.G. Familial heart disease. *Br. Heart J.* **14**: 206–212, 1952.
21. Teare, D. Asymmetrical hypertrophy of the heart in young adults. *Br. Heart J.* **20**: 1–18, 1958.
22. Brock, R. Functional obstruction of the left ventricle (acquired aortic subvalvular stenosis). *Guy's Hosp. Rep.* **106**: 221–238, 1957.
23. Bercu, B.A., Diettert, G.A., Danforth, W.H., Pund, E.E. Jr., Ahlvin, R.C., and Belliveau, R.R. Pseudoaortic stenosis produced by ventricular hypertrophy. *Am. J. Med.* **25**: 814–818, 1958.
24. Morrow, A.G. and Braunwald, E. Functional aortic stenosis: a malformation characterized by resistance to left ventricular outflow without anatomic obstruction. *Circulation* **20**: 181–189, 1959.
25. Brent, L.B., Aburano, A., Fisher, D.L., Moran, T.J., Myers, J.D., and Taylor, W.J. Familial muscular subaortic stenosis. An unrecognized form of "idiopathic heart disease," with clinical and autopsy observations. *Circulation* **21**: 167–180, 1960.
26. Goodwin, J.F., Hollman, A., Cleland, W.P., and Teare, D. Obstructive cardiomyopathy simulating aortic stenosis. *Br. Heart J.* **22**: 403–414, 1960.
27. Menges, H., Brandenburg, R.O., and Brown, A.L. The clinical, hemodynamic and pathologic diagnosis of muscular subvalvular aortic stenosis. *Circulation* **24**: 1126–1136, 1961.
28. Daoud, G., Gallaher, M.E., and Kaplan, S. Muscular subaortic stenosis. *Am. J. Cardiol.* **7**: 860–864, 1961.
29. Paré, J.A.P., Fraser, R.G., Pirozynski, W.J., Shanks, J.A., and Stubington, D. Hereditary cardiovascular dysplasia. A form of familial cardiomyopathy. *Am. J. Med.* **31**: 37–62, 1961.
30. Wigle, E.D., Heimbecker, R.O., and Gunton, R.W. Idiopathic ventricular septal hypertrophy causing muscular subaortic stenosis. *Circulation* **26**: 325–340, 1962.
31. Cohen, J., Effat, H., Goodwin, J.F., Oakley, C.M., and Steiner, R.E. Hypertrophic obstructive cardiomyopathy. *Br. Heart J.* **26**: 16–32, 1964.
32. Dinsmore, R.E., Sanders, C.A., and Harthorne, J.W. Mitral regurgitation in idiopathic hypertrophic subaortic stenosis. *N. Engl. J. Med.* **275**: 1225–1228, 1966.
33. Simon, A.L., Ross, J. Jr., and Gault, J.H. Angiographic anatomy of the left ventricle and mitral valve in idiopathic hypertrophic subaortic stenosis. *Circulation* **36**: 852–867, 1967.
34. Abbasi, A.S., MacAlpin, R.N., Eber, L.M., and Pearce, M.L. Echocardiographic diagnosis of idiopathic hypertrophic cardiomyopathy without outflow obstruction. *Circulation* **46**: 897–904, 1972.
35. Henry, W.L., Clark, C.E., and Epstein, S.E. Asymmetric septal hypertrophy (ASH): Echocardiographic identification of the pathognomonic anatomic abnormality of IHSS. *Circulation* **47**: 225–233, 1973.
36. Henry, W.L., Clark, C.E., and Epstein, S.E. Asymmetric septal hypertrophy (ASH): The unifying link in the IHSS disease spectrum. Observations regarding its pathogenesis, pathophysiology, and course. *Circulation* **47**: 827–832, 1973.
37. Maron, B.J. and Epstein, S.E. Hypertrophic cardiomyopathy. Recent observations regarding the specificity of three hallmarks of the disease: Asymmetric septal hypertrophy, septal disorganization and systolic anterior motion of the anterior mitral leaflet. *Am. J. Cardiol.* **45**: 141–154, 1980.
38. Sakamoto, T., Tei, C., Murayama, M., Ichiyasu, H., Hada, Y., Hayashi, T., and Amano, K. Giant T wave inversion as a manifestation of asymmetrical apical hypertrophy (AAH) of the left ventricle. Echocardiographic and ultrasonocardiotomographic study. *Jpn. Heart J.* **17**: 611–629, 1976.
39. Nishiyama, S., Yamaguchi, H., Ishimura, T., Nayasaki, F., Takatsu, F., Umeda, T., and Machii, K. Echocardiographic features of apical hypertrophic cardiomyopathy. *J. Cardiogr.* **8**: 177–183, 1978.
40. Yamaguchi, H., Ishimura, T., Nishiyama, S., Nagasaki, F., Nakanishi, S., Takatsu, F., Nishigo, T., Umeda, T., and Machii, K. Hypertrophic non-obstructive cardiomyopathy

with giant negative T waves (apical hypertrophy): ventriculographic and echocardiographic features in 30 patients. *Am. J. Cardiol.* **44**: 401–412, 1979.

41. Fujiwara, H., Kawai, C., and Hamashima, Y. Myocardial fascicle and fiber disarray in 25 μ-thick sections. *Circulation* **59**: 1293–1298, 1979.
42. Kinoshita, N., Nimura, Y., Okamoto, M., Miyatake, K., Nagata, S., and Sakakibara, H. Mitral regurgitation in hypertrophic cardiomyopathy. Non-invasive study by two-dimensional Doppler echocardiography. *Br. Heart J.* **49**: 574–583, 1983.
43. Hoshino, T., Fujiwara H., Kawai, C., and Hamashima, Y. Myocardial fiber diameter and regional distribution in the ventricular wall of normal adult hearts, hypertensive hearts and hearts with hypertrophic cardiomyopathy. *Circulation* **67**: 1109–1116, 1983.
44. Koga, Y., Itaya, K.-I., and Toshima, H. Prognosis in hypertrophic cardiomyopathy. *Am. Heart J.* **108**: 351–359, 1984.
45. Fujii, J., Saihara, S., Sawada, H., Aizawa, T., and Koto, K. Distribution of left ventricular hypertrophy and electrocardiographic findings in patients with so-called apical hypertrophic cardiomyopathy. *J. Cardiogr.* **15** (suppl. VI): 23–33, 1985.
46. Sakurai, S., Tanaka, H., Yoshimura, H., Nakao, S., and Tahara., M. Production of systolic anterior motion of the mitral valve in dogs. *Circulation* **71**: 805–812, 1985.
47. Koga, Y., Itaya, M., Takahashi, H., Koga, M., Ikeda, H., Itaya, K-I., and Toshima, H. Apical hypertrophy and its genetic and acquired factors. *J. Cardiogr.* **15** (suppl. VI): 65–74, 1985.
48. Morimoto, S., Sekiguchi, M., Hasumi, M., Inagaki, Y., Takimoto, H., Ohtsubo, K., Hiroe, M., Hirosawa, K., Matsuda, M., and Komatsu, Y. Do giant negative T waves represent apical hypertrophic cardiomyopathy? Left ventriculographic and cardiac biopsy studies. *J. Cardiogr.* **15** (suppl. IV): 35–51, 1985.
49. Nagata, S., Park, Y.-D., Minamikawa, T., Yutani, C., Kamiya, T., Nishimura, T., Kozuka, T., Sakakibara, H., and Nimura, Y. Thallium perfusion and cardiac enzyme abnormalities in patients with familial hypertrophic cardiomyopathy. *Am. Heart J.* **109**: 1317–1322, 1985.
50. Tanaka, M., Fujiwara, H., Onodera, T., Wu, D.-J., Hamashima, Y., and Kawai, C. Quantitative analysis of myocardial fibrosis in normal, hypertensive hearts, and hypertrophic cardiomyopathy. *Br. Heart J.* **55**: 575–581, 1986.
51. Onodera, T., Fujiwara, H., Tanaka, M., Wu, D.-J., Hamashima, Y., and Kawai, C. Familial hypertrophic cardiomyopathy mimicking typical dilated cardiomyopathy. *Jpn. Circ. J.* **50**: 614–617, 1986.
52. Tanaka, M., Fujiwara, H., Onodera, T., Wu, D.-J., Matsuda, M., Hamashima, Y., and Kawai, C. Quantitative analysis of narrowings of intramyocardial small arteries in normal hearts, hypertensive hearts, and hearts with hypertrophic cardiomyopathy. *Circulation* **75**: 1130–1139, 1987.
53. Maron, B.J. and Epstein, S.E. Hypertrophic cardiomyopathy: A discussion of nomenclature. *Am. J. Cardiol.* **43**: 1242–1244, 1979.
54. Maron, B.J. Structural features of the athlete heart as defined by echocardiography. *J. Am. Coll. Cardiol.* **7**: 190–203, 1986.
55. Yock, P.G., Hatle, L., and Popp, R.L. Patterns and timing of Doppler-detected intracavitary and aortic flow in hypertrophic cardiomyopathy. *J. Am. Coll. Cardiol.* **8**: 1047–1058, 1986.
56. Maron, B.J., Gottdiener, J.S., Arce, J., Rosing, D.R., Wesley, Y.E., and Epstein, S.E. Dynamic subaortic obstruction in hypertrophic cardiomyopathy: Analysis by pulsed Doppler echocardiography. *J. Am. Coll. Cardiol.* **6**: 1–8, 1985.
57. Pollick, C., Morgan, C.D., Gilbert, B.W., Rakowski, H., and Wigle, E.D. Muscular subaortic stenosis. The temporal relationship between systolic anterior motion of the anterior mitral leaflet and the pressure gradient. *Circulation* **66**: 1087–1094, 1982.
58. Stewart, W.J., Schiavone, W.A., Salcedo, E.E., Lever, H.M., Cosgrove, D.M., and Gill, C.C. Intraoperative Doppler echocardiography in hypertrophic cardiomyopathy: correlations with the obstructive gradient. *J. Am. Coll. Cardiol.* **10**: 327–335, 1987.

59. Spirito, P. and Maron, B.J. Patterns of systolic anterior motion of the mitral valve in hypertrophic cardiomyopathy: assessment by two-dimensional echocardiography. *Am. J. Cardiol.* **54**: 1039–1046, 1984.
60. Panza, J.A. and Maron, B.J. Valvular aortic stenosis and asymmetric septal hypertrophy: Diagnostic considerations and clinical and therapeutic implications. *Eur. Heart J.* **9**: (suppl. C): 71–76, 1988.
61. Hess, O.M., Schneider, J., Turina, M., Carroll, J.D., Rothlin, M., and Krayenbuehl, H.P. Asymmetric septal hypertrophy in patients with aortic stenosis: An adaptive mechanism or a coexistence of hypertrophic cardiomyopathy? *J. Am. Coll. Cardiol.* **1**: 783–789, 1983.
62. Wicker, P., Roudaut, R., Haissaguere, P., Villega-Arino, P., Clementy, J., and Dallocchio, M. Prevalence and significance of asymmetric septal hypertrophy in hypertension: an echocardiographic and clinical study. *Eur. Heart J.* **4**: (suppl. G): 1–5, 1983.
63. Savage, D.D., Drayer, J.I.M., Henry, W.L., Mathews, E.C., Ware, J.H., Gardin, J.M., Cohen, E.R., Epstein, S.E., and Laragh, J.H. Echocardiographic assessment of cardiac anatomy and function in hypertensive subjects. *Circulation* **59**: 623–632, 1979.
64. Doi, Y.L., Deanfield, J.E., McKenna, W.J., Dargie, H.J., Oakley, C.M., and Goodwin, J.F. Echocardiographic differentiation of hypertensive heart disease and hypertrophic cardiomyopathy. *Br. Heart J.* **44**: 395–400, 1980.
65. Shapiro, L.M., Kleinebenne, A., and McKenna, W.J. Distribution of left ventricular hypertrophy in hypertrophic cardiomyopathy: comparison to athletes and hypertensives. *Eur. Heart J.* **6**: 967–974, 1985.
66. Maron, B.J., Edwards, J.E., and Epstein, S.E. Prevalence and characteristics of disproportionate ventricular septal thickening in patients with systemic hypertension. *Chest* **73**: 466–470, 1978.
67. Maron, B.J., Epstein, S.E., and Roberts, W.C. Hypertrophic cardiomyopathy and transmural myocardial infarction without significant atherosclerosis of the extramural coronary arteries. *Am. J. Cardiol.* **43**: 1086–1102, 1979.
68. Maron, B.J., Spirito, P., Wesley, Y., and Arce, J. Development and progression of left ventricular hypertrophy in children with hypertrophic cardiomyopathy. *N. Engl. J. Med.* **315**: 610–614, 1986.

[illegible]

PATHOLOGY

Gross Morphology and Light Microscopic Features of Hypertrophic Cardiomyopathy

E.G.J. Olsen

National Heart Hospital and Cardiothoracic Institute, London, U.K.

INTRODUCTION

Following the World Health Organization/International Society and Federation of Cardiology task force recommendation on nomenclature on cardiomyopathies,[1] "with or without obstruction" has been omitted from the term hypertrophic cardiomyopathy.

In 1957, Lord Brock, then Sir Russell Brock, reported on patients believed to have aortic valve stenosis and illustrated this by a case which was, on inspection of the valve at surgery, found to be normal. A muscular subvalvular bulge of the septum was however noted, resulting in functional subvalvular stenosis.[2] The following year, there were eight reported cases of what was long considered the first morphological description of this condition.[3] Subsequently, however, research has shown that two Frenchmen, Liouvillc, in 1889, and Hallopeau, in the same year, can be credited with the first description of hypertrophic cardiomyopathy.[4]

Following Teare's report, other studies soon followed. As is often the case with "new diseases," after the initial description, features are added, association with other diseases claimed, and diagnostic characteristics of the condition described. These are often recanted later, so that in the end, doubt as to the very existence of the disease has been expressed. Hypertrophic cardiomyopathy is no exception, and indeed may well be cited as a typical example.

There is no doubt that hypertrophic cardiomyopathy exists and that it is a distinct entity.

MACROSCOPIC APPEARANCES

When patients with this condition die—not infrequently, unexpectedly and suddenly—the hearts are overweight, globular in shape, and firm to the touch. On opening the heart, asymmetric hypertrophy of the interventricular septum can be striking. Measurements of the bulge of the disproportionately thickened septum are often double the normal values, compared with the often severely hypertrophied free left ventricular wall.[3,5] The myocardium of the cut surface of the affected septum has a whorled appearance likened to watered silk (Fig. 1). Cutting the area has also been likened to slicing an unripe pear. The septal bulge may be diffuse or maximal at the apex, in the mid-region, or in the vicinity of the aortic valve. Displacement of the anterior papillary muscle, which contributes to the classic angiographic and echocardiograph appearances of the left ventricular cavity, interferes with the normal closure of the mitral valve, resulting in mitral insufficiency, a condition not infrequently diagnosed during life. As a result of insufficiency, thickening of the mitral valve leaflet is found. The valve is usually

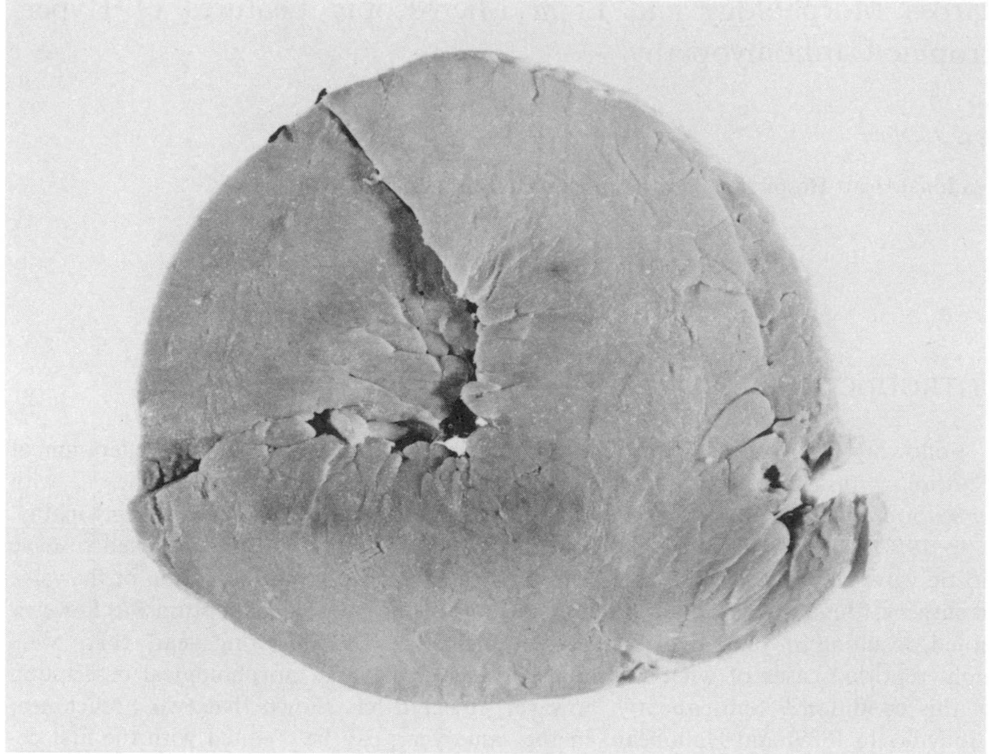

Fig. 1. Cross section of the ventricles showing a whorled appearance of the myocardial muscle in the slightly asymmetrically thickened interventricular septum.

in normal position, although abnormalities have been noted: the anterior mitral valve leaflet is related to the posterior aortic valve leaflet instead of the normal arrangement when continuity with the right aortic valve leaflet is present.[6]

Endocardial thickening may be found, but this is not confined to any specific region in the left (or right) ventricle. The anterior mitral valve leaflet may however impinge on the septum, resulting in a mirror image of the valve, often leading to extremely thickened endocardium[7] (Fig. 2).

The extramural coronary arteries are usually normal, but occasionally some plaques of arteriosclerosis may be noted; narrowing of the vascular lumina is, however, not present in any form. Despite the normality of the coronary arteries, infarct-like lesions—even extending transmurally—have been described.[8]

Heart failure is usually rare in patients with hypertrophic cardiomyopathy; when it occurs it is often a preterminal event, but the characteristic macroscopic features remain.

Recent experience has shown that symmetric hypertrophic cardiomyopathy occurs (Fig. 3). In this form macroscopic diagnosis is impossible. Echocardiographic analysis has suggested an incidence as high as 31%.[9] Death may be sudden or unexpected, but no specific changes have been identified in these cases.

Reference to measuring the interventricular septum has already been made. Ratios exceeding unity are common.[10] Values as high as three are not infrequently found,

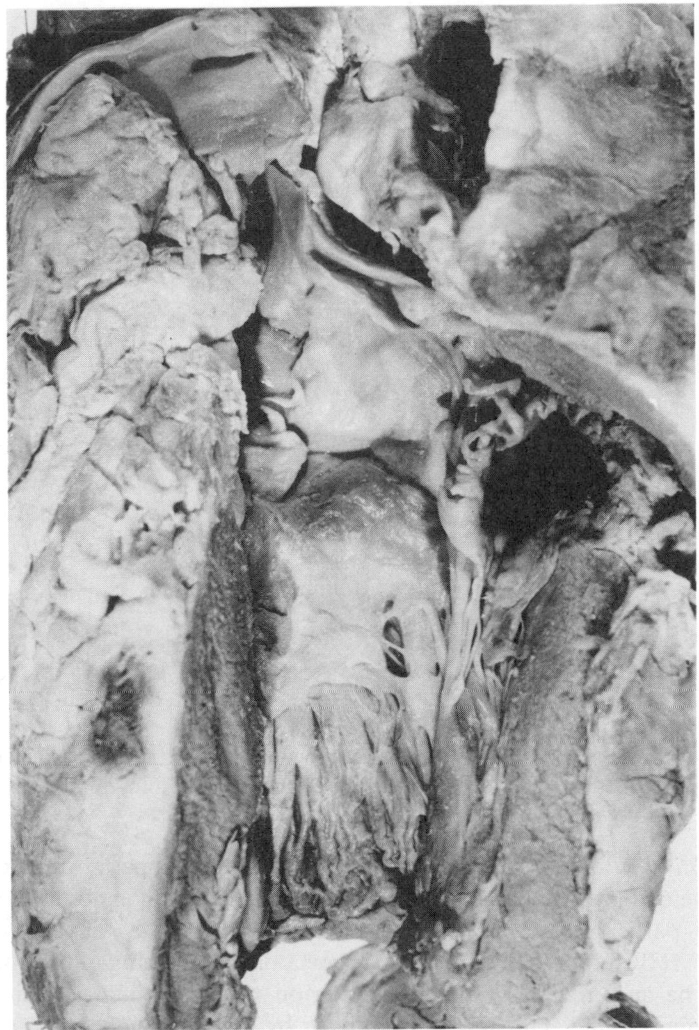

Fig. 2. "Mirror image" of the anterior mitral valve leaflet which has resulted in severe endocardial thickening beneath the aortic valve.

compared with other conditions in which, even if hypertrophy is severe, unity of septal and free wall ratios is maintained. Analyses of echocardiographic measurements of the septum and left posterior wall have established a ratio exceeding 1.3 in patients with hypertrophic cardiomyopathy, compared with 1.03 in normal individuals and control cases.[11)]

There is no doubt that if the ratio clearly exceeds 1.3 this constitutes a characteristic feature of hypertrophic cardiomyopathy; however, caution in interpreting this is necessary. This is emphasized by a study of 125 infants of two years of age or less with congenital heart disease. In 25% of patients the interventricular septum/left ventricular free wall ratio exceeded 1.3.[12)] Assessment of asymmetric hypertrophy alone can therefore be unreliable if the changes are mild.

The reliability of diagnosis based on the macroscopic appearance has been challenged,

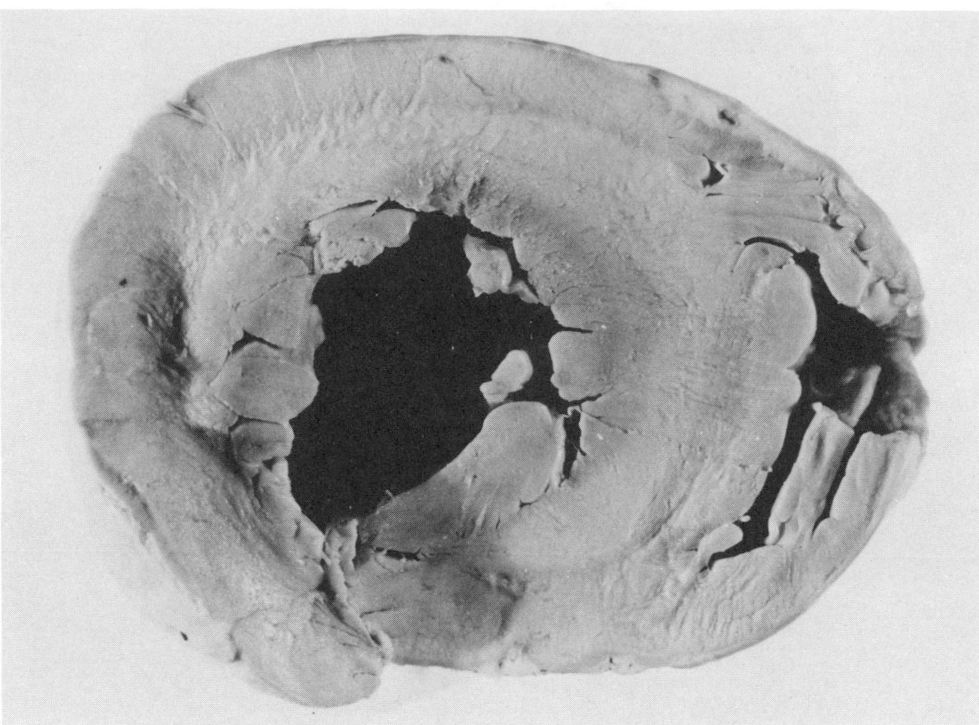

Fig. 3. Cross section of the ventricles showing symmetric myocardial hypertrophy in a histologically proven case of hypertrophic cardiomyopathy.

particularly in view of the fact that hypertrophic cardiomyopathy can occur to some degree in developing normal fetuses and in the normal newborn in addition to congenital heart disease, particularly when the right ventricle is involved, as well as in other cardiac conditions.[13] It therefore follows that disproportionate thickening of the interventricular septum can be an unreliable diagnostic criterion when taken in isolation, especially when thickening is mild. This was substantiated by another study which reported eight patients with asymmetric thickening, among whom histology confirmed the diagnosis of hypertrophic cardiomyopathy in only two.[14] This emphasizes the importance of histological examination.

The disproportionately thickened interventricular septum may also bulge into the right ventricular cavity, and experience of obtaining endomyocardial biopsies from the septum of that chamber has shown positive results.[15]

LIGHT MICROSCOPIC APPEARANCES

Histology

Although this aspect will also be discussed in the next section, some personal experiences of the author will be detailed. After the initial description of the histological appearance by Teare, who drew attention to "bizarre and disorganised arrangement of muscle bundles" as well as severe hypertrophy and clefts, descriptive details of the changes have been expanded. Endomyocardial tissue, obtained at surgical operation

TABLE Comparison of histological features of surgical biopsies from 67 patients with hypertrophic cardiomyopathy (solid colums) and "ordinary" hypertrophy from 67 patients with aortic valve stenosis (open colums). A plus system has been used. The height of the column is determined by the number of patients showing these features expressed as a percentage.

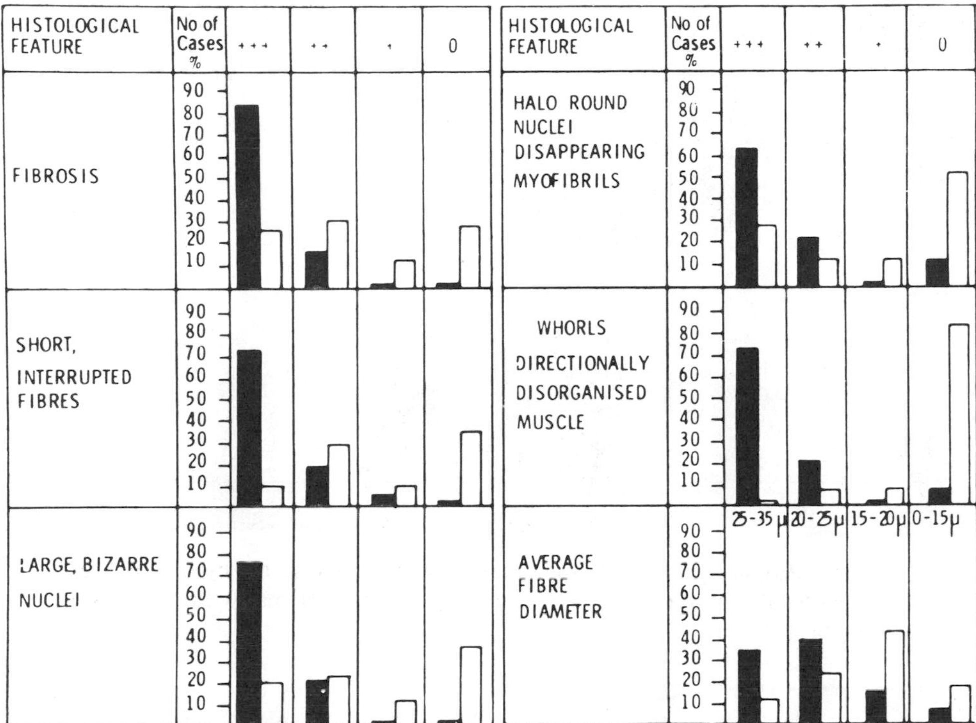

forming part of the procedure of relieving the "obstruction" in patients with hypertrophic cardiomyopathy, was assessed and compared with tissue from identical sites from patients with aortic valve stenosis showing what was referred to as "ordinary hypertrophy" (see Table). This comparative study permitted the histological HOCM index to be formulated.[16] Extreme hypertrophy of individual myocardial fibers was encountered (the diameter exceeding 100 μm) in hypertrophic cardiomyopathy, whereas in ordinary hypertrophy the maximum diameter measured 35 μm. Disarray dominated the histological picture (Fig. 4). Short runs of severely hypertrophied myocytes interrupted by connective tissue that frequently showed some chronic inflammatory cells were typical. The interstitial clefts described by Teare were also seen and contributed to the cellularity of the interstitial connective tissue (Fig. 5). The nuclei of the myocytes were large and vesicular, frequently assuming bizarre outlines. Varying degrees of interstitial fibrosis were also encountered. Degenerative changes in the myocytes were frequent and took the form of "disappearing" myofibrils, which even at this level of investigation could clearly be identified. The clear spaces thus created were referred to as perinuclear halos.[16,17] The myofibers were often arranged in whorls, contributing to the disarray. This whorling could also be seen within individual myocytes when hydropic change separating individual myofibrils was present. A maximum of three points was awarded to each of five of the histological features (short runs of fibers interrupted by connective tissue, large bizzare nuclei, fibrosis, degenerating muscle with disappearing myofibrils,

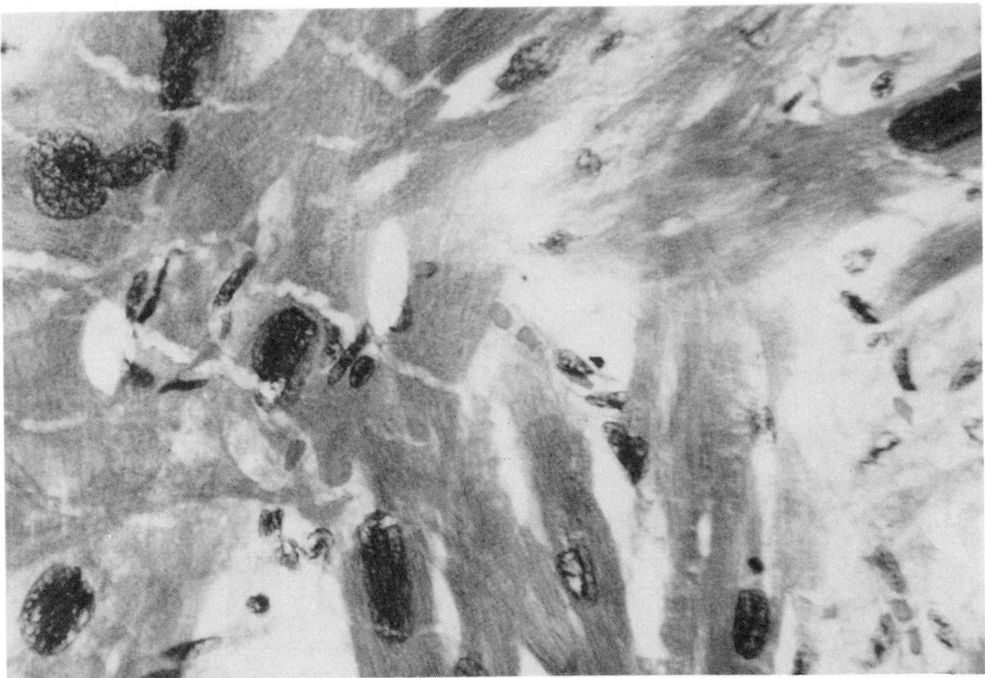

Fig. 4. Photomicrograph showing severe disarray and severe hypertrophy of myocardial fibers together with bizarre shaped nuclei. Hematoxylin and eosin stain; × 400.

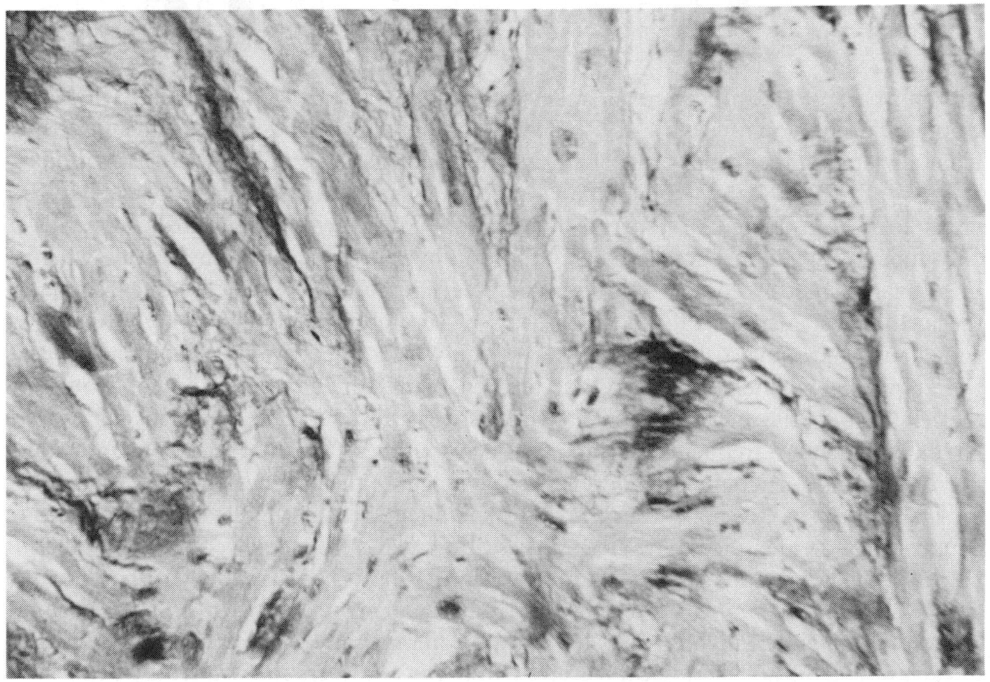

Fig. 5. Photomicrograph illustrating interstitial collagen (in black) from an area of disarray. Miller's elastic van Gieson stain × 300.

disorganized myofibril "whorling" muscle) and the total was expressed as 100%. This constituted the histological HOCM index. Overlap of individual parameters with ordinary hypertrophy was encountered.

It was found that if values exceeded 50% a firm diagnosis of hypertrophic cardiomyopathy could be made. Although the tissue was obtained in the initial study at surgery, it has now been applied to analyzing tissues obtained by bioptome, where lower values (between 35% and 50%) have shown good correlation between the suspected clinical diagnosis and the morphological appearance.

The intramyocardial vessels have, in my experience and that of other workers, either been normal or shown some intimal thickening of concentrically arranged fibroelastic tissue. These vessels were usually located within areas of interstitial fibrosis or areas of fibrous replacement of myocytes, rarely narrowing the lumina by more than 50%.[5,18] More extensive changes have, however, been reported. In 40 of 48 patients with hypertrophic cardiomyopathy, medial and/or intimal thickening was found reducing the lumina. The areas in which these vessels were found were located especially in the septum, anterior left ventricular wall, and areas of fibrosis. An underlying congenital component contributing to the disease was suggested as a result of these findings; this also explains the ischemic symptoms these patients frequently have.[19]

The epicardium is unremarkable and the endocardium is usually nonspecifically thickened to a mild degree except in the area of the septum beneath the aortic valve, where, due to mitral valve impingement, immense thickening can be found. This consists of fibroelastic tissue only and is occasionally covered with a thin layer of fibrin. Smooth muscle hypertrophy is usually not evident, but if heart failure has been present, some foci of smooth muscle prominence can be found.

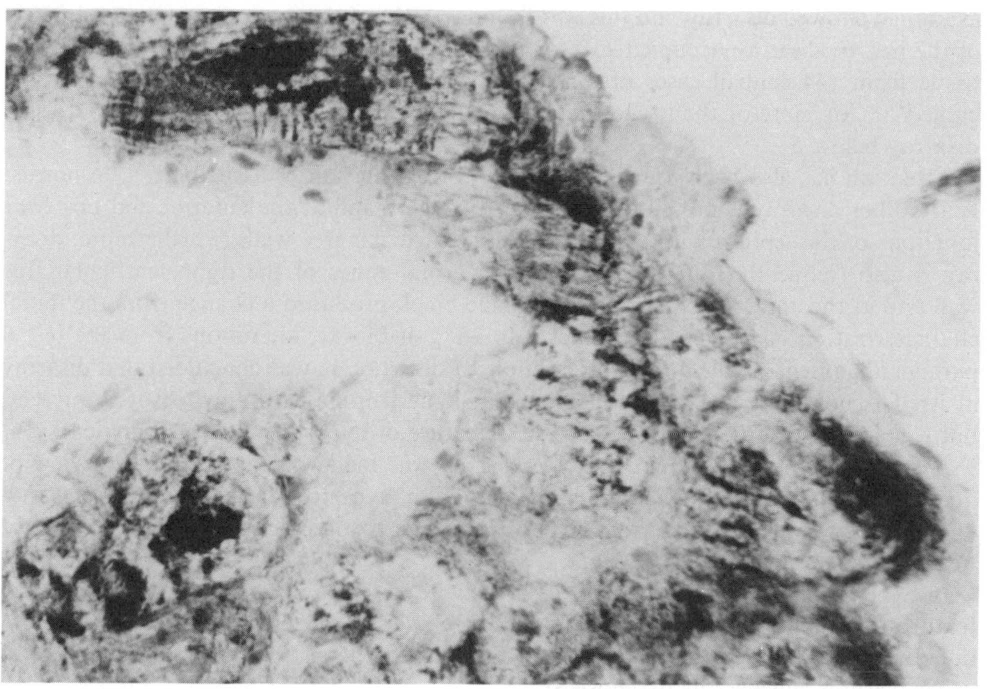

Fig. 6. Glycogen accumulation in myocytes in hypertrophic cardiomyopathy showing "pooling" in the centre of the fibres. PAS × 400.

Histochemistry

Extensive histochemical investigation has also been undertaken on tissue obtained from endomyocardial biopsies or material obtained at surgery. Glycogen, neutral fat, lipofuscin, dehydrogenases including succinate and lactate dehydrogenase, oxidases, lysosomal hydrolases, cholinesterase, alkaline phosphatase, phosphorylase, glycogen synthetase, and leucine aminopeptidase have been investigated.[20] Among these, glycogen accumulation has been found to be of diagnostic value. This accumulation can often be immense, forming lakes and producing smudging at microscopic examination instead of retaining the granular appearance found in ordinary hypertrophy (Fig. 6). The accumulation appears to be unrelated to the degree of hypertrophy. The other substances enumerated above frequently show increases. Such increases can be severe, but appear to be related to the degree of hypertrophy present.

At this level of investigation, patients who have died suddenly or unexpectedly have also shown no specific features.

DIAGNOSIS OF HYPERTROPHIC CARDIOMYOPATHY

Caution is necessary in interpreting disproportionate thickening of the interventricular septum at the macroscopic level only. If, however, ratios or measurements are great, this alone permits diagnosis. Histological evaluation is often necessary. Application of the histological HOCM index, which takes various histological parameters into consideration, permits firm diagnosis. Singling out any particular feature can be misleading. Disarray has been singled out as being a "sensitive and specific marker of the disease," having been substantiated by persuasive evidence obtained by examining the hearts of 54 patients at necropsy. In 94% of these 54 patients, at least 5% or more of the area examined showed disarray and this was found in 89% of the sections examined. In 56% of the hearts, disarray occupied 25% or more of the tissue sections. In a comparison of tissue from 144 control cases obtained from normal or diseased hearts, only 7% occupied 5% or more of the tissue slides, though 26% of the control cases showed some disarray below 5%.[21]

Attention has also been drawn to the effect of orientation of tissue blocks. In normal hearts fiber disarray is present in the subaortic region and at the anterior and posterior junctions of the septum with the right or left ventricular free walls. Furthermore, disarray is also frequently found in the subendocardial zones of the right ventricular free wall and at the apex. Orientation of the tissue block produced a change from the initial characterization in 52 out of 60 blocks. In 38% of blocks, alterations from the initial parallel alignment changed on reorientation to disarray. It was concluded that disarray in itself is not necessarily an indication that hypertrophic cardiomyopathy is present, but it is not denied that it may constitute a feature of hypertrophic cardiomyopathy.[22]

A strong case for the importance of disarray was made on the basis of a review of quantitative analyses of tissue from patients with hypertrophic cardiomyopathy that distinguished this condition from hypertrophy due to other causes and from normal hearts.[23]

In hypertrophic cardiomyopathy, the areas with disarray also show other histological features, including severe hypertrophy, bizarre shaped nuclei, and other features detailed above. Although there is no doubt that disarray is characteristic, the presence of other features clinches the diagnosis.[24]

The criteria have been applied to endomyocardial biopsies. Indications for biopsy are rarely as strong as, for example, in dilated cardiomyopathy; only if serious doubt as to the diagnosis exists are patients subjected to this form of investigation. In recent years endomyocardial biopsy, a technique first described in Japan,[25] has gained increasing usage throughout the world. My own experience dates back to 1971, and up to the present only 150 cases suspected of having hypertrophic cardiomyopathy have thus been investigated (out of a total of 2,700 patients so far analyzed),[26] the reason being that the clinical and noninvasive investigations usually permit diagnosis. The histological and histochemical criteria above have been strictly applied, but the histological HOCM index is lower (33–50%) due to the small size of the tissue samples. Diagnosis has been confirmed on biopsy in 40% of the cases; in 50% of the cases other pathology was found (in 5% of patients amyloid was found). Disarray forms the main diagnostic criterion on endomyocardial biopsies, and even right ventricular biopsies yield good results.[15]

HYPERTROPHIC CARDIOMYOPATHY "WITH OR WITHOUT OBSTRUCTION"

Doubt as to the presence of true obstruction has already been expressed,[1] and from a morphological point of view, differences between patients "with obstruction" and those "without" was believed to be present.

Macroscopically no differences have been noted, but the distribution of abnormal fibers in the two clinical settings were thought to be different. In hypertrophic cardiomyopathy "with obstruction," the abnormal fibers were believed to be located in the disproportionate thickening of the interventricular septum extending to a variable extent into the anterior and posterior left ventricular walls.[17,27] In patients where obstruction did not occur clinically, identical abnormal fibers were found, but these were focally distributed in the left or right ventricular wall. Further experience has shown that complete overlap exists, as exemplified by a report on two siblings suffering from hypertrophic cardiomyopathy "with obstruction" in whom the nonobstructive pattern was noted morphologically.[28] These findings tend to support the suggestion that true obstruction may not exist.

HYPERTROPHIC CARDIOMYOPATHY WITH OTHER CONDITIONS

Well-documented cases of hypertrophic cardiomyopathy occurring in association with other diseases have appeared in the literature, including conditions such as hyperthyroidism,[29] Friedreich's ataxia,[30,31] and lentigenosis.[32,33]

Mandatory to laying claim to such association is not only clinical evaluation by noninvasive investigation, but also morphological evaluation, which is easily achieved by endomyocardial biopsy. Unless this has been done, critical assessment of the cases having been observed is necessary.

ETIOLOGY

The etiology is unknown. There is no doubt that genetic factors play an important role, and evidence that inheritance is by an autosomal dominant trait with almost complete penetrance is well established.[34] Embryonic growth disturbance, hamartoma, increased noradrenaline, primary disorder of myocardial muscle metabolism, myopathic disease, hypertension, relationship of catecholamines, abnormal contraction toward the end of systolic isometric contraction interfering with normal muscle alignment, small vessel disease, and the contributory role of the HLA system have all been suggested.[35]

A possible endogenous mechanism has been explored experimentally, based on the clinical observation that hyperthyroidism can occur together with hypertrophic cardiomyopathy.[29,36] In the circulation of one patient with covert thyrocardiac disease, tri-iodothyroacetic acid (triac) and tetra-iodothyroacetic acid (tetrac), the acetic analogues of tri-iodothryronin and thyroxin, have been found. This finding was explored experimentally by administering triac to pregnant rats and studying the effect on the hearts of the newborn offspring. When high doses of triac had been administered to the pregnant rats, disarray of myofibrils dominated the ultrastructural picture. Subsequent experiments showed that triac was found to act on the cell membrane, where it interfers with calcium flux, and, as has previously been suggested,[37] leads to an extra isometric contraction during fetal life that results in malalignment of myocytes. This experimental model and the experiments that have been performed have been detailed in *Cardiomyopathy Update 1: Pathogenesis of Myocarditis and Cardiomyopathy,* Kawai and Abelmann (eds.) University of Tokyo Press, 1987.

CONCLUSIONS

There is no doubt that hypertrophic cardiomyopathy is a distinct entity and that morphological diagnosis can be achieved. Criteria for such a diagnosis must however be observed. Pronouncements based on insufficient experience must be shunned, otherwise controversey will continue to exist.

REFERENCES

1. Report of the WHO/ISFC Task Force on the definition and classification of cardiomyopathies. *Br. Heart J.* **44**: 672–673, 1980.
2. Brock, R.C. Functional obstruction of the left ventricle (Acquired aortic sub-valvar stenosis). *Guy's Hosp. Rep.* **106**: 221–238, 1957.
3. Teare, D. Asymmetrical hypertrophy of the heart in young adults. *Br. Heart J.* **20**: 1–8, 1958.
4. Wigle, E.D. and Silver, M.D. Myocardial fiber disarray and ventricular septal hypertrophy in asymmetrical hypertrophy of the heart (editorial). *Circulation* **58**: 398–402, 1978.
5. Olsen, E.G.J. Anatomic and light microscopic characterisation of hypertrophic obstructive cardiomyopathy and non-obstructive cardiomyopathy. *Eur. Heart J.* **4**: (suppl. F) 1–8, 1983.
6. Bjork, V.O., Hultquist, G., and Lodin, H. Subaortic stenosis produced by an abnormally placed anterior mitral leaflet. *J. Thorac. Cardiovasc. Surg.* **41**: 659–669, 1961.
7. Davies, M.J., Pomerance, A., and Teare, R.D. Pathological features of hypertrophic obstructive cardiomyopathy. *J. Clin. Pathol.* **27**: 529–535, 1974.
8. Maron, B.J., Epstein, S.E., and Roberts, W.C. Hypertrophic cardiomyopathy and transmural myocardial infarction without significant atherosclerosis of the extramural coronary arteries. *Am. J. Cardiol.* **43**: 1086–1102, 1979.
9. Shapiro, L.M. and McKenna, W.J. Distribution of left ventricular hypertrophy in hypertrophic cardiomyopathy: A two-dimensional echocardiographic study. *J. Am. Coll. Cardiol.* **2**: 437–444, 1983.
10. Menges, J.H., Brandenburg, R.D., and Brown, A.L. Jr. The clinical, hemodynamic and pathologic diagnosis of muscular subvalvular aortic stenosis. *Circulation* **24**: 1126–1136, 1961.

11. Henry, W.L., Clark, C.E., and Epstein, S.E. Asymmetric septal hypertrophy (ASH): Echocardiographic identification of the pathognomonic anatomic abnormality of IHSS. *Circulation* **47**: 225–233, 1973.
12. Maron, B.J., Edwards, J.E., Moller, J.H., and Epstein, S.E. Prevalence and characteristics of disproportionate ventricular septal thickening in infants with congenital heart disease. *Circulation* **59**: 126–133, 1979.
13. Bulkley, B.H., Weisfelt, M.L., and Hutchins, G.M. Asymmetric septal hypertrophy and myocardial fiber disarray. Features of normal, developing and malformed hearts. *Circulation* **56**: 292–298, 1977.
14. Maron, B.J., Henry, W.L., Roberts, W.C., and Epstein, S.E. Comparison of echocardiographic and necropsy measurements of ventricular wall thickness in patients with and without disproportionate septal thickening. *Circulation* **55**: 341–346, 1977.
15. Alexander, C.S. and Gobel, F.L. Diagnosis of idiopathic hypertrophic subaortic stenosis by right ventricular septal biopsy. *Am. J. Cardiol.* **34**: 142–151, 1974.
16. Van Noorden, S., Olsen, E.G.J., and Pearse, A.G. Hypertrophic obstructive cardiomyopathy. A histological, histochemical and ultrastructural study of biopsy material. *Cardiovasc. Res.* **5**: 118–131, 1971.
17. Olsen, E. G.J. Morbid anatomy and histology in hypertrophic obstructive cardiomyopathy. In: Hypertrophic Obstructive Cardiomyopathy, Wolstenholme, G.E.W. and O'Connor, M. (eds.), Ciba Foundation Study Group No. 37, J. & A. Churchill, London, 1971, pp. 183–191.
18. James, T.N. and Marshall, T.K. De subitaneis mortibus. XII: Asymmetrical hypertrophy of the heart. *Circulation* **51**: 1149–1166, 1975.
19. Maron, B.J., Wolfson, J.K., Epstein, S.E., and Roberts, W.C. Intramural ("small vessel") coronary artery disease in hypertrophic cardiomyopathy. *J. Am. Coll. Cardiol.* **8**: 545–557, 1986.
20. Van Noorden, S. and Pearse, A.G.E. Histochemistry and electron microscopy of the heart in hypertrophic obstructive cardiomyopathy. In: Hypertrophic Obstructive Cardiomyopathy. Wolstenholme, G.E.W. and O'Connor, M. (eds.), Ciba Foundation Study Group No. 37, J. & A. Churchill, London, 1971, pp. 192–121.
21. Maron, B.J. and Roberts, W.C., Quantitative analysis of cardiac muscle cell disorganization in the ventricular septum of patients with hypertrophic cardiomyopathy. *Circulation* **59**: 689–706, 1979.
22. Becker, A.E. and Caruso, G. Myocardial disarray. A critical review. *Br. Heart J.* **47**: 527–538, 1982.
23. Maron, B.J. Myocardial disorganization in hypertrophic cardiomyopathy. *Br. Heart J.* **47**: 1–8, 1983.
24. Olsen, E.G.J. Myocardial disarray revisited (Leader). *Br. Med. J.* **285**: 991–992, 1982.
25. Sakakibara, E. and Konno, S. Endomyocardial biopsy. *Jpn. Heart J.* **3**: 537 543, 1962.
26. Olsen E.G.J., personal observation.
27. Maron, B.J., Ferrans, V.J., Henry, W.L., Clark, C.E., Redwood, D.R., Roberts, W.C., Morrow, A.G., and Epstein, S.E. Differences in distribution of myocardial abnormalities in patients with obstructive and non-obstructive asymmetric septal hypertrophy (ASH): Light and electron microscopic findings. *Circulation* **50**: 436–446, 1974.
28. Edwards, W.D., Zakheim, R., and Mettioli, L. Asymmetric septal hypertrophy in childhood. Unreliability of histologic criteria for differentiation of obstructive and nonobstructive forms. *Human Pathol.* **8**: 277–284, 1977.
29. Symons, C., Richardson, P.J., and Feizi, O. Hypertrophic cardiomyopathy and hyperthyroidism. A report of 3 cases. *Thorax* **29**: 713–719, 1974.
30. Smith, E.R., Sangalang, V.E., Hefferman, L.P., Welch, J.P., and Flemington, C.S. Hypertrophic cardiomyopathy: The heart disease of Friedreich's ataxia. *Am. Heart J.* **94**: 428–434, 1977.
31. Leading Article: Cardiac involvement in Friedreich's ataxia. *Br. Med. J.* **1**: 261, 1978.

32. Polani, P.E., and Moynihan, E.J. Progressive cardiomyopathic lentigenosis. *Q. J. Med.* **41**: 205, 1972.
33. Somerville, J. and Bonham-Carter, R.E. The heart in lentigenosis. *Br. Heart J.* **34**: 58–66, 1972.
34. Henry, W.L., Clark, C.E., and Epstein, S.E. Asymmetric septal hypertrophy (ASH): The underlying link in the IHSS disease spectrum. Observations regarding pathogenesis, pathophysiology and course. *Circulation* **47**: 827–832, 1973.
35. Olsen, E.G.J. The Pathology of the Heart (2nd edition), Macmillan Press Ltd., London and Basingstoke. 1980, pp. 324–325.
36. Bell, R., Barber, P.V., Bray, C., and Beton, D.C. Incidence of thyroid disease in cases of hypertrophic cardiomyopathy. *Br. Heart J.* **40**: 1306–1309, 1979.
37. Bulkley, B.H., Weisfeldt, M.L., and Hutchings, G.M. Isometric cardiac contraction. A possible cause of the disorganised myocardial pattern of idiopathic hypertrophic subaortic stenosis. *New Engl. J. Med.* **295**: 135–139, 1977.

Light and Electron Microscopic Features of Hypertrophic Cardiomyopathy

Victor J. Ferrans

Ultrastructure Section, Pathology Branch, National Heart, Lung and Blood Institute, National Institutes of Health, Bethesda, Maryland, U.S.A.

This chapter describes the histology and ultrastructure of the heart in hypertrophic cardiomyopathy. The most important microscopic features of the myocardium in this disorder are: 1) hypertrophy of the cardiac myocytes; 2) foci of disarray involving bundles of myocytes, individual myocytes, and myofibrils (Figs. 1–4); 3) variable degrees of interstitial fibrosis; 4) alterations in the structure of the small intramural coronary arteries (Figs. 5 and 6), and 5) a plaque-like area of endocardial thickening overlying the left ventricular surface of the ventricular septum in the region of the ventricular outflow tract.[1] The last of these features is considered to be caused by contact between the anterior mitral leaflet and the ventricular septal surface, thus being a consequence of obstruction to left ventricular outflow; the other features occur regardless of the presence or absence of such obstruction.

Myocyte Hypertrophy

Myocyte hypertrophy, a cardinal manifestation of the disorder, is present to a very severe degree, as shown by a marked increase in the total mass of the heart. Microscopically, the increase in cardiac mass is manifested by an increase in the sizes of the individual myocytes, by alterations in their nuclear morphology, and by an increase in the amount of fibrous connective tissue. As discussed below, it seems likely that the number of myocytes is also increased (hyperplasia). On microscopic examination, the transverse diameters of the myocytes are increased.[2–5] The lengths of the myocytes also are increased, but this is more difficult to evaluate in tissue sections. Both in sections and in isolated myocyte preparations, it is evident that many myocytes have unusual degrees of branching or otherwise have distorted shapes, and under such circumstances the transverse diameters do not always constitute accurate indices of the degree of myocyte enlargement.[2]

The nuclei of the myocytes are greatly enlarged, hyperchromatic and bizarre-shaped, often having blunt rather than pointed ends. The hyperchromasia represents a manifestation of polyploidy of nuclear DNA.[6] The nuclear membranes often show markedly increased degrees of convolutions;[7] intranuclear tubules derived from the nuclear membranes occur as extreme manifestations of nuclear abnormalities. The myofibril-free perinuclear areas also are enlarged and may contain large amounts of glycogen and numerous mitochondria.[4,8] These areas characteristically appear lightly stained in preparations stained with hematoxylin-eosin. We also have observed (unpublished observations) accumulation of basophilic degeneration material, which is related to glycogen,[9] in septal myocardium from several patients with hypertrophic cardiomyopathy.

Other ultrastructural changes[1,2,8] in myocardium of patients with hypertrophic cardiomyopathy include: extensive side-to-side intercellular junctions (which correlate

A

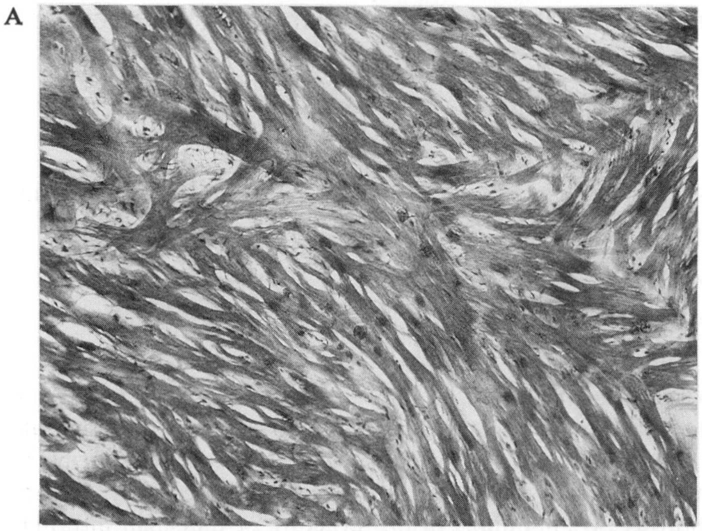

B

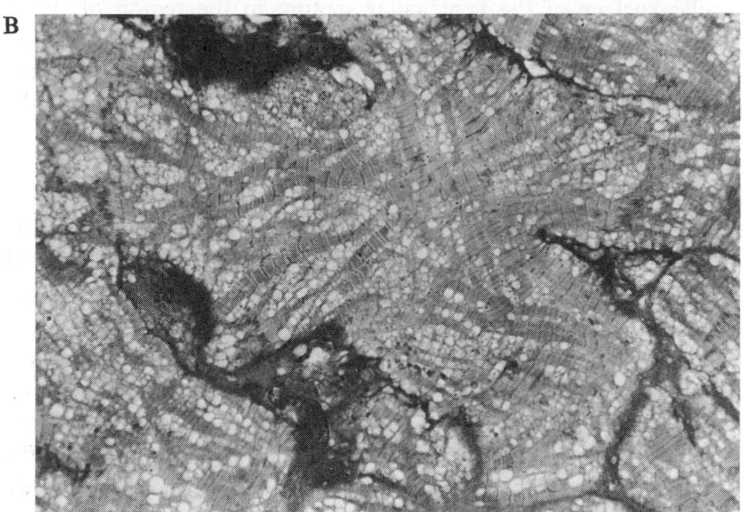

Fig. 1. A. Extensive disarray of myocytes in ventricular septum of patient with hypertrophic cardiomyopathy. Masson trichrome, × 200. B. One micron thick section of tissue embedded in plastic and stained with toluidine blue, showing highly abnormal shape of a myocyte in ventricular septum of patient with hypertrophic cardiomyopathy. Note divergent directions of the myofibrils. × 750.

with the abnormalities of cell shape and orientation), large cisterns of rough-surfaced endoplasmic reticulum increased numbers of lysosomes and lipofuscin granules, mild to moderate dilatation of T tubules, increased amounts of 10 nm filaments (cytoskeletal filaments), widened Z bands, evidence of formation of new sarcomeres, and alterations in the orientation and alignment of myofibrils. The mitochondria and the sarcoplasmic reticulum do not show distinctive changes, although the mitochondria often appear increased in number, particularly in the perinuclear areas. In areas of disarray, the myofibrils show crisscrossing and branching (Figs. 3 and 4), in which myofilaments originat-

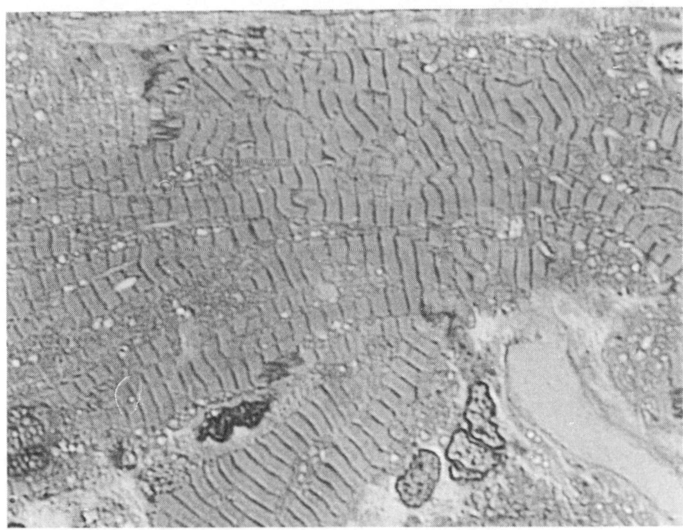

Fig. 2. Disarray involving myofibrils and sarcomeres in ventricular septal myocyte of patient with hypertrophic cardiomyopathy. Plastic section, Nomarski interference microscopy, × 1,200.

ing from a single Z band course in widely diverging directions.[2] The preceding changes are nonspecific in a qualitative sense; however, as described below, the alterations related to disarray of the muscle cells and their contractile elements are very prominent in hypertrophic cardiomyopathy, and important observations have been made on the quantitation of these findings.[10–15]

The occurrence of asymmetric septal hypertrophy in most patients with hypertrophic cardiomyopathy has served as a stimulus for investigations of the regional distribution of the myocardial hypertrophy, which has been evaluated by counting cell layers and measuring myocyte diameters in different areas of the heart. These studies have shown that the asymmetrically hypertrophied septum in hypertrophic cardiomyopathy contains an abnormally large number of layers of myocytes, and that these myocytes are not larger than those in other areas of these hearts.[10] Fujiwara *et al.*[12] found that the number of layers of myocytes in ventricular septum (630 ± 80) was increased in comparison to that in normal subjects (490 ± 70) and in patients with hypertensive heart disease (510 ± 80), that in patients with hypertrophic cardiomyopathy there was a good correlation between the numbers of layers of myocytes and the degree of asymmetric septal thickening, and that the diameters of the myocytes did not differ significantly in ventricular septum (19 ± 3 μm) and posterior left ventricular free wall (21 ± 2 μm). Fujiwara *et al.*[12] also found that the numbers of cell layers in the left ventricular free wall in patients with hypertrophic cardiomyopathy were reduced in comparison to those in control patients (360 ± 70 vs. 480 ± 50). Other studies[14,15] did not agree with this finding.

Another study[13] also compared the number and size of myocytes, the amount of interstitial space, and the extent of the disarray in the ventricular septum and the left ventricular free wall in 6 patients with chronic systemic hypertension and asymmetric septal hypertrophy and in 25 control individuals, including 15 with no cardiac disease and 10 with systemic hypertension not associated with asymmetric septal hypertrophy.

A

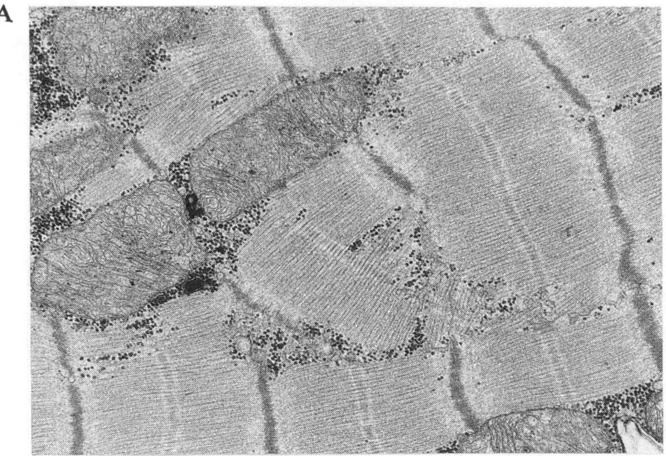

B

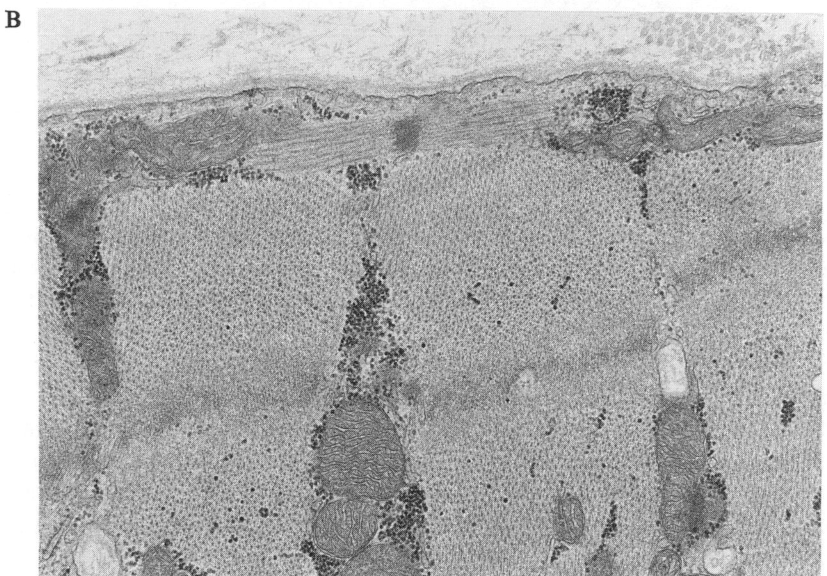

Fig. 3. Myofibrillar disarray. A. Electron micrograph of ventricular septal muscle from patient with hypertrophic cardiomyopathy, showing area (center) of divergent orientation of a myofibril. Uranyl acetate and lead citrate stain, × 28,000. B. Electron micrograph of subsarcolemmal area, showing small, narrow myofibril that courses perpendicular to axis of adjacent myofibrils. Uranyl acetate and lead citrate stain, × 34,000.

The numbers of layers of myocytes in the septum and left ventricular free wall were 680 ± 90 and 440 ± 40, respectively, in the patients with asymmetric septal hypertrophy and hypertension, and 500 ± 60 and 490 ± 60, respectively, in the control patients.

Unverferth *et al.*[14] also quantified myocyte diameters, percentage of fibrous tissue and numbers of cell layers in right ventricular free wall, left ventricular free wall and ventricular septum in 8 patients who died of complications of hypertrophic cardiomyopathy and in 8 age-matched controls without heart disease. In these two groups of pa-

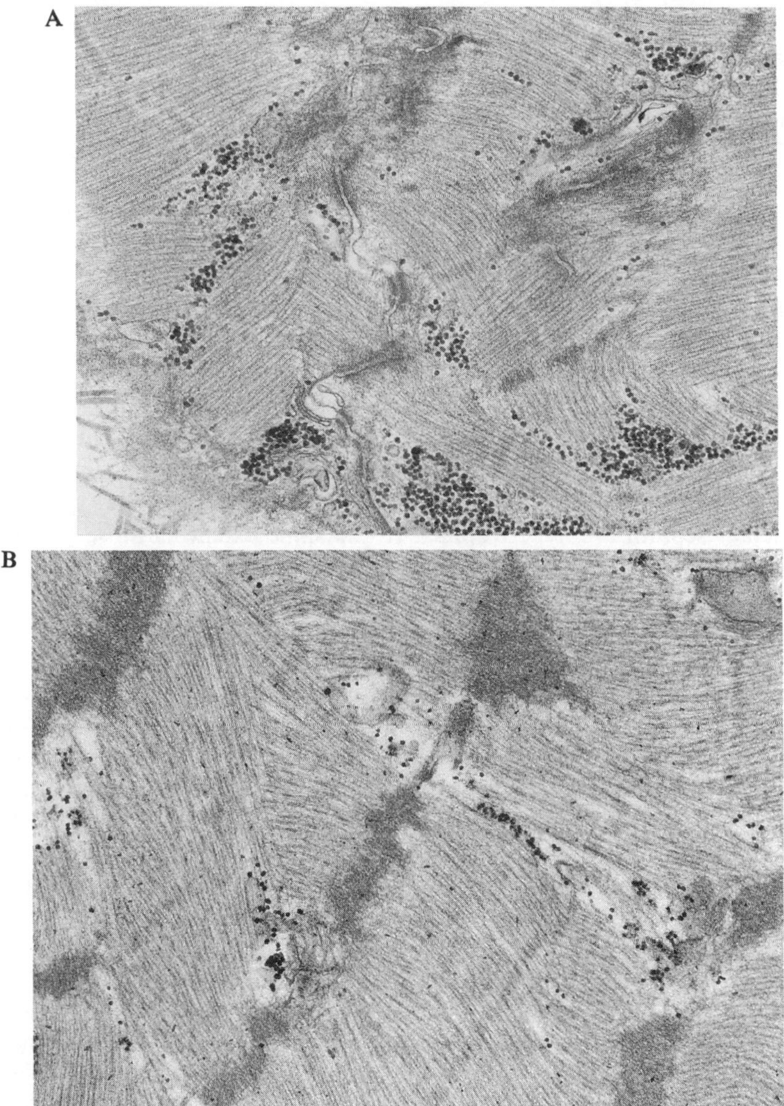

Fig. 4. Severe disarray of myofibrils and myofilaments. A. Crisscrossing of myofibrils and myofilaments in the region of an intercalated disc in ventricular septal muscle of patient with hypertrophic cardiomyopathy. Uranyl acetate and lead citrate stain, ×38,000.

tients, the numbers of cell layers were as follows: right ventricular free wall, 185 ± 44 and 193 ± 20; ventricular septum, 572 ± 154 and 444 ± 74; and left ventricular free wall, 439 ± 115 and 406 ± 84, respectively. The cell diameters were largest in those layers of the ventricular septum and of the left ventricular free wall that were closest to the left ventricular cavity. This finding was in contrast to that of Hoshino *et al.*,[11] who found the greatest cell diameters in the midportion of the ventricular septum. Unverferth *et al.*[14] found the diameters of myocytes to be similar in ventricular septum and in other areas of left ventricle.

Frenzel *et al.*[15] evaluated tissue samples from 3 groups of patients with respect to size of ventricular septal myocytes, volume density of interstitium and fibrous tissue, and number of layers of myocytes. On the basis of data obtained from right ventricular endomyocardial biopsies, the number of myocyte layers in the septum was calculated to be 715 ± 93 in 7 patients with normal cardiac morphology and 1,242 ± 149 in one group of 7 patients with hypertrophic cardiomyopathy. In another 7 patients, data obtained from right ventricular endomyocardial biopsies and left ventricular myectomy specimens from the same patients were used to calculate the numbers of cell layers in ventricular septum; these were estimated to be 1,119 ± 177 and 810 ± 232, respectively. These calculated numbers of layers of septal myocytes were larger than those obtained by actual cell counts in other studies [ref. 12–14, including Linzbach's study[16] of the number of layers in normal hearts ($n = 520$)].

The studies just reviewed clearly indicate that the number of layers of myocytes in the asymmetrically hypertrophied ventricular septum of patients with hypertrophic cardiomyopathy is larger than normal. The increase in mass of the septum is proportional to the increased number of layers of myocytes in this region, and the myocytes in the ventricular septum are hypertrophied to the same extent as those in the left ventricular free wall.[11,12] Increased amounts of fibrous tissue also contribute to the increased thickness of the ventricular septum, but the increase in septal thickness cannot be accounted for only on the basis of larger amounts of fibrous tissue.

It remains to be determined whether the increased number of cell layers in the ventricular septum of patients with hypertrophic cardiomyopathy is due to: 1) abnormal amounts of cell division (hyperplasia) during development and/or later in life; 2) abnormal patterns of myocyte migration during development; 3) failure of regression of the pattern of disproportionate septal thickening that is seen normally[17] during fetal life (and which seems to have a delayed regression in infants of diabetic mothers,[18–20] or 4) a combination of two or more of these factors.

Hyperplasia of myocytes normally occurs during the prenatal phase of cardiac development and stops soon after birth, at which time hypertrophy becomes the main mechanism by which cardiac mass increases. The transition from a hyperplastic to a hypertrophic type of growth can be delayed by mechanical overloading of the neonatal heart. Under certain circumstances, the ability of cardiac myocytes to synthesize DNA and undergo mitotic division can be restored after the neonatal period; however, it is uncertain to what extent this results in complete cell division or only in either polyploidy or bi- or multinucleation, which are known to occur normally in human hearts, and which can be greatly increased in hypertrophy.[21] It has been suggested that in hypertrophic cardiomyopathy there is increased hyperplasia of cardiac myocytes early in life, and that this hyperplasia leads to permanently disturbed patterns of cardiac gross anatomy, with abnormal numbers of layers of myocytes in the ventricular septum. These changes would be followed by a phase of progressive hypertrophy after the switch from hyperplastic to hypertrophic growth.[21] Recent evidence suggests that there is an acceleration of the process of asymmetric septal hypertrophy after the onset of puberty, but the microscopic changes that accompany this change remain unknown.[22,23]

Myocardial Disarray

Foci of disarray of bundles of myocytes, of individual myocytes, and of contractile elements within cells, have been demonstrated in the hearts of patients with hypertrophic cardiomyopathy by techniques of 1) light microscopic examination of thin (5 μm) and thick (25 μm) histologic sections,[5,24–30] 2) transmission electron microscopy of ultrathin sections,[1-4,31-33] and 3) scanning electron microscopy of partially dissociated myocardium.[31-33]

Myocardial disarray in hypertrophic cardiomyopathy was first described by Teare[24] in his initial report of the cardiac anatomic findings in this disorder. Since then, other investigators have confirmed these findings, and shown: 1) that some degree of dissarray is present in the hearts of normal individuals[26,29,34] and of individuals with heart diseases other than hypertrophic cardiomyopathy,[35-40] and 2) that the extent and severity of the disarray are much greater in hypertrophic cardiomyopathy than in other conditions,[29,39,40] and 3) that disarray is also extensive in patients with right-sided hypertrophic obstructive cardiomyopathy,[41] in patients with nonobstructive apical hypertrophic cardiomyopathy,[42] and patients with symmetric hypertrophic cardiomyopathy.[43] These findings have led to contradictory conclusions (see ref. 34 for review). Some investigators have concluded that the diagnostic usefulness of the finding of myocardial disarray in biopsy specimens is very limited,[29] while others believe that the diagnosis of hypertrophic cardiomyopathy can be made accurately on the basis of qualitative observations of myocardial disarray in endomyocardial biopsies taken from the right side of the ventricular septum.[44]

Variations in the definition of what constitutes myocardial disarray constitute a most important element of this controversy. This is specially true with respect to the importance given to minor deviations from a parallel arrangement, particularly when bundles of myocytes follow curving paths around blood vessels. Based on study of transverse sections of ventricular septum (i.e., cut along a plane perpendicular to the long axis of the left ventricle). Maron and Roberts[39] recognized 4 major types of cardiac muscle cell disorganization. Type I-A disorganization, the most common, consisted of areas in which adjacent cardiac myocytes were aligned perpendicularly or obliquely to each other, usually forming tangled masses or "pinwheel" configurations. Although most of these lesions were small, the size of individual foci of type I-A disorganization varied greatly. In type I-B disorganization, relatively broad bundles of muscle cells were oriented at oblique or perpendicular angles to each other; however, cells within these bundles were normally arranged. Both type I-A and I-B exclusively involved areas of septum in which the muscle cells were cut longitudinally (as is the case in the middle third of the ventricular septum). Type II-A disorganization consisted of narrow, longitudinally cut bundles of cells that were interlaced in various directions among larger groups of transversely cut cells. This type of disorganization gave the myocardium a swirled appearance. Type II-B was similar to type II-A disorganization, except that the narrow, longitudinally cut bundles of cells were more linear. A fifth type of disorganization was observed in three control patients, none of whom had hypertrophic cardiomyopathy. This pattern consisted of relatively small islands of disorganized, longitudinally cut cells within much larger areas of transversely cut cells.

According to Maron and Roberts,[39] abnormally arranged cardiac muscle cells were not considered to represent true disorganization if present in the following areas where cells normally converge at acute angles: 1) at or near the junction of the ventricular septum with the left and right ventricular free walls, where adjacent muscle cells are joined at acute angles because of the interlacing, interweaving, fanning out or changing course of bundles; 2) intrabeculations; 3) in, or at the edges of, areas of fibrosis; 4) at points of convergence of major muscle bundles, and 5) adjacent to interstitial spaces containing blood vessels. Artifactual disarray also occurs as the result of buckling or waviness of bundles of muscle cells. In addition, variable degrees of cellular and/or myofibrillar disarray occur normally in atrial myocardium,[44] atrioventricular node,[45,46] and Purkinje fibers.[47–49] A disorderly arrangement of cells and myofibrils is characteristic of embryonic cardiac muscle, in which myofibrils in early stages of development have myofilaments that radiate in different directions from a single Z band.[48,49] Branching of cells and myofibrils is found in primitive hearts such as those of crustaceans, in which the cardiac walls are spongy and highly trabeculated.[50,51] Thornell *et al.*[47] described disarray of cells and myofibrils in branching false tendons of the cat heart, and attributed it to the multidirectional mechanical forces to which the false tendons are subjected. Ross and Streeter[52] found disarray in the myocardium of the macaque, not only in the interventricular septum but also in the entire subendocardium, wherever there was trabeculation. Myocardial fiber disarray has been described as a purely qualitative finding in the hearts of patients with idiopathic dilated cardiomyopathy, alcoholic cardiomyopathy, hypertensive heart disease, coronary heart disease, cor pulmonale, and various congenital heart diseases including tetralogy of Fallot and aortic and mitral atresia[26,29,35–40]; however, except in aortic and mitral atresia,[57] the amount of disarray is considerably smaller in these conditions than in hypertrophic cardiomyopathy. Thus, hypertrophic cardiomyopathy cannot be diagnosed solely on the bais of the qualitative observation of myocardial disarray in biopsy specimens, even though it is often possible to demonstrate such a disarray in biopsies and in operatively removed fragments of septal muscle from patients with this disease. Isner *et al.*[53] showed that the disarray in hypertrophic cardiomyopathy is much more easily demonstrable in large histologic sections of ventricular septum than in small, operatively removed samples from this area. The disarray usually is most pronounced in the central third of the ventricular septum[30,58]; however, endomyocardial biopsy specimens include only very superficial layers of septal muscle, and at myotomy-myectomy the tissue is resected mainly from the one-third of the septum facing the left ventricular cavity.

Quantitative Aspects of Myocardial Disarray

Maron and Roberts used a quantitative video planimetry system to determine the percentage area of myocardium that was occupied by disorganized cells in transverse sections of ventricular septum in 54 patients with hypertrophic cardiomyopathy.[39] Septal disorganization was present in 94% of these patients; and involved 5% or more of the section in 89% of the patients and 25% or more of the section in 56% of the patients. Septal disorganization was present in only 26% of 144 control patients with other heart diseases or normal hearts, in which it usually was limited in extent. In only 7% of the controls studied did abnormally arranged cells occupy 5% or more of the tissue section. The average area of septum disorganized was 31 ± 3% (mean ± S.E.M.) in patients with hypertrophic cardiomyopathy and only 1.5 ± 0.6% in the control patients ($P < 0.001$).

Using the same technique, Maron *et al.* studied the distribution of cardiac musle cell disorganization in different regions of the left ventricular wall in 52 patients with hypertrophic cardiomyopathy.[40] Cellular disorganization in the ventricular septum was both common and extensive (involving a mean of 35 4%). Disorganization was also substantial, but less marked (24 ± 3%) in the left ventricular free wall. Disorganization in anterior left ventricular free wall was particularly extensive (32 ± 4%) and did not differ significantly from that present in the ventricular septum. Marked disorganization (> 5% of the tissue section) was diffusely distributed in the ventricular septum and left ventricular free wall in 33 of the 52 patients (63%). Of the four histologic types of disorganization described by Maron and Roberts, type I (particularly type I-A) was most often the predominant form in ventricular septum and left ventricular free wall;

only in one patient did the extent of type II disorganization exceed that of type I.

Maron and Roberts[39] found no relation between the extent of disorganization of septal muscle and sex, presence or absence of symptoms, duration of symptoms, presence of coronary artery disease or atrial fibrillation, mode of death, magnitude of the left ventricular outflow tract obstruction or left ventricular end-diastolic pressure, heart weight, ventricular septal thickness, septal-free wall ratio, or whether myotomy-myectomy had been performed. Septal disorganization was greater in patients who were younger than 18 years of age at the time of death than in older patients (although a linear relationship did not exist between extent of septal disorganization and age). Septal disorganization also was more marked in patients who were members of families with malignant hypertrophic cardiomyopathy[58] and less extensive in patients with a history of systemic hypertension. No clinical or anatomic parameter appeared to be characteristic of either the 6 patients with hypertrophic cardiomyopathy who showed no or minimal (less than 3%) septal disorganization or the 5 patients who had marked (70% or greater) disorganization. Particularly marked left ventricular free wall and combined free wall and septal disorganization were present in 14 patients without functional limitation in whom sudden death occurred early in life ($>$ 25 years of age) and was the initial manifestation of cardiac disease. In contrast, although abnormally arranged cardiac muscle cells were identified in the left ventricular free wall in 47% of patients with other congenital or acquired heart diseases, or with normal hearts, this disorganization was usually limited in extent (mean, $2 \pm 0.5\%$ of the tissue area). The extent of free wall and combined septal and free wall disorganization was also greater in 5 patients with nonobstructive hypertrophic cardiomyopathy than in 24 patients with obstruction to left ventricular outflow under basal conditions; however, this difference did not achieve statistical significance. Free wall and combined septal and free wall disorganization were absent or particularly focal in 4 patients with associated systemic hypertension (mean, 0.5% of tissue area).

Three limitations are inherent to the morphometric studies of Maron *et al.*[39,40,54]

1. For all practical purposes, evaluation of myocyte disarray is possible only when the majority of the cells in a histologic section are cut longitudinally. In transverse sections of ventricular septum, longitudinally sectioned myocytes appear as a band in the middle of the septum, and these myocytes account for most of the disarray present in the septum. In longitudinal sections of septum, myocytes in the two subendocardial regions appear longitudinally sectioned; disarray in these two areas is less prominent than in the central area, in which the myocytes appear sectioned transversely (thus making it difficult to evaluate disarray in this area). For this reason, transverse sections of the septum are preferred over longitudinal sections for study of disarray; however, in either plane of section there is a certain percentage of cells in which disarray cannot be evaluated. Actually, this problem is more severe in evaluating disarray of the free walls of the ventricles than it is in evaluating septal disarray, because the arrangement of the myocytes in the free walls is much more complex and irregular than in the septum.

2. No provision has been made in these studies for evaluation of the disarray of myofibrils (for this reason, the relationship between cellular and myofibrillar disarray has not been evaluated quantitatively) or for evaluation of the actual severity of the dissarray of cells (as opposed to only its presence).

3. These studies have been used for only limited mapping of the disarray. Maron *et al.*[59] have shown that several different patterns of anatomic distribution of left ventricular hypertrophy are distinguishable in these patients according to the degree to which they involve various regions of the ventricular septum and left ventricular free

wall. Detailed studies have not yet been made correlating these patterns of hypertrophy with observations on the histologic architecture of the heart. Similarly, quantitative studies of myocardial disarray have not been made in any of the "secondary" forms of hypertrophic cardiomyopathy (see Perloff[60] for review) in which this disease coexists with other cardiac lesions or with various systemic disorders.

Interstitial Fibrosis

Interstitial fibrosis often is a prominent feature of hypertrophic cardiomyopathy, particularly in the asymmetrically hypertrophied ventricular septum, and is manifested either by bands of fibrous connective tissue which encircle the myocytes, separating them from adjacent structures, or by large areas of replacement fibrosis. The latter lesions are thought to result from myocardial necrosis due to narrowing of small, intramural coronary arteries.[61,62] The percentage area of septal and left ventricular myocardium occupied by fibrous tissue in patients with hypertrophic cardiomyopathy is greater than that in control patients. According to Unverferth *et al.*,[14] this increase tends to be maximal in the ventricular septum (up to about 20% compared to about 6% in normals). Extensive myocardial fibrosis has also been found in myocardium of patients with right-sided hypertrophic obstructive cardiomyopathy. The fibrosis tends to be maximal in patients with the late stage of the disease, in which ventricular dilatation and vascular lesions occur.

Vascular Lesions

As mentioned above, patients with hypertrophic cardiomyopathy often show narrowing of intramural coronary arteries, which tends to be maximal in the ventricular septum and which is related to intimal and medial thickening by increased amounts of fibrous connective tissue, elastic tissue and smooth muscle cells, and adventitial fibrosis (Figs. 5 and 6). These lesions can be of considerable clinical significance in the late stages of the disease, in which they can be the cause of cardiac dilatation, fibrosis and thinning of the left ventricular free wall. Their precise relationship to the cardiomyopathic process is unknown. They are not specific for hypertrophic cardiomyopathy, as they also occur in various other conditions.[62–65]

Tanaka *et al.*[66] made quantitative studies of the diameter and percentage of the total vessel area occupied by the lumen in small intramyocardial arteries of 15 patients with typical hypertrophic cardiomyopathy, 4 patients with hypertrophic cardiomyopathy and cavity dilatation, 10 patients with systemic hypertension and 15 normal adult individuals. The relationships between narrowings of the intramyocardial coronary arteries and myocyte hypertrophy, myocardial fiber disarray, and fibrosis were also examined. The external caliber and the ratio of the luminal area to the total cross-sectional area of the vessel were calculated, using an image analyzer, in 85 to 203 intramyocardial small arteries from each patient. The external calibers of these vessels were similar among groups of hearts with hypertrophic cardiomyopathy, hypertensive hearts and normal hearts, but were greater in those with hypertrophic cardiomyopathy associated with cavity dilatation. The mean % of the cross-sectional area occupied by the lumen in intramyocardial small arteries was similarly reduced in the hearts with hypertrophic cardiomyopathy (29 ± 5% in the ventricular septum and 31 ± 5% in the left ventricular free wall) and in hypertensive hearts (30 ± 8% and 31 ± 7%) compared with that in normal hearts (40 ± 5% and 38 ± 5%) and was the lowest in the ventricular septum of hearts with hypertrophic cardiomyopathy and cavity dilatation (17 ± 3%). The mean % of cross-sectional area occupied by the lumen in small intramural coronary

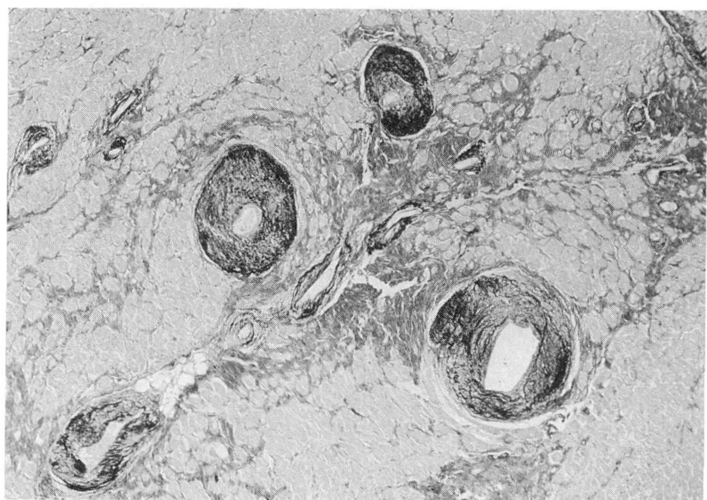

Fig. 5. Histologic section showing abnormally thick small arteries in ventricular septum of patient with hypertrophic cardiomyopathy. Elastica-van Gieson stain, ×150.

arteries was inversely correlated with heart weight (r = −0.59), the mean size of myocytes (r = −0.66 in the ventricular septum, r = −0.63 in the free wall), and percent fibrotic area in the septum (r = −0.68), but did not correlate with the presence or absence of myocyte disarray.

Maron *et al.*[67] made histological analyses of left ventricular myocardium obtained at autopsy from 48 patients with hypertrophic cardiomyopathy and 68 patients with either normal hearts or acquired heart disease. In hypertrophic cardiomyopathy, abnormal intramural coronary arteries were characterized by thickening of the vessel wall and an apparent decrease in luminal size (external arterial diameter < 1500 μm; average 300 μm). The wall thickening was due to proliferation of medial and/or intimal components, particularly smooth muscle cells and collagen. Of the 48 patients with hypertrophic cardiomyopathy, 40 (83%) had abnormal intramural coronary arteries located in the ventricular septum (33 patients), anterior left ventricular free wall (20 patients), or posterior free wall (9 patients). Altered intramural coronary arteries were significantly more common in tissue sections having considerable myocardial fibrosis (31 out of 42, 74%) than in those with no or mild fibrosis (31 of 102, 30%; $p < 0.001$). Abnormal intramural coronary arteries were also identified in 3 out of 8 infants who died of HCM before 1 year of age. In contrast, altered intramural coronary arteries were identified only rarely in 6 (9%) of the 69 control patients, and those arteries showed only mild thickening of the wall and minimal luminal narrowing. Moreover, of those patients who did show abnormal intramural coronary arteries, such vessels were about twenty times more frequent in patients with HCM (0.9 ± 0.2/cm^2 myocardium) than in control patients (0.04 ± 0.02/cm^2 myocardium).

Maron *et al.*[67] concluded that intramural coronary arteries with markedly thickened walls and narrowed lumina are present in increased numbers in most patients with hypertrophic cardiomyopathy at necropsy, and that these vascular lesions may represent a congenital component of the underlying cardiomyopathic process. Although the clini-

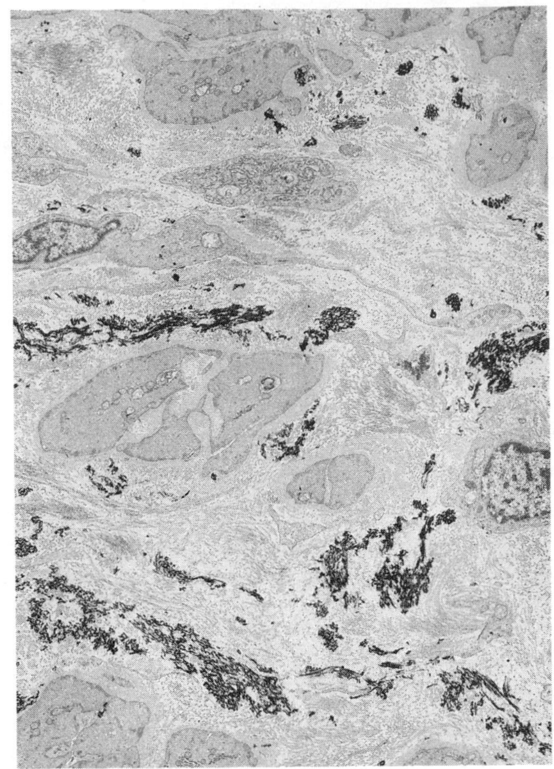

Fig. 6. Electron micrograph of part of small artery similar to those showin in Fig. 5. The wall of the vessel is composed of smooth muscle cells, collagen and abundant elastin (stained black). Tannic acid stain, × 8,000.

cal significance of "small vessel coronary artery disease" in hypertrophic cardiomyopathy is unclear, the occurrence of structurally altered intramural coronary arteries within or adjacent to areas of substantial myocardial necrosis and/or fibrosis suggests a causal role for these arteries in producing ischemia.

Endocardial Thickening

The area of endocardial thickening on the ventricular septal surface of the left ventricular outflow tract is composed of fibrous and elastic connective tissue and smooth muscle cells. This lesion is often found in apposition to a similar area of fibroelastic thickening in the anterior mitral leaflet. It is thought that both of these changes are consequences of contact between the anterior mitral leaflet and the septal surface. Accordingly, this lesion is regarded as evidence of present or previous obstruction to left ventricular outflow.[1)]

Neural Elements

An early study of hypertrophic cardiomyopathy reported an increase in the fluorescence, induced by treatment of tissue with paraformaldehyde and attributed to the presence of catecholamines, in sympathomimetic nerves in myocardium in the left ventricular outflow tract of patients with hypertrophic obstructive cardiomyopathy. Subsequent studies did not confirm this finding, and biochemical studies led to the conclusion that myocardium from these patients showed depletion of catecholamines that was proportional to the degree of cardiac failure (see ref. 2 for review). The ultrastructure of cardiac nerves in patients with hypertrophic cardiomyopathy has not been reported in detail.

Hypertrophic Cardiomyopathy Associated with Other Disorders

It is now well known that hypertrophic cardiomyopathy can occur in association with a number of cardiac and systemic disorders.[60] However, little information is available on details of the pathology of the heart (i.e., quantification of disarray, presence of unusual morphological findings) in patients having such combined disorders. Some interesting observations that have been made on some of these unusual forms of hypertrophic cardiomyopathy include the demonstration of amyloid deposits in hearts of patients with amyloidosis and asymmetric septal hypertrophy[68,69] and deposits of glycolipid material (presumed to be ceramide trihexoside) in cardiac myocytes and coronary arteries of patients with hypertrophic cardiomyopathy and Fabry's disease.[70-72] Recent studies also have shown that certain patients with hypertrophic cardiomyopathy also have unusual systemic abnormalities of mitochondrial structure and function. Prominent among these disorders is Leigh's disease (progressive subacute necrotizing encephalomyelopathy), an autosomal recessive condition with clinical mainfestations which appear in infancy and are mainly neurological.[73-76] The biochemical defect is thought to be heterogeneous, with low levels of pyruvate decarboxylase in the CNS, liver, skeletal muscle and heart; in some cases there is also deficiency of cytochrome oxidase. The disease is usually fatal in infancy; however, some patients have survived to adolescence or adulthood. The heart in Leigh's disease shows masive hypertrophy, with an increase in weight of up to twice that expected for the patient's age. Grossly, the hypertrophy may resemble that seen in the usual form of hypertrophic cardiomyopathy. Asymmetric septal hypertrophy and myocardial fiber disarray have been observed.

Ultrastructurally, there is a paucity of myofibrils and a marked increase in the numbers of mitochondria, which may be abnormally shaped and have tubular cristae. This disease has been thought to represent a "mitochondrial cardiomyopathy". However, quantitative parameters for establishing this diagnosis have not been established. Also associated with hypertrophic cardiomyopathy is a syndrome of congenital cataracts, mitochondrial myopathy affecting skeletal muscle and cardiac muscle and exercise-induced lactic acidosis. Some of the patients with this syndrome have been found to have asymmetric septal hypertrophy and a marked degree of myocardial fiber disarray.[77-79] Furthermore, other disorders of unknown etiology, including some rare cases of dilated cardiomyopathy occurring in small children, also are characterized by marked increases in the numbers of mitochondria in cardiac myocytes.[80-82] Abnormalities of cardiac mitochondria also occur in the Kearns-Sayre syndrome.[83-85] Thus, the relationship between mitochondrial cardiomyopathies and hypertrophic cardiomyopathy remains to be clarified.

Hypertrophic Cardiomyopathy in Animals

Several studies have reported the sporadic occurrence of hypertrophic cardiomyopathy in cats, dogs and pigs (see ref. 86 for review). Most of these studies have described the nonobstructive type, and in most cases the degree of asymmetric septal hypertrophy and of myocardial fiber disarray have been minimal. The disease appears to be relatively frequent in cats, but to date no colony of affected animals has been established. Histologic and electron microscopic studies have been made of the morphology of the heart in hypertrophic cardiomyopathy occurring in cats. In this species, the disease tends to affect middle-aged males most frequently, and is 3 times more frequent in males than in females. However, the age range of affected cats may be wide, as seen in a large series (n = 128) of affected cats that ranged from 8 months to 16 years of age. The occurrence of cases in related cats suggests a role for heredity. Clinically, affected cats generally present with sudden onset of congestive heart failure with dyspnea, anorexia, and lethargy. Approximately half of affected cats will have aortic thromboembolism and posterior paresis. Some cats may have sudden, unexpected death without previous clinical signs. At necropsy, extracardiac findings include aortic thromboembolism, renal infarction, and pulmonary congestion and edema. Affected hearts are enlarged and have diffuse hypertrophy of the left ventricular free wall, ventricular septum and left ventricular papillary muscles, marked dilatation and hypertrophy of the left atrium, and a narrow left ventricular cavity. In a few cats, asymmetric septal hypertrophy is observed, as manifested by a septal/free wall thickness ratio of 1.1 or greater (rather than by the 1.3 or greater ratio used to classify the human cases). Histologically, diffuse hypertrophy, myocyte disarray (disarray occurs mostly in association with asymmetric septal hypertrophy), interstitial fibrosis, and fibromuscular hyperplasia of small intramural coronary arteries are seen. Of 129 cat hearts with hypertrophic cardiomyopathy, 44% had foci of myocyte disarray in the ventricular septum; in 31% the disarray involved at least 5% of the myocytes in the section.[86)]

Cardiac histopathologic and ultrastructural alterations in 10 cats with hypertrophic cardiomyopathy consisted of hypertrophy and disarray of cardiac muscle cells (most severe in left ventricle and ventricular septum), interstitial fibrosis, and fibromuscular hyperplasia of small intramural coronary arteries. The hypertrophied fibers had large nuclei, prominent Golgi complexes, and numerous polysomes; some fibers had crisscrossing myofibrils. Degenerative alterations in hypertrophied myocytes were: perinuclear distension of elements of sarcoplasmic reticulum, focal myofibrillar lysis, numerous thick clumps of Z-band material, and abundant lipofuscin granules. The interstitium showed accumulations of collagen fibrils, increased numbers of fibroblasts, and scattered remnants of basement membrane. One cat had dilated chambers, but also had typical histologic and ultrastructural alterations of hypertrophic cardiomyopathy and was considered to have a late stage of this disorder.

Hypertrophic cardiomyopathy in dogs predominates in males. German shepherds are most frequently affected, but cases in dogs of small breeds have also been reported.[86)] Aproximately 50% of the dogs had sudden unexpecte ddeath (which occurred in some dogs during routine surgical procedures); the remaining dogs had evidence of congestive cardiac failure with dyspnea and cough. At necropsy, the hearts were enlarged and showed ventricular hypertrophy, decreased left ventricular cavity size, and left atrial dilatation. Asymmetric septal hypertrophy (septal/free wall thickness ratio, > 1.1) was often present. Microscopically, myocyte disarray was seen in the ventricular septum of 20% of the dogs.

In a series of 1906 necropsy cases of pigs at the Pig Research Institute of Taiwan, 32 cases of hypertrophic cardiomyopathy were reported.[87)] Twenty-three of these had the symmetric form, and 9 the asymmetric form (which was defined by a septal/free wall thickness ratio of 1.1 rather than by the 1.3 ratio used in classifying the human disorder). Relative heart weights were increased by 50%. The ventricular walls were severely thickened, and the left ventricular cavity was small in size and abnormal in shape. Microscopic study revealed consistent myocyte hypertrophy; however, only some cases had disarray of myocytes. Thus, it seems that hypertrophic cardiomyopathy in pigs (and also in dogs and cats) is more frequently of the symmetric type and is less frequently associated with myocyte disarray than is the case in humans.

REFERENCES

1. Roberts, W.C. and Ferrans, V.J. The pathologic anatomy of the cardiomyopathics (idiopathic dilated and hypertrophic types, infiltrative types and endomyocardial disease with and without eosinophilia). *Hum. Pathol.* **6**: 287–342, 1975.
2. Ferrans, V.J., Morrow, A.G., and Roberts, W.C. Myocardial ultrastructure in idiopathic hypertrophic subaortic stenosis. A study of operatively excised left ventricular outflow tract muscle in 14 patients. *Circulation* **45**: 769–792, 1972.
3. Olsen, E.G.J. The pathology of idiopathic hypertrophic subaortic stenosis (hypertrophic cardiomyopathy). A critical review. *Am. Heart J.* **100**: 533–562. 1980.
4. Van Noorden, S., Olsen, E.G.J., and Pearse, A.G.E. Hypertrophic obstructive cardiomyopathy: A histological, histochemical and ultrastructural study of biopsy material. *Cardiovasc. Res.* **5**: 118–131, 1971.
5. Maron, B.J. and Roberts, W.C. Hypertrophic cardiomyopathy and cardiac muscle cell disorganization revisited: Relation between the two and significance. *Am. Heart J.* **102**: 95–110, 1981.
6. Adler, C.P. Ploidiemuster und Zellzahl in Herzen mit Kardiomyopathie. *Verh. Dtsch. Ges. Pathol.* **62**: 516, 1978.
7. Ferrans, V.J., Jones, M., Maron, B.J., and Roberts, W.C. The nuclear membranes in hypertrophied human cardiac muscle cells. *Am. J. Pathol.* **78**: 427–460. 1975.
8. Maron, B.J., Ferrans, V.J., and Roberts, W.C. Ultrastructural features of degenerated cardiac muscle cells in patients with cardiac hypertrophy. *Am. J. Pathol.* **79**: 387–434, 1975.
9. Ferrans, V.J. and Butany, J.W. Ultrastructural pathology of the heart. In: Diagnostic Electron Microscopy, Vol. 4, Trump, B.F. and Jones, R.T. (eds.) John Wiley & Sons. Inc. pp. 319–473, 1983.
10. Ferrans, V.J. and Rodriguez, E.R. Specificity of light and electron microscopic features of hypertrophic obstructive and nonobstructive cardiomyopathy. Qualitative, quantitative and etiologic aspects. *Eur. Heart J.* **4** (Suppl F): 9–22, 1983.
11. Hoshino, T., Fujiwara, H., Kawai, C., and Hamashima, Y. Myocardial fiber diameter and its regional distribution throughout the ventrical wall in normal adult hearts, hypertensive hearts and hearts with hypertrophic cardiomyopathy. *Circulation* **67**: 1109–1116, 1983.
12. Fujiwara, H., Hoshino, T., Yamana, K., Fujiwara, T., Furuta, M., Hamashima, Y., and Kawai, C. Number and size of myocytes and amount of interstitial space in the ventricular septum and in the left ventricular free wall in hypertrophic cardiomyopathy. *Am. J. Cardiol.* **52**: 818–823. 1983.
13. Fujiwara, H., Fujiwara, T., Hamashima, Y., and Kawai, C. Number and size of myocytes, amount of interstitial space and extent of disarray of the hearts in patients with systemic hypertension and asymmetric septal hypertrophy. *Jpn. Circ. J.* **49**: 406–414, 1985.
14. Unverferth, D.V., Baker, P.B., Pearce, L.I., Lautman, J., and Roberts, W.C. Regional myocyte hypertrophy and increased interstitial myocardial fibrosis in hypertrophic cardiomyopathy. *Am. J. Cardiol.* **59**: 932–936. 1987.
15. Frenzel, H., Schwartzkopff, B., Reinecke, P., Kamoni, K., and Losse, B. Evidence for muscle fiber hyperplasia in the septum of patients with hypertrophic obstructive cardiomyopathy. Quantitative examination of endomyocardial biopsies and myectomy specimens. *Z. Kardiol.* **76**. Suppl 3. 14–19. 1987.
16. Linzbach, A.J. Hypertrophy, hyperplasia and structural dilatation of the human heart. *Adv. Cardiol.* **18**: 1–14, 1976.
17. Maron, B.J., Verter, J., and Kapur, S. Disproportionate ventricular septal thickening in the developing normal human heart. *Circulation* **57**: 520–526. 1978.

18. Gutgesell, H.P., Mullins, C.E., Gillette, P.C., Speer, M., Rudolph, A.J., and McNamara, D.G. Transient hypertrophic subaortic stenosis in infants of diabetic mothers. *J. Pediat.* **89**: 120–125, 1976.
19. Gutgesell, H.P., Speer, M., and Rosenberg, H.S. Characterization of the cardiomyopathy in infants of diabetic mothers. *Circulation* **61**: 441–450, 1980.
20. Way, G.L., Ruttenberg, H.D., Eshaghpour, E., Nora, J.J., and Wolfe, R.R. Hypertrophic obstructive cardiomyopathy in infants of diabetic mothers. *Circulation* 53–54 Suppl II: II-105, 1976.
21. Ferrans, V.J. and Rodriguez, E.R. Evidence of myocyte hyperplasia in hypertrophic cardiomyopathy and other disorders with myocardial hypertrophy? *Z. Kardiol.* **76**, Suppl 3: 20–25, 1987.
22. Maron, B.J., Spirito, P., Wesley, Y., and Arce, J. Development and progression of left ventricular hypertrophy in children with hypertrophic cardiomyopathy. *N. Engl. J. Med.* **315**: 610–614, 1986.
23. Spirito, P. and Maron, B.J. Absence of progression of left ventricular hypertrophy in adult patients with hypertrophic cardiomyopathy. *J. Am. Coll. Cardiol.* **9**: 1013–1017, 1987.
24. Teare, D. Asymmetrical hypertrophy of the heart in young adults. *Br. Heart J.* **20**: 1–8, 1958.
25. Fujiwara, H., Kawai, C. and Hamashima, Y. Myocardial fascicle and fiber disarray in 25 μ-thick sections. *Circulation* **59**: 1293–1298. 1979.
26. Van der Bel-Kahn, J. Muscle fiber disarray in common heart diseases. *Am. J. Cardiol.* **40**: 355–364, 1977.
27. Wigle, E.D. and Silver, M.D. Myocardial fiber disarray and ventricular septal hypertrophy in asymmetrical hypertrophy of the heart. *Circulation* **58**: 398–402, 1978.
28. Pomerance, A. and Davies, M.J. Pathological features of hypertrophic obstructive cardiomyopathy (HOCM) in the elderly. *Br. Heart J.* **37**: 305–312, 1975.
29. Becker, A.E. and Caruso, G. Myocardial disarray. A critical review. *Br. Heart J.* **49**: 527–538, 1982.
30. Tazelaar, H.D. and Billingham, M.E. The surgical pathology of hypertrophic cardiomyopathy. *Arch. Pathol. Lab. Med.* **111**: 257–260, 1987.
31. Izumi, T., Miura, K., and Hattori, A. Myofiber branching in hypertrophic human heart. *Biomed. Res.* 2 Suppl: 265–271, 1981.
32. Izumi, T. Myofiber branching in idiopathic cardiomyopathy under the scanning electron microscope. *Jpn. Circ. J.* **46**: 443–449, 1982.
33. Kawamura, K., Uehara, H., Noda, S., and Takatsu, T. Scanning electron microscope study on normal or hypertrophied myocardial cells isolated from autopsied human hearts. In: Cardiomyopathy, Clinical, Pathological and Theoretical Aspects. Sekiguchi M, Olsen EGJ, (eds.) Baltimore, MD: University Park Press, 165–184, 1978.
34. Ferrans, V.J. and Roberts, W.C. Myocardial biopsy: A useful diagnostic procedure or only a research tool? *Am. J. Cardiol.* **41**: 965–967, 1978.
35. Somerville, J. and Becu, L. Congenital heart disease associated with hypertrophic cardiomyopathy. *Johns Hopkins Med. J.* **140**: 151–162, 1977.
36. Somerville, J. and Becu, L. Congenital heart disease associated with hypertrophic cardiomyopathy. *Br. Heart J.* **40**: 1034–1039, 1978.
37. Becú, L., Somerville, J., and Gallo, A. "Isolated" pulmonary valve stenosis as part of more widespread cardiovascular disease. *Br. Heart J.* **38**: 472–482, 1976.
38. Jones, M., Ferrans, V.J., Morrow, A.G., and Roberts, W.C. Ultrastructure of crista supraventricularis muscle in patients with congenital heart disease associated with right ventricular outflow tract obstruction. *Circulation* **51**: 39–67, 1975.
39. Maron, B.J. and Roberts, W.C. Quantitative analysis of the distribution of cardiac muscle cell disorganization in the ventricular septum of patients with hypertrophic cardiomyopathy. *Circulation* **59**: 689–706, 1979.
40. Maron, B.J., Anan, T.J., and Roberts, W.C. Quantitative analysis of the distribution of

cardiac muscle cell disorganization in the left ventricular wall of patients with hypertrophic cardiomyopathy. *Circulation* **63**: 882–894, 1981.
41. Fukuhara, M., Koyama, O., Hinami, F., and Tanemoto, K. Echocardiographic and endomyocardial biopsy findings of right-sided hypertrophic obstructive cardiomyopathy. *J. Cardiography* **15**: 347–357, 1985.
42. Nakanishi, S., Nishiyama, S., Nishimura, S., and Yamaguchi, H. Histological features of apical hypertrophic cardiomyopathy. *J. Cardiography* **15** (Suppl. VI): 3–11, 1985.
43. Tanaka, M., Fujiwara, H., and Kawai, C. Pathological features of hypertrophic cardiomyopathy without asymmetrical septal hypertrophy. *Br. Heart J.* **56**: 294–297, 1986.
44. Hibbs, R.G. and Ellison, J.P. The atrioventricular valves of the guinea pig. II. An ultrastructural study. *Am. J. Anat.* **138**: 374, 1973.
45. Challice, C.E. Microstructure of specialized tissues in the mammalian heart. *Ann. N.Y. Acad. Sci.* **156**: 14–33, 1969.
46. Virágh, S. and Challice, C.E. Variations in filamentous and fibrillar organization, and associated sarcolemmal structures, in cells of the normal mammalian heart. *J. Ultrastruct. Res.* **28**: 321–324, 1969.
47. Thornell, L-E., Sjöström, M., and Andersson, K-E. The relationship between mechanical stress and myofibrillar organization in heart Purkinje fibres. *J. Mol. Cell. Cardiol.* **8**: 689–695, 1976.
48. Manasek, F.J. Histogenesis of the embryonic myocardium. *Am. J. Cardiol.* **25**: 149–168, 1970.
49. Manasek, F.J. Some comparative aspects of cardiac and skeletal myogenesis. In: Development Regulation Aspects of Cell Differentiation. Caward StJ, (ed.) New York, London: Academic Press, 193–217, 1973.
50. Howse, H.D., Ferrans, V.J., and Hibbs, R.G. A light and electron microscopic study of the heart of a crayfish, *Procambarus clarkii* (Giraud): I. Histology and histochemistry. *J. Morph.* **131**: 237–252, 1970.
51. Howse, H.D., Ferrans, V.J., and Hibbs, R.G. A light and electron microscopic study of the heart of a crayfish *Procambarus clarkii* (Giraud): II. Fine structure. *J. Morph.* **133**: 353–373, 1971.
52. Ross, A.A. and Streeter, D.D. Jr. Nonuniform subendocardial fiber orientation in the normal macaque left ventricle. *Eur. J. Cardiol.* **3**: 29, 1975.
53. Isner, J.M., Maron, B.J., and Roberts, W.C. Comparison of amount of myocardial cell disorganization in operatively exercised septectomy specimens with amount observed at necrospsy in 18 patients with hypertrophic cardiomyopathy. *Am. J. Cardiol.* **46**: 42–47, 1980.
54. Maron, B.J., Sato, N., Roberts, W.C., Edwards, J.E., and Chandra, R.S. Quantitative analysis of cardiac muscle cell disorganization in the ventricular septum. Comparison of fetuses and infants with and without congenital heart disease and patients with hypertrophic cardiomyopathy. *Circulation* **60**: 685–696, 1979.
55. Maron, B.J., Edwards, J.E., Moller, J., and Epstein, S.E. Prevelance and characteristics of disproportionate ventricular septal thickening in infants with congenital heart disease. *Circulation* **59**: 126–133, 1979.
56. Maron, B.J., Edwards, J.E., Ferrans, V.J., Clark, C.E., Lebowitz, E.A., Henry, W.L., and Epstein, S.E. Congenital heart malformations associated with disproportionate ventricular septal thickening. *Circulation* **52**: 926–932, 1975.
57. Bulkley, B.H., D'Amico, B., and Taylor, A.L. Extensive myocardial fiber disarray in aortic and pulmonary atresia. Relevance to hypertrophic cardiomyopathy. *Circulation* **67**: 191–198, 1983.
58. Maron, B.J., Lipson, L.C., Roberts, W.C., Savage, D.D., and Epstein, S.E. "Malignant" hypertrophic cardiomyopathy: Identification of a subgroup of families with unusually frequent premature death. *Am. J. Cardiol.* **41**: 1133–1140, 1978.
59. Maron, B.J., Gottdiener, J.S., and Epstein, S.E. Patterns and significance of distribution

of left ventricular hypertrophy in hypertrophic cardiomyopathy. A wide angle, two-dimensional echocardiographic study of 125 patients. *Am. J. Cardiol.* **48**: 418–428, 1981.

60. Perloff, J.K. Pathogenesis of hypertrophic cardiomyopathy: Hypotheses and speculations. *Am. Heart J.* **101**: 219–226, 1981.
61. Maron, B.J., Epstein, D.E., and Roberts, W.C. Hypertrophic cardiomyopathy and transmural myocardial infarction without significant atherosclerosis of the extramural coronary arteries. *Am. J. Cardiol.* **43**: 1086–1102, 1979.
62. James, T.N. and Marshall, T.K. De Subitaneis Mortibus XII. Asymmetric hypertrophy of the heart. *Circulation* **51**: 1166, 1975.
63. Lalich, J.J., Allen, J.R., and Pik, W.C.W. Myocardial fibrosis and smooth muscle cell hyperplasia in coronary arteries of allylamine-fed rats. *Exp. Mol. Pathol.* **21**: 29–39, 1974.
64. James, T.N. Small arteries of the heart. *Circulation* **56**: 2–14, 1977.
65. Geer, J.C., Bishop, S.P., and James, T.N. Pathology of small intramural coronary arteries. *Pathol. Annu.* **2**: 125–154, 1979.
66. Tanaka, M., Fujiwara, H., Onodera, T., Wu, D-J., Matsuda, M., Hamashima, Y., and Kawai, C. Quantitative analysis of narrowings of intramyocardial small arteries in normal hearts, hypertensive hearts, and hearts with hypertrophic cardiomyopathy. *Circulation* **75**: 1130–1139, 1987.
67. Maron, B.J., Wolfson, J.K., Epstein, S.E., and Roberts, W.C. Morphologic evidence for "small vessel disease" in patients with hypertrophic cardiomyopathy. *Z. Kardiol.* **76** (Suppl 3): 91–100, 1987.
68. Sedlis, S.P., Saffitz, J.E., Schwob, V.S., and Jaffe, A.S. Cardiac amyloidosis simulating hypertrophic cardiomyopathy. *Am. J. Cardiol.* **53**: 969–970, 1984.
69. Griffiths, B.E., Hughes, P., Dowdle, R., and Stephen, M.R. Cardiac amyloidosis with asymmetrical septal hypertrophy and deterioration after nifedipine. *Thorax* **37**: 711–712, 1982.
70. Fritz, P., Schneider, H., Heimburg, P., and Wegner, G. Sekundare hypertrophe obstruktive Kardiomyopathie bei Morbus Fabry. *Med. Welt.* **29**: 1851–1854, 1978.
71. Kuhn, H., Kohler, E., Hort, W., and Frenzel, H. Concealed myocardial storage disease (Fabry's disease): Pitfalls in the diagnosis of hypertrophic nonobstructive cardiomyopathy. *Circulation* **66** (suppl 2): II-117, 1982.
72. Colucci, W.S., Lorell, B.H., Schoen, F.J., Warhol, M.J., and Grossman, W. Hypertrophic obstructive cardiomyopathy due to Fabry's disease. *N. Engl. J. Med.* **307**: 926–928, 1982.
73. Rutledge, J.C., Haas, J.E., Monnat, R., and Milstein, J.M. Hypertrophic cardiomyopathy is a component of subacute necrotizing encephalomyelopathy. *J. Pediat.* **101**: 706–710, 982.
74. Miyabayashi, S., Ito, T., Narisawa, K., Iinuma, K., and Tada, K. Biochemical study in 28 children with lactic acidosis, in relation to Leigh's encephalomyelopathy. *Eur. J. Pediat.* **143**: 278–283, 1985.
75. Langes, K., Frenzel, H., Seitz, R.J., and Kluitmann, G. Cardiomyopathy associated with Leigh's disease. *Virchows Arch. Pathol. Anat.* **407**: 97–105, 1985.
76. Kluitmann, G., Braumann, H.G., Kratz, H.W., Liersch, R., Langes, K., Seitz, R.J., and Frenzel, H. Akuter Verlauf des Leigh-Syndroms mit hypertropher Kardiomyopathie bei einem weiblichen Saugling. *Monatsschr. Kinderheilkd.* **133**: 688–693, 1985.
77. van Ekeren, G.J., Stadhouders, A.M. Egberink, G.J.M., Sengers, R.C.A., Daniels, O., and Kubat, K. Hereditary mitochondrial hypertrophic cardiomyopathy with mitochondrial myopathy of skeletal muscle, congenital cataract and lactic acidosis. *Virchows. Arch.* **412**: 47–52, 1987.
78. Cruysberg, J.R.M., Sengers, R.C.A., Pinckers, A., Kubat, K., and van Haelst, U.J.G.M. Features of a syndrome with congenital cataract and hypertrophic cardiomyopathy. *Am. J. Ophthalmol.* **102**: 740–749, 1986.
79. Sengers, R.C.A., Stadhouders, A.M., van Lakwijk-Vondrovicova, E., Kubat, K., and Ruitenbeek, W. Hypertrophic cardiomyopathy associated with a mitochondrial myopathy of voluntary muscles and congenital cataract. *Br. Heart J.* **54**: 543–547, 1985.

80. Grantzow, R. and Hübner, G. Mitochondrial cardiomyopathy with a high degree of heart muscle hypertrophy. *Monatsschr. Kinderheikld.* **130**: 909–910, 1982.
81. Hübner, G. and Grantzow, R. Mitochondrial cardiomyopathy with involvement of skeletal muscles. *Virchows Arch.* **399**: 115–125, 1983.
82. Kajihara, H., Oda, N., Tahara, E., Tsuchioka, Y., Matsuura, H., Kajiyama, G., Matsuura, H., Hiramoto, T., and Sato, H. Histopathological observation of the heart with diffuse and abnormal proliferation of mitochondria in the myocardial cells: Report of an adult case. *Heart Vessels* **2**: 233–238, 1986.
83. Schwartzkopff, B., Frenzel, H., Lösse, B., Borggrefe, M., Toyka, K.V., Hammerstein, W., Seitz, R., Deckert, M., and Breithardt, G. Heart involvement in progressive external ophthalmoplegia (Kearns-Sayre syndrome): Electrophysiologic, hemodynamic and morphologic findings. *Z. Kardiol.* **75**: 161–169, 1986.
84. Hübner, G., Gokel, J.M., Pongratz, D., Johannes, A., and Park, J.W. Fatal mitochondrial cardiomyopathy in Kearns-Sayre syndrome. *Virchows Arch.* **408**: 611–621, 1986.
85. Kleber, F.X., Park, J.W., Hubner, G., Johannes, A., Pongratz, D., and Konig, E. Congestive heart failure due to mitochondrial cardiomyopathy in Kearns-Sayre syndrome. *Klin. Wochenschr.* **65**: 480–486, 1987.
86. Van Vleet, J.F. and Ferrans, V.J. Myocardial diseases of animals. *Am. J. Pathol.* **124**: 98–178, 1986.
87. Hsu, F.S. and Du, S-J. Cardiac diseases in swine. In: Pig Model for Biomedical Research, Roberts, H.R. Dodds W.J. (eds.) Pig Research Institute, Taiwan, Republic of China, pp. 134–143, 1982.

Intramural Coronary Artery Disease in Hypertrophic Cardiomyopathy

Hisayoshi Fujiwara and Chuichi Kawai

The Third Division, Department of Internal Medicine, Faculty of Medicine, Kyoto University, Kyoto, Japan

ABSTRACT

Intramyocardial small artery (IMSA) disease has been reported in hearts with hypertrophic cardiomyopathy (HCM). In the present study, stenosis of IMSA in HCM was quantitatively analyzed and compared with that in other cardiac diseases. The relationship between IMSA disease and coronary reserve, fibrosis, disarray, cardiac hypertrophy, and chest pain is discussed. A case report of HCM showing features mimicking dilated cardiomyopathy (DCM) in the late stage, probably due to marked stenosis of IMSA, is presented. We concluded that IMSA disease is of pathophysiologic importance in patients with HCM, DCM-like HCM in particular.

INTRAMURAL MYOCARDIAL SMALL ARTERY IN HEARTS WITH HYPERTROPHIC CARDIOMYOPATHY AND OTHER CARDIAC DISEASES

Stenosis of the intramyocardial small arteries (IMSA) has been reported in hearts with hypertrophic cardiomyopathy (HCM) and other cardiac diseases (Fig. 1).[1–7] IMSA (external diameter $<1,500$ μm; average 300 μm) are abnormal in about 80% of patients with HCM studied at autopsy.[5,6] The walls are thickened due to an increase in intimal or medial components, and frequently the lumens appear to be narrowed. IMSA with stenosis are most commonly found in the ventricular septum, but are often present in the left ventricular free wall. However, stenosis of IMSA is not unique to HCM. IMSA stenosis occurs in a minority of patients with systemic hypertension, aortic valvular stenosis, dilated cardiomyopathy, and coronary artery disease.[5] According to Opherk *et al.*,[8] endomyocardial biopsy specimens taken from patients with systemic hypertension did not show any structural changes of IMSA. In these specimens, luminal narrowing of IMSA was qualitatively examined. Since the degree of IMSA narrowing varies considerably within the left ventricular wall, analysis of small biposy samples may not have been sufficient. Moreover, slight-to-moderate narrowing of IMSA in these hearts may have been overlooked by qualitative evaluation. Therefore, we quantitatively analyzed the degree of IMSA narrowing in large transverse sections using an image analyzer (Fig. 2).[7]

The mean percent lumen (%lumen) of IMSA in the ventricular septum was 17+3% in hearts with DCM-like HCM, 29+5% in hearts with HCM, 30+8% in hypertensive hearts, and 40+5% in normal hearts (Fig. 3). DCM-like HCM refers to patients with HCM whose features mimic dilated cardiomyopathy in the late stage. The mean % lumen values of IMSA with an extenal caliber of more than 60 μm and less than 60 μm were 16+3% and 19+4% in hearts with DCM-like HCM, 31+6% and 27+4% in hearts with HCM, 31+8% and 28+9% in hypertensive hearts, and 42+6% and 36+

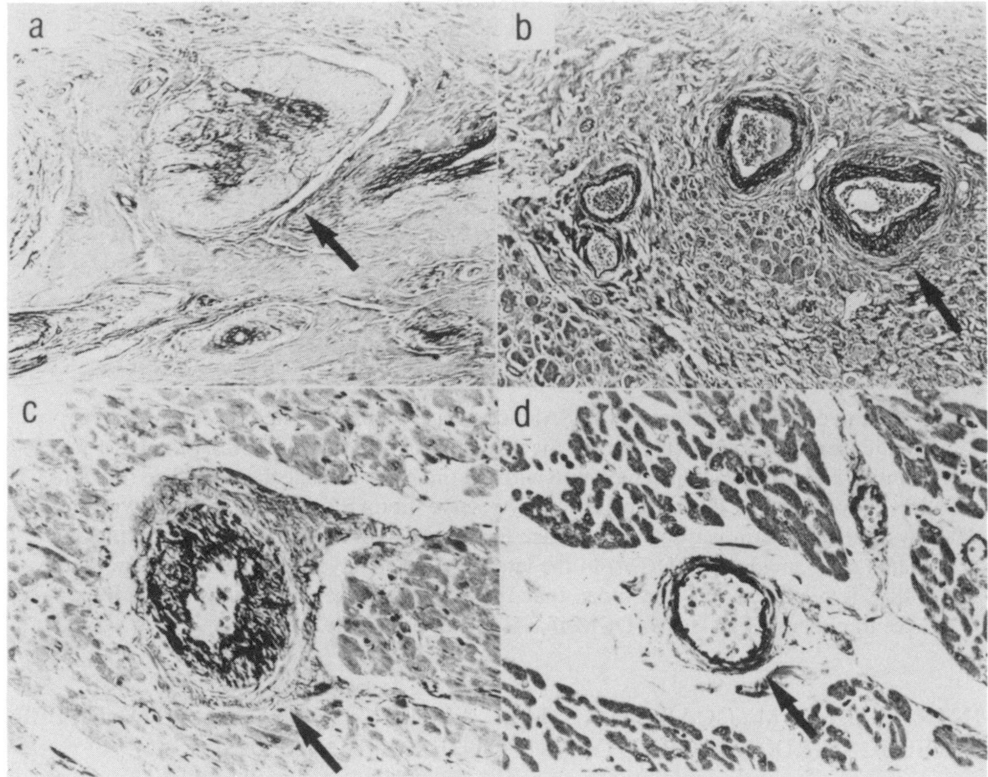

Fig. 1. Photomicrographs of IMSAs with various degree of narrowing. a, Photomicrograph of numerous markedly narrowed IMSAs and massive fibrosis in the ventricular septum of a heart with DCM-like HCM. b, Photomicrograph of the free wall of a heart with DCM-like HCM. By comparison with the ventricular septum, both the narrowing of the IMSAs and the extent of fibrosis are mild. c, Photomicrograph of a moderately narrowed IMSA in a hypertensive heart. d, Photomicrograph of the IMSA without narrowing in a normal control. The %lumen values of the IMSAs labeled by arrows were 0.7% (a), 23% (b), 9% (c), and 54% (d). (Elastic van Gieson stain; ×40 [a], ×100 [b], ×200 [c and d].) Reproduced from Tanaka, Fujiwara, *et al.*[7] with the permission of the publisher.

6% in normal hearts, respectively (Fig. 4). Regardless of the size of the IMSA, the mean %lumen in hearts with DCM-like HCM was significantly less than that in any other group; the mean %lumen in hearts with HCM and that in hypertensive hearts were similar, and both were significantly less than that in normal hearts.

The mean %lumen values of IMSA in the right, middle, and left thirds of the ventricular septum were 18±5%, 18±3%, and 16±2% in hearts with DCM-like HCM, 29±6%, 29±6%, and 29±6% in hearts with HCM, and 30±7%, 28±10%, and 28±11% in hypertensive hearts, respectively (Fig. 5). There was no difference in mean %lumen values among these three regions of the ventricular septum in any group.

The mean %lumen of IMSAs in the free wall was 33±4% in hearts with DCM-like

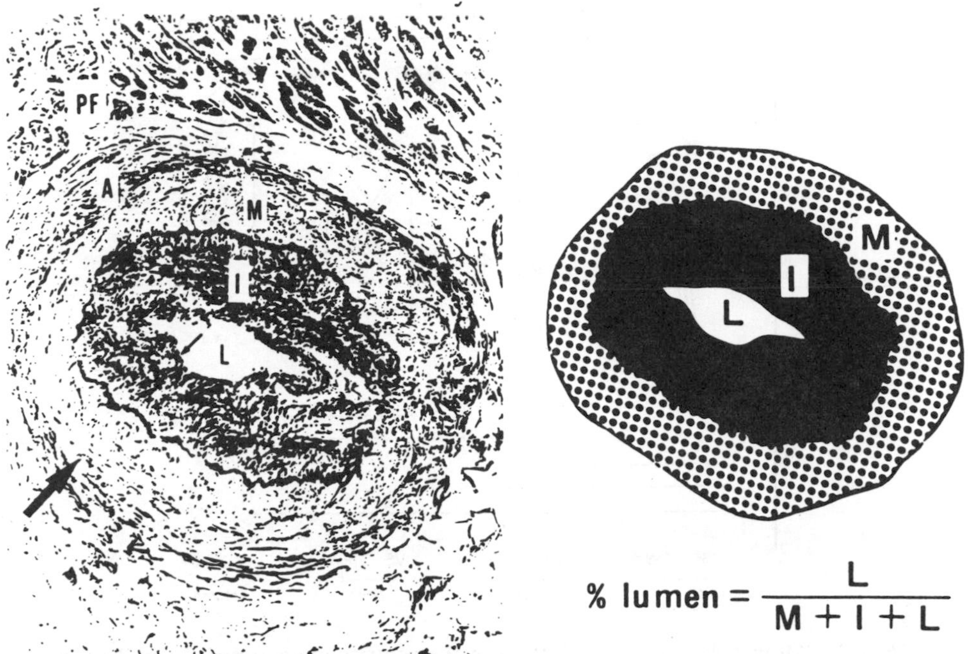

Fig. 2. Method for quantifying narrowings of IMSAs. The inner border of the intima (I) (small arrow) and the outer border of the media (M) (large arrow) are traced, and the ratio of the areas encircled by these tracings is calculated as the percent luminal area (%area): luminal area (L) divided by the summed areas of the media, intima, and lumen. Adventitia (A) was excluded because it was often continuous with perivascular fibrosis (PF), which made it difficult to distinguish the border between these two. Reproduced from Tanaka, Fujiwara *et al.*[7] with the permission of the publisher.

HCM, 31±5% in hearts with HCM, 31±7% in hypertensive hearts, and 38±5% in normal hearts (Fig. 3). The mean %lumen values of IMSAs with an external caliber of more than 60 μm and less than 60 μm were 38±6% and 31±4% in hearts with DCM-like HCM, 34±5% and 28±4% in hearts with HCM, 31±8% and 30±6% in hypertensive hearts, and 42+4% and 36+5% in normal hearts, respectively (Fig. 4). Regardless of the size of the IMSA, the mean %lumen was significantly less in hearts with DCM-like HCM, HCM, and hypertensive disease than in normal hearts, but no differences were found among the three disease groups.

The mean %lumen values of IMSA in the inner, middle, and outer thirds of the free wall were 31±7%, 36±4%, and 34±3% in hearts with DCM-like HCM, 28±6%, 31±5%, and 33±6% in hearts with HCM, 27±9%, 31±8%, and 35±7% in hypertensive hearts, and 34±4%, 38±6%, and 42±5% in normal hearts (Fig. 5). The mean %lumen was less in the subendocardium than in the subepicardium in hearts with HCM, hypertensive hearts, and normal hearts.

In hearts with DCM-like HCM, the mean %lumen of the IMSA was significantly less in the ventricular septum than in the free wall (Figs. 1 a and b, and 3). However, no such difference was evident in any other group.

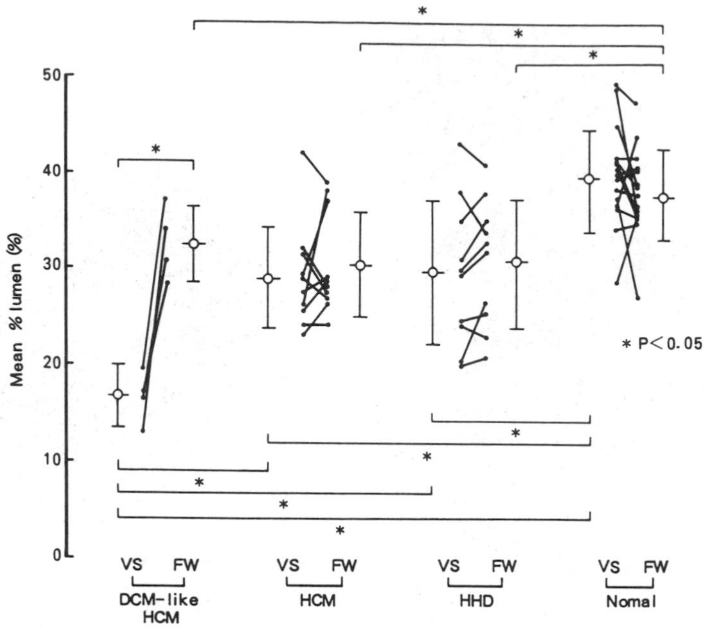

Fig. 3. Mean % lumen of the IMSAs in the ventricular septum (VS) and left ventricular free wall (FW) of hearts with DCM-like HCM, hypertrophic cardiomyopathy (HCM), and hypertensive heart disease (HHD), and in normal controls. In the septum, the mean % lumen in DCM-like HCM was the lowest. The mean % lumen values were less in DCM-like HCM, HCM, and HHD than in the normal controls both in the septum and free wall. The mean % lumen was less in the septum than in the free wall in DCM-like HCM. Reproduced from Tanaka, Fujiwara, *et al.*[7] with the permission of the publisher.

CASE REPORT OF DCM-LIKE HCM WITH MARKED INTRAMYOCARDIAL SMALL CORONARY ARTERY DISEASE

A Japanese man aged 38 years at the time of death had had exertional dyspnea of 18 years' duration. His two sisters had HCM, one with and one without obstruction. Six years before his death, the echocardiogram revealed marked asymmetric septal hypertrophy (ASH), systolic anterior motion of the anterior mitral leaflet, and lack of dilatation of the left ventricular end-diastolic dimension (47 mm) (Fig. 6). The wall thickness was 19 mm in the ventricular septum and 10 mm in the left ventricular posterior wall. Left ventricular hypertrophy was noted on ECG and chest X-ray (CTR = 62%). Thereafter, the signs and symptoms of congestive heart failure, including dyspnea, palpitation, edema, congestion of the lungs, and pleural effusion in the chest X-ray, worsened, although the patient had been treated with digitalis and diuretics. Four years before his death, echocardiogram showed mild ASH (ventricular septum/left ventricular posterior wall = 13 mm/8 mm), disappearance of systolic anterior motion of the anterior mitral leaflet, and mild dilatation of the left ventricular cavity (left ventricular end-diastolic dimension = 51 mm) with poor motion (Fig. 6). Intact coronary arteries, diffuse poor contraction of the left ventricular wall, increased left ventricular end-diastolic pressure (23 mmHg), and lack of systolic pressure gradient in the left ventricular cavity were evident at the time of cardiac catheterization.

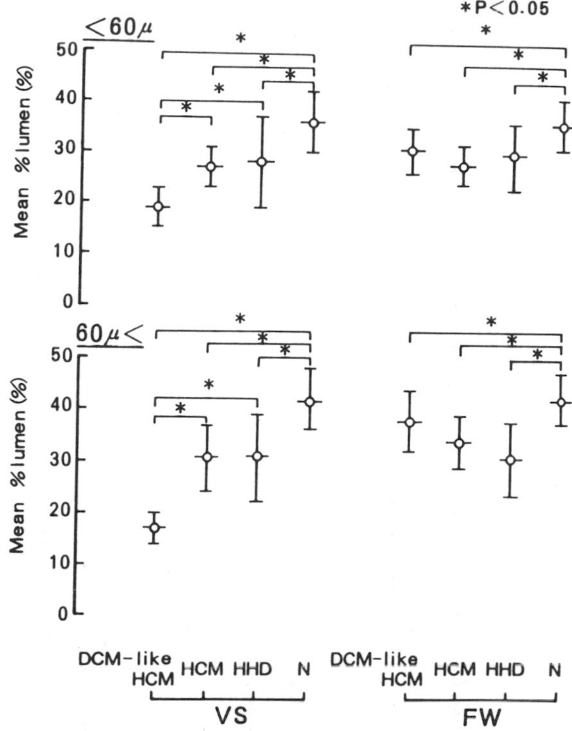

Fig. 4. Mean % lumen of IMSAs with an external caliber of < 60μm (top) and > 60μm (bottom) in the ventricular septum (VS) and left ventricular free wall (FW) of hearts with DCM-like HCM, HCM, and hypertensive heart disease (HHD), and in normal controls (N). Regardless of the size of the IMSA, the mean % lumen in DCM-like HCM was the lowest among all groups in the septum; the mean % lumen was less in DCM-like HCM, HCM, and HHD than in the normal controls in both the septum and free wall. Reproduced from Tanaka, Fujiwara, *et al.*[7] with the permission of the publisher.

Two months before his death, multiple thromboemboli suddenly appeared in the cerebral and renal arteries. Echocardiogram revealed moderate dilatation of the left ventricular cavity (left ventricular end-diastolic dimension = 55 mm), disappearance of ASH (ventricular septum/left ventricular posterior wall = 7 mm/9 mm), paradoxical movement of the ventricular septum, poor contraction of the left ventricular posterior wall, and absence of systolic anterior motion (Fig. 6). The patient died of cerebral infarction and acute renal failure. He had had no chest pain, syncopal attack, or hypertension.

At autopsy, the heart weighed 480 g and showed dilated hypertrophy in the left ventricle, right ventricle, and left atrium (Fig. 6). The wall thickness was 9 mm in the ventricular septum and 13 mm in the left ventricular posterior wall. The left ventricular diameter was 42 mm. These data coincided with the echocardiographic findings in the end-systole two months before his death. The extent of fibrosis and disarray is shown in Figs. 6 and 7. Massive transmural fibrosis (30% in the venticular septum), diffuse disarray (18% in the ventricular septum), and marked narrowing of the IMSA (Figs. 6 and 7) were localized in the ventricular septum and the anterior left ventricular wall. Mural

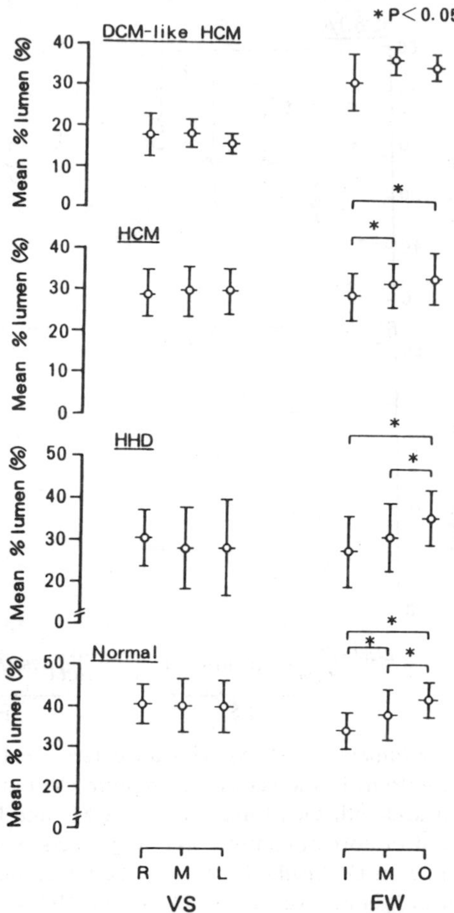

Fig. 5. Mean % lumen of IMSAs in the right (R), middle (M), and left (L) thirds of the ventricular septum (VS) and in the inner (I), middle (M), and outer (O) third of the left ventricular free wall (FW) in hearts with DCM-like HCM, HCM, and hypertensive heart disease (HHD) and in normal controls. The mean % lumen decreased from the outer to the inner third of the free wall in HCM, HHD, and normal hearts. Reproduced from Tanaka, Fujiwara, *et al.*[7] with the permission of the publisher.

thrombi were present in the left atrium, but coagulation necrosis was not evident and the extramural coronary arteries were not stenosed.

The clinical and macroscopic pathological findings at the end stage were typical of those seen in DCM. However, the family history, echocardiographic findings observed for six years, and the diffuse disarray of 18% in the ventricular septum indicated that this man had HCM with obstruction.[9,10] Massive transmural fibrosis is unusual in HCM and DCM.[11,12] We reported that an increase of transmural muscle layers in the ventricular septum is pathogenetic for ASH.[13] The insidious disappearance of ASH and dilatation of the left ventricular cavity with progressive congestive heart failure were related to the decrease in transmural muscle layers following necrosis of myocytes and

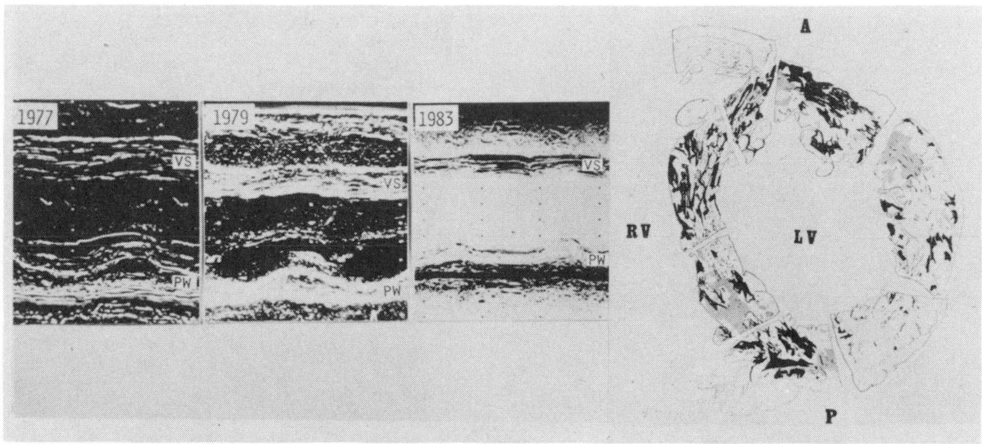

Fig. 6. Echocardiographic findings and macroscopic findings of the autopsied heart, in which distribution of fibrosis and disarray was traced, in DCM-like HCM. Left: Echocardiogram at the age of 32 years (1977) showed marked asymmetric septal hypertrophy (ASH) and no dilatation of the left ventricular (LV) cavity. The degree of ASH decreased and the LV dimension increased slightly at the age of 34 years (1979). Echocardiogram at the age of 38 years (1983) revealed disappearance of ASH, paradoxical movement of the ventricular septum (VS), and dilatation of the LV cavity. PW = left ventricular posterior wall. Right: Transverse section of the LV at the level of the mitral leaflets, showing the extents of fibrosis (dark areas) and disarray (dotted areas). Transmural massive fibrosis and diffuse disarray are seen in the ventricular septum (VS) and the anterior LV wall. Note that the most of the fibrosis is present in the middle and outer thirds of the LV wall. In the VS, fibrosis was accounted for 30% and disarray for 18%.

the chronic progression of fibrosis in the ventricular septum and anterior left ventricular wall.

Systemic thromboembolism, probably thrombi from the left atrium, was first noted two months before the patient's death. The hypertrophy of the ventricular septum was not marked, even six years before death, compared with usual cases of HCM. The patient had no syncopal attack or chest pain, and extramural coronary arteries were not stenosed. These findings indicated that thromboembolism, a brief period of hypoxia or hypotension, and hypertrophy in the ventricular septum are untenable for the pathogenesis of chronic progressive massive fibrosis. Spasm of major coronary arteries was also excluded because massive fibrosis was mostly present in the middle and outer thirds of the left ventricular wall. The most plausible cause of the massive fibrosis in the ventricular and anterior left ventricular wall was multiple ischemia in those regions, following marked narrowing of the IMSA, which is sometimes seen in the patients with HCM. Vasospasm of IMSA was also considered. The distribution of massive fibrosis in this case coincided with that of disarray seen in usual HCM.[9,10] Therefore, it is likely that the tissue areas with disarray contained the stenosed IMSA and the myocytes were replaced by massive fibrosis.

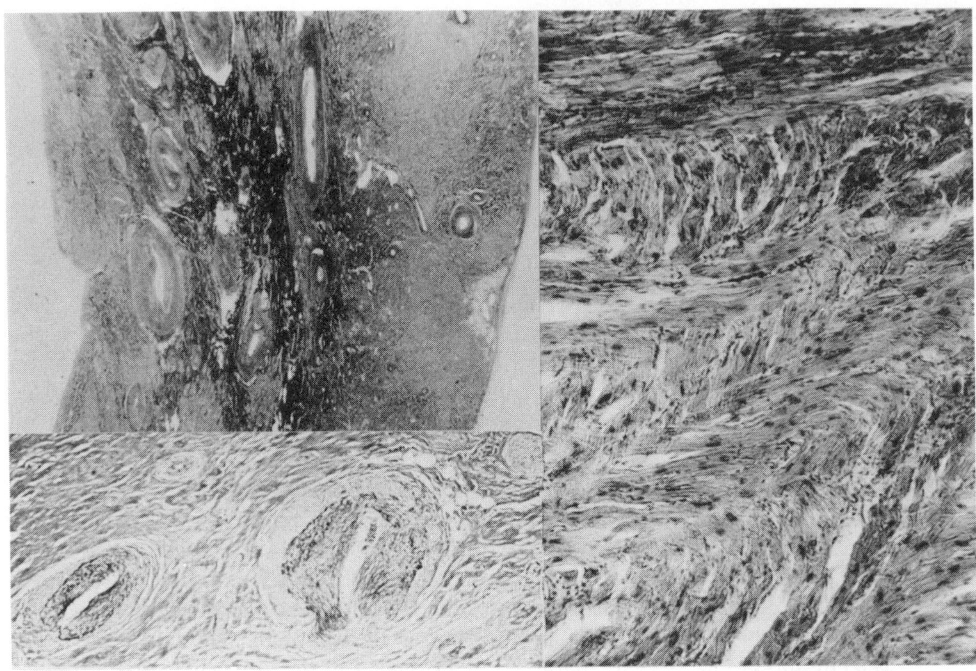

Fig. 7. Microscopic finding of the autopsied heart in DCM-like HCM. Left upper: Ventricular septum. Note massive fibrosis and stenosis of IMSAs (elastic van Gieson stain, ×20). Left lower: Arterioles with stenosis in the ventricular septum (elastic van Gieson stain, ×100). Right: Myocardial fascicular disarray in the ventricular septum (25μm thick section, hematoxylin and eosin stain, ×100).

INTRAMYOCARDIAL SMALL ARTERY DISEASE AS A PATHOGENETIC MECHANISM FOR THE REDUCED CORONARY RESERVE IN HCM

Chest pain is a common symptom of patients with HCM,[14,15] or systemic hypertension[8] despite angiographically normal epicardial coronary arteries. Moreover, these patients often demonstrate abnormal findings on myocardial ^{201}Ti imaging[16-18] or abnormal lactate metabolism during pacing.[19] Reduction in coronary flow reserve in hearts with HCM and normal epicardial coronary arteries has been reported.[8,19-22] A variety of possible mechanisms have been suggested: augmentation of the extravascular component of coronary resistance, inadequate capillary density in relation to the increased myocardial mass,[23-25] coronary artery spasm,[26] septal perforator artery compression,[27] abnormal arteriovenous oxygen difference,[19] and IMSA disease.[1-7]

Our quantitative analysis (described above) revealed that in both hearts with HCM and hypertensive hearts the luminal area was narrowed despite the marked hypertrophy of myocytes. Coronary reserve has been reported to decrease more in the subendocardium than in the subepicardium.[28-30] Our data revealed that this was also the case for the mean %lumen of IMSA, indicating that IMSA disease is a possible pathogenetic mechanism for the reduced coronary reserve in both hearts with HCM and hypertensive hearts.

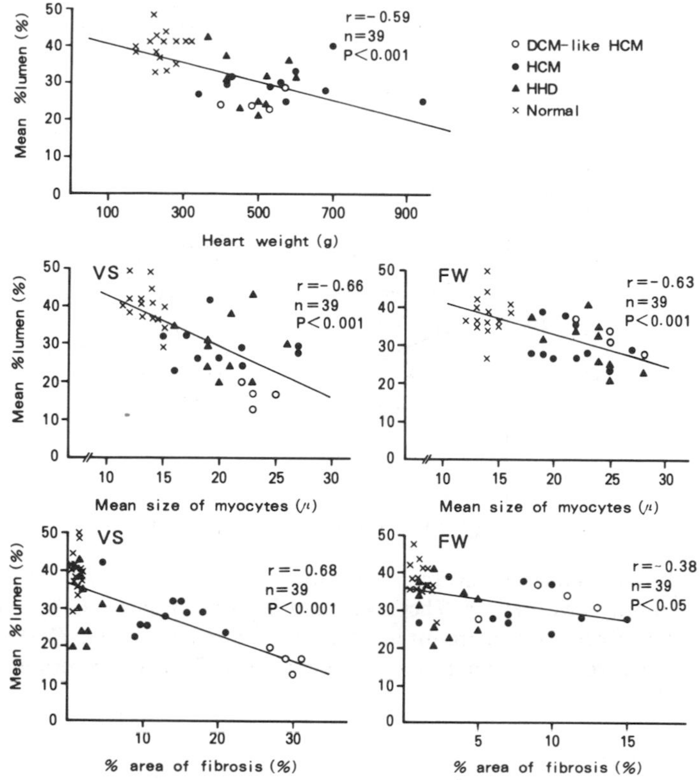

Fig. 8. Relationship of the mean %lumen of IMSAs to heart weight (top), mean size of myocytes (middle), and percent fibrotic area (bottom). Correlation coefficients and regression lines were obtained from the values of hearts with DCM-like HCM, HCM, hypertensive heart disease (HHD), and normal controls. VS = ventricular septum; FW = left ventricular free wall. Reproduced from Tanaka, Fujiwara, *et al.*[7] with the permission of the publisher.

RELATIONSHIP BETWEEN INTRAMYOCARDIAL SMALL ARTERY DISEASE AND FIBROSIS, DISARRAY, AND CARDIAC HYPERTROPHY

Hearts with DCM-like HCM have massive fibrosis, particularly in the ventricular septum.[2–4] Previously, we reported that the extent of fibrosis is greater in hearts with HCM ($10.5 \pm 4.3\%$) and hypertensive hearts ($2.6 \pm 1.5\%$) than in normal hearts ($1.1 \pm 0.5\%$); the extent of fibrosis increases from the epicardial to the endocardial layer of the left ventricular free wall.[11]

The mean %lumen of IMSA was lowest in the ventricular septum of hearts with DCM-like HCM, was less in hearts with HCM and hypertensive hearts than in normal hearts, decreased from the epicardial to the endocardial layer of the free wall, and was inversely correlated with the percent area of fibrosis (Fig. 8). These observations indicate that narrowing of IMSA is associated with an increased level of fibrosis in hearts with HCM and hypertensive hearts, particularly in the ventricular septum of hearts with DCM-like HCM. However, the increase of fibrosis in hearts with HCM compared with hypertensive hearts cannot be explained by narrowing of the IMSA, since the mean %lumen values were similar in these groups. Other factors such as myocardial fiber

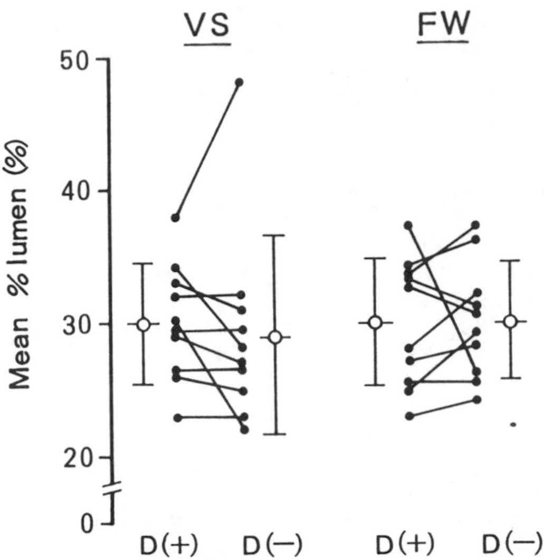

Fig. 9. Mean %lumen of IMSAs in tissues with [D(+)] and without [D(−)] disarray in hearts with HCM. There was no difference in the mean %lumen of the IMSA between the two groups in either the ventricular septum (VS) or free wall (FW). Reproduced from Tanaka, Fujiwara, *et al.*[7] with the permission of the publisher.

disarray are also important in the pathogenesis of extensive fibrosis in hearts with HCM.[31]

Our study showed that there was no difference in the mean %lumen of IMSA between tissues with and without disarray (Fig. 9). This indicates that myocardial fiber disarray is not important in the pathogenesis of IMSA disease. The mean %lumen was inversely correlated with heart weight and mean size of myocytes (Fig. 8). The myocardial fiber diameter has been reported to increase from the epicardial to the endocardial layer of the left ventricular free wall.[32] Our study revealed that the mean %lumen of the IMSA decreases from the epicardial to the endocardial layer. Cardiac hypertrophy is probably one of the pathogenetic factors involved in narrowing of the IMSA in these hearts. However, the pathogenesis of marked narrowing of IMSA in hearts with DCM-like HCM remains unclear because there was no significant difference in heart weight or mean size of myocytes between hearts with DCM-like HCM and those with HCM or hypertensive disease.

RELATIONSHIP BETWEEN INTRAMYOCARDIAL SMALL ARTERY DISEASE AND CHEST PAIN

The relationship between IMSA disease and chest pain was not clear in hearts with HCM or hypertensive disease.[7] Even in patients with DCM-like HCM whose septa were occupied by many severely narrowed IMSA, typical anginal chest pain was not observed. Thus the pathogenetic role of IMSA disease in anginal pain clinically observed in patients with HCM or hypertension is equivocal.

Acknowledgments

We thank M. Jinnai and S. Tomita for assistance in preparing this paper and D. Mrozek for reading it.

This work was supported in part by a Research Grant for Cardiomyopathy from the Ministry of Health and Welfare of Japan.

REFERENCES

1. James, T.N. and Marshall, T.K. De Suitaneis Morbitus. XII. Asymmetrical hypertrophy of the heart. *Circulation* **51**: 1149–1166, 1975.
2. Maron, B.J., Epstein, S.E., and Roberts, W.C. Hypertrophic cardiomyopathy and transmural myocardial infarction without significant atherosclerosis of the extramural coronary arteries. *Am. J. Cardiol.* **43**: 1086–1102, 1979.
3. Fujiwara, H., Onodera, T., Tanaka, M., and Kawai, C. Progression from hypertrophic obstructive cardiomyopathy to typical dilated cardiomyopathy like features in the end stage. *Jpn. Circ. J.* **48**: 1210–1214, 1984.
4. Onodera, T., Fujiwara, H., Tanaka, M., Wu, D.J., Hamashima, Y., and Kawai, C. Familial hypertrophic cardiomyopathy mimicking typical dilated cardiomyopathy. *Jpn. Circ. J.* **50**: 614–618, 1986.
5. Maron, B.J., Wolfson, J.K., Epstein, S.E., and Roberts, W.C. Intramural "small vessel" coronary artery disease in hypertrophic cardiomyopathy. *J. Am. Coll. Cardiol.* **8**: 545–557, 1986.
6. Maron, B.J., Bonow, R.O., Cannon, R.O., Leon, M.B., and Epstein, S.E. Hypertrophic cardiomyopathy—Interrelations of clinical manifestations, pathophysiology and therapy. *N. Engl. J. Med.* **316**: 780–789, 1987.
7. Tanaka, M., Fujiwara, H., Onodera, T., Wu, D.J., Matsuda, M., Hamashima, Y., and Kawai, C. Quantitative analysis of narrowings of intramyocardial small arteries in normal hearts, hypertensive hearts, and hearts with hypertrophic cardiomyopathy. *Circulation* **75**: 1130–1139, 1987.
8. Opherk, D., Mall, G., Zebe, H., Schwarz, F., Weihe, E., Manthey, J., and Kubler, W. Reduction of coronary reserve: A mechanism for angina pectoris in patients with arterial hypertension and normal coronary arteries. *Circulation* **69**: 1–7, 1984.
9. Fujiwara, H., Kawai, C., and Hamashima, Y. Myocardial fascicle and fiber disarray in 25μ-thick sections. *Circulation* **59**: 1293–1298. 1979.
10. Fujiwara, H., Hoshino, T., Fujiwara, T., Kawai, C., and Hamashima, Y. Classification and distribution of myocardial fascicle and fiber disarray in 14 hearts with hypertrophic cardiomyopathy in 25μ-thick sections. *Jpn. Circ. J.* **46**: 225–234, 1982.
11. Tanaka, M., Fujiwara, H., Onodera, T., Wu, D.J., Hamashima, Y., and Kawai, C. Quantitative analysis of myocardial fibrosis in normals, hypertensive hearts and hypertrophic cardiomyopathy. *Br. Heart J.* **55**: 575–581, 1986.
12. Onodera, T., Fujiwara, H., Tanaka, M., Wu, Wu, D.J., Hamashima, Y., and Kawai, C. Quantitative analysis of cardiac fibrosis in normal hearts, hearts with secondary eccentric hypertrophy and hearts with dilated cardiomyopathy. *Card. Bull. Acta. Cardiol.* **23**: 53–59, 1986.
13. Fujiwara, H., Hoshino, T., Yamana, K., Fujiwara, T., Furuta, M., Hamashima, Y., and Kawai, C. Number and size of myocytes and amount of interstitial space in the ventricular free wall in hypertrophic cardiomyopathy. *Am. J. Cardiol.* **52**: 818–823, 1983.
14. Frank, S., and Braunwald, E. Idiopathic hypertrophic subaortic stenosis: Clinical analysis of 126 patients with emphasis on the natural history. *Circulation* **37**: 759–788, 1968.
15. Goodwin, J.F. Hypertrophic disease of the myocardium. *Prog. Cardiovasc. Dis.* **16**: 199–200, 1973.
16. Hanrath, P., Mathey, D., Montz, R., Thiel, U., Vorbringer, H., Kupper, W., Schneider,

C., and Bleifeld, W. Myocardial thallium-201 imaging in hypertrophic obstructive cardiomyopathy. *Eur. Heart J.* **2**: 177–185, 1981.

17. O'Gara, P.T., Bonow, R.O., Damske, B.A., Maron, B.J., Spirito, P., Bacharach, S.L., Green, M.B., Larson, S.M., and Epstein, S.E. Myocardial perfusion abnormalities in patients with hypertrophic cardiomyopathy and normal coronary arteries. *J. Am. Coll. Cardiol.* **7**: 95A, 1986 (abst.).
18. Legand, V., Hodgson, J.M., Bates, E.R., Aueron, F.M., Mancini, G.B.J., Smith, J.S., Gross, M.D., and Vogel, R.A. Abnormal coronary flow reserve and abnormal radionuclide exercise test results in patients with normal coronary angiograms. *J. Am. Coll. Cadiol.* **6**: 1245–1253, 1985.
19. Cannon, R.O. III, Rosing, D.R., Maron, B.J., Leon, M.B., Bonow, R.O., Watson, R.M., and Epstein, S.E. Myocardial ischemic in patients with hypertrophic cardiomyopathy: contribution of inadequate vasodilator reserve and elevated left ventricular filling pressures. *Circulation* **71**: 234–243, 1985.
20. Wangler, R.D., Peters, K.G., Marcus, M.L., and Tomanek, R.J. Effects of duration and severity of arterial hypertension and cardiac hypertrophy on coronary vasodilator reserve. *Circ. Res.* **51**: 10–18, 1982.
21. Pichard, A.D., Gorlin, R., Smith, H., Ambrose, J., and Meller, J. Coronary flow studies in patients with left ventricular hypertrophy of the hypertensive type: evidence for an impaired coronary vascular reserve. *Am. J. Cardiol.* **47**: 547–553, 1981.
22. Weiss, M.D., Ellis, K., Sclacca, R.R., Johnson, L.L., Schmitt, D.H., and Cannon, P.J. Myocardial blood flow in congestive and hypertrophic cardiomyopathy. *Circulation* **54**: 484–493, 1976.
23. Linzbach, A.J. Heart failure from the point of view of quantitative anatomy. *Am. J. Cardiol.* **5**: 370–382, 1960.
24. Rakusan, K. Quantitative morphology of capillaries of the heart: Number of capillaries in animal and human hearts under normal and pathological conditions. *Methods Achiev. Exp. Pathol.* **5**: 272–000, 1971.
25. Breish, E.A., Houser, S.R., Carey, R.A., Spann, J.F., and Bove, A.A. Myocardial blood flow and capillary density in chronic pressure overload of the feliac left ventricle. *Cardiovasc. Res.* **14**: 469–475, 1980.
26. Nishimura, K., Nosaka, H., Saito, T., and Nobuyoshi, M. Another possible mechanism of angina in hypertrophic cardiomyopathy. *Circulation* **68** (suppl. III): III–162, 1983 (abst.).
27. Pichard, A.D., Meller, J., Teichholz, L.E., Lipnik, S., Gorlin, R., and Herman, M.V. Septal perforator compression (narrowing) in idiopathic hypertrophic subaortic stenosis. *Am. J. Cardiol.* **40**: 310–314, 1977.
28. Griggs, D.M. Jr. and Nakamura, Y. Effects of coronary constriction on myocardial distribution of iodoantipyrine 131I. *Am. J. Physiol.* **215**: 1082, 1968.
29. Buckberg, G.D., Fixler, D.E., Archie, J.P., and Hoffman, J.I.E. Experimental subendocardial ischemia in dogs with normal coronary arteries. *Circ. Res.* **30**: 67–81, 1972.
30. Hoffman, J.I.E. and Buckberg, G.D. Transmural variations in myocardial perfusion. In: Progress in Cardiology, Yu, P.N., Goodwin, J.F. (eds), Philadelphia, Lea & Febiger, 1976, vol. 5, p.38.
31. Tanaka, M., Fujiwara, H., Onodera, T., Wu, D.J., Matsuda, M., Hamashima, Y., and Kawai, C. Pathogenetic role of myocardial fiber disarray in the progression of cardiac fibrosis in normal hearts, hypertensive hearts and hearts with hypertrophic cardiomyopathy. *Jpn. Circ. J.* **51**(6): 624–630, 1987.
32. Hoshino, T., Fujiwara, H., Kawai, C., and Hamahsima, Y. Myocardial fiber diameter and regional distribution in the ventricular wall of normal adult hearts, hypertensive hearts and hearts with hypertrophic cardiomyopathy. *Circulation* **67**: 1109–1116, 1983.

The Value of Endomyocardial Biopsy in Diagnosing Hypertrophic Cardiomyopathy

*Morie Sekiguchi**, *Shin-ichi Nunoda, and Michiaki Hiroe***

* The Heart Institute of Japan Tokyo Women's Medical College, Tokyo, Japan.
** Department of Radiology, Tokyo Women's Medical College, Tokyo, Japan.

ABSTRACT

To investigate whether bizarre myocardial hypertrophy with disorganization (BMHD) is characteristic of hypertrophic cardiomyopathy (HCM) at the biopsy level, the histopathology of the biopsied left ventricular (LV) myocardium in 18 patients with essential hypertension (HT) and 14 patients with HCM was studied. A "biopsy score" was devised for a more quantitative evaluation of the BMHD and a comparative study on the biopsy score of the LV biopsied specimen was also performed.

BMHD was defined as myocardial cells showing hypertrophy, disorganization, and bizarre nuclei. "Disorganization" of myocardial cells was distinguished by both the terminology and histopathological characteristics from "disarrangement" of myocardial cells. BMHD was found in 2 of 18 patients with HT (11%) and in 10 of 14 patients with HCM (71%) in the LV biopsied specimens ($P<0.005$). A similar study was done in the right ventricular (RV) specimens in which the incidence of BMHD was only 2.8% (2/72 patients) with chronic RV overload as compared to 66% (33/50 patients) with HCM ($P<0.001$).

INTRODUCTION

Endomyocardial biopsy[1,2] is now widely used in diagnosing specific heart muscle diseases and myocarditis and in assessing myocardial dysfunction or prognosis.[3-7] When a clinical or autopsy diagnosis of hypertrophic cardiomyopathy(HCM) is made, abnormal architecture of myocardial cells is accepted[8-21] as an important diagnostic element, in addition to asymmetric septal hypertrophy and systolic anterior motion of the anterior mitral leaflet. However, abnormal architecture of myocardial cells, termed "disarray", has been found by various investigators[18,20,22-25] in other myocardial disorders, including hypertension, the tetralogy of Fallot, and pulmonary and/or aortic valvular diseases, and is regarded as a nonspecific finding for HCM. An important element of this controversy is the lack of consensus regarding what constitutes abnormal cellular arrangement in the ventricular myocardium. This problem of definition is accentuated by the fact that some nondiseased hearts or hearts with cardiac diseases other than hypertrophic cardiomyopathy contain areas of myocardium in which adjacent cardiac muscle cells are not arranged in a precisely parallel alignment.

The definition of the deviation from parallel cellular arrangement has differed considerably among investigators. Sekiguchi *et al.*[26] and Nunoda *et al.*[7] reported that bizarre myocardial hypertrophy with disorganization(BMHD) is a characteristic finding for HCM. In their view, BMHD is different from the mere "disarray" of myocardial cells.

In order to ascertain whether BMHD is characteristic of and diagnostic for HCM, we examined histologically biopsy specimens from the left and right ventricular myocardium of patients with HCM and compared them with those from patients with essential hypertension (HT) or chronic right ventricular overloading (CRVO). Further, we devised a "biopsy score" for the quantitative histological diagnosis of HCM and the biopsy score of the left ventricular biopsied specimens from patients with HCM and HT was compared.

In this article, our view of the significance of BMHD which is based on our systematic investigations[4,6,7,26] will be introduced and discussed.

SUBJECTS AND METHODS

Eighteen adult cases of essential hypertention (HT) (mean age 50 ± 7 years) in stage I or II of the WHO criteria and 14 cases of HCM (46 ± 10 years) were studied for the left ventricular biopsy analysis.[7]

For the right ventricular study, 72 adult cases of chronic right ventricular overloading (CRVO) (mean age 34 ± 11 years) and 50 cases of HCM (mean age 40 ± 14 years) were analyzed. The 72 cases were broken down into mitral valvular disease (n = 36), primary pulmonary hypertension (n = 3), cor pulmonale (n = 1), patent ductus arteriosus associated with pulmonary hypertension (n = 1), tetralogy of Fallot (n = 7), pulmonary stenosis (n = 5), atrial septal defect (n = 14), and ventricular septal defect (n = 5).[6]

A routine histopathological analysis using 4 μm-thick paraffin-embedded specimens was made. The two investigators who examined the specimens were not informed about the clinical background of the patients.

Definitions Used in Diagnosing Hypertrophic Cardiomyopathy

The word "disarray" was not used to define the characteristics of HCM because it

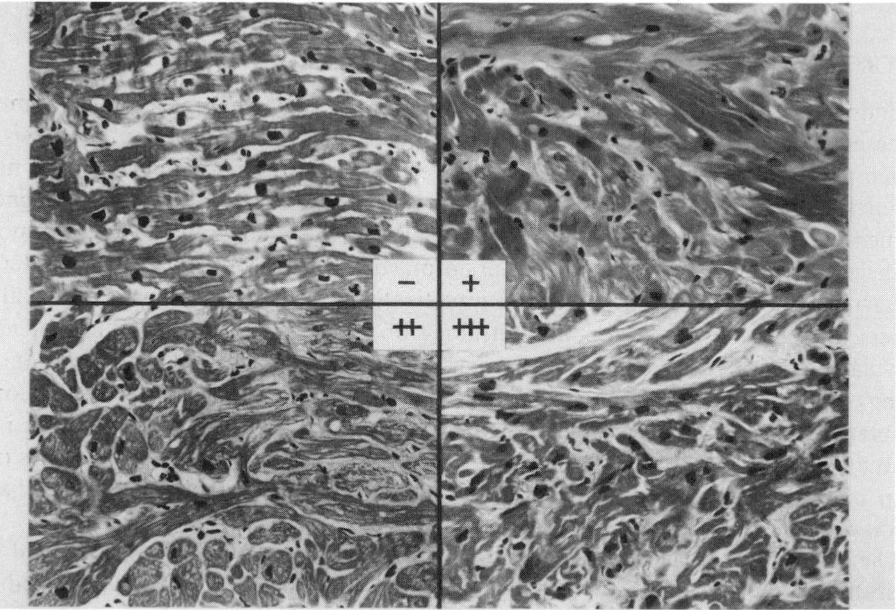

Fig. 1. Model micrographs of the disarrangement of myocardial grading (−) to (+ + +). The bar indicates 40 m (From Nunoda *et al.*[7], reproduced with permission)

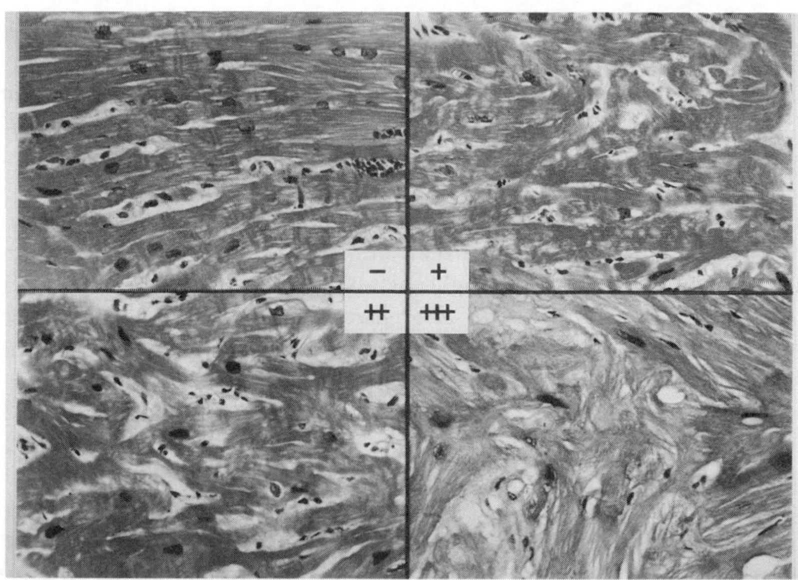

Fig. 2. Model micrographs of bizarre myocardial hypertrophy with disorganization (BMHD) grading (−) to (+++). The bar indicates 40 m (From Nunoda *et al.*[7], reproduced with permission)

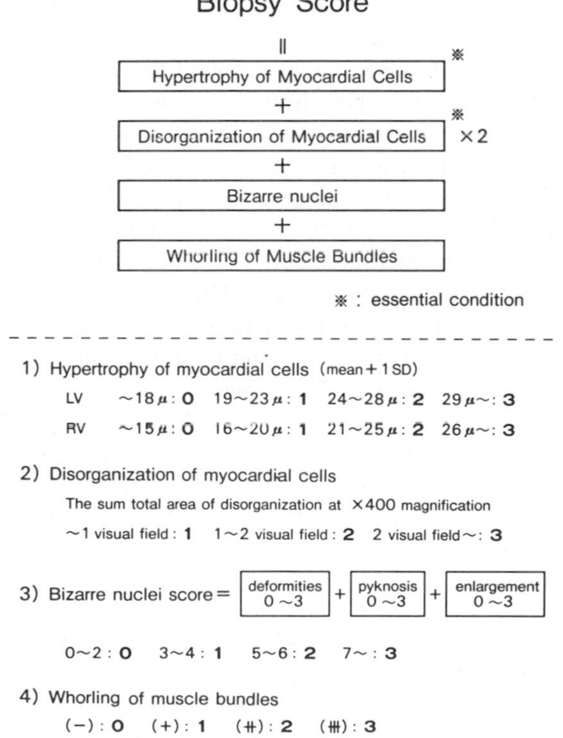

Biopsy Score
‖
Hypertrophy of Myocardial Cells ※
+
Disorganization of Myocardial Cells ※ ×2
+
Bizarre nuclei
+
Whorling of Muscle Bundles
※ : essential condition
1) Hypertrophy of myocardial cells (mean + 1 SD)
LV ~18μ : 0 19~23μ : 1 24~28μ : 2 29μ~ : 3
RV ~15μ : 0 16~20μ : 1 21~25μ : 2 26μ~ : 3
2) Disorganization of myocardial cells
The sum total area of disorganization at ×400 magnification
~1 visual field : 1 1~2 visual field : 2 2 visual field~ : 3
3) Bizarre nuclei score = deformities 0~3 + pyknosis 0~3 + enlargement 0~3
0~2 : 0 3~4 : 1 5~6 : 2 7~ : 3
4) Whorling of muscle bundles
(−) : 0 (+) : 1 (++) : 2 (+++) : 3

Fig. 3. Method of biopsy score determination of bizarre myocardial hypertrophy with disorganization (BMHD) (From Nunoda *et al.*[7], reproduced with permission)

has been used by different investigators in both HCM and non-HCM conditions. We devised the following definitions for clarification.

Disarrangement of myocardial cells: There is a multidirectional arrangement of the myocardial cells, but individual cells do not show a tight connection at the light-microscopic level. Model photomicrographs of disarrangement of myocardial cells are depicted in Fig. 1.

Disorganization of myocardial cells: The myocardial arrangement shows a criss-cross architecture and a tight connection of the cells. This is in contrast to disarrangement, where the connection is loose at the light-microscopic level.

Bizarre myocardial hypertrophy with disorganization (BMHD): There is hypertrophy of myocardial cells, disorganization of myocardial cells, and bizarre nuclei. The significance of these features has been discussed by many investigators, including Teare,[8] Olsen,[29] Maron *et al.*[10,13,14,16,17] and Sekiguchi *et al.*[26] and Nunoda *et al.*[6,7] Figure 2 demonstrates the grading (−) to (+ + +) of the BMHD which is used to determine the severity of the disease.

Biopsy score: The biopsy score we devised consists of four factors: 1) hypertrophy of myocardial cells, 2) disorganization of myocardial cells, 3) bizarre nuclei, and 4) whorling of the muscle bundles (Fig. 3). These four factors are considered to be the most characteristic histopathological features of HCM. Hypertrophy and disorganization of myocardial cells are defined as essential conditions for the biopsy score, and the disorganization score is doubled as it is more important than the other factors. The explanation of each factor is as follows.

Hypertrophy of myocardial cells: The diameter of the myocardial cell is determined by measuring the distance across the cell at the narrowest plane across the nucleus on longitudinally cut myocytes, according to the methods of Sekiguchi *et al.*[30] and Baandrup and Olsen.[31] The sections are examined through a ×40 objective lens and a ×10 eyepiece with an ocular micrometer disc. At least 50 cells from each biopsy are measured and the diameters averaged to determine the size of the myocardial cells for each patient. Myocardial cells just below the endocardium, those with severe contraction bands or many degenerative substances, and those in which nuclei are located at branching portions are excluded from the measurement. The score of hypertrophy of myocardial cells is determined by reference to the criteria of Hiroe *et al.*[32] who reported that there was no difference in the mean value of myocardial cells between HCM and other hypertrophied human hearts, including mitral and/or aortic valvular diseases, but there was considerable variation in size in HCM when compared with other heart disease. For these reasons, they reported that the hypertrophy of myocardial cells was graded by the mean value plus one standard deviation(SD) of the diameter of myocardial cells, not by mean value only. In accordance with their criteria,[32] the hypertrophy of the left or right ventricular myocardial cells score is determined (see Table 1).

The quantitative estimation of the disorganization of myocardial cells is based on the sum total areas of disorganization at high magnification (×400). The score of disorganization of myocardial cells is determined as follows: The sum total area of the disorganization of myocardial cells is smaller than one visual field, score 1; larger than one visual field and smaller than two visual fields, score 2; larger than two visual fields, score 3.

Bizarre nuclei: We define bizarre nuclei as those showing deformity, pyknosis, and enlargement. The score of bizarre nuclei is determined by the total score of the three factors, which are graded 0–3, as follows: When the total score of each nuclear factor is 0–2, the bizarre nuclei score is 0; total score of 3–4, bizarre nuclei score is 1; total score of 5–6, bizarre nuclei score is 2; total score of over 7, bizarre nuclei score is 3.

TABLE 1. Method of Grading and Scoring of the Hypertrophy of Myocardial Cells (from Hiroe *et al.*[32]) and Nunoda *et al.*[7])

Left ventricle		Right ventricle	
m±IS.D	score		score
–18μm	0	–15μm	0
19–23μm	1	16–20μm	1
24–28μm	2	21–25μm	2
29– μm	3	26– μm	3

The Whorling of Muscle Bundles

The score of the whorling of muscle bundles is determined by the model micrographs which are graded (–) to (+ + +), as follows: (–), score 0; (+), score 1; (+ +), score 2; (+ + +) score 3.

As mentioned above, the biopsy score comprises four factors (the hypertrophy of myocardial cells, the disorganization of myocardial cells, bizarre nuclei, and the whorling of muscle bundles), and if all four are present to a marked degree, then 15 points would be assigned.

RESULTS OF THE BIOPSY ANALYSIS WITH REGARD TO THE DIAGNOSTIC VALUE OF BIZARRE MYOCARDIAL HYPERTROPHY WITH DISORGANIZATION (BMHD)

BMHD was found in the left ventricular biopsied specimens in 2 of 18 patients with HT(11%) and in 10 of 14 patients with HCM(71%). The incidence of BMHD in the left ventricle in patients with HCM was significantly higher than that in patients with HT($p < 0.005$), as shown by the χ^2 contingency test. The sensitivity, specificity, and predictive accuracy of BMHD in the left ventricular biopsy were calculated according to the following formulae[33]:

$$\text{Sensitivity of BMHD} = \frac{\textit{true positive}}{\textit{true positive} + \textit{false negative}} \times 100$$

$$= \frac{10}{10 + 4} \times 100 = 71(\%)$$

$$\text{Specificity of BMHD} = \frac{\textit{true negative}}{\textit{false positive} + \textit{true negative}} \times 100$$

$$= \frac{16}{2 + 16} \times 100 = 89(\%)$$

$$\text{Predictive accuracy of BMHD} = \frac{\textit{true positive}}{\textit{true positive} + \textit{false positive}} \times 100$$

$$= \frac{10}{10 + 2} \times 100 = 83(\%)$$

The disarrangement of myocardial cells was found in the left ventricular biopsied specimens in 13 of 18 patients with HT(72%) and 10 of 14 patients with HCM(71%).

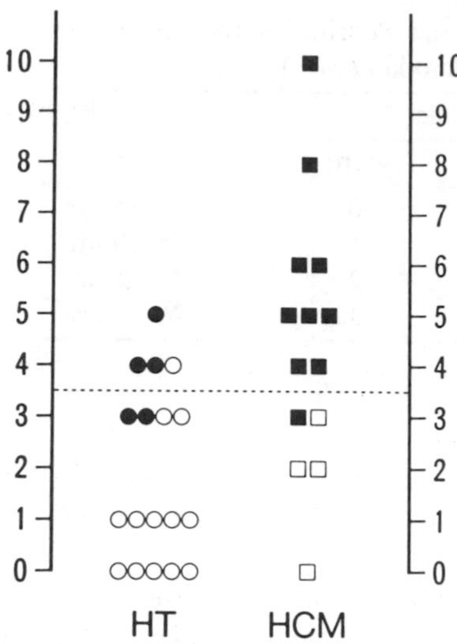

●, ■ : having hypertrophy and disorganization

○, □ : having hypertrophy and no disorganization; having no hypertrophy and disorganization; having no hypertrophy and no disorganization

Fig. 4. The distribution of biopsy score in patients with essential hypertension and hypertrophic cardiomyopathy. HT essential hypertension, HCM hypertrophic cardiomyopathy (From Nunoda *et al.*[7], reproduced with permission)

The incidence of disarrangement of myocardial cells in patients with HCM was not statistically different from that found in patients with HT according to the χ^2 contingency test.

The biopsy score in the left ventricle was lower in patients with HT than in those with HCM (Fig. 4). The borderline zone, which divided the two groups, seemed to be between scores 3 and 4.

The results of our semiquantitative comparative study of the right ventricular biopsy specimens between CRVO and HCM are shown in Table 2. The sensitivity, specificity, and predictive accuracy of BMHD in the right ventricular biopsy were calculated in the same manner as in the left ventricular biopsy analysis.

$$\text{Sensitivity of BMHD} = \frac{33}{33 + 17} \times 100 = 66\%$$

$$\text{Specificity of BMHD} = \frac{70}{2 + 70} \times 100 = 97\%$$

$$\text{Predictive accuracy of BMHD} = \frac{33}{33 + 2} \times 100 = 94\%$$

TABLE 2. Incidence of the Right Ventricular Biopsy Findings in Chronic Right Ventricular Overloading (CRVO) and in Hypertrophic Cardiomyopathy (HCM)

		CRVO (n = 72)					HCM (n = 50)				
		−	+	++	+++	incidence	−	+	++	+++	incidence
Hypertrophy of myocytes		10 (13.9)	41 (56.9)	17 (23.6)	4 (5.6)	62 (86.1)	4 (8.0)	26 (52.0)	18 (36.0)	2 (4.0)	46 (92.0)
	disorganization	69 (95.8)	2 (2.8)	1 (1.4)	0 (0.0)	3 (4.2)	16 (32.0)	17 (34.0)	9 (18.0)	8 (16.0)	34 (68.0)***
Abnormal	whorling	70 (97.2)	2 (2.8)	0 (0.0)	0 (0.0)	2 (2.8)	45 (60.0)	5 (10.0)	0 (0.0)	0 (0.0)	5 (10.0)
structural	disarrangement	14 (19.4)	48 (66.7)	9 (12.5)	1 (1.4)	58 (80.6)	4 (8.0)	35 (70.0)	11 (22.0)	0 (0.0)	46 (92.0)
abnormalities	fragmentation	49 (68.1)	23 (31.9)	0 (0.0)	(00.0)	23 (31.9)	16 (32.0)	28 (56.0)	5 (10.0)	1 (2.0)	34 (68.0)
	abnormal branching	32 (44.4)	36 (50.0)	4 (5.6)	0 (0.0)	40 (55.6)	10 (20.0)	33 (66.0)	7 (14.0)	0 (0.0)	40 (80.0)**
Degeneration of myocytes		39 (54.1)	29 (40.3)	4 (5.6)	0 (0.0)	33 (45.8)	6 (12.0)	39 (68.0)	4 (8.0)	1 (2.0)	44 (88.0)***
Interstitial fibrosis		15 (20.8)	51 (70.9)	6 (8.3)	0 (0.0)	57 (79.1)	7 (14.0)	39 (78.0)	4 (8.0)	0 (0.0)	43 (86.0)
B M H D		70 (97.2)	1 (1.4)	1 (1.4)	0 (0.0)	2 (2.8)	17 (34.0)	20 (40.0)	11 (22.0)	2 (4.0)	33 (66.0)

*: $p < 0.05$ **: $p < 0.01$ ***: $p < 0.001$ BMHD: Bizarre myocardial hypertrophy with disorganization ( ) indicates % incidence

DISCUSSION

Since the first pathological description of HCM by Teare in 1958,[8] many of the clinical and morphological facets of this disease have become a source of controversy. Teare originally described eight patients at necropsy who showed "bizarre and disorganized arrangement of muscle bundles" in an asymmetrically thickened ventricular septum, and it has been considered that disorganized arrangement of the cardiac muscle cells in the myocardium is a characteristic morphological feature of patients with HCM. Maron *et al.*[13,14,17,19] reported that the majority of patients with HCM (about 95%) showed cardiac muscle cell disorganization, and this abnormal cellular architecture occupied particularly large areas of the myocardium. In contrast, cellular disorganization was uncommon in patients with other cardiac diseases or with normal hearts. For this reason, they stated that the cardiac muscle cell disorganization had an important diagnostic role as a morphological marker for HCM.[13,14,17,19] However, other authors[18,20,22–25] have taken the view that disorganized cardiac muscle cells are neither typical of nor particularly specific for HCM. An important element of this controversy is the lack of consensus regarding what constitutes abnormal cellular arrangement.

We consider[26] that bizarre myocardial hypertrophy with disorganization (BMHD) is a more characteristic and diagnostic histopathological finding in HCM, and that "disorganization" of myocardial cells is different from "disarrangement" of myocardial cells. We hold that both disorganization and disarrangement involve a random arrangement of the myocytes. Disarrangement, however, does not show the tight connection of myocardial cells as is seen in disorganization. BMHD, which we have stressed as being a characteristic and diagnostic finding of HCM, consists of hypertrophy and disorganization of myocardial cells and bizarre nuclei, and BMHD is considered a more characteristic finding of HCM than disorganization only.

In the study from the left ventricular biopsy, BMHD was found in 10 of 14 patients with HCM(71%), whereas it was found in only 2 of 18 patients with HT(11%). These results indicate the high specificity(89%) and predictive accuracy(83%) of BMHD for HCM. Also, right ventricular biopsy analysis revealed similar results (Table 2).

The frequency of the "disarrangement" of the muscle bundles was 92% in HCM and 81% in the CRVO. It is suggested, therefore, that the disarrangement does not characterize HCM. However, the "disorganization" was seen only in 2 (2.8%) among the 72 cases with CRVO, whereas of the 50 HCM cases, 33(66%) showed the disorganization($P < 0.001$).

In our study, we also devised a biopsy score in order to diagnose HCM quantitatively.[7] The biopsy score consists of four factors, i.e., hypertrophy of myocardial cells, disorganization of myocardial cells, bizarre nuclei, and whorling of muscle bundles. According to the report of Van Noorden *et al.*[9] who devised the histological HOCM index(HHI), the HHI consisted of five factors, i.e., short runs of fibers interrupted by connective tissue, large bizarre nuclei, fibrosis, degenerating muscle with disappearing myofibrils, and disorganized, whorling muscle. Of these five factors, short runs of fibers interrupted by connective tissue, fibrosis, and degenerating muscle with disappearing myofibrils are present not only in HCM but also in other heart diseases, such as dilated cardiomyopathy and myocarditis. For this reason, our biopsy score was made up of the most characteristic factors for HCM. The results of biopsy score determination in patients with HT and HCM showed a similar tendency to the results of semiquantitative gradings of BMHD, and we believe that the biopsy score is pertinent in diagnosing HCM quantitatively.

From the results of this study, we conclude that BMHD is a highly specific finding for HCM at the biopsy level; however, the disarrangement of myocardial cells is not specific or diagnostic for HCM. Furthermore, a biopsy score of more than four points is considered indicative of HCM at the biopsy level.

In our laboratory, we use the BMHD as one of the hallmarks of HCM, and important data was obtained which revealed that patients with either giant negative T waves in the electrocardiogram or apical hypertrophy of the left ventricle do not always show BMHD in the LV and RV biopsies. The incidence of BMHD in patients with GNT was 21/57 (36.8%) and was significantly less than in patients with HCM without GNT (40/57 cases, 70.1%) ($P < 0.001$).[34] These results led us to conclude that the apical hypertrophy does not always signify the presence of HCM but is often a sign of hypertensive heart disease.

REFERENCES

1. Sakakibara, S. and Konno, S. Endomyocadial biopsy. *Jpn. Heart J.* **3**: 537–543, 1962.
2. Sekiguchi, M. and Konno, S. Histopathological differentiation employing endomyocardial biopsy in the clinical assessment of primary myocardial disease. *Jpn. Heart J.* **10**: 30–46, 1969.
3. Sekiguchi, M. and Konno, S. Diagnosis and classification of primary myocardial disease with the aid of endomyocardial biopsy. *Jpn. Circ. J.* **35**: 737–754, 1971.
4. Sekiguchi, M., Hiroe, M., Ogasawara, S., and Nishikawa, T. Practical aspects of endomyocardial biopsy. *Ann. Acad. Med. Singapore* **10** (Suppl): 115–128, 1981.
5. O'Connell, J.H., Robinson, J.A., Subramanlian, R., and Scanlon, P.J. Endomyocardial biopsy: Technique and applications in heart disease of unknown cause. *Heart Transplantation* **3**: 132–143, 1984.
6. Nunoda, S., Sekiguchi, M., Morimoto, S., Nishikawa, T., Hiroe, M., Hirosawa, K., Genda, A., and Takeda, R. Biopsy assessed BMHD (bizarre myocardial hypertophy with disorganization) as a hallmark of hypertrophic cardiomyopathy—A concept through a study of biopsied right ventricular myocardium in valvular and congenital heart diseases and corpulmonale——. *Jpn. Circ. J.* **46**: 858–859, 1982. (abstract)
7. Nunoda, S., Genda, A., Sekiguchi, M., and Takeda, R. Left ventricular endomyocardial biopsy findings in patients with essential hypertension and hypertrophic cardiomyopathy with special reference to the incidence of bizarre myocardial hypertrophy with disorganization and biopsy score. *Heart Vessels* **1**: 170–175, 1985.
8. Teare, D. Asymmetrical hypertrophy of the heart in young adults. *Br. Heart J.* **20**: 1–8, 1958.
9. Van Noorden, S., Olsen, E.G.J. and Pearse, A.G.E. Hypertrophic obstructive cardiomyopathy, a histological, a histochemical and ultrastructural study of biopsy material. *Cardiovasc. Res.* **5**: 118–131, 1971.
10. Maron, B.J., Ferrans, V.J., Henry, W.L., Clark, C.E., Redwood, D.R., Roberts, W.C., Morrow, A.G., and Epstein, S.E. Differences in distribution of myocardial abnormalities in patients with obstructive and nonobstructive asymmetric septal hypertrophy (ASH). Light and electron microscopic findings. *Circulation* **50**: 436–446, 1974.
11. Alexander, C.S. and Gobel, F.L. Diagnosis of idiopathic hypertrophic subaortic stenosis by right ventricular septal biopsy. *Am. J. Cardiol.* **34**: 142–151, 1974.
12. Pomerance, A. and Davies, M.J. Pathological features of hypertrophic obstructive cardiomyopathy (HOCM) in the elderly. *Br. Heart J.* **37**: 305–312, 1975.
13. Maron, B.J. and Roberts, W.C. Quantitative analysis of cardiac muscle cell disorganization in the ventricular septum of patients with hypertrophic cardiomyopathy. *Circulation* **59**: 689–706, 1979.
14. Maron, B.J., Sato, N., Roberts, W.C., Edwards, J.E., and Chandra, R.S. Quantitative

analysis of cardiac muscle cell disorganization in the ventricular septum. Comparison of fetuses and infants with and without congenital heart disease and patients with hypertrophic cardiomyopathy. *Circulation* **60**: 685–696, 1979.
15. Sutton, M.S.J., Lie, J.T., Anderson, K.R., O'Brien, P.C., and Erye, R.L. Histopathological specificity of hypertrophic obstructive cardiomyopathy. Myocardial fibre disarray and myocardial fibrosis. *Br. Heart J.* **44**: 433–443, 1980.
16. Maron, B.J., Anan, T.J., and Roberts, W.C. Quantitative analysis of the distribution of cardiac muscle cell disorganization in the left ventricular wall of patients with hypertrophic cardiomyopathy. *Circulation* **63**: 882–894, 1981.
17. Maron, B.J. and Roberts, W.C. Hypertrophic cardiomyopathy and cardiac muscle cell disorganization revisited: Relation between the two and significance. *Am. Heart J.* **102**: 95–110, 1981.
18. Becker, A.E. and Caruso, G. Myocardial disarray. A Critical review. *Br. Heart J.* **47**: 527–538, 1982.
19. Maron, B.J. Myocardial disorganization in hypertrophic cardiomyopathy. Another point of view. *Br. Heart J.* **50**: 1–3, 1983.
20. Becker, A.E. Myocardial disorganization in hypertrophic cardiomyopathy. *Br. Heart J.* **51**: 466–468, 1984.
21. Davies, M.J. The current status of myocardial disarray in hypertrophic cardiomyopathy. *Br. Heart J.* **51**: 361–363, 1984.
22. Bulkley, B.H., Weisfeldt, M.L., and Hutchins, G.M. Asymmetric septal hypertrophy and myocardial fiber disarray. Features of normal, developing, and malformed hearts. *Circulation* **56**: 292–298, 1977.
23. Van Der Bel-Kahn, J. Muscle fiber disarray in common heart diseases. *Am. J. Cardiol.* **40**: 355–364, 1977.
24. Hoshino, T., Fujiwara, H., Kawai, C., and Hamashima, Y. Diagnostic value of disarray in endomyocardial biopsy specimens in hypertrophic cardiomyopathy. A critical report based on distribution of disarray in the subendocardial region of autopsied hearts. *Jpn. Circ. J.* **46**: 1281–1291, 1982.
25. Noda, S., Nakayama, Y., Yamamoto, S., Kitaura, Y., Kawamura, K. and Takatsu, T. Myofiber disarray in the myocardial biopsies from patients with common heart diseases and idiopathic cardiomyopathy. *Jpn. Circ. J.* (abstract) **45**: 946–947, 1981.
26. Sekiguchi, M., Hiroe, M., Morimoto, S., and Kawagoe, Y. The contribution of endomyocardial biopsy to the diagnosis and assessment of cardiomyopathies. In: International Congress Series No. 470. Proceedings of the VIII World Congress of Cardiology. Hayase, S. and Murao, S. (eds.) Amsterdam; Excerpta Medica, pp. 583–590, 1979.
27. Report of a WHO Expert Committee. Arterial hypertension. Technical Report Series No. **628**: 7–58, 1978.
28. Hiroe, M., Sekiguchi, M., Matsuda, M., and Abe, H. A colour review of endomyocardial biopsy: Practical method and histopathological pictures. *Nippon-Rinsho* **38**: 2040–2042, 1980. (in Japanese)
29. Olsen, E.G.J. Morbid anatomy and histology in hypertrophic obstructive cardiomyopathy. In: Hypertrophic Obstructive Cardiomyopathy. Wolstenholm, G.E.W., O'Connor, M.J. and Churchill, A. (eds.) London. pp. 183–191, 1971.
30. Sekiguchi, M., Hiroe, M., and Morimoto, S. On the standardization of histopathological diagnosis and semiquatitative assessment of the endo-myocardium obtained by endomyocardial biopsy. Bulletin of the Heart Institute, Japan. pp. 55–85, 1979–1980.
31. Baandrup, U. and Olsen, E.G.J. Critical analysis of endomyocardial biopsies from patients suspected of having cardiomyopathy: I. Morphological and morphometric aspects. *Br. Heart J.* **45**: 475–486, 1981.
32. Hiroe, M., Sekiguchi, M., Haze, K., and Hirosawa, K. Clinical assessement of the severity of cardiomyopathic patients employing endomyocardial biopsy. *Saishin-Igaku* **32**: 78–90, 1977. (in Japanese)

33. Ong, Y.S., Quaife, M.A., Dzindzio, B.S., Emery, J.F., Kotlyarov, E.V., and Forker, A.D. Clinical decision-making with treadmill testing and thallium 201. *Am. J. Med.* **69**: 31–38, 1980.
34. Morimoto, S., Sekiguchi, M., Hasumi, M., Inagaki, Y., Takimoto, H., Ohtsubo, K., Hiroe, M., Hirosawa, K., Matsuda, M., and Komatsu, Y. Do giant negative T waves represent apical hypertrophic cardiomyopathy? Left ventriculographic and cardiac biopsy studies. *J. Cardiography* **15** (Suppl. VI): 35–51, 1985.

BASIC MECHANISMS FOR CARDIAC HYPERTROPHY

α_1-Adrenergic-Stimulated Hypertrophy in Neonatal Rat Heart Muscle Cells

Paul C. Simpson

Cardiology Section (111C), Veterans Administration Medical Center, and Cardiovascular Research Institute and Department of Medicine, University of California, San Francisco, California, U.S.A.

ABSTRACT

The molecular mechanisms of myocardial hypertrophy must be identified, if inadequate, excessive, and pathological hypertrophy are to be understood and treated. A cell culture model system is required for identification of the extracellular signals and intracellular pathways that regulate myocardial cell growth. A model employing neonatal rat ventricular myocytes maintained in low-density, serum-free culture is described. By use of this cell culture system, the α_1-adrenergic receptor has been shown to regulate myocardial cell hypertrophy, development of contractile activity, and expression of specific genes, including messenger RNAs encoding the c-*myc* proto-oncogene and embryonic/neonatal isoforms of contractile proteins (skeletal α-actin and β-myosin heavy chain). Increased RNA expression is mediated in part at the level of transcription. The intracellular pathway(s) linking surface receptor activation with nuclear RNA synthesis are under investigation. A possible role of protein kinase C is suggested by α_1-stimulated phosphoinositide turnover and protein kinase C activation, as well as by the hypertrophic effect of phorbol esters. The specific proteins found in hypertrophied cells vary with the hypertrophic stimulus, and certain cells appear to be "pathologically" hypertrophied, in that they contain a reduced fraction of myosin heavy chain. The overall relevance of α_1-adrenoceptor-stimulated hypertrophy is unknown. However, considerable indirect evidence implicates this α_1 receptor system in the genesis of certain types of hypertrophy *in vivo*.

OVERVIEW AND STATEMENT OF THE PROBLEM

Myocardial hypertrophy is a major problem in clinical cardiology. For example, myocardial hypertrophy is seen in the dilated and hypertrophic cardiomyopathies, valve disease, hypertension, and following myocardial infarction. Hypertrophy is also an integral part of normal development and occurs as a response to vigorous exercise training.

Hypertrophy and Hemodynamic Loading

Hypertrophy can be generally viewed as an adaptive response to an increase in hemodynamic loading. However, it is clear that the hypertrophic response varies considerably with respect to apparent loading conditions. The idiopathic hypertrophic cardiomyopathies, the subject of this monograph, demonstrate hypertrophy excessive for load in the most dramatic form. Conversely, clinical studies have suggested that the hypertrophic response can be inadequate for the imposed hemodynamic load, with consequent pump failure.[1] Furthermore, it appears that the hypertrophy of disease often, if not invariably, results in pump dysfunction, so-called pathological hypertrophy.[1] This situation in disease is in striking contrast to the hypertrophy of normal development or exercise training. Normal pump function is seen in the hypertrophy of exercise, despite similar absolute magnitude of heart enlargement.[2]

A major challenge is to identify the molecular mechanisms of heart growth, so that excessive, inadequate, and pathological hypertrophy can be treated. A central issue is the identity of the signals that initiate and maintain growth. For example, hypertrophy in aortic stenosis appears to be clearly related to increased load. However, it is not known if some mechanical factor, such as cell stretch, is a direct growth signal, or whether there is some intermediary extracellular signal, such as catecholamines. An interaction between both factors is also possible. Studies in clinical, experimental, and genetic hypertension have shown clearly that there is no simple relationship between hypertrophy and blood pressure.[3] Many studies have suggested that catecholamines may regulate myocardial hypertrophy *in vivo* in some circumstances.[4] Furthermore, in the idiopathic hypertrophic cardiomyopathies, and perhaps in hypertensive hypertrophy treated with hydralazine[5] and in the young spontaneously hypertensive rat,[6,7] potential mechanical or loading stimuli appear to be absent. It is unknown whether hypertrophy in these instances results from inappropriate growth stimulation by extracellular molecules such as catecholamines, or from some intrinsic abnormality of cell growth, perhaps analogous to cancer.

Cell Growth Regulation

In the broadest sense, myocardial hypertrophy of all types is a problem of cardiac muscle cell growth regulation. Tremendous progress has been made over the past several years in understanding the control of growth of cells from tissues other than the heart. The study of isolated cells in culture has revealed the fundamental principle that growth can be regulated by extracellular molecules interacting with cell receptors and activating intracellular pathways. Although the full identity and inter-relationships of these three elements are far from being understood, it has also become clear that uncontrolled growth, as in cancer, can result from inappropriate amounts or activities of growth factors, their receptors, or intracellular transducing elements.[8–10] Unless heart muscle cells are fundamentally different from all other types of cells, it can be predicted that their growth will also prove to be regulated by these same three components. The total number of growth factor-receptor-transduction systems in heart muscle cells is obviously not known, since this type of study is in its infancy. However, analogy with other types of cells and the observed diversity of the hypertrophic response *in vivo* both suggest that there could be multiple growth factors with their cognate receptors. Since the complete pathway for intracellular transduction has not been completely defined for any growth factor in any cell, it remains an open question whether growth factors and their receptors will couple to a few or many intracellular pathways. Therefore, the challenge in heart muscle cell biology is to identify growth-transducing systems. It can then be asked whether some element of a system is altered in a given type of myocardial hypertrophy, such as idiopathic hypertrophic cardiomyopathy. This chapter will review the identification of one such system, that involving the interaction of catecholamines with the α_1-adrenergic receptor.

RATIONALE FOR STUDY OF HYPERTROPHY IN CULTURE

In order to identify the extracellular molecules and mechanical factors that might regulate myocardial growth, a model system that permits control of all potential variables is required. Furthermore, hypertrophy *in vivo* is a complex process, produced variably by cardiac muscle cell hypertrophy, fibroblast proliferation and collagen production, endothelial cell hyperplasia, and smooth muscle cell hypertrophy and/or proliferation.[11,12] With models of hypertrophy *in vivo*, there are too many uncontrollable potential stimuli for growth and too many different responding cells. Thus, *in vivo* models cannot be used to dissect out individual growth stimuli and the responses of specific cell populations. However, a cell culture model system is ideally suited for this task. In cell culture, individual potential growth factors can be systematically manipulated, and the response of a defined population of cells can be observed.

Signal-Response Identification in vivo: *Catecholamines*

Catecholamines illustrate very well the problem of signal identification in *in vivo* models. Experimental manipulations producing hypertrophy, including exercise, cold, aortic coarctation, renal hypertension, mineralocorticoid-induced hypertension, hypoxia, and pulmonary hypertension, are all accompanied by increased cardiac sympathetic nerve activity.[4] Therefore, norepinephrine (NE) is a potential extracellular signal in many forms of hypertrophy associated with changes in hemodynamic loading. NE is an effective agonist for all adrenergic receptor subtypes (α_1, α_2, β_1, and β_2). In addition to myocyte α_1, β_1, and β_2 receptors, NE can stimulate neuronal α_2 and β_2 receptors. NE release is decreased by stimulation of neuronal α_2-adrenergic receptors, and increased by stimulation of sympathetic β_2-adrenergic receptors.[13–16] Thus β_2-adrenergic regulation of NE release might be implicated in the hypertrophic effect of isoproterenol,[17] or in the hypertrophy regression with β-adrenergic antagonists.[3,18]

Since angiotensin can also stimulate NE release,[14,19] inhibition of angiotensin-stimulated NE release could be important in the regression of hypertrophy with angiotensin-converting enzyme inhibitors.[20] In fact, a recent study indicates that the enhancement of noradrenergic neurotransmission in renovascular hypertension of the rat is mediated in part by angiotensin II-induced facilitation of NE release.[19] The precise role of calcium channels (and thus of calcium channel antagonists) in NE release has been insufficiently evaluated.[21] Myocardial and/or plasma catecholamine levels are often measured to quantify sympathetic activities, but it is unclear that these values provide an adequate index of myocardial NE turnover or of adrenergic receptor stimulation in the myocardium. For example, pithed rats regain near normal chronotropic responsiveness to neural stimulation within one week after denervation with 6-hydroxydopamine, despite persistent 90% depeletion of cardiac norepinephrine levels.[22] This issue is addressed by others in this volume.

NE synthesis, as well as release and reuptake, needs to be considered. Environmental stress, reserpine, and electrical stimulation all induce the mRNA coding for tyrosine hydroxylase, the rate-limiting enzyme in NE synthesis, in rat superior cervical ganglion sympathetic neurons.[23] Short stimulation can produce a lasting effect on this enzyme.[23] Uptake of NE and epinephrine (EPI) from arterial blood may be another important variable.[24] Sympathetic neurons contain polypeptide transmitters such as substance P and somatostatin, and these cotransmitters can be regulated by stimulation in directions opposite to NE.[23] The possible functional significance for postsynaptic responses is unknown. Little attention has been given to the site and functional role of myocardial EPI stores; these stores persist after denervation.[25–27] Changes in myocyte adrenergic receptors following denervation require investigation.[28] Regional differences in sympathetic innervation have been described, but little is known about similar differences in adrenergic receptor expression.[29] Very little is known about the intrasynaptic vs extrasynaptic distribution of heart muscle cell adrenergic receptors, or the extent of their accessibility to exogenous agonists and antagonists. If there is a heart myocyte α_1-adrenoceptor functionally dedicated primarily to chronic trophic support of the cell (as described below), then independent documentation of its activation or inhibition may prove to be difficult. (That is, study of acute hemodynamic[30] or contractile responses may not be adequate.) Recent work has revealed the possibility of an important muscle cell-sympathetic neuron interaction. Nerve growth factor (NGF), an essential trophic factor for sympathetic neurons, is synthesized by the target cells of those neurons.[31] Thus, there may be an important interaction between a nerve product which is trophic for muscle (NE), and a muscle product which is trophic for nerve (NGF). Could this interaction be altered in hypertrophy or cardiomyopathy? All of these considerations can be summarized by saying that experimental isolation and evaluation of potentially relevant growth signals *in vivo* is extraordinarily difficult at the present time, just considering catecholamines.

Heterogeneity of Cell Types

Catecholamines and adrenergic receptors also illustrate the problem of cell heterogeneity in the samples collected with intact organ or tissue experiments. There have been several studies of adrenergic receptors and postreceptor mechanisms in various forms of hypertrophy. However, very few studies have been done using isolated cells. In the rat heart, less than 25–35% of the cells are myocytes.[12,32] Most of the cells in the intact heart are not striated muscle cells. The numerically greater cells, which include[32] smooth muscle cells, pericytes, macrophages and other blood-borne cells, fibroblasts, and endothelial cells, can express adrenergic receptors and postreceptor mechanisms. Their numbers may well vary during hypertrophy and development. A careful comparison of the characteristics (e.g., numbers per cell) of adrenergic receptors on the various cell types in the heart has not been done, to my knowledge. Furthermore, assays of receptor numbers and other variables are typically normalized to total protein. Since the proportion of protein derived from striated muscle cells (versus other types of cells and extracellular protein) and the amount of protein in each muscle cell may vary in different settings (development, hypertrophy), normalization to total protein is not ideal. Although the experiments are technically more difficult, it would seem that the best strategy is to perform studies on isolated cells. Methods for isolation of adult cardiac myocytes have been developed.[33]

Other Tissue Models

It should be mentioned that study of the intact heart *in vitro* (e.g., the isolated perfused heart) offers some advantages over *in vivo* models with respect to control of variables.[34] However, the problem of cell heterogeneity is not avoided, and growth does not occur. In the model using myocardium transplanted to the ocular chamber or other locations, there is growth as well as enhanced control of potential variables.[35–37]

Cell Culture

The limitations of a cell culture model also need to be recognized. The system that permits control of variables and study of defined cells is an artificial one. For example, the myocyte-myocyte interactions pertaining in intact tissue are altered; cell shape changes as the isolated cells adapt to the culture substrate; the culture medium is not nearly so complex as tissue fluid; and neurons are absent in most cultures, although nerve-muscle cocultures are being studied.[38] For these and other reasons, direct extrapolation of findings in culture to the heart *in vivo* is not appropriate. However, if the cell population and the culture conditions are carefully and completely defined, then potentially important biologic properties can be identified.

There has been no success in the development of transformed cell lines of heart myocytes. Therefore, primary cultures must be used. This has the disadvantage that genetic studies cannot be done and that cells must be obtained from the intact organ for each experiment. However, the use of primary cultures has the advantage of studying normal, nontransformed heart myocytes. Therefore, one can be confident that findings in the culture system do in fact reflect biologic potential that may be realized *in vivo*. The goal in our laboratory is to understand one growth signal-response system that is as simple as possible. The effect of other hormones and growth factors can then be evaluated, singly and in combination. Once potential growth factors, receptors, and intracellular transducing mechanisms have been identified by studies in culture, it will be necessary, and possible, to return to *in vivo* models to test whether and how integration occurs in the intact organ.

CHARACTERISTICS OF A CELL CULTURE MODEL SYSTEM[39–42]

The cell culture system developed in our laboratory over the past several years is the first to be used for study of myocardial cell hypertrophy.[41] Primary cultures are obtained from the ventricles of day-old Sprague-Dawley rats by gentle enzymatic and mechanical dissociation. It is absolutely essential that the resulting cell population be accurately defined. Therefore, cells are maintained at low density in culture, so that individual cells can be identified and counted through the microscope. As in all primary cultures, proliferating fibroblasts are a potential complication. The numbers of these nonmuscle mesenchymal cells (nonmyocytes), the exact identity of which is not clear,[42] are reduced by an initial differential attachment procedure; and their proliferation is prevented by pulse treatment with an inhibitor of DNA synthesis, bromodeoxyuridine. Less than 20% of the muscle cells incorporate this thymidine analogue into their DNA, versus 80% of the nonmyocytes.[42] The resultant cultures are documented to contain $\geq 90\%$ myocytes and $\leq 10\%$ nonmyocytes, and cell numbers do not change as a function of time.

Absence of Cell Division

It should be emphasized that rat myocytes do not divide in the low-density cultures under any condition so far tested, even in the absence of bromodeoxyuridine.[42,43] There is DNA synthesis in $\leq 20\%$ of myocytes, as measured by autoradiography; and mitosis in approximately 10% of cells, as determined by binucleate cells.[42] However, cytokinesis does not occur. This is an intriguing observation in light of the fact that myocytes may divide in the intact heart during the first few days after birth.[6,12,44] The reason(s) for the loss of cell division in culture is (are) unknown. However, the absence of cell proliferation in culture, intrinsic for the myocytes and imposed by bromodeoxyuridine for the nonmyocytes, does provide an experimental advantage. One can routinely obtain at least 5×10^6 myocytes from each neonatal heart. The cells from 20 hearts can be seeded into 35-mm culture dishes at a plating density of 500 cells/mm^2. With a plating efficiency of 30%, the final cell density is 150/mm^2, or 0.12×10^6 cells/dish (800 mm^2 total dish surface area), and the number of dishes available for experiments is 250. There are 36 dishes of 100-mm size (5500 mm^2 surface area/dish with 0.825×10^6 cells/dish).

If care is taken in the procedure, all dishes will contain the same number of cells and the same proportion of myocytes (>90%) for the duration of experiments lasting over many days. Cell counts over time can be used to evaluate possible toxic effects, depending on the experiment. One can then determine cell number in a limited number of dishes, and normalize multiple replicates of biochemical or other assays on a per-cell basis. Normalization on a per-cell basis is an essential feature of the study of hypertrophy in culture.

Serum-Induced Trophic Effects[41)]

Although the myocytes do not divide in culture, they do undergo hypertrophy or enlargement when maintained in medium containing serum. The increase in cell size in response to serum is time dependent and dose related. Hypertrophy is a chronic response that develops over many hours to one or two days. Cell size and its increase (hypertrophy) are defined by three assays: total cell protein content, cell surface area, and cell volume. Cell protein is measured by a chemical or isotopic method.[39)] Surface area is determined by an image analysis technique used on cells attached in the dishes. Volume is assayed using microscopy (or a cell counter), after removal of myocytes from the dishes by selective trypsinization.[41)] As noted, the result of a protein determination in a dish of cells can be divided by the number of cells in that dish to give per-cell content. Since nonmyocyte contamination is ≤10%, their contribution can generally be ignored. Pure cultures of nonmyocytes are easily prepared from the dishes used for differential attachment, and are used for control studies.[39,41)] The surface area and volume assays are entirely specific for the myocytes, and these two indices maintain a constant relationship over time.[41)] The use of three separate size assays provides definite confirmation of the hypertrophic response.

Hypertrophic growth in culture is easily observed and measured and is, in the broad sense at least, the same general process that produces hypertrophy of the intact heart *in vivo*, that is, cardiac myocyte enlargement.[11,12)] *In vivo*, all hypertrophied cells are not the same, as exemplified by differences in the relative proportions of V1 and V3 myosins or by differences in the myofibrillar and nonmyofibrillar volume fractions. Similar observations have been made in the culture system, as will be discussed subsequently. It is therefore desirable to define hypertrophy using an unequivocal but general index, such as total protein, area, or volume. One can then ask whether the hypertrophic phenotype varies as a function of the stimulus, as defined by the expression in the hypertrophied cells of specific proteins, whether contractile, receptor, or channel, for example.

A second response induced in the cultured myocytes by addition of serum to the medium is spontaneous contractile activity or beating, at a rate of 50–100/min at 37°C. Beating, like growth, is a chronic response that requires hours to appear. Beating and morphological features indicate that the myocytes retain the differentiated phenotype when put into culture.

Serum-Free, Single-Cell Cultures[41)]

Hypertrophy and beating are designated "trophic" effects. When serum is removed, these two effects are not seen: cell size remains the same as at isolation and the myocytes are quiescent (not beating). However, in serum-free medium supplemented with transferrin and insulin, the myocytes survive, as documented by cell counts, and respond with hypertrophy and beating to the subsequent addition of serum. Thus the serum-free cultures provide an excellent control population, without baseline hypertrophy or contractile activity, for defined testing of potential trophic factors. This strategy of using a culture medium that is the minimal required for survival and that does not induce growth or contractile activity deserves emphasis. The use of this approach provides the great sensitivity for detection and analysis of regulatory factors, singly and in combination.

Serum-free medium provides the additional advantage that nonmyocyte proliferation is drastically reduced. Thus control cultures without bromodeoxyuridine can be studied.[41,45] Since myocytes do not readily attach to untreated culture dishes in the absence of serum, cells are plated in the presence of serum and switched to serum-free medium on day 1 of culture. Experiments are generally begun after three to five days in defined medium. Unpublished studies with radiolabeled serum proteins suggest that carryover from the initial plating is trivial. This may not be the case when cells are maintained for prolonged times (five days) in serum-containing medium.[46]

It is also critical to recognize that the system described above is a single-cell culture system, allowing unequivocal distinction and counting of myocytes and nonmyocytes. The usual confluent heart cell cultures are actually multilayers,[47] and the cell population under study cannot be defined. The single-cell cultures avoid the problem of an uncertain cell population. However, potentially important cell-cell interactions are also minimized, and this fact needs to be recognized. For example, in our serum-free medium, cell size increases as a function of cell density, and spontaneous contractility develops at a sufficiently high density (unpublished observations). These density-related changes may be due to myocyte-myocyte or myocyte-nonmyocyte interactions. In cultures with a high nonmyocyte fraction ($\sim 50\%$), there is a reduction in the maximal chronotropic response to β-adrenergic stimulation, as compared with cultures containing only 15% nonmyocytes.[42] Nonmyocytes may also produce a factor or factors that stimulates myocyte growth.[48]

Serum and Catecholamines[41]

The dose-related effects of serum on growth and contractility clearly show that myocyte size and function can be regulated by extracellular molecules in the absence of hemodynamic factors. However, serum is enormously complex, containing multiple defined and undefined nutrients, hormones, and growth factors. We have not attempted to isolate the active substance(s) in serum, although we know that serum trophic effects are not inhibited by adrenergic antagonists. Furthermore, stimulation of hypertrophy by catecholamines through a non-β-adrenergic mechanism, as described in the next section, is observed in the presence of serum. However, the response develops over a considerably longer time period than in the absence of serum, and the magnitude of the change versus control is less.[41] One possible explanation for the longer time and lesser magnitude of the response to catecholamines in the presence of serum is that the control cells in this situation are already hypertrophied by the growth stimulants in serum. Therefore, specific compounds have been tested for induction of hypertrophy and/or beating by adding them to the nongrowing, quiescent, serum-free cultures. These studies have revealed previously unsuspected trophic roles for the α_1-adrenergic receptor, as described in the following section. Technical details regarding the pharmacological manipulation of the cultured myocytes have been summarized recently.[40]

ALPHA$_1$-ADRENERGIC TROPHIC EFFECTS IN CULTURE[39,45,49]

Stimulation of the serum-free cultured myocytes with NE or EPI produces a gradual

1.5- to 2.0-fold increase in cell size. NE or EPI also induce spontaneous contractility in essentially all of the cells. The protracted time course of these two trophic responses (many hours) raises the possibility that their intracellular transduction is different from the usually studied acute (seconds to minutes) adrenergic responses. Both of these responses are mediated through the α_1-adrenergic receptor, but they differ in important respects. First, hypertrophy is produced by α_1 stimulation alone, whereas beating requires concomitant β_1-adrenergic activation. In other words, cells stimulated through only the α_1 receptor (as with methoxamine or with NE in the presence of β-adrenergic antagonists) are enlarged but quiescent. This indicates that hypertrophy can occur in the absence of contractile activity. The phenomenon of hypertrophy without contractile activity is also seen during stimulation with phorbol esters[50,51] or with NE in the presence of calcium channel antagonists.[52] Therefore, hypertrophic growth does not *require* contractile activity.

A second major difference between the two α_1 trophic responses is that hypertrophy requires RNA and protein synthesis (it is blocked by cycloheximide or actinomycin D), whereas beating does not. That is, beating can be induced even when hypertrophy is blocked. The fact that beating and hypertrophy can be separately induced raises the possibility that these two responses are mediated by different intracellular pathways, both of which are activated by α_1 receptor stimulation.

These and other characteristics of α_1-adrenergic trophic effects are outlined in Table 1. Note that the EC_{50} for the NE responses is within the range estimated for an active sympathetic nerve-muscle junction.[53]

It requires emphasis that the trophic responses defined are chronic, unlike the acute adrenergic effects that have been studied for many years. The observation that the α_1 receptor can regulate a chronic process such as growth is a new one.[54,55] However,

TABLE 1. Characteristics of α_1-Adrenergic Trophic Effects in Serum-free Culture

	Hypertrophy	Beating
Stimulus	Norepinephrine or epinephrine[a]	
Response	1.5- to 2-fold increase in cell size[b]	>95% of cells vs <5% in control
EC_{50}	200 nM	20 nM
Time course	Detect: 3–6 hr Half-max: 12–18 hr Plateau: 24–36 hr	Slightly more rapid
Receptor specificity	α_1	Combined α_1 & β_1
Inhibitors of protein or RNA synthesis (cycloheximide or actinomycin D)	Inhibition	No effect
Inhibitor of DNA synthesis (bromodeoxyuridine)	No effect	No effect
Calcium channel antagonists	Little effect	Inhibition
Pertussis toxin	No effect	No effect

[a] These agonists are stable in the medium under the conditions used, and the responses are not reproduced by known metabolites or unknown degradation products.[39]

[b] There is no increase in DNA synthesis by autoradiography (unpublished), in DNA concentration,[43] or in cell number.[39,41]

subsequent evidence has indicated that a growth-promoting role of the α_1 receptor is not limited to heart muscle cells. Although the cultured rat heart nonmyocytes do not respond to NE under the conditions tested,[39,41,43,45,56] other types of cultured cells do grow in response to α_1 stimulation, as outlined in Table 2. Note that DNA synthesis and cell division are induced in these other types of cells, whereas the myocyte response is limited to hypertrophy. These other types of cells undergo hypertrophy prior to division.[57] Why the heart myocyte response is arrested at hypertrophy is unknown.

The primary focus of our subsequent work has been on the hypertrophic response to α_1 stimulation. The beating response has not been fully characterized. For example, we do not know whether the induction of spontaneous contractility reflects the development of a membrane potential,[58] increases in energy stores,[59] alterations in calcium or other currents,[60,61] or other events. Meidell *et al.* found that long-term treatment with NE does not change ATP concentration,[43] and our preliminary studies support this. The beating phenomenon and the respective contributions to it of α_1 and β_1-adrenergic stimulation require study. Potentially similar chronotropic responses to α_1-adrenergic stimulation are under investigation by others.[38] It is possible that the α_1 contribution to spontaneous contractility is relevant to the clinical problem of α_1-mediated arrhythmias during ischemia.[62]

TABLE 2. Growth Regulation by the α_1-Adrenergic Receptor in Culture

Cell type	Assay	Reference
Rat heart myocytes (neonatal)	Cell size	45
Rat aortic myocytes (adult)	Cell number	63
3T3 fibroblasts	Cell number, DNA synthesis	64
Bovine aortic endothelial cells	Cell number, DNA synthesis	64
Rat hepatocytes (adult)	DNA synthesis	65
FRTL-5 thyroid cells	DNA synthesis	66

GENE EXPRESSION IN α_1-STIMULATED HYPERTROPHY

A major aim of our work is to unravel the intracellular mechanism(s) whereby α_1 stimulation produces hypertrophy. One approach is to investigate the changes in the RNAs and proteins expressed during hypertrophy. The expectation is that these studies will define the intracellular events subject to regulation by the α_1 receptor, i.e., whether RNA synthesis (transcription), RNA degradation, protein synthesis (translation), or protein degradation. Regulation of any one or a combination of these events could in theory produce the increases in general and specific protein contents that define the hypertrophic state. Recall that the α_1 receptor does not alter DNA synthesis in these cells, nor is heart muscle cell DNA synthesis a part of the myocyte hypertrophic response *in vivo*.[11,12]

α_1-Stimulated increases in the content of total RNA and of specific messenger RNAs (mRNAs) indicate that the intracellular mechanism includes pretranslation regulation. Indeed, the transcription of total RNA and of a subset of mRNAs is induced. Furthermore, different hypertrophic stimuli are associated with a distinctive pattern of gene expression. That is, the "phenotype" of hypertrophied cells varies as a function of the stimulus; all hypertrophied cells are not the same.

c-myc *Proto-Oncogene mRNA*[67]

Induction of the c-*myc* proto-oncogene mRNA is an early and transient response to

α_1 stimulation, with an increase in mRNA content detectable at 30 min, a peak at two hours, and a return to baseline by six hours. The c-*myc* mRNA codes for a nuclear protein, and its induction has been previously associated with cell division. Increased c-*myc* expression in hypertrophy suggests that hypertrophy and division share common mechanistic pathways. Proto-oncogene expression in hypertrophy is reviewed in more detail elsewhere.[68]

Total RNA[56]

A later response to α_1 stimulation is an increase in total RNA content, measured by spectrophotometry or ^{14}C-uridine incorporation. The magnitude of this increase is similar to that for total cell protein, and the time course is slightly more rapid (compare Table 1). These measurements of total RNA largely reflect ribosomal RNA (rRNA). Inhibition by actinomycin D suggests that the increase in rRNA content could be due to an increase in synthesis. Direct transcription assay supports this notion (see below).

Actin mRNAs[56]

Concomitant with the increase in total RNA, α_1 stimulation increases the per-cell contents of the mRNAs coding for sarcomeric (α) and cytoskeletal (β/γ) actins. The increase in cytoskeletal actin mRNA is proportional to that in total cell protein or RNA (two-fold), whereas the increase in sarcomeric actin mRNA is disproportionately large (>four-fold). There are two isoforms of sarcomeric or α-actin, the skeletal isoform, expressed predominantly in adult skeletal muscle and immature heart, and the cardiac isoform, expressed predominantly in adult heart. During pressure-load hypertrophy of the adult rat heart *in vivo*, there is increased expression of skeletal α-actin mRNA, the immature isoform.[69] When the neonatal rat cells, which contain equal amounts of both cardiac and skeletal α-actin mRNA, are placed in culture, skeletal α-actin mRNA expression is markedly decreased. That is, the cells assume a more adult-like phenotype. The reason for this down-regulation of the neonatal skeletal α-actin isoform in the neonatal cultured myocytes is unknown, but a similar phenomenon has been noted in another system.[70] α_1 Receptor stimulation of the cultured myocytes results in a selective increase (11-fold) in the per-cell content of skeletal α-actin mRNA. The increase in the adult or cardiac α-actin mRNA is only three-fold. The proportion of total sarcomeric actin mRNA which is the skeletal isoform increases from 20% in control cultured cells to near 50% after α_1 stimulation, a value similar to that found in the intact neonatal heart. Thus, α_1-stimulated hypertrophy in culture and pressure-load hypertrophy *in vivo* appear to be similar, in that both are associated with re-expression of a developmentally immature α-actin isoform. In fact, the α_1 receptor is the first identified molecular mediator of this type of isoform switching.[56]

Myosin Heavy Chain mRNA and Protein

Additional studies suggest similar isoform switching with respect to myosin heavy chain. α_1 Receptor stimulation increases myosin heavy chain protein through a selective increase in V3 myosin,[71] and the augmentation of V3 myosin is mediated by an increase in the content of β-myosin heavy chain mRNA (Waspe *et al.*, unpublished).

Isoform Switching in Hypertrophy

The studies of c-*myc*, skeletal α-actin, and β-myosin heavy chain appear consistent in suggesting that α_1-stimulated hypertrophy is associated with selective expression of genes associated with growth and early development. In some forms of hypertrophy *in vivo*, in both experimental animals and humans, there is re-expression of genes associated with growth and early development.[69,72-78] These observations may provide a clue to the general relevance of α_1-stimulated hypertrophy.

The studies of gene expression also provide a definition of the "phenotype" of hypertrophied cells. The phenotype can differ, depending on the hypertrophic stimulus. For example, thyroid hormone induces hypertrophy of cultured myocytes,[71] but does not increase the mRNAs coding for c-*myc*, skeletal α-actin, or β-myosin heavy chain, all in direct contrast with α_1 stimulation (unpublished).

Transcriptional Regulation

The described increases in the per-cell contents of rRNA and specific mRNAs could provide the basis for augmentation of protein synthesis, and thus of total and specific protein contents. Indeed, Meidell *et al.* have confirmed directly an α_1-mediated stimulation of total and contractile protein synthesis in this model system, with no change seen in protein degradation.[43] The increases in RNA contents could themselves be due to increases in RNA synthesis (transcription) or to decreases in RNA degradation. We are using the nuclear run-on assay to quantify the rate of RNA transcription.[79] α_1-Adrenergic receptor stimulation increases total RNA transcription by 1.5-fold and skeletal α-actin mRNA transcription by six-fold.[79a] These results suggest that the increased steady-state levels of total RNA and skeletal α-actin mRNA are mediated by alterations in RNA synthesis, at least in part. Chien and colleagues have shown that α_1 stimulation increases total RNA and myosin light chain mRNA transcription in the same model, with no change in mRNA degradation.[80]

SIGNAL TRANSDUCTION PATHWAYS FOR α_1-STIMULATED TROPHIC EFFECTS

The previous studies begin to define intracellular events for which mechanisms must be sought. Specifically, what intracellular transduction system(s) is (are) set in motion by α_1 receptor activation that result in RNA transcription? How does the surface receptor transmit a signal to the cell nucleus?

Phospholipase C and Protein Kinase C

Initial work is focused on the phosphoinositide-protein kinase C postreceptor system.[81] Stimulation of the α_1 receptor acutely activates a phospholipase C that catalyzes phosphoinositide hydrolysis, as measured by production of inositol phosphates.[82] In our hands, this phospholipase C activation appears to be insensitive to pertussis toxin, as are the trophic effects. However, there is considerable evidence for guanine nucleotide regulatory (G) protein(s) in the coupling of various receptors, including the α_1-adrenoceptor, to phospholipase C.[83] In the myocytes, there is also acute activation of protein kinase C, as quantified by translocation of enzyme activity from the soluble to the particulate fraction.[84] Translocation of protein kinase C is presumably mediated by diacylglycerol. Diacylglycerol is known to activate protein kinase C and to be a product of phospholipase C activation. Phosphatidylcholine may also be an important source of diacyglycerol, rather than, or in addition to, phosphoinositides.[85]

α_1 Trophic effects require continuous receptor occupancy.[86] The effects are reversed if NE is removed or if an antagonist is added. This behavior implies that the postreceptor system is continuously active. Measurements made after 48-hr treatment with NE do suggest that activation of protein kinase C might be sustained: there is no down-regulation of the α_1 receptor number or desensitization of α_1-stimulated inositol phosphate production, and there is an increase in the total cell activity and amount of protein kinase C.[84]

Tumor-promoting phorbol esters, such as tetradecanoyl phorbol acetate (TPA), stimulate hypertrophy with a potency that parallels their ability to activate protein kinase C in the cells.[50,84] The time course and magnitude of this growth response are remarkably similar to those for α_1-stimulated hypertrophy, but beating is not induced.[51]

Thus considerable indirect evidence implicates protein kinase C in the hypertrophic response. The critical substrates are unknown, but might be one or more DNA-binding proteins that modulate transcription. DNA-binding proteins that activate transcription are modulated by TPA in other types of cells, probably at the post-translational level.[87-89] Thus, protein kinase C may phosphorylate a protein or protein that binds to DNA and activates mRNA transcription. However, there are confusing features about the behavior of protein kinase C in the cultured heart myocytes. First, α_1-induced translocation of protein kinase C activity is a transient response (minutes), unlike α_1 trophic effects. Second, down-regulation of protein kinase C activity by TPA does not abolish the hypertrophic response to NE or TPA (ref. 80 and Henrich and Simpson, unpublished). These findings may be clarified by ongoing studies using monoclonal antibodies to protein kinase C (Mochly-Rosen *et al.*, unpublished). In these studies, more than one form of protein kinase C is revealed by immunofluorescence with monoclonal antibodies, consistent with the evidence from cloning the enzyme that multiple PKC isoforms exist.[90-92] Furthermore, apparent loss of protein kinase C enzyme activity in the myocytes is not accompanied by absence of immunoreactive protein kinase C. The implications of these findings remain to be determined.

Two long-range approaches to the role of protein kinase C in hypertrophy and gene expression are potentially rewarding. First, microinjection of monoclonal antibodies that block activity. Second, identification of the protein(s) that activate RNA transcription and study of their regulation by protein kinase C.[10,93,94]

Other Growth Factors and Mechanisms and Their Integration

This focus on protein kinase C should not obscure the possibility that other protein kinases could be activated by α_1-adrenergic stimulation and play a role in the regulation of transcription. For example, there is a report that inositol-1, 4, 5-triphosphate can activate a protein kinase, independent of an effect on intracellular calcium.[95] Furthermore, there is little direct evidence for the importance of a protein kinase in transcriptional activation. The possibility that a nuclear signal is delivered by some other mechanism than protein phosphorylation needs to be kept in mind.

It is also possible that the α_1 receptor may regulate growth and gene expression at other level(s) in addition to transcription, although we have no direct evidence for this at present. Two recent reports provide an interesting perspective on multilevel regulation from a single receptor system. First, calcium may regulate protein synthesis at the level of translational initiation.[96] Inositol-1, 4, 5-trisphosphate, mentioned above, can release calcium from intracellular stores[97] (see discussion in Ref. 98). Second, protein kinase C may induce an mRNA encoding a protein involved in the initiation of translation.[99]

If activation of a single receptor could potentially transfer information to multiple foci that regulate the overall growth response, then how is the information from multiple receptors integrated? (See Florini[100] and Lichtstein and Rodbard[101] for recent summations of potential muscle growth factors.) For example, receptors for extracellular matrix proteins have recently been recognized.[102] These receptors, called integrins, have an important functional role in muscle cells[103,104] and are themselves regulated by other growth factors.[105] It is possible that integrins are related to "stretch" receptors, which also have a trophic role.[34,106–109] An analysis similar to that underway for the α_1-adrenergic receptor will be required for these receptors and the others that remain to be identified. It may then be possible to decipher how information is normally integrated within the cell and how this integration might be altered in disease.

A MODEL FOR PATHOLOGICAL HYPERTROPHY

The effect of TPA to increase overall cell size without an increase in contractile protein content may provide a model for pathological hypertrophy. *In vivo*, cells from pathologically hypertrophied hearts show a selective reduction in the amount or volume fraction of myofibrils.[110–113] These pathologically hypertrophied cells *in vivo* appear to be similar to TPA-treated cells in culture, in that both have reduced contractile protein as compared with their normally hypertrophied counterparts. TPA stimulation of the cultured myocytes increases the per-cell content of total protein, but not of myosin heavy chain (MHC) protein. Thus there is a reduction in the fraction of total protein which is myosin.[51] In striking contrast, β-MHC iso-mRNA is increased by TPA. Therefore, the failure of MHC protein to accumulate in TPA-treated cells reflects uncoupling of β-MHC iso-protein with expression from the increase in β-MHC iso-mRNA expression.[113a] A similar reduction of myofibrillar proteins by TPA has been observed in cultured skeletal muscle cells.[114]

We and others have evidence that contractile activity can regulate contractile protein expression.[115–117] This effect of contractility to increase myosin synthesis may be mediated at the translational level.[116,118] However, contractile activity may not be the determining factor in the effect of TPA. Cells treated with both NE and TPA undergo hypertrophy, accumulate myosin heavy chain mRNA, and exhibit contractile activity, but still do not maximally accumulate myosin heavy chain (ref. 51 and Waspe *et al.*, unpublished). Note that myosin heavy chain constitutes only a small fraction of total myocardial protein ($\sim 15\%$ in the rabbit),[119] so that a selective reduction in myosin might not be detected when assaying total protein.

The reason(s) for the failure of contractile protein accumulation in TPA-induced growth may become clear as more is learned about regulation and the role of protein kinase C. Myocyte protein kinase C activity responds differently to NE and TPA. Unlike NE, TPA acutely causes *persistent* translocation, accompanied by generation of the catalytic subunit, and chronically causes *down*-regulation of activity.[84] These kinetic differences may be explained in part by more rapid cellular metabolism of diacylglycerol, the endogenous protein kinase C activator, than of TPA. TPA and NE may also differentially modulate different isoforms of protein kinase C, as assessed by immunofluorescence (Mochly-Rosen *et al.*, unpublished). It is possible that muscle myosin heavy chain phosphorylation could alter its rate of degradation[120,121] and that phosphorylation of the substrate could depend on the extent or kinetics of activation of a particular isoform. Recent immunochemical studies have shown that one isoform of protein kinase C is translocated to myofibrils by α_1-adrenergic agonists and TPA (Mochly-Rosen *et al.*, unpublished). Thus, protein kinase C may be physically associated with substrates in the sarcomere. It is interesting to speculate whether a similar phenomenon might occur in pathological hypertrophy *in vivo*.

GENERAL RELEVANCE OF α_1-STIMULATED HYPERTROPHY

The observation of α_1-adrenergic-stimulated hypertrophy of cultured neonatal rat heart muscle cells has been confirmed in other laboratories.[43,117,122] Several other types of cultured cells grow in response to α_1 stimulation (Table 2), although neonatal rat heart nonmuscle cells do not.[39,43] The response of cultured neonatal or fetal heart myocytes from other mammalian species has not been examined, to my knowledge. There is a preliminary report of β-adrenergic stimulation of growth of cultured embryonic chick heart muscle cells.[123]

Cultured Adult Myocytes

The role of α_1-adrenergic stimulation in the growth of cultured adult myocytes is unclear. One laboratory has found both trophic[124] and toxic[106] effects of NE in cultured adult cat heart myocytes; however, the receptor specificities of these responses have not been reported. Preliminary data from another group suggest that α_1 stimulation does produce hypertrophy in cultured adult rat heart myocytes.[125] Our own unpublished observations suggest that cultured adult rat heart myocytes have a blunted response to NE, relative to that seen in neonatal cells. Growth stimulation of cultured adult rat heart myocytes by TPA has been observed by Claycomb.[126] If further work supports the observations of growth stimulation by TPA, but not (or less) by α_1 agonists, it would raise the interesting possibility that the α_1 receptor is not coupled or is poorly coupled to a growth-transducing pathway in cultured normal adult myocytes.

Stimulation of the α_1 receptor does activate phospholipase C in the adult cells.[127] Coupling of the α_1 receptor to growth may require re-expression of some protein (e.g., a G protein or an isoform of protein kinase C) that is not expressed in normal (non-growing) adult cells. This would imply that the α_1 growth pathway is a fetal/neonatal phenotype that is expressed in the adult only with a stimulus to hypertrophy, perhaps analogous to the re-expression of early developmental isoforms of contractile and other proteins during pressure-load hypertrophy. It is also relevant to note that the concentration of α_1-adrenergic receptors and protein kinase C in the normal myocardium decreases with age.[128–130] This might be expected if these elements are primarily involved in growth regulation. Clarification of the role of an α_1-adrenergic growth mechanism in the adult heart requires more information on the growth-transducing intracellular pathway(s) activated by α_1 stimulation and the response of cultured adult myocytes from normal and hypertrophied hearts, in the rat and in other species.[131]

In vivo

There is considerable evidence for a role of catecholamines in myocardial hypertrophy *in vivo*. It has been thought for some time, and recently confirmed,[132] that long-term catecholamine treatment can produce hypertrophy, without changing hemodynamic determinants. This area is discussed by Laks, a pioneer in the field.[133] Circumstantial evidence, including studies of catecholamine turnover and depletion, and of adrenergic antagonists, implicates catecholamines in the genesis of several different forms of hypertrophy, both clinical and experimental.[3–5,18,37,134–139] In a recent preliminary report, aortic banding in guinea pigs increased myocardial α_1 receptor number prior to the development of hypertrophy, and an α_1 antagonist, but not a β-adrenergic antagonist, attenuated the hypertrophic response.[140] There is certainly no unanimity on the role of catecholamines,[30] and the experimental difficulty of correctly assessing and controlling all relevant variables needs to be recalled. Furthermore, the receptor specificity

(α- vs β-adrenergic) has received insufficient attention until recently. Certainly there is a basis and need for further investigation.

Spontaneously Hypertensive Rat

The spontaneously hypertensive rat (SHR) may provide a model for human hypertrophic cardiomyopathy, since there is evidence that hypertrophy in this animal can be independent of hypertension.[6,7] Toshima, Koga, and colleagues at Kurume have shown that cultured cells from the neonatal SHR heart express a greater number of α_1-adrenergic receptors and exhibit a significantly greater hypertrophic response to NE than control cells from the Wistar-Kyoto (WKY) rat.[141,142] Similarly, Scholz and colleagues have found a selectively enhanced inotropic response to α_1 stimulation in isolated papillary muscles from the SHR (and cardiomyopathic hamster).[143,144] Cultured neurons from the brains of the SHR express more α_1-adrenergic receptors than similar cells from the WKY.[145] In addition, there are several reports of hyperactivity of phospholipase C and protein kinase C in other tissues of the SHR.[146–151] These observations all raise the possibility of genetic activation of an α_1-adrenergic/protein kinase C growth-transducing mechanism in the SHR. Experiments to distinguish cause from effect are required.

Human Hypertrophic Cardiomyopathy

There is, to my knowledge, no direct evidence for a role of the α_1 receptor in human hypertrophic cardiomyopathy, although α_1-adrenergic receptors and contractile responses are known to be present in human myocardium.[152] It has been suggested that adrenergic mechanisms are important in the genesis of this disease.[153] The evidence available is reviewed by Maisel, Toshima, Sugishita, and others in this volume. If the α_1-adrenergic receptor system is important, the primary defect could reside in the growth factor (catecholamines), the α_1 receptor, or a postreceptor transducing mechanism (e.g., protein kinase C). It is noteworthy that hypertrophic cardiomyopathy develops or progresses in childhood and adolescence, when the rate of normal growth is also accelerated, but does not progress in adult patients.[154,155] This finding may imply that the disease reflects the abnormal expression of a normal growth-transducing mechanism.

Growth Factor Interactions

Thus there is sufficient evidence that an α_1 growth mechanism may be important in hypertrophy to warrant further study. However, it seems unlikely that any single growth factor will be dominant in all forms of hypertrophy in all circumstances. Rather, given the phenotypic variability of the hypertrophic response seen *in vivo* and in culture, and the response of many cells, including heart cells, to several growth factors, it seems more likely that multiple and interacting growth stimuli will prove to be important. The primary influence may vary in different circumstances, e.g., exercise hypertrophy as compared with hypertensive hypertrophy or hypertrophic cardiomyopathy.

An example from hypertrophy *in vivo* may clarify this point. In the rat, hypothyroidism is associated with relative upregulation of myocardial β-myosin heavy chain (MHC) mRNA and down-regulation of α-MHC mRNA. β- and α-MHC mRNA encode the proteins which constitute V3 and V1 myosin, respectively. Thyroid hormone treatment induces α-MHC and decreases β-MHC mRNA, an effect that is also seen in cultured myocytes.[36,156,157] Thus thyroid hormone positively regulates α-MHC mRNA and negatively regulates β-MHC mRNA, probably at the transcriptional level.[158] In pressure-load hypertrophy *in vivo*, there is induction of β-MHC mRNA, and this upregulation is not explained by decreases in circulating levels of thyroid hormones.[73] However, high-dose thyroid hormone treatment of pressure-loaded animals can down-regulate β-MHC and up-regulate α-MHC mRNA, despite a progressive increase in the overall magnitude of hypertrophy.[73] One interpretation of these results is that the normal negative coupling between thyroid hormone and β-MHC can be loosened or relaxed during pressure-load hypertrophy, perhaps allowing a tighter coupling between β-MHC and some factor that produces its up-regulation. It is interesting to speculate whether this other factor positively regulating β-MHC could be the α_1-adrenergic receptor.

CONCLUSIONS

The studies reviewed above permit two major conclusions: (1) the α_1-adrenergic receptor may have an important role in heart muscle cell growth, gene expression, and development of function; and (2) a cell culture model system is a vital tool for identifying the growth factors, receptors, and intracellular mechanisms that produce myocardial hypertrophy.

Acknowledgments

The studies reviewed here have been done in collaboration with J.S. Karliner, C.P. Ordahl, D. Mochly-Rosen, L.T. Williams and colleagues, N.H. Bishopric, C.J. Henrich, C.S. Long, L.E. Waspe, and N.W. White. Support for the author's work was provided by the Veterans Administration Research Service and the United States Public Health Service (HL 31113, HL 35561). The author is a clinical investigator of the Veterans Administration.

REFERENCES

1. Grossman, W. Cardiac hypertrophy: Useful adaptation or pathologic process? *Am. J. Med.* **69**: 576–584, 1980.
2. Schaibel, T.E., Ciambrone, G.J., Capasso, J.M., and Scheuer, J. Cardiac conditioning ameliorates cardiac dysfunction associated with renal hypertension in rats. *J. Clin. Invest.* **73**: 1086–1094, 1984.
3. Tarazi, R.C. The heart in hypertension. *N. Engl. J. Med.* **312**: 308–309, 1985.
4. Ostman-Smith, I. Cardiac sympathetic nerves as the final common pathway in the induction of adaptive cardiac hypertrophy. *Clin. Sci.* **61**: 265–272, 1981.
5. Leenen, F.H.H., Smith, D.L., Farkas, R.M., Reeves, R.A., and Marquez-Julio, A. Vasodilators and regression of left ventricular hypertrophy: hydralazine versus prazosin in hypertensive human. *Am. J. Med.* **82**: 969–978, 1978.
6. Clubb, F.J. Jr., Bell, P.D., Kriseman, J.D., and Bishop, S.P. Myocardial cell growth and blood pressure development in neonatal spontaneously hypertensive rats. *Lab. Invest.* **56**: 189–197, 1987.
7. Cutilletta, A.F., Erinoff, L., Heller, A., Low, J., and Oparil, S. Development of left ventricular hypertrophy in young spontaneously hypertensive rats after peripheral sympathectomy. *Circ. Res.* **40**: 428–434, 1977.
8. Heldin, C.-H. and Westermark, B. Growth factors: mechanism of action and relation to oncogenes. *Cell* **37**: 9–20, 1984.
9. Marshall, C.J. Oncogenes and growth control 1987. *Cell* **49**: 723–725, 1987.
10. Varmus, H.E. Oncogenes and transcriptional control. *Science* **238**: 1337–1339, 1987.
11. Fanburg, B.L. Experimental cardiac hypertrophy. *N. Engl. J. Med.* **282**: 723–732, 1970.

12. Zak, R. Development and proliferative capacity of cardiac muscle cells. *Circ. Res.* **34/35** (suppl. II): 17–26, 1974.
13. Dahlof, C. Studies on β-adrenoceptor mediated facilitation of sympathetic neurotransmission. *Acta Physiol. Scand. Suppl.* **500**: 1–147, 1981.
14. Langer, S.Z. Presynaptic regulation of the release of catecholamines. *Pharmacol. Rev.* **32**: 337–362, 1981.
15. Starke, K. Regulation of noradrenaline release by presynaptic receptor systems. *Rev. Physiol. Biochem. Pharmacol.* **77**: 1–124, 1977.
16. Westfall, T.C., Peach, M.J., and Tittermary, V. Enhancement of the electrically induced release of norepinephrine from the rat portal vein: Mediation by β_2-adrenoceptors. *Eur. J. Pharmacol* **58**: 67–74, 1979.
17. Stanton, H.C., Brenner, G., and Mayfield, E.D. Jr. Studies on isoproterenol-induced cardiomegaly in rats. *Am. Heart J.* **77**: 72–80, 1969.
18. Strauer, B.E., Bayer, F., Brecht, H.M., and Motz, W. The influence of sympathetic nervous activity on regression of cardiac hypertrophy. *J. Hypertension* **3** (suppl. 4): S39–S44, 1985.
19. Zimmerman, J.B., Robertson, D., and Jackson, E.K. Angiotensin II-noradrenergic interactions in renovascular hypertensive rats. *J. Clin. Invest.* **80**: 443–457, 1987.
20. Pfeffer, J.M., Pfeffer, M.A., Mirsky, I., and Braunwald, E. Regression of left ventricular hypertrophy and prevention of left ventricular dysfunction by captopril in the spontaneously hypertensive rat. *Proc. Natl. Acad. Sci. USA* **79**: 3310–3314, 1982.
21. Hirning, L.D., Fox, A.P., McCleskey, E.W., Oliyera, B.M., Thayer, S.A., Miller, R.J., and Tsien, R.W. Dominant role of N-type Ca^{2+} channels in evoked release of norepinephrine from sympathetic nerves. *Science* **239**: 57–61, 1988.
22. Fluharty, S.J., Vollmer, R.R., Meyers, S.A., McCann, M.J., Zigmond, M.J., and Stricker, E.M. Recovery of chronotropic responsiveness after systemic 6-hydroxydopamine treatment. *J. Pharm. Exp. Ther.* **243**: 415–423, 1987.
23. Black, I.B., Adler, J.E., Dreyfus, C.F., Friedman, W.F., LaGamma, E.F., and Roach, A.H. Biochemistry of information storage in the nervous system. *Science* **236**: 1263–1268, 1987.
24. Honda, T., Ninomiya, I., and Azumi, T. Cardiac sympathetic nerve activity and catecholamine kinetics in cat hearts. *Am. J. Physiol.* **252**: H879–H885, 1987.
25. Ellison, J.P. and Hibbs, R.G. Catecholamine-containing cells of the guinea pig heart: an ultrastructural study. *J. Mol. Cell. Cardiol.* **6**: 17–26, 1974.
26. Pollack, G.H. Cardiac pacemaking: an obligatory role of catecholamines? *Science* **196**: 731–738, 1977.
27. Spurgeon, H.A., Priola, D.V., Montoya, P., Weiss, G.K., and Alter, W.A. III Catecholamines associated with conductile and contractile myocardium of normal and denervated dog hearts. *J. Pharm. Exp. Ther.* **190**: 466–471, 1974.
28. Williams, K., Strange, P.G., and Bennett, T. Alterations in β-adrenoceptor number and catecholamine content of chick atria after reversible sympathetic denervation with 6-hydroxydopamine. *Naunyu-Schmiedeberg's Arch. Pharmacol* **336**: 64–69, 1987.
29. Upsher, M.E. and Weiss, H.R. Heterogeneous distribution of beta adrenoceptors in the dog left ventricle. *J. Mol. Cell Cardiol.* **18**: 657–660, 1986.
30. Cooper, G. I.V., Kent, R.L., Uhob, C.E., Thompson, E.W., and Marino, T.A. Hemodynamic versus adrenergic control of cat right ventricular hypertrophy. *J. Clin. Invest.* **75**: 1403–1414, 1985.
31. Bandtlow, C.E., Heumann, R., Schwab, M.E., and Thoenen, H. Cellular localization of nerve growth factor synthesis by *in situ* hybridization. *EMBO J.* **6**: 891–899, 1987.
32. Nag, A.C. Study of non-muscle cells of the adult mammalian heart: a fine structural analysis and distribution. *Ctyobios* **28**: 41–61, 1980.
33. Clark, W.A., Decker, R.S., and Borg, T.K., eds., Biology of Isolated Adult Cardiac Myocytes. Elsevier Science Publishing Co., Inc. 1988, p. 441.
34. Kira, Y., Kochel, P.J., Gordon, E.E., and Morgan, H.E. Aortic perfusion pressure as

a determinant of cardiac protein synthesis. *Am. J. Physiol.* **246**: C247–C258, 1984.
35. Klein, I. and Hong, C. Effects of thyroid hormone on cardiac size and myosin content of the heterotopically transplanted rat heart. *J. Clin. Invest.* **77**: 1694–1698, 1986.
36. Korecky, B., Zak, R., Schwartz, K., and Aschenbrenner, V. Role of thyroid hormone in regulation of isomyosin composition, contractility, and size of heterotopically isotransplanted rat heart. *Circ. Res.* **60**: 824–830, 1987.
37. Tucker, D.C. and Gist, R. Sympathetic innervation alters growth and intrinsic heart rate of fetal rat atria maturing *in oculo*. *Circ. Res.* **59**: 534–544, 1986.
38. Steinberg, S.F., Drugge, E.D., Bilezikian, J.P., and Robinson, R.B. Acquisition by innervated cardiac myocytes of a pertussis toxin-specific regulatory protein linked to the α_1 receptor. *Science* **230**: 186–188, 1985.
39. Simpson, P. Stimulation of hypertrophy of cultured neonatal rat heart cells through an alpha$_1$-adrenergic receptor and induction of beating through an alpha$_1$- and beta$_1$-adrenergic receptor interaction: Evidence for independent regulation of growth and beating. *Circ. Res.* **56**: 884–894, 1985.
40. Simpson, P.C. Measurement of pharmacological effects in isolated myocytes. In: Biology of Isolated Adult Cardiac Myocytes. Clark, W.A., Decker, R.S., and Borg, T.K., (eds.), Elsevier Science Publishing Co., Inc., 1988, pp. 108–117.
41. Simpson, P., McGrath, A., Savion, S. Myocyte hypertrophy in neonatal rat heart cultures and its regulation by serum and by catecholamines. *Circ. Res.* **51**: 787–801, 1982.
42. Simpson, P. and Savion, S. Differentiation of rat myocytes in single cell cultures with and without proliferating nonmyocardial cells: Cross striations, ultrastructure, and chronotropic response to isoproterenol. *Circ. Res.* **50**: 101–116, 1982.
43. Meidell, R.S., Sen, A., Henderson, S.A., Slahetka, M.F., and Chien, K.R. α_1-adrenergic stimulation of rat myocardial cells increases protein synthesis. *Am. J. Physiol.* **251**: H1076–H1084, 1986.
44. Clubb, F.J., Jr. and Bishop, S.P. Formation of binucleated myocardial cells in the neonatal rat: An index for growth hypertrophy. *Lab. Invest.* **50**: 571–577, 1984.
45. Simpson, P. Norepinephrine-stimulated hypertrophy of cultured rat myocardial cells is an alpha$_1$-adrenergic response. *J. Clin. Invest.* **72**: 732–738, 1983.
46. Grynberg, A., Athias, P., and Degois, M. Effect of change in growth environment on cultured myocardial cells investigated in a standardized medium. *In vitro Cell Develop. Biol.* **22**: 44–50, 1986.
47. Hyde, A., Blondel, B., Malter, A., Cheneval, J.P., Filloux, B., and Girardier, L. Homo- and heterocellular junctions in cell cultures: An electrophysiological and morphological study. *Prog. Brain. Res.* **31**: 283–311, 1969.
48. Henrich, C.J. and Simpson, P.C. Neonatal rat heart nonmuscle cells produce factor(s) causing muscle cell hypertrophy. *J. Cell Biochem.* (suppl. 12A): 132, 1988.
49. Simpson, P., Bishopric, N., Coughlin, S., Karliner, J., Ordahl, C., Starksen, N., Tsao, T., White, N., and Williams, L. Dual trophic effects of the alpha$_1$-adrenergic receptor in cultured neonatal rat heart muscle cells. *J. Mol. Cell. Cardiol.* **18** (suppl. 5): 45–58, 1986.
50. Simpson P.C. and Karliner, J.S. Regulation of cardiac myocyte hypertrophy by a tumor-promoting phorbol ester. *Clin. Res.* **33**: 229A, 1985.
51. White, N., Tsao, T., and Simpson, P. Contractile protein content is increased in hypertrophy stimulated by norepinephrine but not by a phorbol ester: An example of pathological hypertrophy in cultured neonatal rat heart muscle cells. *J. Am. Cell. Cardiol.* **7**: 122A, 1986.
52. Simpson, P. Calcium entry blockers inhibit catecholamine-induced beating but not catecholamine-stimulated hypertrophy of cultured rat heart cells. *Clin. Res.* **33**: 90A, 1984.
53. Bevan, J.A. Norepinephrine and the presynaptic control of adrenergic transmitter release. *Fed. Proc.* **39**: 187–190, 1978.
54. Benfey, B.G. Function of myocardial α_1-adrenoceptors. *Life Sci.* **31**: 101–112, 1982.

55. Bruckner, R., Mugge, A., and Scholz, H. Existence and functional role of alpha$_1$-adrenoceptors in the mammalian heart. *J. Mol. Cell. Cardiol.* **17**: 639–645, 1985.
56. Bishopric, N.H., Simpson, P.C., and Ordahl, C.P. Induction of the skeletal α-actin gene in α_1 adrenoceptor-mediated hypertrophy of rat cardiac myocytes. *J. Clin. Invest.* **80**: 1194–1199, 1987.
57. Baserga, R. Growth in size and cell DNA replication. *Exp. Cell Res.* **151**: 1–5, 1984.
58. Tohse, N., Hattori, Y., Nakaya, H., and Kanno, M. Effects of α-adrenoceptor stimulation on electrophysiological properties and mechanics in rat papillary muscles. *Gen. Pharmacol.* **18**: 539–546, 1987.
59. Clark, M.G., Patten, G.S., and Filsell, O.H. Evidence for an α-adrenergic receptor-mediated control of energy production in heart. *J. Mol. Cell. Cardiol.* **14**: 313–321, 1982.
60. Lindemann, J.P. α-adrenergic stimulation of sarcolemmal protein phosphorylation and slow responses in intact myocardium. *J. Biol. Chem.* **261**: 4860–4867, 1986.
61. Presti, C.F., Scott, B.T., and Jones, L.R. Identification of an endogenous protein kinase C activity and its intrinsic 15-kilodalton substrate in purified canine cardiac sarcolemmal vesicles. *J. Biol. Chem.* **260**: 13879–13889, 1985.
62. Heathers, G.P., Yamada, K.A., Kanter, E.M., and Corr, P.B. Long-chain acylcarnitines mediate the hypoxia-induced increase in α_1-adrenergic receptors on adult canine myocytes. *Circ. Res.* **61**: 735–746, 1987.
63. Blaes, N. Boissel, J.-P. Growth-stimulating effect of catecholamines on rat aortic smooth muscle cells in culture. *J. Cell Physiol.* **116**: 167–172, 1983.
64. Sherline, P. and Mascardo, R. Catecholamines are mitogenic in 3T3 and bovine aortic endothelial cells. *J. Clin. Invest.* **74**: 483–487, 1984.
65. Cruise, J.L., Houck, K.A., and Michalopoulous, G.K. Induction of DNA synthesis in cultured rat hepatocytes through stimulation of α_1 adrenoceptors by norepinephrine. *Science* **227**: 749–751, 1985.
66. Burch, R.M., Luini, A., Mais, D.E., Corda, D., Vanderhoek, J.Y., Kohn, L.D., and Axelrod, J. α_1-adrenergic stimulation of arachidonic acid release and metabolism in a rat thyroid cell line: mediation of cell replication by prostaglandin E_2. *J. Biol. Chem* **261**: 11236–11241, 1986.
67. Starksen, N.F., Simpson, P.C., Bishopric, N., Coughlin, S.R., Lee, W.M.F., Escobedo, J.A., and Williams, L.T. Cardiac myocyte hypertrophy is associated with c-*myc* proto-oncogene expression. *Proc. Natl. Acad. Sci. USA* **83**: 8348–8350, 1986.
68. Simpson, P.C. Proto-oncogenes and cardiac hypertrophy. *Ann Rev. Physiol.*, **51**, 1989 (in press).
69. Schwartz, K., de la Bastie, D., Bouveret, P., Oliveriro, P., Alonso, S., and Buckingham, M. α-skeletal muscle actin mRNAs accumulate in hypertrophied adult rat hearts. *Circ. Res.* **59**: 551–555, 1986.
70. Silbertstein, L., Webster, S.G., Travis, M., and Blau, H.M. Developmental progression of myosin gene expression in cultured muscle cells. *Cell* **46**: 1075–1081, 1986.
71. White, N., Tsao, T., and Simpson, P. Differential regulation of myosin isoenzymes in alpha-1 and thyroid hormone stimulated hypertrophy in cultured neonatal rat heart muscle cells. *Clin. Res.* **34**: 16A, 1986.
72. Charlemagne, D., Maixen, J.-M., Preteseille, M., and Lelievre, L.G. Ouabain binding sites and (Na^+, K^+)-ATPase activity in rat cardiac hypertrophy: Expression of the neonatal forms. *J. Biol. Chem.* **261**: 185–189, 1986.
73. Izumo, S., Lompre, A.-M., Matsuoka, R., Koren, G., Schwartz, K., Nadal-Ginard, B., and Mahdavi, M. Myosin heavy chain messenger RNA and protein isoform transitions during cardiac hypertrophy: Interaction between hemodynamic and thyroid hormone-induced signals. *J. Clin. Invest.* **79**: 970–977, 1987.
74. Izumo, S., Isoyama, S., Nadal-Ginard, B., and Mahdavi, V. Acute pressure overload causes rapid induction of the proto-oncogenes and a stress protein gene in the myocardium. *Circulation* **76** (suppl. IV): IV–477, 1987.

75. Komuro, I., Kurabayashi, M., and Takaku, F. Expression of cellular oncogenes during development and pressure-overload hypertrophy of the rat hearts. *Circulation* **76** (suppl. IV): IV–476, 1987.

76. Mulvagh, S.L., Michael, L.H., Perryman, M.B., Roberts, R., and Schneider, M.D. A hemodynamic load in vivo induces cardiac expression of the cellular oncogene, c-*myc*. *Biochem. Biophys. Res. Commun.* **147**: 627–636, 1987.

77. Tsuchimochi, H., Yazaki, Y., Kawana, M., Kimata, S., and Takaku, F. The existence of a fetal type myosin heavy chain (MHC) in the human heart and its abnormal expression in the ventricles of dilated cardiomyopathy. *Circulation* **76** (suppl. IV): IV–262, 1987.

78. Tsuchimochi, H., Kuro-o.M., Takaku, F., Yoshida, K., Kawana, M., Kimata, S.-I., and Yazaki, Y. Expression of myosin isozymes during the developmental stage and their redistribution induced by pressure overload. *Jpn. Circ. J.* **50**: 1044–1052, 1986.

79. McKnight, G.S. and Palmiter, R.D. Transcriptional regulation of the ovalbumin and conalbumin genes by steroid hormones in chick oviduct. *J. Biol. Chem.* **254**: 9050–9058, 1979.

79a. Long, C.S., Ordahl, C.P., and Simpson, P.C. Alpha-1 adrenergic receptor stimulation of gene transcription in neonatal rat myocardial cells in culture. *Circulation* **78**: II–562, 1988.

80. Lee, H.R., Henderson, S.A., Meidell, R.S., Yuan, D., and Chien, K.R. Alpha adrenergic regulation of cardiac gene transcription during hypertrophy in cultured myocardial cells. *Circulation* **74**: II–156, 1986.

81. Exton, J.H. Mechanisms involved in alpha-adrenergic phenomena. *Am. J. Physiol.* **248**: E633–E647, 1985.

82. Karliner, J.S., Simpson, P.C., Braun, L., Honbo, N., and Woloszyn, W. Alpha$_1$-adrenoceptor regulation of phosphoinositide turnover in hypertrophied myocardial cells. *Circulation* **72**: III–182, 1985.

83. Lo, W.W.Y. and Hughes, J. Receptor-phosphoinositidase C coupling: Multiple G-proteins? *FEBBS Lett.* **224**: 1–3, 1987.

84. Henrich, C.J. and Simpson, P.C. Differential acute and chronic response of protein kinase C in cultured neonatal rat heart myocytes to α_1-adrenergic and phorbol ester stimulation. *J. Mol. Cell Cardiol.* **20**: (in press), 1988.

85. Besterman, J.M., Duronio, V., and Cuatrecasas, P. Rapid formation of diacylglycerol from phosphatidylcholine: a pathway for generation of a second messenger. *Proc. Natl. Acad. Sci. USA* **83**: 6785–6789, 1986.

86. Simpson, P. Norepinephrine-stimulated hypertrophy of cultured rat heart cells requires continuous alpha$_1$-adrenergic receptor occupancy. *Circulation* **70**: II–198, 1984.

87. Angel, P., Imagawa, M., Chin, R., Stein, B., Imbra, R.J., Rahmsdorf, H.J., Jonat, C., Herrlich, P., and Karin, M. Phorbol ester-inducible genes contain a common *cis* element recognized by a TPA-modulated *trans*-acting factor. *Cell* **49**: 729–739, 1987.

88. Chiu, R., Imagawa, M., Imbra, R.J., Bockoven, J.R., and Karin, M. Multiple *cis*- and *trans*-acting elements mediate the transcriptional response to phorbol esters. *Nature* **329**: 648–651, 1987.

89. Lee, W., Mitchell, P., and Tjian, R. Purified transcription factor AP-1 interacts with TPA-inducible enhancer elements. *Cell* **49**: 741–752, 1987.

90. Coussens, L., Parker, P.J., Rhee, L., Yang-Feng, T.L., Chen, E., Waterfield, M.D., Francke, U., and Ullrich, A. Multiple, distinct forms of bovine and human protein kinase C suggest diversity in cellular signalling pathways. *Science* **233**: 859–866, 1986.

91. Knopf, J.L., Lee, M.-H., Sultzman, L.A., Kriz, R.W., Loomis, C.R., Hewick, R.M., and Bell, R.M. Cloning and expression of multiple protein kinase C cDNAs. *Cell* **46**: 491–502, 1986.

92. Parker, P.J., Coussens, L., Totty, N., Rhee, L., Young, S., Chen, E., Stabel, S., Waterfield, M.D., and Ullrich, A. The complete primary structure of protein kinase C—the major phorbol ester receptor. *Science* **233**: 853–859, 1986.

93. Maniatis, T., Goodbourn, S., and Fischer, J.A. Regulation of inducible and tissue-specific gene expression. *Science* **236**: 1237–1245, 1987.
94. Ordahl, C.P., Mar, J., Clyne, J., and Simpson, P. Gene transfer into myogenic cells in primary culture. In: Molecular Biology of Muscle Development. UCLA Symposium on Molecular and Cellular Biology, New Series, vol. 29. Emerson, C., Fischman, D.A., Nadal-Ginard, B., and Siddiqui, M.A.Q. (eds.), Alan R. Liss, Inc., 1985, pp. 547–558.
95. Whitman, M.R., Epstein, J., and Cantley, L. Inositol 1,4,5-trisphosphate stimulates phosphorylation of a 62,000-dalton protein in monkey fibroblast and bovine brain cell lysates. *J. Biol. Chem.* **259**: 13652–13655, 1984.
96. Chin, K.-V., Cade, C., Brostrom, C.O., Galuska, E.M., and Brostrom, M.A. Calcium-dependent regulation of protein synthesis at translational initiation in eukaryotic cells. *J. Biol. Chem.* **262**: 16509–16514, 1987.
97. Nosek, T.M., Williams, M.F., Zeigler, S.T., and Godt, R.E. Inositol trisphosphate enhances calcium release in skinned cardiac and skeletal muscle. *Am. J. Physiol.* **250**: C807–C811, 1986.
98. Woodcock, E.A., White, L.B.S., Smith, A.I., and McLeod, J.K. Stimulation of phosphatidylinositol metabolism in the isolated, perfused rat heart. *Circ. Res.* **61**: 625–631, 1987.
99. Brostrom, M.A., Chin, K.-V., Cade, C., Gmitter, D., and Brostrom, C.O. Stimulation of protein synthesis in pituitary cells by phorbol esters and cyclic AMP: Evidence for rapid induction of a component of translational initiation. *J. Biol. Chem.* **262**: 16515–16523, 1987.
100. Florini, J.R. Hormonal control of muscle growth. *Muscle Nerve* **10**: 577–598, 1987.
101. Lichtstein, D. and Rodband, D. A second look at the second messenger hypothesis. *Life Sci.* **40**: 2041–2051, 1987.
102. Hynes, R.O. Integrins: A family of cell surface receptors. *Cell* **48**: 549–554, 1987.
103. Borg, T.K., Rubin, K., Lundgren, E., Borg, K., and Obrink, B. Recognition of extracellular matrix components by neonatal and adult cardiac myocytes. *Develop. Biol.* **104**: 86–96, 1984.
104. Foster, R.F., Thompson, J.M., and Kaufman, S.J. A laminin substrate promotes myogenesis in rat skeletal muscle cultures: Analysis of replication and development using antidesmin and anti-BrdUrd monoclonal antibodies. *Develop. Biol.* **122**: 11–20, 1987.
105. Ignotz, R.A. and Massague, J. Cell adhesion protein receptors as targets for transforming growth factor -β action. *Cell* **51**: 189–197, 1987.
106. Mann, D.L., Vinciguerra, S., Kent, R.L., Rozich, J., and Cooper, G. Load regulation vs adrenoceptor activation of cardiocytes in culture: the primacy of load. *Circulation* **76** (suppl. IV): IV–477, 1987.
107. Sachs, F. Biophysics of mechanoreception. *Membr. Biochem.* **6**: 173–195, 1986.
108. Vandenburg, H.H. and Kaufman, S. Stretch-induced growth of skeletal myotubes correlates with activation of the sodium pump. *J. Cell Physiol.* **109**: 205–214, 1981.
109. Vandenburgh, H.H. Cell shape and growth regulation in skeletal muscle: Exogenous versus endogenous factors. *J. Cell Physiol.* **116**: 363–371, 1983.
110. Katagiri, T., Kitsu, T., Akiyama, K., Takeyama, Y., and Niitani, H. Alterations in fine structures of myofibrils and structural proteins in patients with dilated cardiomyopathy—studies with biopsied heart tissue. *Jpn. Circ. J.* **51**: 682–688, 1987.
111. Kozlovskis, P.L., Fieber, L.A., Pruitt, D.K., Smets, M.J., Bassett, A.L., Kimura, S., and Myerburg, R.J. Myocardial changes during the progression of left ventricular pressure-overload by renal hypertension or aortic constriction: myosin, myosin ATPase, and collagen. *J. Mol. Cell. Cardiol.* **19**: 105–114, 1987.
112. Maron, B.J., Ferrans, V.J., and Roberts, W.C. Myocardial ultrastructure in patients with chronic aortic valve disease. *Am. J. Cardiol.* **35**: 725–729, 1975.
113. Schwarz, F., Schaper, J., Kittstein, D., Flameng, W., Walter, P., and Schaper, W. Reduced

volume fraction of myofibrils in myocardium of patients with decompensated pressure overload. *Circulation* **63**: 1299–1304, 1981.

113a. Waspe, L.E., Ordahl, C.P., Simpson, P.C. Altered myosin gene expression in phorbol ester-induced hypertrophy of cultured heart cells. *Circulation* **78**: II–562, 1988.

114. Lin, Z., Eshelman, J.R., Forry-Schaudies, S., Duran, S., Lessard, J.L., and Holtzer, H. Sequential disassembly of myofibrils induced by myristate acetate in cultured myotubes. *J. Cell Biol.* **105**: 1365–1376, 1987.

115. Bishopric, N., Tsao, T., Ordahl, C., and Simpson, P. Contractile activity modulates contractile protein gene expression in norepinephrine-stimulated myocardial cell hypertrophy. *Circulation* **72**: III–26, 1985.

116. McDermott, P., Daood, M., and Klein, I. Contraction regulates myosin synthesis and myosin content of cultured heart cells. *Am. J. Physiol.* **249**: H763–H769, 1985.

117. McDermott, P.J., Xenophontos, X.P., and Morgan, H.E. Contraction stimulates myocyte growth in culture. *Circulation* **76** (suppl. IV): IV–477, 1987.

118. MeDermott, P., Whitaker-Dowling, P., and Klein, I. Regulation of cardiac myosin synthesis: studies of RNA content in cultured heart cells. *Exp. Cell Res.* **173**: 183–192, 1987.

119. Samarel, A.M., Ferguson, A.G., and Burgess, L. Quantitative analysis of myofibrillar protein subunits: Demonstration of large molar excesses of myosin light chains in rabbit ventricular myocardium. *J. Mol. Cell. Cardiol.* **19**: 699–707, 1987.

120. Kuczmarski, E.R. and Spuclich, J.A. Regulation of myosin self-assembly: phosphorylation of *Dictyostelium* heavy chain inhibits formation of thick filaments. *Proc. Natl. Acad. Sci. USA* **77**: 7292–7296, 1980.

121. Pontremoli, S., Melloni, E., Michetti, M., Sparatore, B., Salamino, F., Sacco, O., and Horecker, B.L. Phosphorylation by protein kinase C of a 20-kDa cytoskeletal polypeptide enhances its susceptibility to digestion by calpain. *Proc. Natl. Acad. Sci. USA* **84**: 398–401, 1987.

122. Inuzuka, S., Chiba, M., Nakata, M., Shida, M., Miyazaki, Y., Norhara, M., Sakai, S., Koga, Y., and Toshima, H. Variable hypertrophic effect of catecholamines on cultured rat myocardial cells. *J. Mol. Cell. Cardiol.* **18** (suppl. I): 331, 1986.

123. Clark, W.A., Waszak, G.A., and Cho, K. β-adrenergic stimulation of chick heart cell growth *in vitro* in defined serum-free medium. *J. Cell Biol.* **105**: 190a, 1987.

124. Simpson, P. Comments on "Load regulation of the properties of adult feline cardiocytes: The role of substrate adhesion" which appeared in *Circ. Res.* **58**: 692–705, 1986. *Circ. Res.* **62**: 864–866, 1988.

125. Yokota, S. and Khairallah, P.A. Transmembrane transduction via α_1-adrenoceptors In isolated cardiac myocytes. *Fed. Proc.* **46**: 1306, 1987.

126. Claycomb, W.C. "Dedifferentiation" of the cultured adult cardiac muscle cell by TPA. In: Biology of Isolated Adult Cardiac Myocytes. Clark, W.A., Decker, R.S., Borg, T.K., (eds.), Elsevier Science Publishing Co., Inc. , 1988, pp. 284–287.

127. Brown, J.H., Buxton, I.L., and Brunton, L.L. α_1-adrenergic and muscarinic cholinergic stimulation of phosphoinositide hydrolysis in adult rat cardiomyocytes. *Circ. Res.* **57**: 532–537, 1985.

128. Girard, P.R., Mazzei, G.J., and Kuo, J.F. Immunological quantitation of phospholipid/Ca^{2+}-dependent protein kinase and its fragments: tissue levels, subcellular distribution, and ontogenetic changes in brain and heart. *J. Biol. Chem.* **261**: 370–375, 1986.

129. Limas, C.J. Characterization of phorbol diester binding to isolated cardiac myocytes. *Arch. Biochem. Biophys.* **238**: 300–304, 1985.

130. Schaffer, W. and Williams, R.S. Age-dependent changes in expression of alpha$_1$-adrenergic receptors in rat myocardium. *Biochem. Biophys. Res. Commun.* **138**: 387–391, 1986.

131. Langer, G.A. Interspecies variation in myocardial physiology: the anomalous rat. *Environ. Health Perspec.* **26**: 175–179, 1978.

132. King, B.D., Sack, D., Kichuk, M.R., and Hintze, T.H. Absence of hypertension despite

chronic marked elevations in plasma norepinephrine in conscious dogs. *Hypertension* **9**: 582–590, 1987.

133. Laks, M.M. and Morady, F. Norepinephrine—the myocardial hypertrophy hormone? *Am. Heart J.* **91**: 674–675, 1976.
134. Corea, L., Bentivoglio, M., Verdecchia, P., and Motolese, M. Plasma norepinephrine and left ventricular hypertrophy in systemic hypertension. *Am. J. Cardiol.* **53**: 1299–1303, 1984.
135. Genovese, A., Chiariello, M., Bozzaotre, M., Latte, S., DeAlfieri, W., and Condorelli, M. Adrenergic activity as a modulating factor in the genesis of myocardial hypertrophy in the rat. *Exp. Mol. Pathol.* **41**: 390–396, 1984.
136. Muiesan, G., Agabiti-Rosei, E., and Muiesan, M.L. Adrenergic activity and myocardial anatomy and function in essential hypertension. *J. Hypertension* **3** (suppl. 4): S45–S50, 1985.
137. Rossi, M.A. and Carillo, S.V. Does norepinephrine play a central causative role in the process of cardiac hypertrophy? *Am. Heart J.* **109**: 622–624, 1985.
138. Tarazi, R.C., Sen, S., Saragoca, M., and Khairallah, P. The multifactorial role of catecholamines in hypertensive cardiac hypertrophy. *Eur. Heart J.* **3** (suppl. A): 103–110, 1982.
139. Trimarco, B., Ricciardelli, B., De Luca, N., De Simone, A., Cuocolo, A., Galva, M. D., Picotti, G.B., and Condorelli, M. Participation of endogenous catecholamines in the regulation of left ventricular mass in progeny of hypertensive parents. *Circulation* **72**: 38–46, 1985.
140. Tamai, J., Hori, M., Iwakura, K., Kagiya, T., Iwai, K., and Kitabatake, A. Role of α_1-adrenoceptor activity in progression of cardiac hypertrophy in guinea pigs with aortic banding. *Circulation* **76** (suppl. IV): IV–195, 1987.
141. Nakata, M., Chiba, M., Inuzuka, S., Shida, M., Miyazaki, Y., Nohara, M., Sakai, S., Koga, Y., and Toshima, H. Increased hypertrophic and chronotropic responses to norepinephrine in the cultured myocardial cells of spontaneous hypertensive rat. *J. Mol. Cell. Cardiol.* **18** (suppl. 1): 181, 1986.
142. Toshima, H., Nakata, M., Nohara, M., Chiba, M., and Koga, Y. Increased adrenergic receptor activity and hypertrophic response to norepinephrine in cultured SHR myocardial cell. *Circulation* **76** (suppl. IV): IV–534, 1987.
143. Bohm, M., Mende, U., Schmitz, W., and Scholz, H. Cardiac alpha-receptors and cardiac hypertrophy in genetic predisposition to hypertension. *Am. Heart J.* **112**: 1347–1349, 1986.
144. Mende, U. and Scholz, H. Increased sensitivity to α-adrenoceptor stimulation in hearts from spontaneously hypertensive rats. *Naunyn-Schmiedeberg's Arch. Pharmacol.* **332** (suppl.): R46, 1986.
145. Feldstein, J.B., Pacitti, A.J., Sumners, C., and Raizada, M.K. α_1-adrenergic receptors in neuronal cultures from rat brain: increased expression in the spontaneously hypertensive rat. *J. Neurochem.* **47**: 1190–1198, 1986.
146. Kato, H. and Takenawa, T. Phospholipase C activation and diacylglycerol kinase inactivation lead to an increase in diacylglycerol content in spontaneously hypertensive rat. *Biochem. Biophys. Res. Commun.* **146**: 1419–1424, 1987.
147. Kawaguchi, H., Okamoto, H., Saito, H., and Yasuda, H. Renal phospholipase C and diglyceride lipase activity in spontaneously hypertensive rats. *Hypertension* **10**: 100–106, 1987.
148. Koutouzov, S., Remmal, A., Marche, P., and Meyer, P. Hypersensitivity of phospholipase C in platelets of spontaneously hypertensive rats. *Hypertension* **10**: 497–504, 1987.
149. MacKay, M.J. and Cheung, D.W. Increased reactivity in the mesenteric artery of spontaneously hypertensive rats to phorbol ester. *Biochem. Biophys. Res. Commun.* **145**: 1105–1111, 1987.
150. Takaori, K., Itoh, S., Kanayama, Y., and Takeda, T. Protein kinase C activity in platelets

from spontaneously hypertensive rats (SHR) and normotensive Wistar Kyoto rats (WKY). *Biochem. Biophys. Res. Commun.* **141**: 769–773, 1986.

151. Turla, M.B. and Webb, R.C. Enhanced vascular reactivity to protein kinase C activators in genetically hypertensive rats. *Hypertension* **9** (suppl. III): 150–154, 1987.

152. Bohm, M., Beuckelmann, D., Diet, F., Feiler, G., Kemkes, B., and Erdmann, E. α-adrenoceptors in the failing heart. *Circulation* **76** (Suppl IV): IV–63, 1987.

153. Perloff, J.K. Pathogenesis of hypertrophic cardiomyopathy: Hypotheses and speculations. *Am. Heart J.* **101**: 219–226, 1981.

154. Maron, B.J., Spirito, P., Wesley, Y., and Arce, J. Development and progression of left ventricular hypertrophy in children with hypertrophic cardiomyopathy. *N. Engl. J. Med.* **315**: 610–614, 1986.

155. Spirito, P. and Maron, B.J. Absence of progression of left ventricular hypertrophy in adult patients with hypertrophic cardiomyopathy. *J. Am. Coll. Cardiol.* **9**: 1013–1017, 1987.

156. Gustafson, T.A., Bahl, J.J., Markham, B.E., Roeske, W.R., and Morkin, E. Hormonal regulation of myosin heavy chain and α-actin gene expression in cultured fetal rat heart myocytes. *J. Biol. Chem.* **262**: 13316–13322, 1987.

157. Umeda, P.K., Darling, D.S., Kennedy, J.M., Jakovcic, S., and Zak, R. Control of myosin heavy chain expression in cardiac hypertrophy. *Am. J. Cardiol.* **59**: 49A–55A, 1987.

158. Darling, D.S., Kennedy, J.M., DeGroot, L.J., Jakovic, S., Zak, R., and Umeda, P.K. Transcriptional regulation of cardiac myosin heavy chain expression by thyroid hormone. *Circulation* **72** (suppl. III): III–25, 1985.

Molecular and Biological Aspects of Cardiac Hypertrophy

Y. Yazaki, H. Tsuchimochi, I. Komuro, U. Kurabayashi, and F. Takaku

The Third Department of Internal Medicine, University of Tokyo School of Medicine, Tokyo, Japan

It is well known that many muscle proteins consist of mutiple molecular forms and are members of multigene families. Polymorphism has been detected even in typical muscle proteins like myosin, actin, tropomyosin, troponin, and certain sarcoplasmic and sarcolemmal proteins. In addition, the biological activity between members of each gene family differs. As a consequence, muscle phenotype is not fixed but continually adapts to the functional and metabolic demands placed on the organ.

During enlargement of the heart due to overload, a significant reconstitution of the organ, including myocytes and intracellular constituents, occurs, as does cellular hypertrophy induced by the increased synthesis of cellular components attempting to meet the increased demand in work. This adaptational phenomenon can be defined at the molecular level in terms of altered transcription of specific genes. Since no activation of mitotic activity of the myocytes is evident, DNA replication is observed mainly in connective tissue cells.

To analyze the process of cardiac hypertrophy due to overload at the molecular level, one must be able to identify individual types of muscle proteins and their specific genes. Since analysis of cardiac myosin isoforms—of which enzymatic activities regulate both contractility and energy efficiency for contraction of the muscle—can provide insight into the process of cardiac hypertrophy, we developed monoclonal antibodies specific for two types of cardiac myosin and characterized these isoforms by immunofluorescence study using these monoclonal antibodies. Furthermore, we cloned specific genes encoding the heavy and light chains of these cardiac myosin isoforms from the human cDNA library and demonstrated the regulation of their expression in the overloaded human heart. We also examined experimentally the transcriptional regulation of specific genes whose early expression was observed in the heart after acute overloading, such as the cellular oncogenes. In this chapter, we review our current study on these subjects. We mainly investigated human materials to obtain clinical implications from our observations.

REDISTRIBUTION OF CARDIAC MYOSIN ISOZYMES IN THE HUMAN HEART DUE TO OVERLOAD

Myosin is a major contractile protein in muscle cells that utilizes enzymatic activity (ATPase) to liberate energy from ATP to cause muscle contraction. Electrophoretic and immunochemical studies indicate that multiple myosin isoforms exist among various muscle tissues and that heterogenous fiber distribution (with respect to myosin composition) varies according to the developmental stage or the physiological or pathological stage of the muscle. Each myosin isoform contains a specific combination of heavy and light chains.

The molecular diversity of cardiac myosins has been revealed by several different experimental approaches. Enzymatic,[1-4] electrophoretic,[5-7] and immunochemical[8-10] analyses have shown the existence of two distinct cardiac myosin heavy chains, HCα and HCβ. It has also been demonstrated by electrophoresis under nondenaturing conditions that cardiac myosin is composed of three different isozymes, referred to as V1, V2, and V3.[5,10,11] V1 and V3 correspond to homodimers of HCα and HCβ, respectively, while V2 is a heterodimer of HCα and HCβ. V1 has higher ATPase activity than V3 and has increased efficiency of force production compared with V1.[12-15] Isozymes of cardiac myosin show characteristic patterns in their distribution according to species,[1,2,16] fiber type,[3,8,10] developmental[8,10,11,16,17] and hormonal state,[2,5,6,10,17,18] and pressure overload.[19-23] Especially, isozymic changes induced by pressure overload are thought to play some role in the pathophysiology of cardiac hypertrophy. However, it has not been conclusively determined that isoforms are present in human cardiac myosin, since nondenaturing pyrophosphate gel electrophoretic analysis failed to separate individual isozymes of human cardiac myosin. On electrophoretic gels, human cardiac myosin is composed of a single band, which appears to be very close to the rat V3 isomyosin.

In order to discriminate human cardiac HCα and HCβ, we have prepared monoclonal antibodies specific for the heavy chains of HCα and HCβ, and revealed immunohistochemically the coexistence of these two types of heavy chains in human atrial and ventricular myocardium.[24-26] We also examined their redistribution in human myocardium hypertrophied because of overload.[24,25] Antimyosin monoclonal antibodies were produced by hybridomas obtained by fusion of myeloma cells (P3X63Ag8U1) with isolated spleen cells of BALB/c mice immunized with bovine atrial and human ventricular myosin as HCα or HCβ antigen, respectively, essentially by the method of Kohlen and Milstein.[27] Two clones (CMA19 and HMC14) of hybrid cells secreting antimyosin antibodies were selected for discriminating the antigenic difference between HCα and HCβ by ELISA tests (Fig. 1). The distribution of myosin isozymes in human atrial and ventricular myocardium was investigated by immunofluorescence assay using these monoclonal antibodies. Human myocardial specimens were obtained from patients with or without valvular disease during open heart surgery or at autopsy. Cryostat tissue sections were stained by the indirect immunofluorescence procedure.

Distribution of Cardiac Myosin Isozymes in Human Atrial and Ventricular Myocardium

By immunofluorescence assay using two types of monoclonal antibodies, CMA19 and HMC14, we showed a heterogenous composition of myocytes with different reactivities with the antibodies in the human myocardium.[24,25] In atrial myocardium, more than 95% of myocytes were strongly stained by CMA19 (Fig. 2). However, wide variation was observed in staining intensity by HMC14 among individual atrial myocytes, ranging from a completely negative to a strongly positive reaction, and myocytes giving a positive reaction comprised from 20% to 40% of total myocytes. They were occasionally grouped, but mainly interspersed, and could not be distinguished from unreactive myocytes by size or other morphological criteria. This observation revealed a distribution of a particular form of myosin heavy chain antigenetically related to ventricular myosin heavy chain in the atrial myocardium, although HCα was a predominant myosin heavy chain isoform.

In the ventricular myocardium, all myocytes were brightly stained by HMC14, and

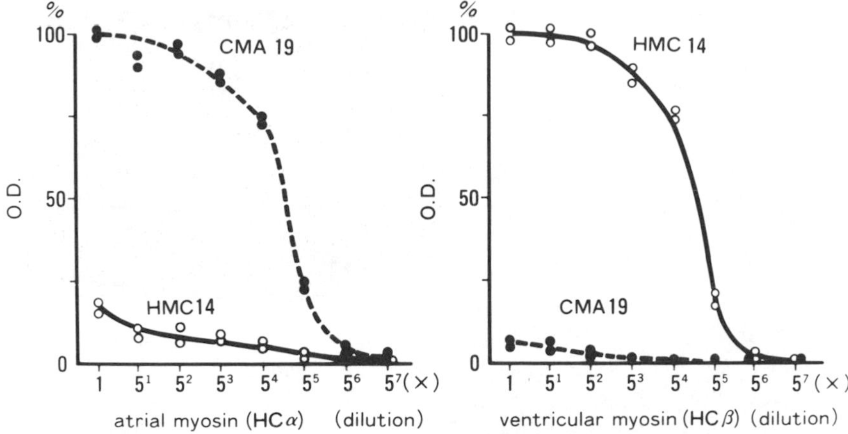

Fig. 1. Reactions of monoclonal antibodies with human atrial (A) and ventricular (B) myosin. Results are expressed as the percentage of maximum optical density at 550 nm. CMA19 (*) and HMC14 (○) reacted specifically with atrial and ventricular myosin, respectively. They showed no reaction with light chains. The negligible reaction between CMA19 and ventricular myosin, and the reduced amount of cross-reactivity between HMC14 and atrial myosin are explained by the presence of a very small quantity of atrial-type myosin in the ventricle, and a significant amount of ventricular-type myosin in the atrium, respectively.[25)]

most of them were completely unreactive to CMA19. Only a few interspersed myocytes gave a positive reaction to CMA19 (Fig. 2), but they showed a characteristic distribution. Hardly any of the ventricular myocytes just under the endocardium were labeled by CMA19. The number of labeled myocytes increased gradually from the subendocardial to the subepicardial region, where up to 15% of the myocytes were stained by CMA19. Interestingly, a considerable number of papillary myocytes were also labeled, even though they are located just next to the subendocardial ventricular myocardium. Figure 3 presents a typical case showing the distribution of labeled myocytes with CMA-19. These observations suggest that the ventricular myocardium comprised almost exclusively V3 isomyosin and that the gene operating the synthesis of HCα was expressed in only a few ventricular myocytes, especially in the epicardial region. Our comparative study of the primary structure of HCα and HCβ fractionated from the canine heart using the monoclonal antibodies revealed that atrial HCα and ventricular HCα were indistinguishable proteins and that atrial HCβ was essentially the same as ventricular HCβ.[28)]

In conclusion, our study demonstrated (a) the existence of two types of myosin isozymes in the human myocardium, (b) a striking difference in their distribution between atrial and ventricular myocardium, and (c) significant regional variation in the number of ventricular myocytes containing HCα. HCβ is the predominant myosin heavy chain isoform in the ventricle, whereas the main isoform in the atrium is HCα. Considering that ventricular pressure is much higher than atrial pressure and that HCβ appears to be suited for pressure work, the difference in the distribution of myosin isozymes between atrial and ventricular myocardium is regarded as a physiological adaptation to their loaded hemodynamic work. Furthermore, the significant difference in the distribution of ventricular myocytes containing HCα between the subendocardial and subepi-

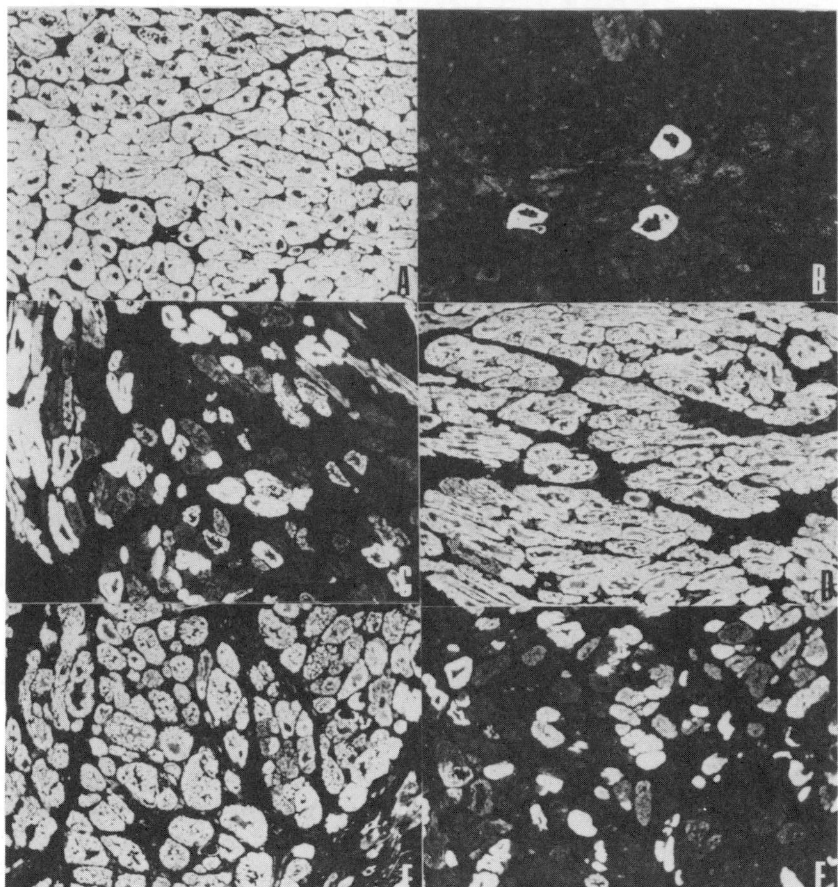

Fig. 2. Immunofluorescence staining patterns of human cardiac tissues. (A) Cryostat section of normal human ventricle stained by HMC14. All fibers reacted strongly and uniformly. (B) As in (A), except that the muscle fibers were stained by CMA19. A small number of fibers was reactive. (C) Cryostat section of normal human atrium stained by HMC14. The staining intensity was highly variable. (D) As in (C), except that the myofibers were stained by CMA19. Almost all fibers were strongly reactive. Note the myofiber that shows a weak reaction (arrow). (E) Cryostat section of a pressure-overloaded atrium stained by HMC14. The specimen was obtained from a patient with mitral stenosis and regurgitation. Almost all fibers became reactive. (F) As in (E), except that the myofibers were stained by CMA19. Unreactive fibers increased significantly.[25)]

cardial regions is considered to correspond to the difference in contractile conditions between them: myocytes in the subendocardial region are required to perform greater pressure work than those in the subepicardial region.[29)] Since V3 myosin shows greater economy of force production than V1 myosin,[12-15)] the regional variation in HCα content is also regarded as a physiological adaptation to the wall stress.

Isozymic Transition of Cardiac Myosin in Overloaded Human Heart

Evidence has been accumulated that the relative proportion of the two basic isoforms

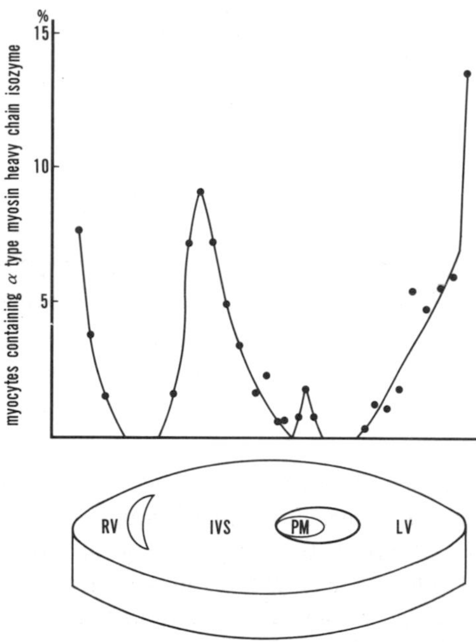

Fig. 3. Scheme of the distribution of ventricular myofibers reactive with CMA19. The number of labeled myofibers is greater in the subepicardial region and the central portion of the interventricular septum than in the subendocardial region. Note that papillary myofibers also show regional variation in the number of labeled fibers. RV, right ventricle; IVS, interventricular septum; LV, left ventricle; PM, papillary muscle.[26]

of myosin change in rat and rabbit ventricles during development[8,10,11,16,17] and during cardiac overload.[19-23] To confirm whether or not redistribution of these isozymes occurs in the human myocardium subjected to overload, we performed an immunohistochemical study using the monoclonal antibodies CMA19 and HMC14 on the overloaded human myocardium.

When pressure-overloaded atria obtained from patients with mitral stenosis and/or regurgitation or tricuspid regurgitation during open heart surgery were stained by each antibody, a striking reversal of the staining pattern was observed (Fig. 2E and F). The number of myocytes reactive with HMC14 were increased significantly, while the number reactive with CMA19 showed a corresponding decrease. To demonstrate the changes in the amount of each myosin isozyme more quantitatively, we counted the number of myocytes that reacted with each antibody, and the total scores per 1,000 myocytes were calculated in each specimen and plotted against each mean atrial pressure or mean pulmonary wedge pressure (Fig. 4). This observation revealed that the degrees of HCα decrement and HCβ increment correlated well with the mean atrial pressure.[25] We also observed a decrease in the number of myocytes reactive with CMA19 in the left ventricular specimens obtained from patients with mitral and/or aortic valvular disease; this decrease corresponded to the increment of peak left ventricular pressure.[30] There was no correlation between the number of myocytes reactive with CMA19 and left ventricular volume or end-diastolic pressure. These results showed that pressure overload may play a major role in the isozymic transition of cardiac myosin.

The isozymic redistribution in pressure-overloaded myocardium may have physiolog-

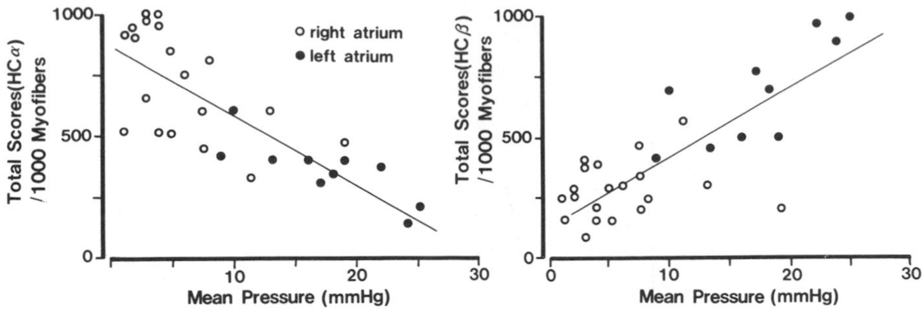

Fig. 4. The total scores per 1,000 myofibers of HCα (A) or HCβ (B) plotted against the mean atrial or pulmonary capillary wedge pressure.[26] ○, right atrium; *, left atrium.

ical implications. Since the low ATPase activity related to the low velocity of shortening improves the efficiency of contraction for an equivalent amount of work, as previously described,[12–15] HCβ appears to be a physiological myosin isozyme for performing pressure work. Overloaded atrial myocytes may promote synthesis of HCβ instead of HCα in order to improve the efficacy of contraction. Thus, the isozymic redestribution can be considered as a physiological adaptive mechanism that responds to increased pressure overload. The isozymic transition from HCα to HCβ in the overloaded atrium seen in our study may participate in a compensatory mechanism by which the mechanical function of the atrium changes from volume work to pressure work. In the ventricular myocardium, the normal myosin isozyme pattern is already an exclusively HCβ-dominant one. Therefore, the physiological importance of isozymic redistribution in the human heart induced by overload seems to be greater in the atrium than in the ventricle, since the content of HCα which could be transformed to HCβ is much larger in the atrial myocardium.

MOLECULAR CLONING AND CHARACTERIZATION OF HUMAN CARDIAC α- AND β-TYPE MYOSIN HEAVY CHAIN cDNA CLONES: REGULATION OF THEIR EXPRESSION DURING PRESSURE OVERLOAD

To understand the molecular basis of the myosin heavy chain isozyme transition in overloaded human myocardium, we investigated the level of expression of individual myosin heavy chain mRNA in pressure-overloaded human atrium. For this purpose, we isolated two cDNA clones encoding either HCα or HCβ from a fetal human heart cDNA library and analyzed different accumulations of these mRNAs in the human heart with Northern blot hybridization using these cDNA as probes.

Our successful cloning of HCα and HCβ cDNAs established the existence of two molecular variants in the human heart.[31] In Fig. 5, the nucleotide sequences of these two types of heavy chain cDNA clones are compared. These cDNAs are quite homologous, exhibiting 96% nucleotide homology within the translated region. Only 77 of the 1,596 nucleotides compared in our study were divergent. In contrast, 3′-untranslated regions show extensive sequence divergence. From available cardiac heavy chain cDNA sequence data obtained from rat,[32] rabbit,[33] and mouse,[34] it is clear that the sequence homology between widely separated species extends into the 3′-untranslated regions when comparing the same heavy chain isotypes. These data provide evidence of isotype-specific presservation of heavy chain 3′-untranslated regions during evolution.

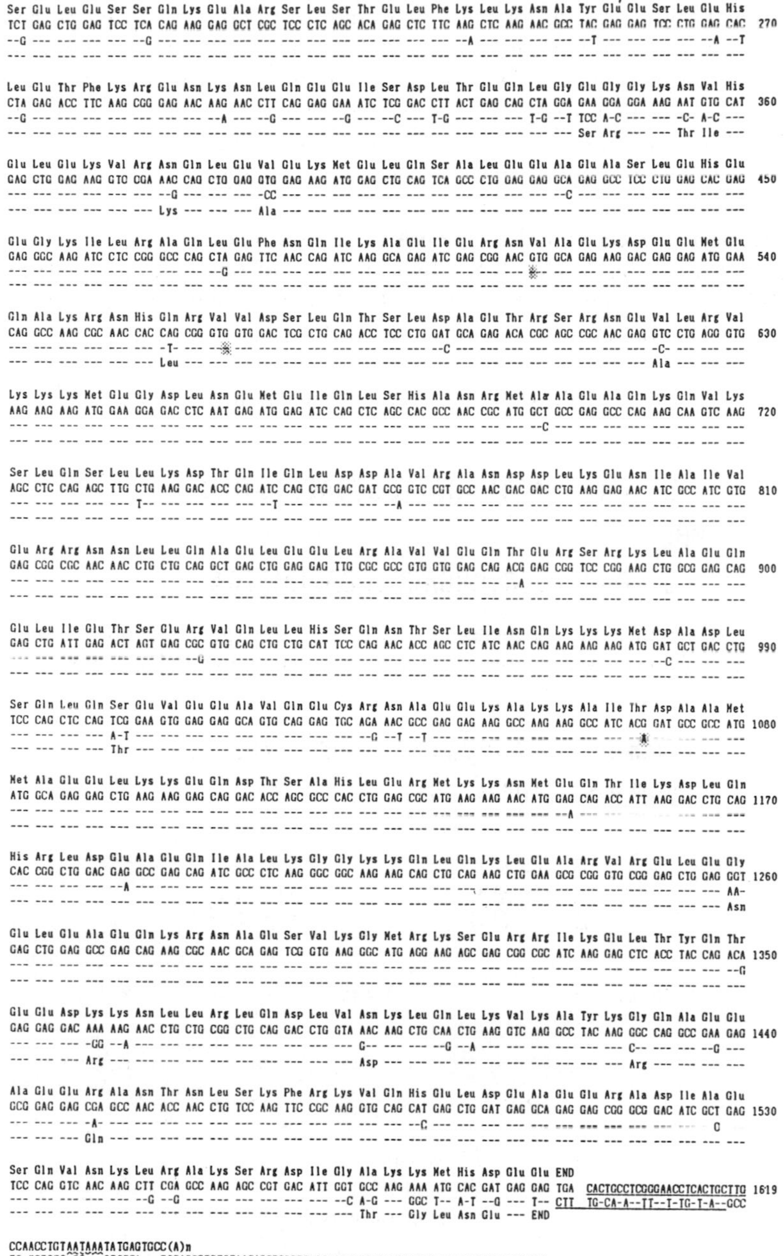

Fig. 5. Nucleotide and deduced amino acid sequences of HCα and HCβ clones.[31] Nucleotides are numbered to the right of each line. Line 1, amino acid sequence of HCα clone; Line 2, nucleotide sequence of HCα clone; Line 3, nucleotide sequence of HCβ clone; Line 4, amino acid sequence of HCβ clone. Nucleotides and amino acids are written only where different from the HCα clone. The dashed line indicates a sequence identical to that of the HCα clone. Underlined 26 bases represent the complementary sequences of the oligonucleotides synthesized for probes. Wavy lines indicate the polyadenylation signal sequence. Shaded boxes show the bases different from the nucleotide sequences reported by Jandreski *et al.*[48]

We examined the expression of these two types of myosin heavy chain genes in the human heart by Northern blot analysis using these cDNAs as probes. Since the nucleotide sequences of these two cDNAs are highly homologous, it is difficult to identify the specific heavy chain mRNA expressed in the myocardium by RNA blot analysis using the cDNA coding sequence. To overcome this difficulty, synthetic oligonucleotide probes complementary to the unique 3′-untranslated regions (Fig. 6) were used in Northern blot analysis.

The expression of HCα and HCβ mRNA in several muscle tissues at fetal and adult stages are shown in Fig. 7. The strong hybridization of fetal and adult atrial mRNAs with the HCα probe indicates that HCα mRNA predominates in the atrium both in fetal and adult life. In contrast, the strong hybridization of fetal and adult ventricular

α-, β-MHC specific oligonucleotide probe (26 mer)

α-MHC

5′ CAAGCAGTGAGGTTCCCGAGGCAGTG 3′

β-MHC

5′ GGCTTTGCTGGCACCTCCAGGGCTGA 3′

Fig. 6. Oligonucleotide sequences of HCα-and HCβ-specific probes. Twenty-six oligonucleotides were synthesized for each heavy chain-specific probe.

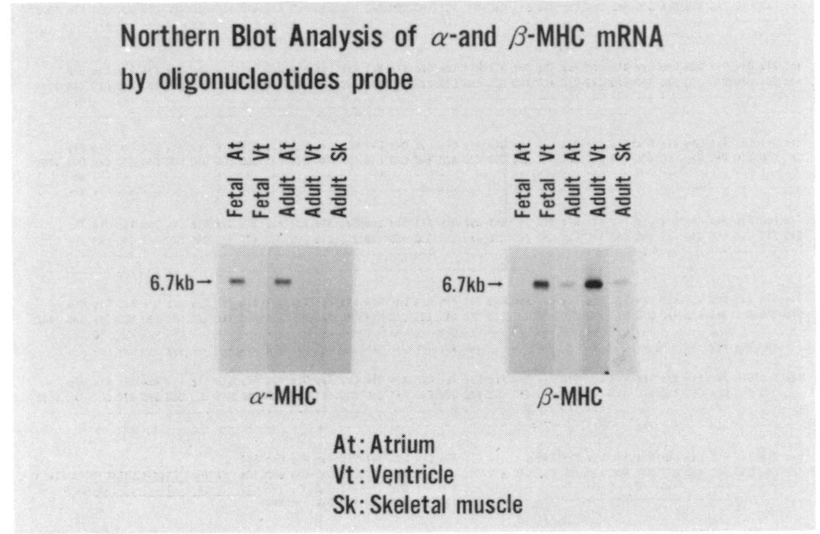

Fig. 7. Autoradiographs of Northern blot analysis showing the tissue and stage specificity of HCα-and HCβ-specific probes. Hybridization of ^{32}P-labeled HC^{2} 3′-UT (panel A) or HCβ 3′-UT oligonucleotide probes (panel B) to Hybond N membranes containing human muscle RNA was performed. Ten micrograms of total RNA was loaded in each lane. The heavy chain mRNA band is marked on the side of the figure. RNA isolated from fetal atrium (lane 1). RNA isolated from fetal ventricle (lane 2). RNA isolated from adult left atrium (lane 3). RNA isolated from adult left ventricle (lane 4). RNA isolated from adult psoas muscle (lane 5).[31]

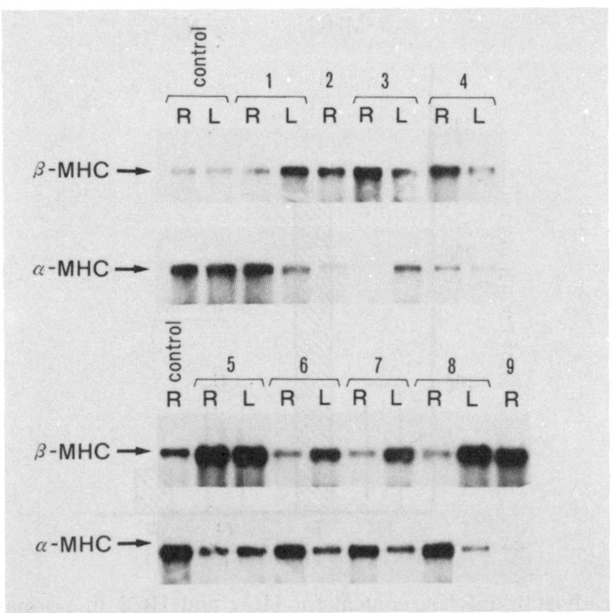

Fig. 8. Detection of HCα and HCβ mRNA in total cellular RNA from normal and diseased human atria. The same RNA blot was sequentially hybridized with labeled oligonucleotides specific for HCβ mRNA: exposure, 24 hr; HCβ mRNA: exposure, 24 hr. Normal atrial RNA controls are shown in the left lanes of the figure. The lanes containing right (R) and left (L) atrial RNA (10 μg) from patients 1–9 are indicated. The heavy chain mRNA band is marked on the side of the figure (IICα, HCβ).[31]

mRNA with the HCβ probe indicates that HCβ mRNA is predominant in the ventricle. However, some accumulation of this mRNA was also observed in adult atrium and skeletal muscle. These results demonstrate that HCβ gene is expressed to some extent in the adult atrium and that this gene is also expressed in the skeletal muscle, probably slow-twitching muscle. These data correlate very well with the observations obtained by immunohistochemical examination using monoclonal antibodies.[24–26] HCα and HCβ coexisted in 20% to 40% of adult atrial myocytes (Fig. 2).

Hybridization patterns of atrial mRNA from patients whose atria suffered from pressure overload caused by valvular disease or pulmonary hypretension are shown in Fig. 8. Nine patients were examined.[31] In the control patient who died from breast cancer, HCα mRNA was predominant in both right and left atria. However, in pressure-overloaded atria, accumulation of HCβ mRNA was observed. Pattern 1 in Fig. 8. shows the hybridization of atrial mRNA from the patient with mitral regurgitation. Strong hybridization of left atrial mRNA was observed with the HCβ probe whereas diminished hybridization was seen with the HCα probe. In this patient, the left atrium suffered from pressure overload. In patient 3, an almost completely reversed hybridization pattern was seen for right atrial mRNA. Strong hybridization was observed with the HCβ probe, whereas very little was seen with the HCα probe. This patient suffered from primary pulmonary hypertension. In this case, the right atrium was submitted to pressure overload. The degree of Northern blotting of atrial mRNA with the probes was analyzed

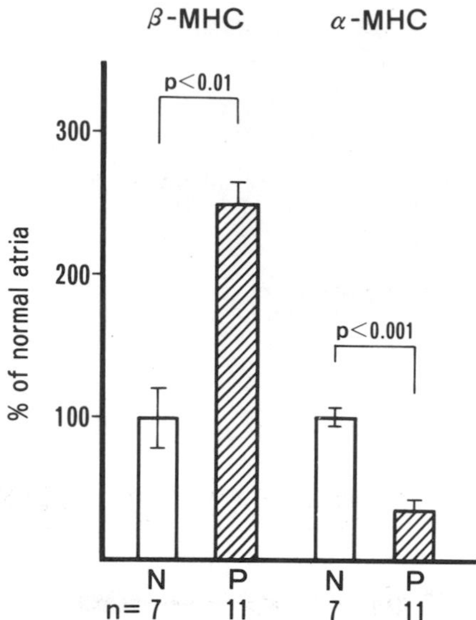

Fig. 9. Steady-state mRNA content for HCα and HCβ in normal (N) and pressure-overloaded (P) atria. Data from each group are presented as mean β SEM. RNA content in each atrium was quantitated by densitometric analysis of autoradiograms of Northern blots hybridized with the appropriate ^{32}P-labeled probes, as described in the text. Results are expressed as percentage of values in normal atria. Student's *t*-test indicated the HCβ mRNA level was significantly higher and HCα mRNA level was significantly lower in pressure-overloaded atria compared with normal atria.[31]

by densitometric scanning, and the results are summarized in Fig. 9. In overloaded atria, the level of HCβ mRNA was significantly elevated, whereas the level of HCα mRNA was markedly decreased. Studies described by Izumo *et al.*[35] demonstrated that heavy chain isozyme transition during hemodynamic overload in the rat ventricle is produced by changes in the level of HCα and HCβ gene expression. One of the important implications of our study centers on whether the HCα and HCβ genes in the human atrium respond to hemodynamic overload in the same fashion as seen in the hypertrophied rat ventricle.

Results of comparative examinations by Northern blot hybridization and immunofluorescence staining indicate that changes in HCα and HCβ mRNA levels are in large part reflected in changes in their respective proteins. Although immunofluorescence staining is not a quantitative determination, translation and post-translational mechanisms, if present, do not appear to play a major role in the production of heavy chain isozyme switches in response to hemodynamic overload.

It would be interesting to determine whether the same isoform transition occurs in cardiac myosin light chain. Using electrophoretic techniques, Cummins *et al.* found that the ventricular type of light chain replaces the atrial type in overloaded human atria.[36] We have isolated essentially full-length cDNA clones encoding atrial or ventricular alkali light chain from the fetal human heart cDNA library and examined the level of each type of myosin light chain mRNA in overloaded atria by Northern blot analysis.[37] Our preliminary data demonstrated an increased level of ventricular light chain mRNA from overloaded atria, suggesting that ventricular myosin light chain gene expression is upregulated by overload, as observed in ventricular heavy chain gene expression. Although the physiological significance of ventricular light chain induction in overloaded atria remains unclear, the concomitant replacement of ventricular heavy and light chains should work against pressure overload.

From the data presented here, the following important question remains to be answered: What is the biochemical signal that regulates HCα and HCβ gene expression in the pressure-overloaded condition? Significant evidence has been accumulated to suggest that sequences in the 5′ flanking regions are important for the regulation of transcription. Gustafson *et al.*[38] have identified the 5′ flanking sequences responsible for the induction by thyroid hormone in the rat HCα gene. Furthermore, Saez *et al.*[39] have shown that the 5′ flanking sequences of rat and human HCα gene are highly homologous. In order to define gene regulation in cardiac hypertrophy, studies of a number of muscle-specific genes whose expression is altered by pressure overload may provide necessary information to identify the sequences in the 5′ flanking regions that are important for the regulation of transcription in pressure overload.

To resolve this question, we examined experimentally the expression of cellular oncogenes that participate in cell proliferation as well as cell transformation, using rat ventricular myocardium placed in the condition of pressure overload by aortic banding.

EXPRESSION OF CELLULAR ONCOGENES DURING CARDIAC HYPERTROPHY

Cardiac myocytes divide only in the fetal period, losing their ability to replicate DNA soon after birth. Then, hearts grow by an increase in cell size (hypertrophy), not cell number (proliferation). In addition to the increase in cell size, structurally and functionally different proteins, isoforms, are expressed in the hypertrophied heart. Cellular hypertrophy and isoform switching were thought to be due to an increase in transcriptional activity. Recently, several peptides have been reported to regulate the transcriptional activity of genes. To determine the molecular mechanism of cardiac hypertrophy and isoform switching, we investigated genes whose level of expression was changed from the early period by pressure overload.

Cellular oncogenes have been presumed to play a role in growth control. Recent evidence that the products of several cellular oncogenes are either growth factors or growth factor receptors strongly suggested this hypothesis. To determine the role of cellular oncogenes in the growth of the heart, the expression pattern of eight cellular oncogenes during the developmental stage and pressure-overloaded hypertrophy of the rat heart were examined.[40] To produce pressure-overloaded cardiac hypertrophy, the upper part of the abdominal aorta of 40-day-old male Wistar rats was constricted with a hemoclip. To investigate developmental changes, hearts of embryos, neonates, and adults were examined. After the animals were killed, RNA was extracted from the ventricles and 3 μg of poly(A) RNA was separated by 1.2% agarose gels. After transfer to a nylon membrane, mRNA was hybridized with eight oncogene probes (*myc, fos, sis, Ha-ras, erbA, erbB, myb,* and *src*). Three oncogenes, c-*myc*, c-*fos*, and c-*Ha-ras*, which are known to play an important role in proliferation, were expressed in the pressure-overloaded hearts. Figure 10 shows the expressed patterns of these three genes. Increased expression of c-*fos*-related sequences was recognized from as early as 30 min after the operation. By densitometric scanning, the peak at 8 hr after the operation showed an eight- to 10-fold increase over the preoperative control level. The level of expression decreased gradually thereafter to the baseline at 48 hr. The expression pattern of c-*myc*

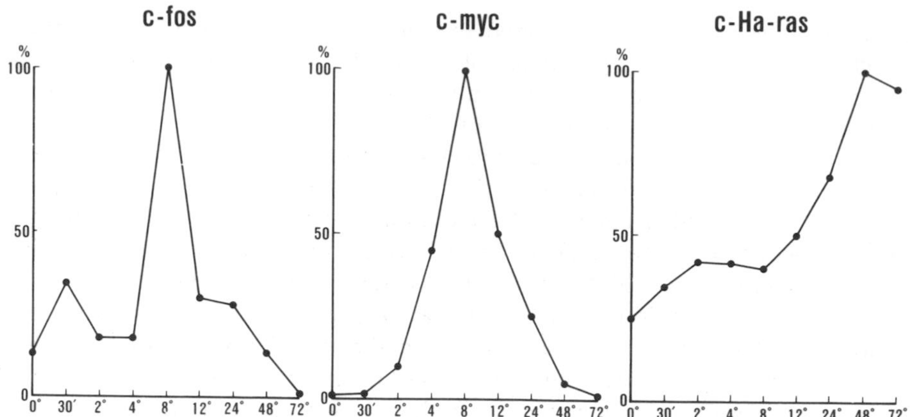

Fig. 10. Relative amounts of c-*onc* expression in pressure-overloaded cardiac hypertrophy. Relative amounts of c-*onc* expression were determined by soft-laser density scanning of the RNA blot autoradiograms. Relative OD was plotted against hour after aortic constriction and values were expressed as percent of the highest level of expression of a given c-*onc*. Average levels from three separate experiments are shown.[40]

was similar to that of c-*fos*. Its expression was detectable by 4 hr after the operation, peaked at 8 hr, and decreased to baseline at 48 hr. Some c-*Ha-ras*-related sequences were expressed in sham-operated hearts, and increased gradually after pressure overload.

C-*fos* is the cellular homologue of the oncogene of two mouse osteosarcoma viruses, FBJ-MSV and FBR-MSV.[41] All *fos* genes encode nuclear proteins and show a complex pattern of tissue-, cell-type, and stage-specific expression,[42] suggesting a correlation with the cellular differentiation process. In the hypertrophic hearts, cellular differentiation should occur actively. For instance, the β myosin heavy chain was expressed by 24 hr after aortic constriction (as previously described), and fetal isoforms were reported to be expressed in the other contractile proteins, actin and tropomyosin, in the hypertrophic hearts. It is of interest that the expression of c-*fos* showed a peak 8 hr after aortic constriction and returned to the uninduced level by 48 hr. The level of c-*fos* expression was very low in the fetal period, and gradually increased during development. Although the role of c-*fos* is unknown, its expression was stage specific, suggesting that c-*fos* might be related to the differentiation process during cardiac hypertrophy and aging.

C-*myc* also encodes nuclear protein, is expressed in relation to the cell cycle,[43] and may play a role in cellular proliferation. Recently, the expression of c-*myc* was reported to be increased in cultured cardiac myocytes in which hypertrophy had been induced by α_1-adrenergic agents.[44] In the present study, the c-*myc* gene was also expressed in pressure-overloaded hearts *in vivo*. Although the α_1-adrenergic mechanism may be activated by aortic constriction, further investigation is necessary to determine the stimuli inducing the expression of the c-*myc* gene and cardiac hypertrophy. The c-*myc* gene was expressed only in the fetal period, which is the proliferative period, suggesting that enhanced expression of the c-*myc* gene may be related to both cardiac cell division and cell hypertrophy.

Ha-ras genes encode 21 kDa proteins (p21) that appear to be involved in the control of cellular growth and differentiation,[45] and mutations affecting *ras* genes and overproduction of normal p21 can induce a transformed phenotype.[46] Recently, p21 was reported to affect the phosphatidylinositol-4,5-biphosphate breakdown pathway and the level of inositol-1,4,5-triphosphate to be elevated in the *ras*-transformed cells.[47] In cultured cardiac myocytes, α_1-adrenergic agonists have been reported to induce hypertrophy via the phosphoinositide/protein kinase C pathway.[44] In this study, mRNA endocing the *ras* gene was highly expressed in the pressure-overloaded heart. These results and observations suggest that enhanced expression of the *ras* gene might be associated with cardiac hypertrophy.

In cardiac hypertrophy, c-*fos* and c-*myc* genes were expressed from the early period, and the expression of c-*Ha-ras* was enhanced, as in cellular proliferation. In normal physiological development, c-*fos*, c-*myc*, and c-*Ha-ras* were expressed in different periods.

These results suggest that cellular oncogenes may participate in the normal developmental process and hypertrophy of hearts.

Acknowledgments

We are grateful to Drs. M. E. Buckingham and A. Weydert for their generous gift of the mouse α-MHC cDNA clone and to Drs. Y. Shibasaki and H. Hirai for their help during the course of our experiment. This investigation was supported in part by a Grant-in-Aid for Scientific Research from the Ministry of Education, Science and Culture of Japan, and grants from the Ministry of Welfare and the research workshop on cell calcium signals in the cardiovascular system.

REFERENCES

1. Yazaki, Y. and Raben, M.S. Cardiac myosin adenosinetriphosphatase of rat and mouse: Distinctive enzymatic properties compared with rabbit and dog cardiac myosin. *Circ. Res.* **35**: 15–23, 1974.
2. Yazaki, Y. and Raben, M.S. Effect of thyroid state on the enzymatic characteristic of cardiac myosin: A difference in behavior of rat and rabbit cardiac myosin. *Circ. Res.* **36**: 208–215, 1975.
3. Yazaki, Y., Ueda, S., Nagai, R., *et al.* Cardiac atrial myosin adenosine triphosphatase of animals and humans: Distinctive enzymatic properties compared with cardiac ventricular myosin. *Circ. Res.* **45**: 522–527, 1979.
4. Mercadier, J.J., Bouveret, P., Gorza, L., *et al.* Myosin isozymes in normal and hypertrophied human ventricular myocardium. *Circ. Res.* **53**: 52–62, 1983.
5. Hoh, J.F.Y., McGrath, P.A., and Hale, P.J. Electrophoretic analysis of multiple forms of rat cardiac myosin: Effect of hypophysectomy and thyroxine replacement. *J. Mol. Cell Cardiol.* **10**: 1053–1076, 1978.
6. Flink, I.L., Raber, J.H., and Morkin, E. Thyroid hormone stimulates synthesis of a cardiac myosin isozyme: Comparison of the two-dimensional electrophoretic patterns of the cyanogen bromide peptides of cardiac myosin heavy chains from euthyroid and thyrotoxic rabbits. *J. Biol. Chem.* **254**: 3105–3110, 1979.
7. Chizzonite, R.A., Everett, A.W., Clark, W.A., *et al.* Isolation and characterization of two molecular variants of myosin heavy chain from rabbit ventricle: Change in the their content during normal growth and after treatment with thyroid hormone. *J. Biol. Chem.* **257**: 2056–2065, 1982.
8. Sartore, S., Gorza, L., Pierobon-Bormioli, S., *et al.* Myosin types and fiber types in cardiac muscle. I. Ventricular myocardium. *J. Cell Biol.* **88**: 226–233, 1981.
9. Gorza, L., Sartore, S., and Schiaffino, S. Myosin types and fiber types in cardiac muscle. II. Atrial myocardium. *J. Cell Biol.* **95**: 838–845, 1982.

10. Clark, W.A. Jr., Chizzonite, R.A., Everett, A.W., *et al.* Species correlations between cardiac isomyosins: A comparison of electrophoretic and immunological properties. *J. Biol. Chem.* **257**: 5449–5454, 1982.
11. Schwartz, K., Lompre, A.M., Bouveret, P., *et al.* Comparison of rat cardiac myosin at fetal stages in young animals and in hypothyroid adults. *J. Biol. Chem.* **257**: 14412–14418, 1982.
12. Alpert, N.R. and Murieri, L.A. Increased myothermal economy of isometric force generation in compensated cardiac hypertrophy induced by pulmonary artery constriction in the rabbit. *Circ. Res.* **50**: 491–500, 1982.
13. Ebrecht, G., Rupp, H., and Jacob, R. Alteration of mechanical parameters in chemically skinned preparations of rat myocarldium as a function of isoenzyme pattern of myosin. *Basic. Res. Cardiol.* **77**: 220–234, 1982.
14. Pagani, E.D. and Julian, F.J. Rabbit papillary muscle myosin isozymes and the velocity of muscle shortening. *Circ. Res.* **54**: 586–594, 1984.
15. Holubarsch, C., Goulette, R.P., Litten, R.Z., *et al.* The economy of isometric force development, myosin isozyme pattern, and myofibrillar ATPase activity in normal and hypothyroid rat myocardium. *Circ. Res.* **56**: 78–86, 1985.
16. Lompre, A.M., Mercardiar, J.J., Winsewsky, C., *et al.* Species and age dependent changes in the relative amounts of cardiac myosin isoenzymes in mammals. *Dev. Biol.* **84**: 286–290, 1981.
17. Chizzonite, R.A., Everett, A.W., Prior, G., *et al.* Comparison of myosin heavy chains in atria and ventricles from hyperthyroid, hypothyroid, and euthyroid rabbits. *J. Biol. Chem.* **259**: 15564–15571, 1984.
18. Dillmann, W.H., Barrieux, A., and Reese, G.S. Effect of diabetes and hypothyroidism on the predominance of cardiac myosin heavy chains synthesized *in vivo* or in a cell-free system. *J. Biol. Chem.* **259**: 2035–2038, 1984.
19. Gorza, L., Pauletto, P., Pessina, A.C., *et al.* Isomyosin distribution in normal and pressure-overloaded rat ventricular myocardium; an immunohistochemical study. *Circ. Res.* **49**: 1003–1009, 1981.
20. Rupp, H. Polymorphic myosin as the common determinant of myofibrillar ATPase in different haemodynamic and thyroid states. *Basic Res. Cardiol.* **77**: 34–46, 1982.
21. Lompre, A.M., Schwartz, L.K., d'Albis, A., *et al.* Myosin isozyme redistribution in chronic heart overload. *Nature* **282**: 105–107, 1979.
22. Mercadier, J.J., Lompre, A.M., Wisnewsky, C., *et al.* Myosin isozymic changes in several models of rat cardiac hypertrophy. *Circ. Res.* **49**: 525–532, 1981.
23. Litten, R.Z., Martin, B.J., Low, R.B., *et al.* Altered myosin isozyme patterns from pressure-overloaded and thyrotoxic hypertrophied rabbit hearts. *Circ. Res.* **50**: 856–864, 1982.
24. Yazaki, Y., Tsuchimochi, H., Kuro-o, M., *et al.* Distribution of myosin isozymes in human atrial and ventricular myocardium: Comparison in normal and overload heart. *Eur. Heart J.* **5** (suppl. F): 103–110, 1984.
25. Tsuchimochi, H., Sugi, M., Kuro-o, M., *et al.* Isozymic changes in myosin of human atrial myocardium induced by overload: Immunohistochemical study using monoclonal antibodies. *J. Clin. Invest.* **74**: 662–665, 1984.
26. Kuro-o, M., Tsuchimochi, H., Ueda, S., *et al.* Distribution of cardiac myosin isozymes in human conduction system: Immunohistochemical study using monoclonal antibodies. *J. Clin. Invest.* **77**: 340–347, 1986.
27. Kohler, G. and Milstein, C. Continuous cultures of fused cells secreting antibody of predefined specificity. *Nature* **256**: 495–497, 1973.
28. Komuro, I., Tsuchimochi, H., Ueda, S., *et al.* Isolation and characterization of two isozymes of myosin heavy chain from canine atrium. *J. Biol. Chem.* **261**: 4504–4509, 1986.
29. Yin, F.C.P. Ventricular wall stress. *Circ. Res.* **49**: 829–842, 1981.
30. Kawana, M., Kimata, S., Taira, A., *et al.* Isozymic changes in myosin human ventricular myocardium induced by pressure overload. *Circulation* **74**: II-82, 1986.

31. Kurabayashi, M., Tsuchimochi, H., Komuro, I., *et al.* Molecular cloning and characterization of human cardiac α- and β-form myosin heavy chain cDNA clones: Regulation of expression during development and pressure overload in human atrium. *J. Clin. Invest.* **82**: 524–531, 1988.
32. Mahdavi, V., Periasamy, M., and Nadal-Ginard, B. Molecular characterization of two myosin heavy chain genes expressed in the adult heart. *Nature* (Lond.) **297**: 659–665, 1982.
33. Shinha, A.M., Umeda, P.K., Kavinsky, C.J., *et al.* Molecular cloning of mRNA sequences for cardiac α and β myosin heavy chains: Expression in ventricles of normal, hypothroid and thyrotoxic rabbits. *Proc. Natl. Acad. Sci. USA* **79**: 5847–5851, 1982.
34. Weydert, A., Daubas, P., Lazaridis, I., *et al.* Genes for skeletal muscle myosin heavy chains are clustered and are not located on the same mouse chromosome as a cardiac myosin heavy chain gene. *Proc. Natl. Acad. Sci. USA* **82**: 7183–7187, 1985.
35. Izumo, S., Lompre, A.M., Matsuoka, R., *et al.* Myosin heavy chain messenger RNA and protein isoform transition during cardiac hypertrophy: interaction between hemodynamic and thyroid homone-induced signals. *J. Clin. Invest.* **79**: 970–977, 1987.
36. Cummins, P. Transition in human atrial and ventricular myosin light-chain isozymes in response to cardiac-pressure-overload-induced hypertrophy. *Biochem. J.* **205**: 195–204, 1982.
37. Kurabayashi, M., Tsuchimochi, H., Komuro, I., *et al.* Molecular cloning and characterization of human atrial and ventricular myosin alkali light chain cDNA clones. *J. Biol. Chem.* **263**: 13930–13936, 1988.
38. Gustafson, T.A., Markham, B.E., Bahl, J.J., *et al.* Thyroid hormone regulates expression of a transfected α-myosin heavy-chain fusion gene in fetal heart cells. *Proc. Natl. Acad. Sci. USA* **84**: 3122–3126, 1987.
39. Seaz, L.J., Gianola, K.M., McNally, E.M., *et al.* Human cardiac myosin heavy chain genes and their linkage in the genome. *Nucleic Acids Res.* **15**: 5443–5459, 1987.
40. Komuro, I., Kurabayashi, M., Takaku, *et al.* Expression of cellular oncogenes in the myocardium during the developmental stage and pressure-overloaded hypertrophy. *Circ. Res.* **62**: 1075–1079, 1988.
41. Curran, T. and Teich, N.M. Candidate product of the FBJ murine osteosarcoma virus oncogene: characterization of a 55,000-dalton phosphoprotein. *J. Virol.* **42**: 114–122, 1982.
42. Muller, R., Muller, D., and Guilbert, L. Differential expression of c-*fos* in hematopoietic cells: correlation with differentiation of monomyelocytic cells *in vitro*. *EMBO J.* **3**: 1887–1890, 1984.
43. Campici, J., Gray, H.E., Pardee, A.B., *et al.* Cell-cycle control of c-*myc* but not c-*ras* expression is lost following chemical transformation. *Cell* **36**: 241–247, 1984.
44. Starksen, N.F., Simpson, P.C., Bishopric, N., *et al.* Cardiac myocyte hypertrophy is associated with c-*myc* protooncogene expression. *Proc. Natl. Acad. Sci. USA* **83**: 8348–8350, 1986.
45. Mulcahy, L.S., Smith, M.R., and Stacey, D.W. Requirement for *ras* proto-oncogene function during serum-stimulated growth of NIT 3T3 cells. *Nature* (Lond.) **313**: 241–243, 1985.
46. Chang, E.H., Furth, M.E., Scolnick, E.M., *et al.* Tumorigenic transformation of mammalian cells induced by a normal human gene homologous to the oncogene of Harvey murine sarcoma virus. *Nature* (Lond.) **297**: 479–483, 1982.
47. Fleischman, L.F., Chahwala, S.B., and Cantley, L. *Ras*-transformed cells: altered levels of phosphatidylinositol-4, 5-biphosphate and catabolites. *Science* **231**: 407–410, 1986.
48. Jandreski, M.A. and Liew, C.C. Construction of a human ventricular cDNA library and characterization of a beta myosin heavy chain cDNA clone. *Hum. Genet.* **76**: 47–53, 1987.

Physiologic and Pathologic Hypertrophy Produced by Chronic Norepinephrine Infusion

Michael M. Laks and William J. Raum***

* Cardiology Division, UCLA School of Medicine, Torrance, California, U.S.A.
** Cardiovascular Research Laboratory and Heart Station, UCLA School of Medicine, Harbor-UCLA Medical Center, Torrance, California, U.S.A.

ABSTRACT

Recent and past evidence from both *in vivo* and *in vitro* studies is summarized to support the concept that norepinephrine produces myocardial cellular hypertrophy. The experimental model consisting of a long-term continuous subhypertensive infusion of norepinephrine in the conscious, free-roaming dog is a method to produce and study physiologic and pathologic hypertrophy. The concept of physiologic and pathologic hypertrophy is outlined, and the tissue markers differentiating them are discussed as to their evolution from structural, functional, and biochemical data. A biochemical clue as to the mechanism of hypertrophic cardiomyopathy has emanated from these studies. After norepinephrine infusion, and before ventricular hypertrophy occurred, the ventricular septum showed a marked increase in myocardial β-receptors with no increase in adenylate cyclase and cAMP content. Consequently, the ventricular septum has a unique biochemical structure to produce myocardial cellular hypertrophy as a response to norepinephrine. The biochemical stimulus for the production of ventricular hypertrophy has been postulated to be a relative decrease in cAMP and/or a stimulation of the alpha-1 receptors. These proposed mechanisms apply specifically to the hypertrophy process in hypertrophic cardiomyopathy and possibly more generally could be applied to the hypertrophy process per se. Finally, biochemical schematic models are presented describing postulated mechanisms for the genesis of hypertrophic cardiomyopathy and congestive cardiomyopathy and the central role of norepinephrine.

INTRODUCTION

An observation published by our group in 1969 has led to a continuing series of studies into the mechanisms of norepinephrine (NE)-induced hypertrophy.[1] We observed that, after banding the canine pulmonary artery for three months or more, myocardial cell lengths increased not only in the right ventricle, as expected, but also in the left ventricle.[1] Because there was no hemodynamic reason for the left ventricle to enlarge its cell size, we hypothesized that a hormone or a substance may be elaborated from the right ventricle and act on the left ventricle to cause its hypertrophy. NE, a major biologically active substance in the ventricle, was proposed as a likely inducer of left ventricular hypertrophy. After a review of studies on myocardial structural, functional, and biochemical alterations produced by the infusions of NE, we will formulate a unifying hypothesis for the fundamental mechanisms involved in myocardial hypertrophy, utilizing both our data and the contributions of several other investigators.

BACKGROUND STUDIES AND CONCEPTS

Evidence that NE Causes Myocardial Cellular Hypertrophy

An important component of our experimental design had been to infuse NE at a rate that would not increase systemic pressure, thereby eliminating an increase in afterload as the etiology for ventricular hypertrophy. In addition, there was no increase in ventricular preload during the first two months of chronic NE infusion, as indicated by the lack of change in cardiac output and heart rate. Since NE infusion produced an increase in ventricular weight without a significant hemodynamic change, NE was considered to be a major inducer of myocardial cellular hypertrophy.[2,3] Most recently, Hintze confirmed our observation that chronic subhypertensive infusion of NE in the conscious dog produces ventricular hypertrophy.[4] Studies by his group also strengthened the concept that NE can produce ventricular hypertrophy by a direct effect on the myocardium. He demonstrated in the conscious dog that the components of wall stress did not increase after chronic NE infusion in that both left ventricular end-diastolic dimensions and end-diastolic pressure did not change. Furthermore, indices of contractility and ventricular function (dP/dT, dD/dt, LV cardiac work, LV stroke work, and double product) did not change. Thus, NE-induced hypertrophy is not secondary to an increased ventricular wall stress, contractility, or ventricular function. These observations give further support to the hypothesis that NE has a direct effect on the myocardium and should therefore be recognized as a hormone which evokes myocardial cellular hypertrophy. Utilizing a different model, Simpson[5] demonstrated that neonatal myocardial rat cells exposed to NE in tissue culture develop significant hypertrophy which is accompanied by a proportional increase in myocardial cellular protein synthesis. Therefore, our *in vivo* and Simpson's *in vitro* studies provide significant support for our hypothesis that NE plays a significant role in the hypertrophy process.

The Concept of Physiologic and Pathologic Hypertrophy

From our group's study of the structure, function, and biochemical mechanisms of the hypertrophy process, we have concluded that ventricular hypertrophy should be divided at least into physiologic hypertrophy and pathologic hypertrophy states.[6–10] In the clinical domain, this distinction has great importance since athletes and many nonprofessional athletic individuals have demonstrated significant electrocardiographic and echocardiographic ventricular hypertrophy which should be considered physiologic hypertrophy. Unfortunately, in the clinical field ventricular hypertrophy has a negative connotation by being frequently associated with the words "pathologic hypertrophy." Since 1970, our group has deemed it necessary to highlight the impact of this dual classification,[6–10] and we have focused upon the role of NE in both ventricular hypertrophy processes.[2,6–10]

Pathologic versus Physiologic Hypertrophy

During our analysis of the effects of NE on the myocardium, we found that two distinctly different types of hypertrophy developed which correlated with the duration of NE infusion. After 3 to 4 months' exposure to subhypertensive levels of NE, cardiac output increased, as did the left ventricular ejection fraction.[6] Light and electron microscopy of the hypertrophied myocardium demonstrated no pathologic alterations. For example, intercalated discs were normal in dimension and configuration[7]; hydroxyproline, an index of collagen content, did not change; and myosin ATPase in the left ventricle was either normal or increased.[8,9] The characteristics of this type of hypertrophy mimicked those seen in well-conditioned athletes and were therefore labelled physiologic hypertrophy. With longer (6 to 8 months) NE infusion, some of the following characteristic features of hypertrophic cardiomyopathy were observed in left ventricular angiograms, ventricular pressure studies, and gross examination of the heart: thickened walls, increased ventricular weight, small ventricular cavity, intracavitary pressure gradients at rest, with vasodilators and inotropic agents, postectopic beat phenomena, and anterior tethering of the mitral valve.[11,12] Electron microscopy revealed a disarray of the myocardial fibers of the left ventricular septum. From these observations, we concluded that infusions of NE over a period of at least six months can produce pathologic hypertrophy. However, in accordance with the studies of Hintze, another important determinant for the production of pathologic hypertrophy appears to be the infusion rate of NE achieved. Although Hintze's time period of infusion of one month was significantly shorter than our six-month period, his infusion rate was at least 10 times as great (0.5 mg/kg/min compared with our rate of 0.003–0.04). The other important difference was that Hintze's route of administration of NE was subcutaneous while our route was intravenous. As previously described in his studies, subhypertensive infusion of NE did not increase ventricular function. Furthermore, he observed a blunting of the baroreceptor reflex and a bradycardia. Even though no tissue studies have been completed, Hintze agrees that the hypertrophy he produced is probably pathologic.[4]

In summary, although the concentration of NE infused is clearly a determinant for the production of pathologic hypertrophy, additional studies are needed to expand and confirm these important observations.

A New Model for Cellular Pathologic Hypertrophy: An in vitro *Study*

As previously presented, Simpson's group has done extensive studies *in vitro* using the rat neonatal heart muscle cell preparation.[5,12] He has demonstrated that NE produces myocardial cellular growth. This myocardial cellular growth or hypertrophy produced by NE is manifested by an increase in protein synthesis.

Simpson's group presented a fascinating model for the production of pathologic hypertrophy.[13] In the rat neonatal heart cell preparation NE increased total protein 56% and myosin heavy chain 102% ($P < 0.01$). Most important, NE increased the heavy chain to total protein ratio 33% ($P < 0.05$). A chemical which is a known tumor-producing agent called phorbol-12-myristate-13-acetate produced an increase in total protein but did not increase myosin heavy chains; it actually decreased the myosin heavy chain to total protein ratio by 20%. The addition of NE to the tumor-producing agent caused the same degree of total protein increase as did NE alone (50%), while the myosin heavy chain to total protein ratio decreased by 22% ($P < 0.01$). The tumor-producing agent combined with norepinephrine increased cell size similar to norepinephrine alone. Because the myocardial cells increased with a concomitant increase in contractile machinery as represented by myosin heavy chain, this experimental design may be a model for pathologic hypertrophy.

In summary, these new studies confirm the direct role that NE plays in the production of myocardial cellular hypertrophy and further substantiates the need to divide the term myocardial hypertrophy into physiologic and pathologic entities. Of course, other factors besides NE may be responsible for the production of pathologic hypertrophy.

To provide a basis for these additional studies, we have proposed that the following characteristics be used to define two major forms of ventricular hypertrophy, physiologic and pathologic.[8-10] Physiologic hypertrophy is a fully compensatory, structural, and functional response to stress on the myocardium which may be produced by an increase in preload, afterload, and/or a direct stimulation of the myocardium by, for example, NE. The major determinant in the definition of physiologic hypertrophy is that ventricular function increases proportionally to, or more than, an increase in myocardial cell size. In contrast, pathologic hypertrophy results in a diminishing degree of ventricular function when correlated to increasing cell size.

Physiologic Hypertrophy: Physiologic hypertrophy occurs as a result of a mild and/or properly timed increase in the periodicity of stress such as that produced by: (1) a mild pulmonary artery banding,[8,10] (2) the early stage of NE infusion,[6] (3) normal ductal closure of the newborn,[8] and (4) normal exercise.[8]

In addition to the stimulus, the extent and growth characteristics of vascular supply and the subjects' age, sex, and species may influence the development and maintenance of physiologic hypertrophy.

While performing a histologic examination of myocardium from dogs and humans who meet the hemodynamic, electrocardiographic, and gross anatomic characteristics for either physiologic or pathologic hypertrophy, we developed the following differential tissue markers as summarized in Fig. 1:

(1) A symmetric increase in myocardial cell size characterizes physiologic hypertrophy, while an asymmetric increase in myocardial cell size would be pathologic hypertrophy.

(2) Myofilaments and myofibers which increase in proportion to an increase in func-

MYOCARDIAL TISSUE MARKERS **DIFFERENTIATING**

PHYSIOLOGICAL FROM PATHOLOGICAL **HYPERTROPHY**

TISSUE MARKERS	**PHYSIOLOGICAL**	PATHOLOGICAL
INCREASE MYOCARDIAL CELL SIZE	**SYMMETRIC**	ASYMMETRIC
MYOFILAMENTS AND MYOFIBER	**PROP ↑**	DISARRAY
INTERCALATED DISC	**NORMAL**	↑ WIDTH, DOUBLE
Z BANDS	**NORMAL**	↑ WIDTH
MITOCHONDRIA	**NORMAL, PROP ↑**	SWOLLEN, ALTERED
SARCOPLASMIC RETICULUM	**NORMAL, PROP ↑**	SWOLLEN, ALTERED
NECROSIS	**NONE**	YES
FIBROSIS (HYDROXYPROLINE)	**PROP ↑ TO CELL**	> ↑ TO CELL
MYOSIN ATPASE	<--> ↑	↓
NOREPINEPHRINE	<--> ↑	↓
GLYCOGEN	<-->	↓ ALTERED
BETA-RECEPTORS	<--> ↑ ?	↓ ?

Fig. 1. Myocardial tissue markers differentiating physiologic from pathologic hypertrophy. See text for more complete description.

tion would be a physiologic change. However, if the fibers are disarrayed, the hypertrophy would be pathologic.[11,12]

(3) In the case of physiologic hypertrophy the intercalated discs would be normal, and in pathologic hypertrophy they would be widened and have cell projections.[14,15] An extreme example of the above pathologic tissue markers is hypertrophic cardiomyopathy in which the myofiber is so disarrayed and accompanied by projections from the cell that the cell simulates the changes seen in a tumor.

(4) We consider that the Z bands are normal in physiologic hypertrophy but are widened in pathologic hypertrophy. Therefore, we do not consider that Z band widening is an indicator of sarcomere genesis. Rather, the widened Z bands are probably a marker for pathologic hypertrophy.

(5) The mitochondria and

(6) the sarcoplasmic reticulum are normal or increased in size in physiologic hypertrophy and are usually swollen and altered in pathologic hypertrophy.

(7) Minimal or no necrosis would be present in physiologic hypertrophy, while necrosis is a well-recognized and logical marker of pathologic hypertrophy.[16,17]

(8) Collagen fibers, as measured by hydroxyproline content, increase in proportion to cell size in physiologic hypertrophy and increase proportionately more than cell size in pathologic hypertrophy.

(9) In physiologic hypertrophy, myosin ATPase increases or may not change; but in pathologic hypertrophy, it decreases.[9]

(10) We have hypothesized that NE content may increase or not change in physiologic hypertrophy. NE levels have been reported to decrease in pathologic hypertrophy.[17] However, since NE content does not represent the true physiologic activity state of NE, its tissue concentration may be decreased, increased, or unchanged in physiologic hypertrophy. Therefore, myocardial NE content measurement alone is of limited value. Figure 1 was created before the study to be presented was started and therefore predicted that the beta-receptor density would increase or not change in physiologic hypertrophy. In contrast, beta-receptor density was hypothesized to decrease in pathologic hypertrophy; a decrease was demonstrated in human hearts.[18]

The unknown effect of NE infusion on myocardial beta-receptors stimulated the following series of studies.

Biochemical Studies on Chronic Subhypertensive Infusion of Norepinephrine

Norepinephrine Infusion Method: Male mongrel dogs (25–29 kg) were implanted with polyvinyl chloride catheters placed under fluoroscopic control in the right jugular with the tip in the right atrium and in the right common carotid with the tip in the mid-thoracic aorta. The catheters were tunneled subcutaneously from the anterior cervical region and exteriorized in the dorsal cervical region. The catheters were housed in a specially designed dog jacket and maintained bimonthly with a saline solution containing heparin (40 U/ml).[2,19,20] An Infusaid pump was implanted subcutaneously in the flank a catheter running subcutaneously from the pump outlet to the circumflex iliac vein with and, under fluoroscopy, positioned in the inferior vena cava. The pump operates on a freon-based pressure system that is precalibrated prior to implantation to deliver 2.1 μl/min at 37°C. The reservoir capacity is 47 ml and is filled biweekly by injection through the skin into a resealable diaphragm. Control dogs also received the catheters, but not the pumps. All hemodynamic measurements were obtained in the conscious dog. Cardiac output was measured by the green dye technique and the ejection fraction by arteriography.[19] The NE infusion was begun at a rate of 0.45 μg/min. The infusion rate was increased weekly for three weeks to a total dose of 1.4 ± 0.2 μg/min. Systemic pressures were maintained in the normal, subhypertensive range. Plasma was obtained for NE determinations at 8 a.m. and 4 p.m. weekly in both the NE-infused and control dogs. After three months of infusion, hemodynamic measurements were again obtained and the dogs killed. The chest was opened rapidly, the heart removed, atria dissected away, and ventricles weighed. A stainless steel punch was used to obtain sections (approximately 2 g wet wt) of the free walls of the right and left ventricles approximately midway between the base and apex. The time lapse between killing and placing the tissue samples in iced buffer was approximately 5 min.

Plasma Norepinephrine Method: Plasma NE was measured by radioimmunoassay (RIA)[21,22] after cold hydrolysis of the sample to yield a measure of the free and sulfate-conjugated NE.[23] Myocardial NE was measured by RIA as previously described.[22] Protein was estimated utilizing reagents from Biorad Laboratories (Richmond, CA).

Assays of Binding of ^{125}Iodohydroxybenzylpindolol to Myocardial Membranes: The procedures are minor modifications of those described by others.[24] Approximately 2 g of myocardium was placed in 40 ml of ice-cold buffer [0.25 M sucrose, 20 mM Tris (hydroxymethyl) amino-methane base, 1 mM $MgSO_4$, and 140 mM NaCl, pH 7.5] and homogenized for 15 sec in a Polytron homogenizer (Brinkman Instruments, Westbury, NY) at a setting of 5. The homogenate was filtered through a single layer of cheesecloth, then centrifuged at 300 × *g* for 10 min at 4°C. The pellet was discarded and the supernatant centrifuged at 30,000 × *g* for 15 min. The supernatant was discarded and the pellet washed with 40 ml of homogenization buffer without sucrose (incubation buffer) and centrifuged at 30,000 × *g* for 15 min. The final pellet was resuspended with incubation buffer to give a final protein concentration of approximately 2.5 mg/ml. The recovery of membrane protein was approximately 20 mg/g of initial tissue wet weight.

Aliquots of membrane protein (100 μg protein) in triplicate were incubated with varying concentrations of (noniodinated) hydroxybenzylpindolol (HYP) (0.5–50 mM), with approximately 90,000 cpm of iodohydroxybenzylpindolol (IHYP) (sp sct 2.2 Ci/mmol) in incubation buffer in a total volume of 300 μl for 60 min at 37°C in the presence or absence of 0.3 M *dl*-propranolol. Following incubation, the samples were diluted with 5 ml buffer (10 mM Tris base, 140 mM NaCl, pH 7.5) and filtered through Whatman GF/C glass fiber filters. The filters were washed with an additional 15 ml of buffer at room temperature, then placed in glass culture tubes and the radioactivity retained on the filters quantitated in a Micromedic 4/600 gamma counter.

Assays of cAMP and Adenylate Cyclase Activity in the Heart: The procedures are modifications of those described by others.[25] Approximately 2 g of myocardial tissue was homogenized in 10 vol of ice-cold buffer (50 mM Tris base, 10 mM $MgSO_4$, pH 7.5) in a Polytron homogenizer for 15 sec at a setting of 5. Aliquots (50 μl, containing approximately 500 μg protein) were incubated at 30°C for 10 min in the reaction mixture containing 50 mM Tris base (pH 7.5), 10 mM $MgSO_4$, 8 mM theophylline, 20 mM phosphocreatine, 50 μg creatinine phosphokinase, 0.2 mM ATP, and 1 mM ascorbic acid in the presence or absence of l-isoproterenol (10^{-9} – 10^{-3} M) in a total volume of 150 μl. The reaction was stopped by immersing the tube in a boiling water bath for 2 min. The tubes were then centrifuged at 10,000 × *g* for 20 min and aliquots of the supernatant were taken directly for RIA measurement of the cAMP formed.

Statistical Methods: Data are presented as means ± SEM. Beta-receptor density is calculated by Scatchard analysis.[24] The sensitivity of adenylate cyclase to isoproterenol stimulation was obtained as the concentration of isoproterenol producing half-maximal adenylate cyclase activity as estimated by Probit analysis.[25] Student's *t*-test, 1- and 2-way analysis of variance, was used for statistical analysis of the data.

RESULTS AND DISCUSSION

Experimental Results: After a three-month infusion of NE, cardiac output did not change, the ejection fraction increased, and, in accordance with the experimental design, systemic pressure did not change (Fig. 2).[26,27] Ventricular weights did not increase

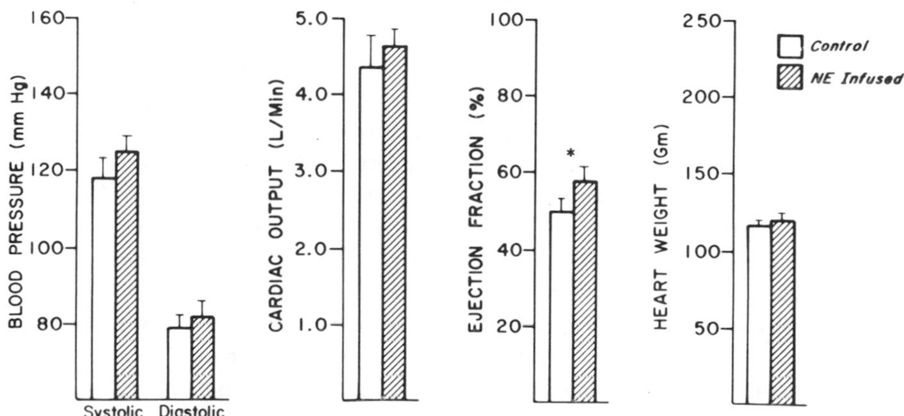

Fig. 2. Effects of three-month infusion of NE on hemodynamic function and heart weight. All values are means ± SEM. *P < 0.05. Note the increase in ejection fraction and no change in heart weight after NE infusion.

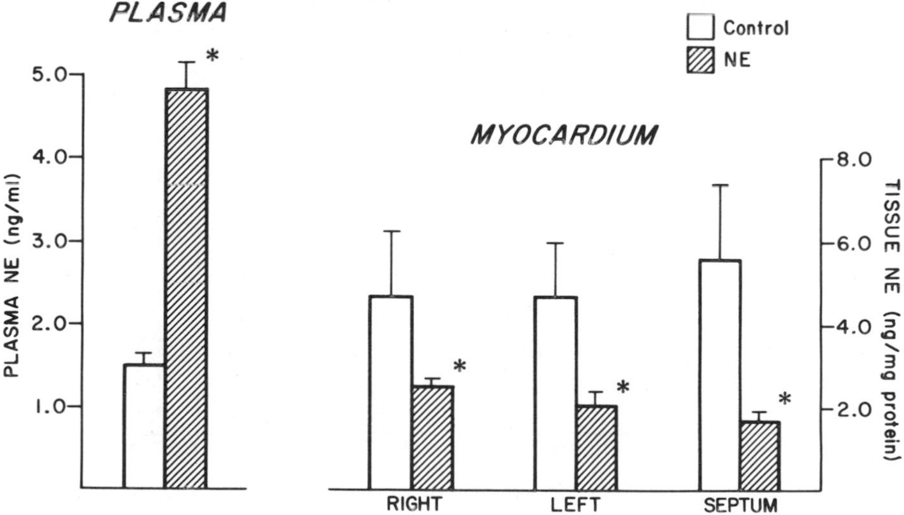

Fig. 3. Plasma and myocardial tissue NE concentration in normal dogs and dogs receiving NE. Controls are represented by the open bars and dogs receiving NE are represented by the hatched bars. *P < 0.05 to < 0.001.

significantly. Therefore, the reported alterations in the myocardium, both physiologically and biochemically, occur just prior to the development of significant hypertrophy.

Figure 3 illustrates that a subhypertensive, incrementally increased dose of NE does markedly increase plasma NE up to about 4.8 ng/ml compared with a normal control of 1.5 ng/ml. Of significant interest, both the right and left ventricular and septal myocardial NE content decreased significantly.

As shown in Fig. 4, the beta-receptor density increased significantly in the left ventricle but the greatest increase occurred in the septum. Adenylate cyclase activity significantly increased in both the right and left ventricles, but no significant change was detected in the septum. Cyclic AMP tissue concentrations were not altered significantly in any portion of the heart.[26]

These results lead to several observations and conclusions. First, because beta-receptor density increased instead of decreasing as receptors usually do in response to an agonist, it was concluded that the relationship between myocardial beta-receptors and infused NE is complex. This relationship is discussed in the next section. Second, beta-receptor density increases before significant hypertrophy develops. Similar observations were reported by other investigators utilizing a variety of experimental models (reviewed in refs. 26,27) Combining the first and second observations, we concluded that changes in beta-receptor density are only related to the stimulus producing hypertrophy or its route of administration and are not due to the process or degree of hypertrophy. In addition, Malik and Geha[28] reported that the beta-antagonist practolol did not prevent hypertrophy induced by banding the rat aorta, which casts further doubt on a direct role for beta-receptor stimulation in the hypertrophy process. However, these observations do not rule out a mechanism in which a lack of beta stimulation is the etiology. Because NE is a mixed alpha-beta-agonist, we suggested that alpha-receptor stimulation by NE could be an alternate pathway to the hypertensive process. At about the same time we published these conclusions, Simpson[12] reported that NE stimulated protein synthesis in rat myocardial cell cultures. This effect was blocked by a specific alpha-1 antagonist, Terazosin, but was not blocked by the beta-antagonist propranolol.[29] Simpson concluded that hypertrophy produced by NE was mediated, at least in part, through alpha-1 receptor stimulation. Our third observation was that the beta-

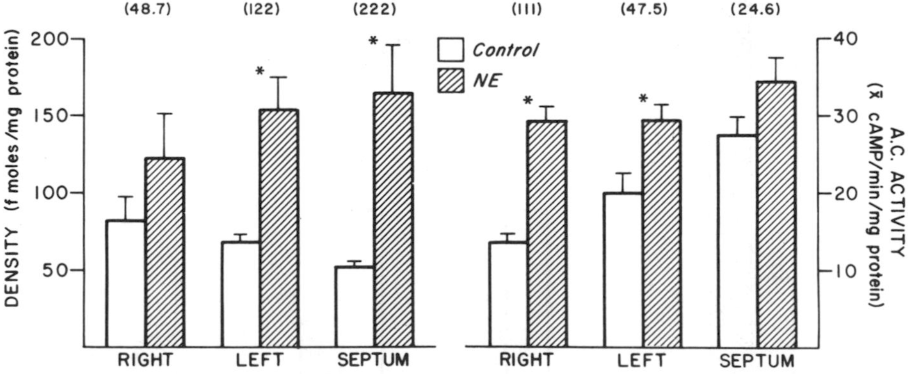

Fig. 4. Effect of NE infusion on beta-receptor density (left) and adenylate cyclase activity (right) is compared among the right and left ventricles and the ventricular septum. The numbers in parentheses refer to the mean percent increase. *$P < 0.05$ to < 0.005 comparing control (open bars) and dogs receiving NE (shaded bars).

receptor adenylate cyclase system in the septum is different from the right and left ventricle in the normal, basal state and also responds to NE infusion differently from the rest of the heart.[26] We concluded these differences may relate to the mechanisms involved in the development of hypertrophic cardiomyopathy specifically, and myocardial hypertrophy in general. Our hypotheses related to this brief outline of our observations and conclusions are discussed in the following sections.

Postulated Mechanism for NE-induced Hypertrophy: Figure 5 illustrates the pathways discussed below. In the proposed model, infused NE can produce increased beta-receptor number in the hypertrophy process by two possible mechanisms. First, NE infusion inhibits synthesis of NE in the sympathetic nerves. As a consequence,[26,27] NE content decreased in the myocardium. If decreased content results in decreased release, there would be less stimulation of beta-receptors producing an up-regulation of receptor numbers. It was reported that beta-receptor density does indeed increase, but no measure of NE release (turnover) was obtained. The second possible pathway involves direct NE stimulation of alpha-1 receptors. It has been suggested that during alpha-agonist stimulation, alpha-receptors go through a conformational change and become beta-receptors.[30] Hence, the observed increase in beta-receptors could come about through these two mechanisms.

Accompanying the increase in beta-receptors, adenylate cyclase activity increased in both the right and left ventricles. The product of adenylate cyclase activity, cAMP con-

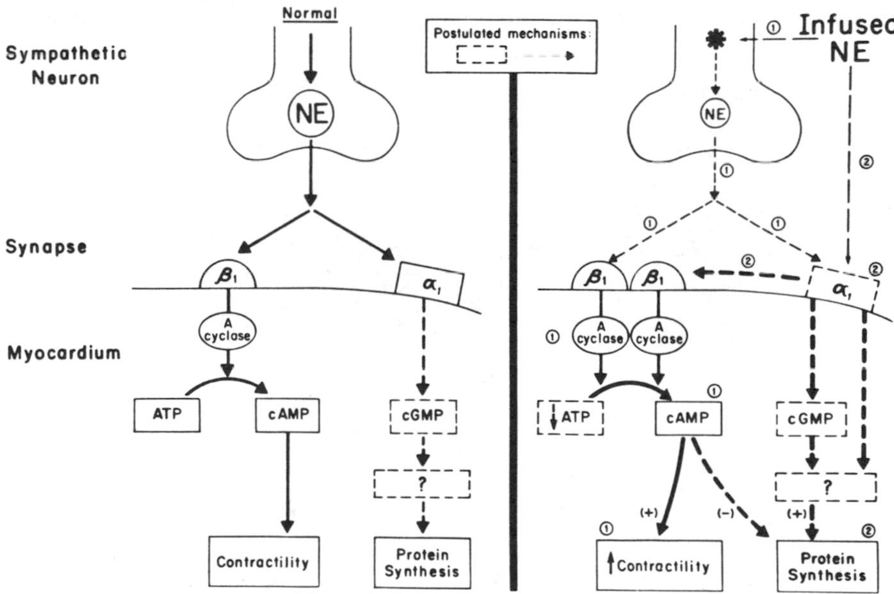

Fig. 5. The normal biochemical relationships are in the left panel. The biochemical results of a three-month infusion of NE are shown in the right panel. These changes occurred in the absence of ventricular hypertrophy and therein preceded the hypertrophy process. Note that protein synthesis is postulated to increase through cAMP diminution and through alpha-1 receptor stimulation. See text for detailed description.

tent, did not increase significantly. There are two possible explanations for this result. Either the breakdown of cAMP was enhanced (phosphodiesterase activity) or the substrate for cAMP synthesis, ATP, was diminished. We consider the latter to be more likely. Although we did not measure ATP content, others have offered this as a reasonable explanation for a similar phenomenon.[31,32]

When ATP concentrations are not limited, cAMP content will increase and contractility will increase (as shown by the solid arrow in Fig. 6). From these studies we postulated that if the myocardial cell contractility decreases because of a decrease in cAMP, protein synthesis is stimulated to produce sarcomeres, and therefore myocardial cellular hypertrophy commences. Consequently, in the heart cAMP increase has a negative effect on protein synthesis, and conversely, a diminution in cAMP is a stimulus for protein synthesis. The ultimate homeostasis is to maintain total ventricular contractility. This hypothesis was formulated after recognizing that a number of seemingly different perturbations to the myocardium all could or do reduce tissue cAMP levels and all result in hypertrophy. For example, isoproterenol- and thyroxine-induced hypertrophy in the rat[31,32] are both associated with decreased tissue cAMP and ATP; beta-receptor blockade,[28] chemical sympathectomy[32] with 6-hydroxydopamine, or nerve growth factor antiserum[33] will all result in decreased cAMP due to lack of beta-receptor stimulation and will not prevent hypertrophy or may even enhance it. The experiment demonstrating that exogenously supplied cAMP will prevent hypertrophy and/or inhibit protein synthesis has not been performed. However, by increasing the ATP stores in the rat heart and thereby providing ample substrate for cAMP synthesis, the development of hypertrophy in response to aortic banding was prevented.[34] An alternate mechanism for hypertrophy evolves from the previously described work of Simpson,[12] who demonstrated that NE increases

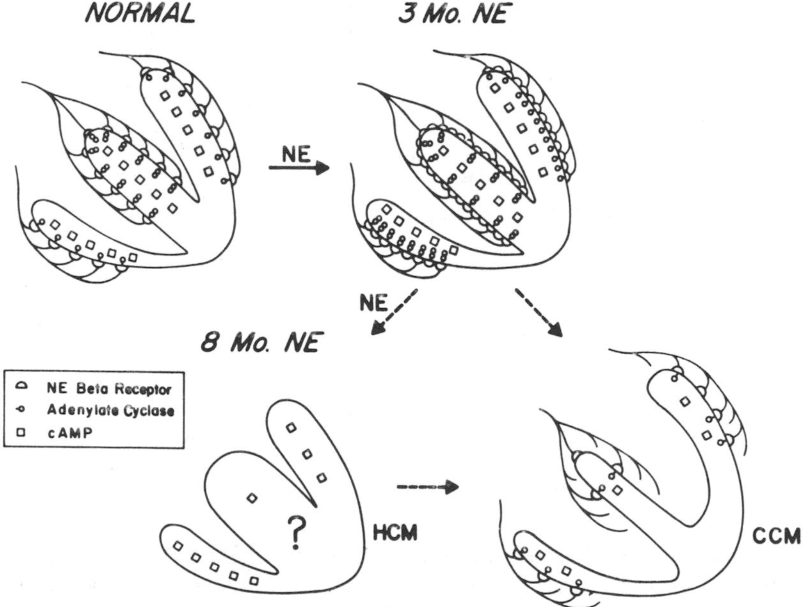

Fig. 6. Schematic drawings of the postulated biochemical mechanisms for the genesis of HCM and CCM. Dashed arrows indicate postulated biochemical changes. See text for detailed description.

protein synthesis via the alpha-1 receptor. The dotted boxes around cGMP indicate that little is known about the relationship of cGMP to NE-induced hypertrophy, but cAMP is being considered as one possible contender in a series of unknown steps between the alpha-1 receptor and protein synthesis. The major new hypothesis offered is that a diminution of cAMP and possibly ATP may be the stimulus for protein synthesis and myocardial cellular hypertrophy.

Norepinephrine-Induced Hypertrophic Cardiomyopathy: Figure 6 summarizes schematically known and postulated relationships among the normal myocardium, hypertrophic cardiomyopathy (HCM), and congestive cardiomyopathy (CCM). We reported that in the normal dog the ventricular septum has biochemical features that make it more sensitive to NE stimulation than either the right or left ventricle. As shown in Fig. 4, adenylate cyclase activity was highest in the ventricular septum compared with the free walls of the right and left ventricle. After a three-month infusion of NE, beta-receptors increased to the greatest degree in the septum. Despite the marked increase in the betareceptors, neither cAMP content nor adenylate cyclase activity increased significantly in the septum. The septum appears to respond more vigorously to NE infusion than the right and left ventricle by producing the greatest increase in beta-receptors, but lacks the reserve of the right and left ventricle to increase its ability to generate cAMP by increasing adenylate cyclase activity. Considering our previous hypothesis that hypertrophy is linked to decreased cAMP levels, one would predict that the septum would be the most vulnerable to the development of hypertrophy (HCM) because of its diminished capacity to generate cAMP under stress (NE infusion). As we have reported, with long-term NE infusion, dogs develop a marked degree of septal hypertrophy, resulting in the tumor-like disarray of myocardial cells in the ventricular septum characteristic of HCM. The data generated from the study of the ventricular and septal adenylate cyclase system complement our hypothesis concerning the relationship between cAMP and the development of hypertrophy and provide a reasonable mechanism for the observed NE-induced HCM in dogs.

Bristow *et al.*[18] demonstrated in human hearts with CCM that both beta-receptors and adenylate cyclase activity are diminished. The pathway directly from the three-month NE-infused myocardium or indirectly through the HCM model is very tentatively drawn (Fig. 6). Considerably more data must be generated to determine if these pathways even exist. The illustration (Fig. 6) is offered to provide a complete spectrum of two pathologic states (HCM and CCM) that have a common bond rooted in marked abnormalities of the adrenergic system. We have speculated that if the intravascular amount of catecholamine is high, CCM may be produced directly from the normal heart. The predicted marked decrease in cAMP is postulated to be the driving stimulus to produce the severe hypertrophy of the myocardial cells, many of which outstrip their blood supply and die, leaving in their wake large grotesque myocardial cells in a sea of fibrosis—the histopathology of a CCM.

In summary, we conclude that:

(A) Chronic infusion of NE produces:

(1) Both a physiologic and pathologic hypertrophy (HCM).

(2) An increase in myocardial beta-receptors with no increase in adenylate cyclase and cAMP content in septum. This change coupled with the presence of a septal increase in adenylate cyclase in the normal heart may be the biochemical clues to the pathogenesis of HCM.

(3) The stimulus for ventricular hypertrophy has been postulated to be a relative decrease in cAMP and/or a stimulation of the alpha-1-receptor.

REFERENCES

1. Laks, M., Morady, F., and Swan, H. Canine right and left ventricular cell and sarcomere lengths after banding the pulmonary artery. *Circ. Res.* **24**: 705–710, 1969.
2. Laks, M., Morady, F., and Swan, H. Myocardial hypertrophy produced by chronic infusion of subhypertensive doses of norepinephrine in the dog. *Chest* **64**: 75, 1973.
3. Laks, M. and Morady, F. Norepinephrine—The myocardial hypertrophy hormone? *Am. Heart J.* **91**: 674–675, 1976.
4. Hintze, T. Personal Communication.
5. Simpson, P., McGrath, A., and Savion, S. Myocyte hypertrophy in neonatal rat heart cultures and its regulation by serum and by catecholamines. *Circ. Res.* **51**: 787–801, 1982.
6. Laks, M., Garner, D., and Wong, W. Increased ejection fraction produced by a long-term subhypertensive infusion of norepinephrine in the conscious dog. *Am. Heart J.* **98**: 732, 1979.
7. Adomian, G., Haeusslein, E., Garner, D., and Laks, M. Comparison of intercalated discs (ID) in the hypertrophied myocardium produced by norepinephrine (NE) and pulmonary arterial banding (PAB). *Fed. Proc.* **36**: 572, 1977.
8. Wikman-Coffelt, J., Laks, M., Riemenschneider, T., and Mason, D. Physiological versus pathological myocardial hypertrophy. *J. Mol. Cell Cardiol.* **10**: 132, 1978.
9. Wikman-Coffelt, J., Laks, M., Riemenschneider, T., and Mason, D. Mechanism of physiologic versus pathologic ventricular hypertrophy process: Enhanced or depressed myosin ATPase activity and contractility governed by type, degree and duration of inciting stress. *Basic Res. Cardiol.* **75**: 149–156, 1980.
10. Wikman-Coffelt, J., Parmley, W., and Mason, D. The cardiac hypertrophy process: Analyses of factors determining pathological vs. physiological development. *Circ. Res.* **45**: 697–707, 1979.
11. Criley, J., Lennon, P., Abbasi, A., and Blaufuss, A. Hypertrophic cardiomyopathy. In: Cardiovascular Disease: Current Status and Advances (monograph). Clinical Cardiovascular Physiology. New York, Grune and Stratton, pp. 771–827, 1976.
12. Blaufuss, A., Laks, M., Garner, D., Ishimoto, B., and Criley, J. Production of ventricular hypertrophy simulating "Idiopathic hypertrophic subaortic stenosis" (IHSS) by subhypertensive infusion of norepinephrine (NE) in the conscious dog. *Clin. Res.* **23**: 77A, 1975.
13. White, N., Tsao, T., and Simpson, P. Contractile protein content is increased in hypertrophy stimulated by norepinephrine but not by a phorbol ester: An example of pathological hypertrophy in cultured neonatal rat heart muscle cells. *J. Am. Coll. Cardiol.* **7**: 122A, 1986.
14. Laks, M., Morady, F., Adomian, G., and Swan, H. Presence of widened and multiple intercalated discs in the hypertrophied canine heart. *Circ. Res.* **27**: 391–402, 1970.
15. Adomian, G., Laks, M., Morady, F., and Swan, H. Significance of the multiple intercalated disc in the hypertrophied canine heart. *J. Mol. Cell. Cardiol.* **6**: 105–110, 1974.
16. Laks, M., French, W., Billingham, M. Toxic effects of drugs on heart muscle. VIII World Congress of Cardiology, p. 68 (S-35). Excerpta Medica, International Congress Series #470, p. 651, 1978.
17. Szakacs, J.E. and Cannon, A. L-norepinephrine myocarditis. *Am. J. Clin. Pathol.* **30**: 425–433, 1958.
18. Bristow, M., Ginsburg, R., Minobe, W., Cubicciotti, R., Sageman, W., Lore, K., Billingham, M., Harrison, D., and Stinson, E. Decreased catecholamine sensitivity and beta-adrenergic-receptor density in failing human hearts. *N. Engl. J. Med.* **307**: 205–211, 1982.
19. Garner, D., Laks, M., and Beazell, J. Technique for the repeated performance of left ventricular cineangiograms and pressures in the conscious dog. *Fed. Proc.* **34**: 435, 1975.
20. Laks, M., Garner, D., Beazell, J., and Piscitelli, J. A new method for internal calibration of left ventricular cineangiography. *Am. J. Physiol.* **232**: H434–H436, 1977.

21. Raum, W.J. Enzymatic radioimmunoassay of epinephrine, norepinephrine, metanephrine, and normetanephrine. *Methods Enzymol.* **142**: 550–571, 1987.
22. Raum, W. and Swerdloff, R. A radioimmunoassay for epinephrine and norepinephrine in tissues and plasma. *Life Sci.* **28**: 2819, 1981.
23. Kuchel, O., Buu, N.T., Fontaine, A., Hamet, P., Beroniade, V., Larochelle, P., and Genest, J. Free and conjugated plasma catecholamines in hypertensive patients with and without pheochromocytoma. *J. Hypertension* **2**: 177–186, 1980.
24. Harden, T.K., Wolfe, B.B., Sporn, J.R., Perkins, J.P., and Molinoff, P.B. Ontogeny of beta-adrenergic receptors in rat cerebral cortex. *Brain Res.* **125**: 99–108, 1977.
25. Goldstein, A., Aronow, L., and Kalman, S.M. The basis of pharmacology (2nd ed.). In: Principles of Drug Action. New York, Wiley, p. 379, 1974.
26. Raum, W., Laks, M., Garner, D., and Swerdloff, R. Beta adrenergic receptor and cyclic AMP alterations in the canine ventricular septum during long-term norepinephrine infusion: Implications for hypertrophic cardiomyopathy. *Circulation* **68**: 693–699, 1983.
27. Raum, W., Laks, M., Garner, D., Ikuhara, M., and Swerdloff, R. Norepinephrine increases beta-receptors and adenylate cyclase in canine myocardium. *Am. J. Physiol.* **15**: H31–H36, 1984.
28. Malik, A. and Geha, A. Role of adrenergic mechanisms in the development of cardiac hypertrophy. *Proc. Soc. Exp. Biol. Med.* **150**: 796–800, 1975.
29. Simpson, P. and McGrath, A. Norepinephrine-stimulated hypertrophy of cultured rat myocardial cells is an alpha-adrenergic response. *J. Clin. Invest.* **72**: 732–738, 1983.
30. Kunos, G., Yong, M.S., and Nickerson, M. Transformation of adrenergic receptors in the myocardium. *Nature (*London*)* **241**: 119–120, 1973.
31. Tse, J., Wrenn, R.W., and Kuo, J.F. Thyroxine-induced changes in characteristics and activities of beta-adrenergic receptors and adenosine 3, 5-monophosphate and guanosine 3′,5′-monophosphate systems in the heart may be related to reputed catecholamine supersensitivity in hyperthyroidism. *Endocrinology* **107**: 6–16, 1980.
32. Cohen, J. Role of endocrine factors in the pathogenesis of cardiac hypertrophy. *Circ. Res.* **35** (suppl. II): 49, 1974.
33. Cutilletta, A., Erinoff, L., Heller, A., Low, J., and Oparil, S. Development of left ventricular hypertrophy in young spontaneously hypertensive rats after peripheral sympathectomy. *Circ. Res.* **40**: 428, 1977.
34. Warbanow, W. Morphologische und funktionelle untersuchungen der hypothermie-bidingten hypertrophie des embryonalen huhnerherzens. *Acta Biol. Med. Ger.* **25**: 281, 1970.

SYMPATHETIC FUNCTION IN HYPERTROPHIC CARDIO-MYOPATHY

Norepinephrine Kinetics in Hypertrophic Cardiomyopathy

*Alan S. Maisel**,**, *Michael Wright***, *Keith D. Wilner***, *and Michael G. Ziegler***

* National Institutes of Health, Bethesda, Maryland, U.S.A.
** Divisions of Cardiology and Nephrology Department of Medicine, Veterans Administration Medical Center, and University of California, San Diego, La Jolla, California, U.S.A.

ABSTRACT

The steady state plasma level of norepinephrine (NE) is the result of two processes; release of NE from the sympathetic nerve terminals into the plasma, and clearance of NE from the circulation. While both an increase in release and a decrease in clearance account for the elevated NE levels in congestive heart failure (CHF), NE kinetics in patients with hypertrophic cardiomyopathy (HCM) have not been studied. We therefore evaluated supine NE levels and NE kinetics in normal volunteers, in 10 patients with HCM, and patients with CHF utilizing a 120 minute 3(H) 1-NE infusion to achieve a steady state plateau concentration. NE clearance was calculated from the infusion rate and 3(H) NE concentration at steady state. NE release rate was determined from the clearance rate and norepinephrine plasma concentration (radioenzymatic technique).

Compared to controls, patients with HCM had higher supine levels of NE (905 ± 137 vs 362 ± 71 pg/ml, $p<0.005$, greater release rate of NE into the plasma (1210 ± 149 ng/min vs 522 ± 98 ng/min $p<0.01$) and similar clearance rates (1.6 ± 0.15 L/min vs 1.35 ± 0.05 L/min, p = ns). Patients with CHF had elevated supine NE levels (1317 ± 160 pg/ml) and a high NE release rate (940 ± 150 ng/min) but had significantly decreased clearance (0.79 ± 0.14 L/min) compared to both control ($p<0.01$) and hypertrophic cardiomyopathy ($p<0.001$). Thus unlike CHF, NE elevation in HCM is due to altered kinetics involving increased release of NE but no change in clearance. This high NE release rate could contribute to the development of HCM.

INTRODUCTION

Evidence derived from animal models suggest that the sympathetic nervous system may have a role in the pathogenesis of hypertrophic cardiomyopathy.[1)] Cardiomyopathic changes resembling hypertrophic cardiomyopathy can be produced by chronic norepinephrine infusion or the administration of nerve growth factor, which enhances sympathetic nerve growth.[2)] Several human conditions such as lentiginosis,[3,4)] Friedreichs ataxia,[5,6)] pheochromocytoma,[7)] von Recklinghausen's disease,[8)] and infants of diabetic mothers[9,10)] have both abnormalities of the sympathetic nervous system and asymmetric septal hypertrophy.

The plasma concentration of norepinephrine, the neurotransmitter of the sympathetic nervous system, has been used as a guide to the activity of that system.[11)] Plasma levels of norepinephrine are the product of two processes: spillover of norepinephrine into the plasma after release from sympathetic nerves and subsequent removal of norepinephrine from blood.[11,12)] As norepinephrine removal is abnormal in some cardiac diseases, biochemical methods that estimate the rate of norepinephrine release and removal should better be able to assess sympathetic tone than plasma norepinephrine measurements alone.[13,14] This study assesses the role of the sympathetic nervous system hypertrophic cardiomyopathy by evaluation of norepinephrine kinetics.

METHODS

Study Population

We studied 10 subjects who have been followed in our cardiomyopathy clinic for an average of 7 years (range 2–10). The diagnosis of hypertrophic cardiomyopathy was based on well known criteria recently reviewed by Epstein *et al.*[15] (Table 1). The subjects had a mean age of 63 years (range 30–88) and a mean left ventricular ejection fraction of 75 percent. All had echocardiograms and 7 of 10 had cardiac catheterization: three of these had a resting systolic pressure gradient in the left ventricular outflow tract and two had gradients provokable by premature ventricular contractions or isoproterenol. Two patients had concomitant coronary artery disease, two had hypertension (pheochromocytoma was excluded), four palpitations, and one patient had been treated with a myomectomy. Five patients complained of chest pain (angina like), two of dizziness, and six of dyspnea. At the time of the study, all patients were New York Heart Association functional class I-III. Their average exercise duration on a treadmill was 9.7 $\pm$ 3 minutes (range 5–14 minutes) using a standard Balke Ware protocol. Three patients were receiving chronic beta blocker treatment and two were taking verapamil. These drugs were difficult to taper in this group of patients, but were held for at least 12 hours prior to the test.

Ten ambulatory subjects (male, aged 22–72 mean age 55 years) with no evidence of cardiac of systemic disease served as controls. In addition, 10 patients with dilated cardiomyopathy and clinical congestive heart failure (NYHA II-IV), with an age of 72 $\pm$ 15, (range 50–82 years) and an ejection fraction of 28 $\pm$ 8 (range 61–90) were studied. All patients were being treated with digitalis and diuretics, and seven were taking vasodilators. All subjects gave written informed consent for the study, which was approved by the Committee on Investigations involving Human subjects for the School of Medicine, UCSD.

Subjects were fasted overnight and remained resting supine in bed. Thirty minutes before infusion an intravenous cannula was inserted in a vein in each forearm, one of which was kept open by infusion and the other with a heparin lock. A blood sample was drawn 5 minutes before the start of the infusion. One-hundred microcurries μCi of 1-^{3}H-norepinephrine (New England Nuclear, specific activity of 25 ci/mmole) was sterilized by passage through a millipore filter and stored at $-70°$C. A sample of this ^{3}H norepinephrine was analyzed by thin layer chromatography with 98% radiochemical purity taken as the minimum acceptable prior to use in humans.

The ^{3}H-norepinephrine was diluted in 50 ml of normal saline containing 100 mg ascorbic acid, and infused in one arm at 30 ml/hr for 10 minutes and then 19 ml/hr for 110 minutes. Plateau levels of ^{3}H-norepinephrine were achieved in less than 60 minutes. Blood was sampled during the infusion at 0, 115, 120 minutes, and 5 minutes after standing. Heparinized blood was immediately placed on ice, centrifuged in the cold and the plasma was separated and frozen at $-70°$C. The blood was assayed for ^{3}H-norepinephrine by alumina chromatography with subsequent washing and elution by acid & scintillation spectrometry of the eluate. Since only catechols bind to the alumina, O-methylated metabolites and free tritium do not interfere with the assay. We checked for the presence of ^{3}H-norepinephrine metabolites derived from the action of mono-

TABLE 1. Patient Characteristics

	Age	RBWD (%)	ECHO ASH/SAM	Murmut Valsalve	CATH	MR (cath or Doppler)	Resting	Gradient
WA	88	70	+/+	+	no	–	–	
LB	70	75	+/+	+	yes	+	+	(30mm)
EB	67	71	+/+	+	yes	–	–	
DG	30	83	+/+	+	yes	–	–	
MH	60	61	+/+	+	yes	+	–	
KH	64	67	+/+	+	yes	–	–	
JT	60	90	+/+	+	no	–	–	
RW	69	80	+/+	+	yes	–	+	(57mm)
LW	63	70	+/+	+	yes	+	+	(67mm)
Wo	72	80	+/+	+	no	–	–	

CAD	Chest pain	ETT-TIME (min)	Syncope/Dizziness	Hypertension	Dyspnea	Palpitations	Myomectomy	MEDICATIONS	NYHA
+	+	8	–	–	+	–	–	–	II
–	+	7	–	+	+	–	–	verapamil	II
–	–	7	–	–	+	+	–	–	II
–		13	–	–	–	–	–	–	II
–	+	6	–	–	–	+	–	propranolol	II
–	–	5	–	–	+	–	–		II
–	–	11	–	+	+	+	–	atenolol	III
+	+	9	+	–	–	–	–	–	I
–	–	9	–	–	+	–	+	verapamil	III
–	+	11	+	–		+	–	metroprolol	I

Abbreviations

ASJ/SAM = asymmetic septal hypertrophy systolic anterior motion.
RNEF = radionucleotide ejection fraction.
CAD = coronary artery disease.
ETT = exercise treadmill test.
CATH = cardiac catheterization.
NYHA = New York Heart Association.
MR = Mitral regurgitation.

amine oxidase by solvent extraction and found none. Thus, the assay was specific for ^{3}H-norepinephrine. Endogenous norepinephrine was measured by radioenzymatic assay as previously described.[14]

Norepinephrine Spillover and Clearance

At steady state during the infusion of ^{3}H-norepinephrine, the total plasma NE clearance and the total spillover rate of NE to plasma can be calculated[11,16–18]:

$$\text{NE Clearance} = \frac{^3\text{H-norepinephrine infusion rate}}{^3\text{H-norepinephrine plasma concentration}}$$

At steady state the amount of NE entering plasma from sympathetic nerves equals the amount of NE cleared from plasma:

$$\text{NE spillover rate} = \text{plasma NE} \times \text{NE clearance}$$

Statistics

Results were expressed in the text as mean ± SEM. To determine statistical significance of norepinephrine levels, clearance, and spillover between groups, we calculated two tailed t-tests.

RESULTS

Norepinephrine Kinetics in Hypertrophic Cardiomyopathy

Figure 1 shows the plasma norepinephrine levels (pg/ml) drawn during 30 minutes of supine rest in normal controls and in patients with hypertrophic cardiomyopathy. The mean levels were 362 pg/ml ± 71 (range 168–770) for controls and 905 pg/ml ± 137 (range 443–1795) for the hypertrophic cardiomyopathy group ($p<0.005$).

Figure 2 shows the rate of spillover in ng/min of norepinephrine into the plasma in control patients and patients with hypertrophic cardiomyopathy. The mean rate of release of norepinephrine into the plasma was over 2 fold greater in the hypertrophic patients than in controls: 1210 ng/min ± 149 versus 522 ng/min ± 98 ($p<0.01$).

Figure 3 shows the norepinephrine clearance in liters/minute in the two groups of patients. The mean value of 1.35 l/min ± 0.05 for control patients was not significantly different from 1.6 l/min ± 0.15 for the patients with hypertrophic cardiomyopathy.

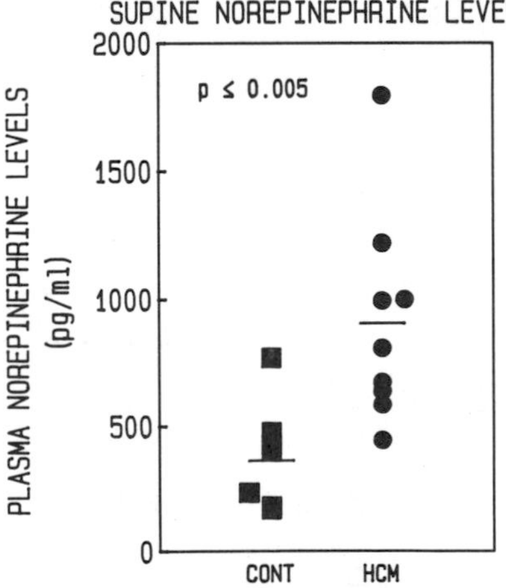

Fig. 1. Supine norepinephrine levels in control patients ($n=10$) and hypertrophic cardiomyopathy ($n=10$).

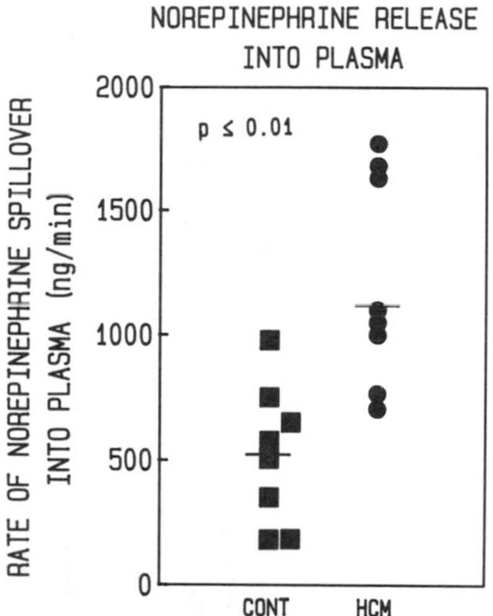

Fig. 2. Norepinephrine release (spillover) into plasma; control ($n=9$) vs. hypertrophic cardiomyopathy ($n=9$).

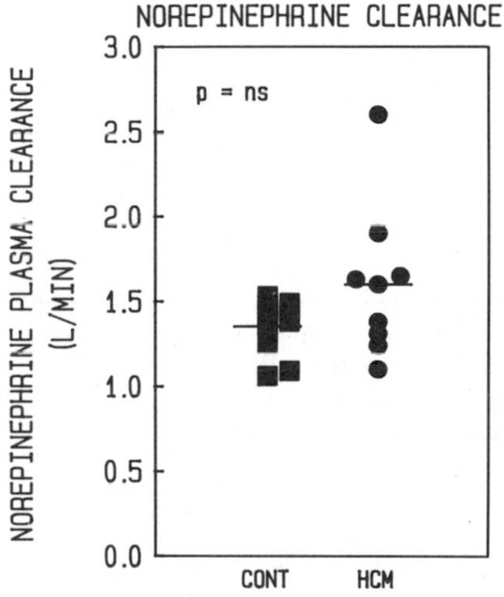

Fig. 3. Norepinephrine clearance, (L/min) control ($n=10$) vs. hypertrophic cardiomyopathy ($n=10$).

Comparison of Hypertrophic Cardiomyopathy with Congestive Heart Failure

We compared norepinephrine kinetic data from the patients with hypertrophic cardiomyopathy to kinetic data in a group of similar aged patients with dilated cardiomyopathy. Figure 4 compares control, heart failure, and hypertrophic cardiomyopathy with respect to supine norepinephrine levels, norepinephrine spillover into the plasma and clearance from the plasma. In heart failure patients, the supine plasma norepinephrine levels were significantly elevated above controls; 1314 pg/ml ± 160 vs 362 pg/ml ± 71 ($p<0.005$), but were not significantly different from hypertrophic cardiomyopathy (Fig. 4A). In patients with congestive heart failure the rate of spillover of norepinephrine (Fig. 4B) was greater than controls, 940 ng/min ± 150 vs 522 ng/min ± 100

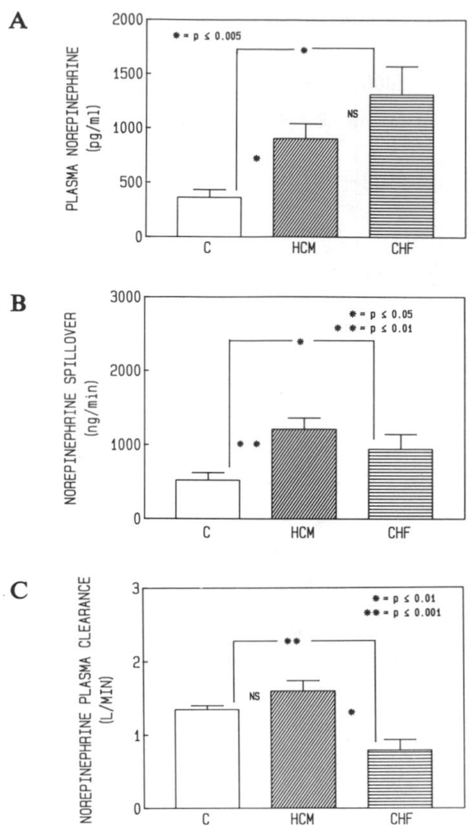

Fig. 4. Comparison of control, ($n=10$) hypertrophic cardiomyopathy ($n=8$) and congestive heart failure with respect to:
A. Supine norepinephrine levels (pg/ml).
B. Norepinephrine spillover (ng/min).
C. Norepinephrine plasma clearance (L/min).

($p<0.05$) but was comparable and not statistically different from patients with hypertrophic cardiomyopathy (1210 ng/min ± 149). The clearance of norepinephrine from the plasma (Fig. 4C) however was significantly decreased in heart failure compared to both control (0.79 1/min ± 0.14 vs 1.35 L/min ± 0.05, $p<0.01$) and hypertrophic cardiomyopathy (0.79 L/min ± 0.14 vs 1.6 L/min ± 0.15, $p<0.001$). Thus, much of the increase in plasma norepinephrine levels seen in heart failure (Fig. 4) is due to impaired clearance of norepinephrine.

Figure 5 shows the plasma norepinephrine levels measured five minutes after assuming the standing position, and is expressed as a percent of supine levels in all three patient groups. While normal controls had over a 2 fold rise in standing norepinephrine level (217% ± 29%), the ability to activate the sympathetic nervous system was diminished in the hypertrophic and heart failure groups. In patients with hypertrophic cardiomyopathy, standing norepinephrine levels were 142% ± 16% of supine levels, significantly less than the control rise ($p<0.025$). In patients with heart failure, standing norepinephrine levels were only 110% ± 7% of supine levels ($p<0.01$ vs controls).

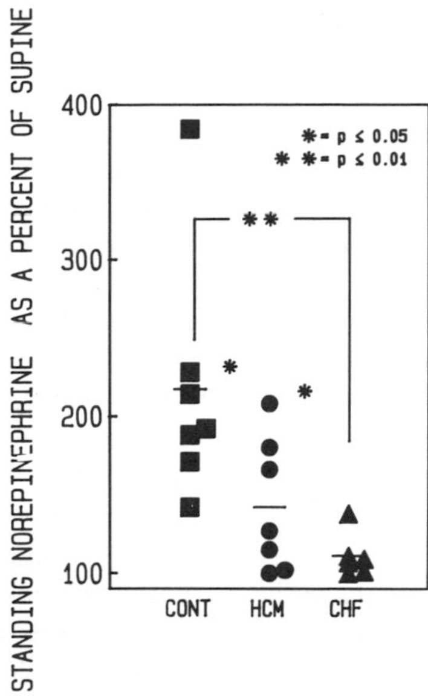

Fig. 5. Standing norepinephrine as a percent of supine norepinephrine in control ($n=8$), hypertrophic cardiomyopathy ($n=8$), and congestive heart failure ($n=7$).

DISCUSSION

The patients with hypertrophic cardiomyopathy spilled norepinephrine into plasma at an average of twice the rate of control subjects, and they cleared norepinephrine at twice the rate of patients with heart failure. The high plasma norepinephrine levels in hypertrophic cardiomyopathy are due to an increased influx of norepinephrine into the bloodstream, not to impaired norepinephrine clearance. The accelerated influx of norepinephrine into the bloodstream could be due to impaired intrasynaptic inactivation of norepinephrine after it is released from sympathetic nerves or to better transport of norepinephrine from the neuronal synapse to the bloodstream. The most straightforward explanation is that it represents increased sympathetic neuronal release of norepinephrine.

Value and Limitations of Kinetic Studies

Plasma norepinephrine levels do not always accurately reflect the amount of sympathetic release of norepinephrine,[19] because only a fraction of the norepinephrine released enters the plasma where it can be measured, and the plasma concentration is the product not only of the rate of diffusion into the plasma, but also the rate of removal, or clearance from the circulation. Thus changes in plasma norepinephrine concentration may result from alterations in plasma clearance, release, or both.

Kinetic techniques for estimating the rate of release of norepinephrine into plasma avoid the influence of norepinephrine plasma clearance.[17,19] Previous studies have shown that during a 90 minute infusion of labeled norepinephrine, a steady state is established, and that any re-release of tracer from sympathetic nerves is negligible in comparison with the rate of infusion.[19,21] Furthermore at typical rates of infusion of radiolabeled norepinephrine, the plasma concentration of ^{3}H-norepinephrine is insufficient to interfere materially with radioenzymatic plasma norepinephrine assays, and the elevation in plasma concentration of unlabeled norepinephrine is trivial (2–3 pg/ml).[18]

Samples for norepinephrine and ^{3}H-norepinephrine were drawn from a forearm vein so the norepinephrine kinetics measured include uptake and release of norepinephrine by the upper limb. The patients with congestive heart failure had a poor ejection fraction and presumably had diminished limb perfusion. Their low ^{3}H-norepinephrine clearance may have been affected by poor perfusion of their limbs.

Effects of Age and Drug Treatment on Norepinephrine Spillover and Clearance

Our hypertrophic cardiomyopathy patients were on average 14 years older than control subjects. Plasma norepinephrine concentration increases with age by about 13% per decade,[13] most likely reflecting reduced clearance.[22–24] While age may affect norepinephrine kinetics to some degree, it is unlikely that the marked changes we have observed are the result of age. Had the hypertrophic cardiomyopathy patients been younger, the clearance of norepinephrine would presumably have been even higher than observed. Additionally, Zeigler *et al.* have shown that beta blockers increase norepinephrine level by reducing clearance.[25] Two patients in the hypertrophic group who had clearances in the lower range (1.31, 1.24) were taking beta blockers at the time of the study, which would have decreased the measured norepinephrine clearance. Another patient whose norepinephrine clearance (1.38) was far below the mean was beginning to show signs of progressing to ventricular dilatation and disappearance of concentric hypertrophy, which once again might decrease clearance. When one takes into account the age and medications taken by the subjects, one could argue that patients with hypertrophic cardiomyopathy may have norepinephrine clearance rates greater than controls.

Norepinephrine Kinetic Differences between Hypertrophic Cardiomyopathy and Congestive Heart Failure

Patients with congestive heart failure consistently demonstrate elevated plasma norepinephrine levels.[26] The prognosis of patients with heart failure is perhaps more clearly linked to plasma norepinephrine concentration then to other variables such as left ventricular dysfunction.[27] Activation of the sympathetic nervous system is a normal response to diminished cardiac output.[28] The catecholamines initially improve cardiac output, but subsequently myocardial beta adrenergic receptors may down-regulate with eventual failure of the compensatory mechanisms.[29] Hasking *et al.* reported results similar to this study in their group of heart failure patients[30]: the increase in plasma norepinephrine concentration was related to increased norepinephrine spillover and reduced clearance. The reported prognostic significance of plasma norepinephrine levels in patients with congestive heart failure may in part reflect that a failing circulation clears norepinephrine from the bloodstream poorly.

Conversely, increased plasma norepinephrine in patients with hypertrophic cardiomyopathy is not caused by decreased cardiac output and does not imply a poor prognosis. Kawai studied myocardial norepinephrine concentration in endomyocardial biopsies both in patients with heart failure and hypertrophic cardiomyopathy.[31] In some of the cases of hypertrophic cardiomyopathy, the concentration of myocardial norepinephrine were extremely high in contrast to the low level present in heart failure. The elevated level of norepinephrine in hypertrophic cardiomyopathy does not appear to cause a significant change in beta adrenergic receptor or adenylate cyclase activity in the heart.[32] Thus while the poor prognosis in patients with heart failure showing high norepinephrine levels may be a manifestation of low cardiac output leading to decrease clearance of norepinephrine, in hypertrophic cardiomyopathy norepinephrine release is increased as well as its clearance, neither appearing to adversely affect prognosis. A prospective study relating norepinephrine levels in patients with hypertrophic cardiomyopathy to their clinical course would be of importance.

On standing, the baroreflexes stimulate norepinephrine release to maintain blood pressure. In congestive heart failure, baroreflexes are activated even while patients are supine, reflecting diminished tissue stores of norepinephrine.[33] These patients barely increased norepinephrine levels on standing. Patients with hypertrophic cardiomyopathy also had a significantly impaired postural norepinephrine response, perhaps because their sympathetic nervous activity is already elevated while they are recumbent.

A deficiency in the method we used for norepinephrine kinetics is the failure of measurements of total body norepinephrine turnover to discriminate between diseases which may alter norepinephrine kinetics in some organs but not others. In their study of heart failure Hasking *et al.*[30] sampled norepinephrine spillover in venous effluent of various organs. They found increased norepinephrine release not only in the heart, but in other organs as well, thereby suggesting a state of generalized increase in global sympathetic nervous system activity. Because the present study was done on outpatients, blood sampling from individual organs was not possible. Thus we cannot say whether the increase in norepinephrine activity we observed in hypertrophic cardiomyopathy is predominantly cardiac origin.

Implication of Norepinephrine Kinetics in the Pathophysiology of Hypertrophic Cardiomyopathy

Over the past 15 years there has been of speculation on the importance of the sympathetic nervous system in the development of hypertrophic cardiomyopathy,[34,35] Catecholamines stimulate hypertrophy of the growing myocardium; in contrast, heart failure usually causes high catecholamine levels later in life. Perloff proposed a possible genetic fault resulting in a disturbance of the interaction between immature, supersensitive adrenergic receptors and extra-cardiac catecholamines during fetal development.[35] The resulting heightened adrenergic stimulation of the developing myocardium might then result in early cellular disarray, and subsequent isometric contractions could then interfere with the normal regression of a disproportionately thickened septum. Clinical observations made in a group of otherwise unrelated diseases support this speculation. Several diseases have in common the occurrence of asymmetric septal hypertrophy with a disorder of the sympathetic nervous system. These include lentiginosis,[3,4] Von Recklinghausen's disease,[8] Friedriechs ataxia[5,6] infants of diabetic mothers,[8,9] and Pheochromocytoma.[7]

Thus it appears possible that altered catecholamine balance is related to the predisposition and or development of hypertrophic cardiomyopathy. This hypothesis could be tested by measuring norepinephrine kinetics in first degree relatives of patients with hypertrophic cardiomyopathy who do not yet have clinical manifestations of the disease.

The role of catecholamines in the causation of hypertrophic cardiomyopathy is speculative. However, there is clear evidence that the catecholamines and drugs that enhance catecholamine release stimulate myocardial hypertrophy. Conversely, catecholamine blocking drugs can lead to regression of myocardial hypertrophy. One would expect these drugs to be most effective in patients with the highest rates of catecholamine release.

Acknowledgments

The authors acknowledge the helpful suggestions and continuing support of Dr. Ralph Shabetai.

This work was supported by grants from the Veterans Administration, the National Institutes of Health, American Heart Association, and Clinical Research Center PHS PR 00827.

REFERENCES

1. Raum, W.J., Laks, M.M., Gainer, D., and Swordloff, R.S. α-adrenergic receptor and cyclic AMP alteration in the canine ventricular septum during long-term norepinephrine infusion: implications for hypertrophic cardiomyopathy. *Circulation* **68**: 693–699, 1983.
2. Witzke, D.J. and Kaye, M.P. Myocardial ultrastructural changes by administration of nerve growth factor. *Surg. Forum* **27**: 295–297, 1976.
3. Polani, P.E. and Myonahan, E.J. Progressive cardiomyopathic lentigenosis. *QJ. Med.* **42**: 295, 1972.
4. Somerville, J. and Bonhan-Carter, R.E. The heart in lentiginosis. *Br. Heart J.* **34**: 58, 1972.
5. Smith, E.R., Sangalang, V.E., Hefferman, L.R., Welch, J.P., and Flemington, C.S. Hypertrophic cardiomyopathy: The heart disease of Friedreichs ataxia. *Am. Heart J.* **94**: 428, 1977.
6. Thosen, C. Cardiomyopathy in Friedreichs ataxia. *J. Acta Paediat.* **153** (suppl): 1, 1964.
7. Serfas, D., Shoback, D.M., and Lorell, B.H. Pheochromocytoma and hypertrophic cardiomyopathy: Apparent suppression of symptoms and noradrenaline secretion by calcium-channel blockade. *Lancet* **2**: 711, 1983.
8. Elliott, C.M., Tajik, A.J., Giulian, E.R., and Gordon, H. Idiopathic hypertrophic subaortic stenosis associated with cutaneous neurofibromatosis. *Am. Heart J.* **92**: 368, 1976.
9. Way, G.L., Wolfe, R.R., Eshaghpour, E., Bender, R.L., Jaffee, R.B., and Rultenberg, H.B. The natural history of hypertrophic cardiomyopathy in infants of diabetic mothers. *J. Pediat.* **95**: 1020, 1979.
10. Gutgesell, H., Speer, M.E., and Rosenberg, H.S. Characterization of the cardiomyopathy in infants of diabetic mothers. *Circulation* **61**: 441, 1980.
11. Esler, M., Willet, I., Leonard, P., Hasking, G., Johns, J., Little, P., and Jennings, G. Plasma norepinephrine kinetics in humans. *J. Auton. Nerv. Sys.* **11**: 125, 1984.
12. Hoeldtke, R.D., Cilmi, K.M., Reichard, G.A., Jr., Bodin, G., and Oren, V.E. Assessment of norepinephrine secretion and production. *J. Lab. Clin. Med.* **101**: 772, 1983.
13. Esler, M., Skews, H., Leonard, P., Jackman, G., Bobik, A., and Korner, P. Age dependence of noradrenaline kinetics in normal subjects. *Clin. Sci.* **60**: 217, 1981.
14. Cryer, P.E. Physiology and pathophysiology of the human sympathoadrenal neuroendocrine system. *N. Eng. J. Med.* **303**: 136–144, 1980.
15. Maron, B.J., Bonow, R.O., Cannon, R.O., Leon, M.B., and Epstein, S.E. Hypertrophic cardiomyopathy. *N. Engl. J. Med.* **316**: 780, 1987.
16. Kopin, I.J. Biochemical assessment of peripheral adrenergic activity. In: The Release of Catecholamines from Adrenergic Neurons, D.M. Paton (Ed.) Pergamon Press, Oxford, 1979, pp. 355–372.
17. Shipley, R.A. and Clarke, R.E. Tracer Methods for *in vivo* Kinetics. New York: Academia, 145–162, 1972.
18. Esler, M.G., Jackman, G., Bojik, A., Kelleher, D., Jennings, G., Leonard, P., Skews, H., and Korner, P. Determination of norepinephrine apparent release rate and clearance in humans. *Life Sci.* **25**: 1461, 1979.
19. Esler, M. Assessment of sympathetic nervous function in humans from noradrenaline plasma kinetics. *Clin. Sci.* **62**: 247, 1982.
20. Fitzgerald, G.A., Hossman, V., Hamilton, C.A., Reid, J.Z., Davies, D.S., and Dollery, C.T.

Interindividual variation in kinetics of infused norepinephrine. *Clin. Pharmacol. Ther.* **26**: 669, 1979.
21. Watson, R.D.S., Esler, M., Leonard, P., and Korner, P.I. Influence of variation in dietary sodium intake on biochemical indices of sympathetic function in normal man. *Clin. Exp. Physiol. Pharmacia* **11**: 1963, 1984.
22. Rubin, P.C., Scott, P.J.W., McLean, K., and Reid, J.L. Noradrenaline release and clearance in relation to age and blood pressure in man. *Europ. J. Clin. Invest.* **12**: 121, 1982.
23. Lake, C.R., Ziegler, M.G., Coleman, M.D., and Kopin, I.J. Age-adjusted plasma norepinephrine levels are similar in normotensive and hypertensive subjects. *N. Eng. J. Med.* **296**: 208, 1977.
24. Goldstein, D.S., Lake, C.R., Cheinow, B., Ziegler, M.G., Coleman, M.P., Taylor, A.A., Mitchell, J.R., Koin, I.J., and Keiser, H.R. Age-dependence of hypertensive-normotensive differences in plasma norepinephrine. *Hypertension* **5**: 100, 1983.
25. Ziegler, M.G., Chernow, B., Woodson, L.C., Coyle, J., Cruess, D., and Lake, C.R. The effect of propranolol on catecholamine clearance. *Clin. Pharmacol. Ther.* **440**: 116–119, 1986.
26. Thomas, J.A. and Marks, B.H. Plasma norepinephrine in congestive heart failure. *Am. J. Cardiol.*, **41**: 233–243, 1978.
27. Cohn, J.N., Levine, T.B., and Olivari, M.T. Plasma norepinephrine as a guide to prognosis in patients with chronic congestive heart failure. *N. Engl. J. Med.*, **311**: 819, 1984.
28. Gaffney, E.T. and Braunwald, E. Importance of the adrenergic nervous system in the support of circulatory function in patients with congestive heart failure. *Am. J. Med.* **34**: 320, 1983.
29. Bistow, M.R., Ginsburg, R., Minobe W, *et al.*: Decreased catecholamine sensitivity and β-adrenergic-receptor density in failing human hearts. *N. Engl. J. Med.* **307**: 205, 1982.
30. Hasking, G.J., Esler, M.D., Jennings, G.L., Burton, K.D., Johns, J.A., and Korner, P.I. Norepinephrine spillover to plasma in patients with congestive heart failure: evidence of increased overall and cardiorenal sympathetic nervous system activity. *Circulation* **73**: 4: 615, 1986.
31. Kawai, C., Yui, Y., Hoshino, L., Sasayama, S., and Matsumori, A. Myocardial catecholamines in hypertrophic and dilated (congestive) cardiomyopathy: A biopsy study.
32. Golf, S., Myhse, E., Abdelnoor, M., Anderson, P., and Hansson, V. Hypertrophic cardiomyopathy characterized by β-adrenoreceptor density, relative amount of β-adrenoreceptor subtypes and adenylate cyclase activity. *Cardiovasc. Rev.* **19**: 693–699, 1985.
33. Bishop, V.S., Malliani, and Thoren, P. Cardiac mechano receptors. In: Handbook of Physiology, Shepherd, J.T., and Abboud, F.M. (Eds.) Scand, 2, Vol. III, Part 2. Bethesda, American Physiologic Society, 1983, p. 497–555.
34. Goodwin, J.F. Prospects and predictions for cardiomyopathics. *Circulation* **50**: 210, 1974.
35. Perloff, J.K. Pathogenesis of hypertrophic cardiomyopathy: hypothesis and speculations. *A.H.J.* 219–220, 1981.

Increased Cardiovascular Responses to Epinephrine and Norepinephrine in Patients with Hypertrophic Cardiomyopathy

Hironori Toshima and Yoshinori Koga

The Third Department of Medicine, Kurume University School of Medicine, Kurume, Japan

ABSTRACT

Hypertrophic cardiomyopathy (HCM) is generally accepted to be transmitted genetically, although the exact mechanism leading to abnormal ventricular hypertrophy is not yet fully understood. Among various mechanisms previously suggested, a link between abnormal catecholamine metabolism and HCM has long attracted many investigators. Nevertheless, there is insufficient evidence regarding augmented sympathetic activities or increased myocardial and plasma norepinephrine levels in this condition. We therefore investigated the cardiovascular responses to the intravenous infusion of epinephrine or norepinephrine in patients with HCM.

Compared with age- and sex-matched control subjects, patients with HCM responded earlier to the lower dosage of epinephrine in terms of echocardiographic left ventricular systolic dimension, fractional shortening, and peak systolic velocity of the posterior wall. The fall in diastolic blood pressure was greater in HCM. Norepinephrine induced significantly greater increases in mean blood pressure, peripheral vascular resistance, and left ventricular contractility in patients with HCM, while a reduction in fractional shortening was less evident.

These observations indicate that the cardiovascular responses to α_1- or β-adrenergic stimulation are increased in patients with HCM. We accordingly propose that increased activity of the cardiovascular adrenergic receptor systems, rather than enhanced sympathetic activity, may be related to the development of abnormal hypertrophy in HCM.

INTRODUCTION

Although hypertrophic cardiomyopathy (HCM) is generally accepted to be genetically transmitted, the exact mechanism that causes abnormal ventricular hypertrophy is not yet fully understood. Recent studies, however, have demonstrated that abnormal hypertrophy is not always present at or shortly after birth, but may develop later in life.[1,2] Figure 1 illustrates a representative patient who demonstrated asymmetric septal hypertrophy and systolic anterior motion of the mitral valve that developed over the past 10 years. The patient also showed right bundle branch block and left precordial negative T-waves. These observations suggest that elucidation of the underlying mechanism involved in abnormal hypertrophy could be of clinical benefit in helping to provide an effective strategy to prevent morphological expression of the disease.

There is substantial evidence suggesting a link between abnormal catecholamine metabolism and HCM.[3-5] In experimental animals, a condition resembling HCM has been produced by subhypertensive dosages of norepinephrine infusion[6,7] and by the

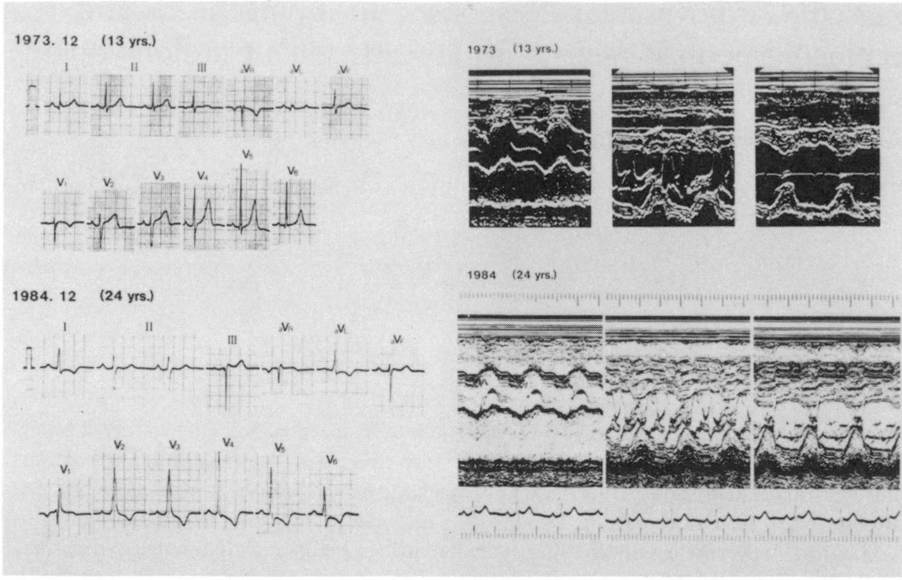

Fig. 1. A representative patient in whom the morphological expression of HCM evolved over 11 years. At age 13, when his older brother was diagnosed as having HCM, he had a family survey but showed no findings characteristic to HCM. After 11 years, at age 24, he developed asymmetric septal hypertrophy and systolic anterior motion of the mitral valve with right bundle branch block and T-wave inversion. Cardiac catheterization confirmed the diagnosis of obstructive HCM by revealing an intraventricular pressure gradient of 25 mmHg.

administration of nerve growth factor,[8] which leads to increased growth of the sympathetic nerve fibers and thereby increases catecholamines. Olsen *et al.*[9,10] administered tri-idothyroacetic acid (triac) to pregnant rats and produced myofibrillar disarray and hypertrophy in the hearts of their offspring. They proposed that the resulting changes were ascribable to indirect adrenergic stimulation rather than to the direct action of triac. Clinical diagnosis of HCM has been reported in such neural crest diseases as neurofibromatosis,[11] lentiginosis,[12-14] and pheochromocytoma.[15] An association of HCM has been further observed with hyperthyroidism[16,17] and hyperinsulinism,[18] conditions with either increased production or increased sensitivity of the myocardial cells to catecholamines. On the basis of this evidence, Goodwin[19] has suggested that HCM is a genetically determined disorder in which catecholamines are handled improperly by the developing fetal heart. More recently, Perloff[3] reviewed the role of catecholamines in the pathogenesis of HCM, and proposed the "cathecholamine hypothesis": faulty interaction between an adrenergic stimulus and the adrenergic receptor sites *in utero* may play a fundamental role in initiating myocardial cellular disarray and in setting the stage for subsequent progression to clinically overt HCM.

We therefore studied plasma catecholamine levels during exercise and the cardiovascular responses to epinephrine and norepinephrine in patients with HCM. This paper summarizes our results and discusses briefly our hypothesis that increased activity of the adrenergic receptor systems may be involved in the pathogenesis of HCM.

SYMPATHETIC NERVE ACTIVITY IN HCM

Despite increasing evidence suggesting a link between HCM and catecholamines, considerable controversy still exists concerning myocardial and plasma catecholamine levels in patients with HCM. In 1964, Pearse[20] reported that norepinephrine content and sympathetic innervation were increased in septal muscle obtained by myectomy in patients with obstructive HCM. Subsequent studies by McCallister and Brown[21] and Van Noorden *et al.*,[22] however, failed to confirm this observation. In a recent study by Kawai *et al.*,[23] who determined the myocardial catecholamine content in biopsy specimens, some patients with HCM showed exceptionally high concentrations of myocardial norepinephrine, while its mean value was not significantly higher than that in those with other types of heart disease who served as a control group. They thus failed to show increased stores of myocardial norepinephrine in patients with HCM.

In work on plasma catecholamines, Dargie *et al.*[24] reported increased norepinephrine levels at rest or standing in patients with HCM. In contrast, Sugishita *et al.*[25] described no differences in plasma norepinephrine levels at rest and at peak exercise between patients with HCM and control subjects, while the level at low-grade exercise was lower in patients with HCM. Myocardial release of norepinephrine in patients with HCM was not increased in the study by Haneda *et al.*[26]

We also compared plasma catecholamine levels at rest and during exercise between 26 patients with nonobstructive HCM and asymmetric septal hypertrophy and 26 age- and sex-matched healthy controls (Fig. 2). There was no difference in the plasma norepinephrine levels at rest between the control subjects and patients with HCM (233 ± 100 vs 201 ± 84 pg/ml). However, the norepinephrine values at rest significantly correlated with age in both groups ($r = 0.63$, $P < 0.001$ for HCM, and $r = 0.73$, $P < 0.001$ for control

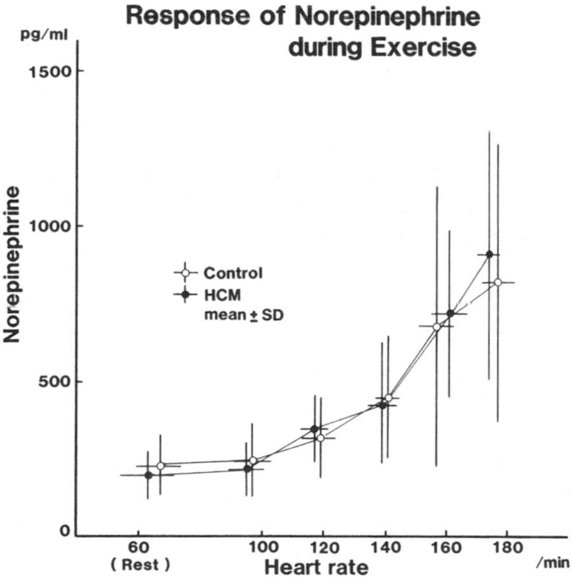

Fig. 2. Plasma norepinephrine levels in patients with hypertrophic cardiomyopathy (●) did not differ from those of controls (○), either at rest or at any time during exercise. Values are expressed as means ± SD.

subjects), in agreement with the previous report[27] showing increased plasma norepinephrine levels with age. During exercise, plasma norepinephrine values increased gradually in both groups, but again no difference between the two groups was observed.

Our results are in contrast with the findings of Dargie *et al.*,[24] but largely compatible with those of Sugishita *et al.*,[25] although we could not demonstrate a depressed increase in norepinephrine levels during low-grade exercise. As our study excluded patients with outflow obstruction, a different patient population may explain the inconsistencies in plasma norepinephrine levels in these studies. Although further studies are needed, our results suggest that sympathetic activity either at rest or during exercise is not higher in patients with HCM.

Hence, there does not seem to be sufficient evidence that myocardial or plasma norepinephrine is increased in patients with HCM. It is postulated therefore that neither augmented sympathetic activity nor increased norepinephrine is a mechanism inducing abnormal hypertrophy in patients with HCM.

RESPONSES TO EPINEPHRINE AND NOREPINEPHRINE IN PATIENTS WITH HCM

When a sympathetic nerve is stimulated, norepinephrine is released from the nerve ending, binds onto the adrenergic receptors of the cell, and activates a chain of intracellular biochemical reactions that lead to the expression of the final cellular response to the stimuli. Enhanced adrenergic function could accordingly be manifested by either an excess release of norepinephrine, increased number or affinity of the adrenergic receptors, or augmented activity in the intracellular biochemical pathway. The lack of sufficient evidence for increased plasma or myocardial catecholamines in patients with HCM has led us to our hypothesis that increased activity in the adrenergic receptors or in the subsequent intracellular pathway might be involved in the pathogenesis of HCM. We[28,29] therefore investigated the cardiovascular responses of patients with HCM to the naturally functioning catecholamines, epinephrine and norepinephrine.

Cardiovascular Responses to Epinephrine

The subjects consisted of 21 patients with nonobstructive HCM, 21 males and five females, with an average age of 37 ± 3 (SE) years. They included 17 patients with asymmetric septal hypertrophy and four with apical hypertrophy who showed the spade-shaped configuration on the left ventriculogram. Patients with intraventricular pressure gradient under basal conditions were excluded from the study, because any outflow obstruction might alter the left ventricular response to epinephrine. Twenty-one healthy volunteers, matched for age and sex, served as control subjects.

After the subjects rested for 20 min in the supine position, epinephrine was infused using a Truth infusion pump Type B-1 (Nakagawa Sekikodo Co., Ltd., Tokyo). The dosage of epinephrine was doubled every 6 min from an initial dose of 0.0185 μg/kg/min to 0.037 μg/kg/min and then to 0.074 μg/kg/min. M-mode echocardiogram, electrocardiogram, and cuff blood pressure were recorded in the baseline period and repeated every 3 min during the infusion. As the initial dose (0.0185 μg/kg/min) of epinephrine did not induce appreciable changes in hemodynamic measurements, the average of the readings at baseline and at 6 min after the initial dose infusion was taken as the baseline value. Readings during the lower (0.037 μg/kg/min) and higher (0.074 μg/kg/min) dose infusions were obtained by averaging the measurements at 3 and 6 min in each stage.

The effects of epinephrine were evaluated by deriving percentage changes from the baseline measurements.

Table 1 summarizes the cardiovascular responses to epinephrine in the patients with HCM and in the control subjects. During the low-dose infusion, the increases in heart rate were comparable in both groups and systolic blood pressure remained unchanged, while the fall in diastolic blood pressure tended to be greater in the patients with HCM. Patients with HCM showed significantly greater responses than control subjects in left ventricular end-systolic dimension, fractional shortening, and peak systolic velocity of the left ventricular posterior wall, while the end-diastolic dimension remained unchanged in both groups. Therefore, the response of the systolic performance of the left ventricle to low-dose epinephrine was increased in patients with HCM.

High-dose infusion of epinephrine further decreased the left ventricular end-systolic dimension and increased fractional shortening and peak systolic velocity of the left ventricular posterior wall. These responses were observed to be greater in the control subjects. The significant differences that were observed during low-dose infusion between the two groups were therefore not found during the high-dose infusion. The greater fall

TABLE 1. Percent Changes in Hemodynamic Measurements during Low (0.037 μg/kg/min) and High (0.074 μg/kg/min) Dose Infusion of Epinephrine

	Total (n = 21)		Younger (n = 9) (<35 years)		Older (n = 12) (≧35 years)	
Dose	HCM	Control	HCM	Control	HCM	Control
Heart rate						
Low	9±3	8±2	11±4	8±1	8±3	9±3
High	17±3	13±2	20±5*	8±2	15±3	17±3
Blood pressure						
Systolic						
Low	0±2	0±1	3±3	0±1	− 3±2	0±1
High	7±2	2±2	11±2	1±5	4±2	2±2
Diastolic						
Low	−18±4	− 8±1	−29±4**	− 7±2	−10±4	− 8±2
High	−26±4*	−12±3	−36±7**	−11±5	−17±4	−13±3
Left ventricular dimension						
End-diastole						
Low	1±1	1±0	2±1	0±0	1±1	1±1
High	3±1	2±1	4±1	1±1	4±1	3+1
End-systole						
Low	− 8±1*	− 4±1	−10±2**	− 3±1	− 7±1	− 5±1
High	−12±2	−12±1	−15±3	−13±2	−10±2	−11±1
Fractional shortening						
Low	12±2*	7±1	15±4	6±1	11±2	8±2
High	19±2	23±2	23±5	28±4	17±2	20±3
Peak PWV						
Low	32±5*	15±4	44±9*	17±6	29±4	16±6
High	61±6	51±7	66±11	53±9	62±7	49±12

Values are means ± SEM.
* $P < 0.05$, ** $P < 0.01$ compared with controls.
HCM = hypertrophic cardiomyopathy, PWV = systolic velocity of the left ventricular posterior wall.

in diastolic blood pressure in patients with HCM attained a statistically significant level during high-dose infusion, while responses of heart rate, systolic blood pressure, and end-diastolic diameter of the left ventricle were similar in the two groups.

The greater response in systolic left ventricular performance of the control subjects during high-dose infusion and the disappearance of the difference (observed during low-dose infusion) were contrary to our expectations. However, it is known that the relationship between the left ventricular pump function and contractility is curvilinear, with increases in stroke volume and ejection fraction becoming smaller after reaching a certain level (usually at around an ejection fraction of 60–70%) despite a constant increase in contractility.[30] Patients with HCM who have augmented pump function at rest could be expected to attain this plateau level easily during epinephrine infusion. The observed response of fractional shortening to epinephrine of patients with HCM was indeed inversely correlated with the baseline value ($r=-0.60$, $P<0.01$ during low-dose infusion, and $r=-0.61$, $P<0.01$ during high-dose infusion). Therefore, the curvilinear relationship between the left ventricular pump function and contractility could explain the disappearance of the significant difference in left ventricular systolic performance between the two groups during high-dose epinephrine. From these considerations, we suggest that during low-dose infusion, the left ventricle of patients with HCM started to respond earlier to epinephrine, which had no appreciable effects on the control subjects. Hence, patients with HCM appear to have a predisposition for increased left ventricular responsiveness to epinephrine.

The response of diastolic blood pressure to epinephrine was again greater in patients with HCM, and the difference attained a statistically significant level during high-dose infusion. The vasodilatory response of the peripheral arteries was thus postulated to be augmented in patients with HCM. These increased responses in the left ventricle and peripheral arteries of patients with HCM may indicate that activity of the β-adrenergic receptor system of the cardiovascular system is increased in this condition.

Another interesting finding in our study was the relationship between the response to epinephrine and age. When the study patients were arbitrarily divided into a younger group (<35 years) and an older group (≥ 35 years), increased responses to epinephrine of patients with HCM in terms of left ventricular systolic function and diastolic blood pressure became more evident in the younger group (Table 1). The younger patients with HCM also showed a greater increase in heart rate during high-dose infusion of epinephrine than age- and sex-matched controls. In contrast, the older patients with HCM presented no appreciable differences from controls in their responses to epinephrine. More advanced myocardial damage in older patients could be one possible explanation for this variance between the two age-groups. However, this seems unlikely, since the younger and older groups did not differ in left ventricular wall thicknesses and dimensions, fractional shortening, peak systolic velocity of the left ventricular posterior wall, or left ventricular end-diastolic pressure. An alternative explanation may be a different clinical profile and possibly different pathogenetic background between the younger and older patients with HCM, as discussed later.

Iida *et al.*[31] similarly investigated the left ventricular response to isoproterenol (0.02 μg/kg/min) in patients with HCM. They again reported that nine HCM patients with asymmetric septal hypertrophy presented a greater increase in the normalized peak rate of change in left ventricular dimension during systole than control subjects (4.5 ± 1.5 vs 2.6 ± 0.8/sec, $P<0.01$), although a further nine patients with symmetric hypertrophy showed no difference in response. They then suggested that the β-adrenergic receptor

TABLE 2. Percent Changes from Baseline Values during Norepinephrine Infusion in Patients with HCM, against Age- and Sex-matched Controls

		Norepinephrine (μg/kg/min)			
		0.06	0.12	0.16	0.20
%△MBP	Control	2±3	5±7	9±4	14±5
	HCM	5±7*	12±8**	20±6***	29±7***
%△PVR	Control	6±4	13±5	20±7	26±7
	HCM	9±8	19±8**	31±5***	39±7***
%△HR	Control	−3±4	−8±4	−11±3	−13±4
	HCM	−5±3	−10±4	−15±3***	−17±5**
%△FS	Control	0.2±0.3	−0.4±1.0	−0.6±1.2	−1.4±1.5
	HCM	0.3±1.0	0.3±1.7	0.4±3.0	0.6±3.0**
%△SBP/ESD	Control	1±5	4±6	7±6	13±6
	HCM	3±4	9±6**	19±8***	31±7***

Values are expressed as means±SD.
* $P<0.05$, ** $P<0.01$, *** $P<0.001$ as compared with controls.
HCM = hypertrophic cardiomyopathy, MBP = mean blood pressure, PVR = peripheral vascular resistance, HR = heart rate, FS = fractional shortening, SBP = systolic blood pressure, ESD = end-systolic dimension.

system is hypersensitive in HCM patients with asymmetric septal hypertrophy, in agreement with our observations. Although they could not show greater responses to isoproterenol in other indices of left ventricular function or in diastolic blood pressure in patients with HCM as we did, it is of note that their subjects included only elderly patients (over 40 years) with HCM, a group that showed no appreciable differences in response to epinephrine in our study.

Cardiovascular Responses to Norepinephrine

The subjects consisted of 26 patients with nonobstructive HCM and asymmetric septal hypertrophy. There were 21 males and five females, with an average age of 39±13 (SD) years. Neither patients with left ventricular outflow obstruction under basal conditions nor those with apical hypertrophy showing the spade-shaped configuration on the left ventriculogram were included in the study. Twenty-six healthy volunteers, matched for age and sex, served as control subjects.

After subjects had 30 min of bed rest, norepinephrine was infused using a Treonic 1P4 infusion pump (Vickers Medical) with stepwise increases every 5 min in doses from the initial 0.06 μg/kg/min to a final 0.20 μg/kg/min. Cuff blood pressure, echocardiogram, and electrocardiogram were recorded twice during the baseline period and repeated at 4 and 5 min at each step of norepinephrine infusion. After the measurements were averaged, the percentage changes from the baseline values were derived to evaluate the response to norepinephrine.

Table 3 summarizes the cardiovascular responses to norepinephrine. Norepinephrine increased systolic, diastolic, and mean blood pressures, and systemic vascular resistance dose dependently both in patients with HCM and control subjects. The increases were greater in the patients with HCM, with significantly different levels at the doses of 0.12 μg/kg/min or more. These observations indicate that the vasoconstrictive response of the peripheral arteries to norepinephrine is augmented in patients with HCM. Heart rate decreased to a greater extent during norepinephrine infusion in the patients with

TABLE 3. Relationship between Responses to Norepinephrine vs Clinical Findings in Patients with HCM

	%△PVR		%△SBP/ESD	
	Normal response	Increased response	Normal response	Increased response
No. of patients	15	11	7	19
Age (years)	37±13	42±13	50±5	35±13**
Family history	9/15	4/11	1/7	12/19*
HR (beats/min)	63±6	64±12	60±6	64±9
MBP (mmHg)	82±13	86±10	89±9	82±12
Norepinephrine (pg/ml)	185±82	224±85	264±69	178±78*
IVST (mm)	18±7	21±4	19±3	20±7
PWT (mm)	12±7	11±3	12±3	12±3
FS (%)	41±7	42±4	43±8	41±6

Values are means ± SD or number of patients.
* $P<0.05$, ** $P<0.01$ as compared with normal response group.
PVR = peripheral vascular resistance, SBP = systolic blood pressure, ESD = end-systolic dimension, HR = heart rate, MBP = mean blood pressure, IVST = interventricular septal thickness, PWT = posterior wall thickness, FS = fractional shortening.

HCM, possibly reflecting a greater elevation in blood pressure. In the echocardiogram, fractional shortening was reduced significantly in control subjects in association with increasing systolic pressure, while it remained unchanged in those with HCM despite a greater increase in systolic pressure. The different responses reached statistically significant levels at 0.20 μg/kg/min of norepinephrine infusion. The ratio of systolic blood pressure to end-systolic dimension of the left ventricle (SBP/ESD), derived as an index approximating left ventricular contractility, increased dose dependently in both groups, though the increase was again greater in the patients with HCM. The inotropic response of the left ventricular muscle to norepinephrine thus seemed to be increased in patients with HCM. As norepinephrine is known to have β_1 activity in addition to α_1 and α_2 stimulation, these findings suggest that patients with HCM have increased sensitivity of the β_1-receptor system of the left ventricular muscle and the α_1-receptor system of the peripheral arteries.

We further investigated the relationship between the responses to norepinephrine and the clinical profile of patients with HCM (Table 3). Eleven patients with HCM showed an increased response in peripheral vascular resistance, exceeding the 95% confidence interval of that of the control subjects. However, those with higher responses did not differ in their clinical profile from the 15 patients with normal responses. In contrast, the 19 patients with increased responses of SBP/ESD to norepinephrine were significantly younger in age and demonstrated more frequent familial occurrence. Although significantly lower in these patients with increased responses, the plasma norepinephrine levels did not differ from those of their age- and sex-matched controls. It therefore seems likely that increased vasoconstrictive response of the peripheral arteries to norepinephrine is a finding common to any patient with HCM, while enhanced inotropic response of the left ventricle is a characteristic of younger patients. These observations were consistent with the results of epinephrine infusion tests which demonstrated increased responses mainly in the younger patients with HCM.

POSSIBLE ROLE OF ADRENERGIC RECEPTOR SYSTEMS IN THE DEVELOPMENT OF HCM

Our observations that responses to epinephrine and norepinephrine are increased in patients with HCM would suggest that such patients have augmented activities in the adrenergic receptor systems of the cardiovascular system. One possible explanation for these observations could be the left ventricular hypertrophy per se, since alterations in the numbers of adrenergic receptors or in responses to catecholamines have been described in various models of left ventricular hypertrophy. An increased number of β-receptors has been reported in left ventricular hypertrophy induced by aortic constriction,[32] two-kidney one-clip renal hypertension,[33,34] or drug-induced hypertension using either guanethidine[35] or 6-hydroxydopamine.[36] In contrast, spontaneously hypertensive rats have been shown to have a decreased number of β-receptors and impaired responses to catecholamine.[34,37–39] Whereas alterations in β-receptors vary with experimental models, Hoffman and Lefkowitz[40] have postulated that myocardial catecholamines may modulate myocardial β-receptors, since the models with increased receptor density have been reported to be associated with depletion in myocardial norepinephrine, while spontaneously hypertensive rats have shown an increased norepinephrine content. Myocardial α_1-receptors have recently been suggested to be similarly modulated by myocardial norepinephrine.[41,42]

In patients with HCM, there seems to be no evidence to suggest alterations in plasma catecholamine and sympathetic activity as discussed before. The myocardial norepinephrine content in patients with HCM was not reduced, and was even higher in some patients, in a study by Kawai *et al.*[23] It seems unlikely therefore that the increased responses to epinephrine and norepinephrine are ascribable to any depletion in myocardial norepinephrine with a consequent up-regulation in adrenergic receptor systems. It might thus be suggested that increased responsiveness in the adrenergic receptor systems is an inherent abnormality of patients with HCM. This postulation is further supported by the increased responses to epinephrine and norepinephrine in the peripheral arteries of these patients, which may not be involved in the disease process of HCM.

Golf *et al.*[43] recently investigated β-receptor density and adenylate cyclase activity in five patients with obstructive HCM, using ventricular septal muscle excised during operation. Although they could not support the hypothesis that HCM is a disorder with an altered β-adrenergic receptor system, their control subjects included those with ventricular hypertrophy who had been shown to have a reduction in myocardial norepinephrine[44] which could lead to up-regulation in the receptors. In contrast, Raum *et al.*[45] and we[46] have demonstrated that myocardial norepinephrine is not increased, but is actually reduced, in experimental ventricular hypertrophy induced by a subhypertensive dose of norepinephrine infusion. We were thus unable to show that direct stimulation of norepinephrine on adrenergic receptors induces myocardial hypertrophy, but rather postulated that the alterations in adrenergic receptor activities observed in this model might be involved in the development of hypertrophy. In cardiomyopathic hamsters, Kajiya *et al.*[47] observed increases in myocardial α_1- and β-receptor numbers and suggested a relation to myocardial hypertrophy prior to the development of heart failure in this animal. Since spontaneously hypertensive rats are another model predisposed to ventricular hypertrophy prior to an elevation of blood pressure,[48,49] we[50] investigated responses to norepinephrine using cultured neonatal cardiomyocytes. As compared with cultured cells from Wistar Kyoto rats, spontaneously hypertensive rats showed increased chronotropic and hypertrophic responses, augmented production of cAMP after exposure to norepinephrine, and a greater number of α_1-receptors. These results again suggest that the predisposition to ventricular hypertrophy in this animal is related to increased activity of the adrenergic receptors. The accumulating evidence thus indicates that it is conceivable that increased activities of adrenergic receptor systems could play an important clinical role in the development of ventricular hypertrophy in patients with HCM.

Although the receptor pathway by which catecholamines induce myocardial hypertrophy is not yet fully understood, recent studies by Simpson *et al.*[51] and Inuzuka[52] from our laboratory have shown that the α_1-receptor cascade can mediate the induction of hypertrophy. An increased vasoconstrictive response in the peripheral arteries to norepinephrine, possibly mediated by α_1-receptors, in patients with HCM was an interesting finding in this respect, although we could not investigate the responsiveness of α_1-receptors in the myocardium. The role of the β-receptor system in ventricular hypertrophy is even less well defined, although β-stimulation is well documented to enhance cardiac function and dilate the peripheral arteries. Inuzuka[52] implied a possibility that β-stimulation could lead to the production of an additional hypertrophic effect in cultured myocardial cells in the presence of α_1-stimulation, while β-stimulation alone could not incuce this. It is of note in this regard that increased β-receptor activity, as suggested by the augmented responses of left ventricular function to epinephrine and norepinephrine and the enhanced vasodilatory responses of the peripheral arteries to epinephrine, was notably observed in the younger patients with HCM. In our clinical experience,[54] these younger patients with HCM generally show familial occurrence and more severe impairment in the diastolic and systolic functions of the left ventricle associated with a higher risk of sudden death. In contrast to these features of younger patients, which are consistent with the classical form of HCM, elderly patients often include those with a history of mild or labile hypertension, but without evidence of familial occurrence. Left ventricular function is usually less impaired and the prognosis is favorable, with rare sudden death. We have therefore suggested that the pathogenetic background may differ between younger and elderly patients with HCM, although the morphological appearance is similar. This clinical experience might be explained by the different responses to epinephrine and norepinephrine: HCM patients with increased activities of both α_1- and β-receptor systems manifest abnormal hypertrophy in earlier life, while those with increased α_1-receptor activity alone may develop the disease more slowly later in life, in association with mild hypertension.

In conclusion, we suggest that increased activities of the myocardial adrenergic receptor systems, rather than increased sympathetic tone, may be the inherent abnormalities of patients with HCM that are involved in the development of excessive hypertrophy. However, it should be noted that these observations were made in patients with HCM who had already developed ventricular hypertrophy. To confirm our hypothesis, we need further prospective studies that investigate sympathetic tone and adrenergic receptor activities, with subsequent echocardiographic follow-up, in relatives of those patients who have yet not manifested the disease.

Acknowledgment

This study was supported in part by a Research Grant for Intractable Diseases from the Ministry of Health and Welfare of Japan.

REFERENCES

1. Maron, B.J., Spirito, P., Wesley Y., and Arce, J. Development and progression of left ventricular hypertrophy in children with hypertrophic cardiomyopathy. *N. Engl. J. Med.* **315**: 610–14, 1986.
2. Shida, M., Miyazaki, Y., Matsuyama, K., Iwami, G., Ooga, M., Chiba, M., Furuta, Y., Toshima, H., and Koga, Y. Hypertrophic cardiomyopathy manifesting different modes of illness. Report of three cases. *J. Cardiology* **17**: 187–97, 1987. (in Japanese)
3. Perloff, J.K. Pathogenesis of hypertrophic cardiomyopathy: Hypotheses and speculations. *Am. Heart J.* **101**: 219–26, 1981.
4. Goodwin, O.K. The frontiers of cardiomyopathy. *Br. Heart J.* **48**: 1–18, 1982.
5. Dargie, H.J. and Goodwin, J.F. Catecholamines, cardiomyopathies and cardiac function. *Prog. Cardiol.* **11**: 93–106, 1982.
6. Laks, M.M., Morady, F., and Swan, H.J.C. Myocardial hypertrophy produced by chronic infusion of subhypertensive doses of norepinephrine in the dog. *Chest* **64**: 75–8, 1973.
7. Blaufuss, A.H., Laks, M.M., Garner, D., Ishimoto, B.M., and Criley, J.M. Production of ventricular hypertrophy simulating "idiopathic hypertrophic subaortic stenosis" (IHSS) by subhypertensive infusion of norepinephrine (NE) in the conscious dog. *Clin. Res.* **23**: 77A, 1975. (abstr.)
8. Witzke, D.J. and Kaye, M.P. Myocardial ultrastructural changes induced by administration of nerve growth factor. *Surg. Forum* **27**: 295–97, 1976.
9. Olsen, E.G.J., Symons, C., and Hawkey, C. Effect of triac on the developing heart. *Lancet* **ii**: 221–23, 1977.
10. Olsen, E.G.J. An endocrine experimental model for myofibrillar disarray. In: Cardiomyopathy Update 1, Pathogenesis of myocarditis and cardiomyopathy, Kawai, C. and Abelmann, W.H. (eds.), University of Tokyo Press, Tokyo 1987, pp. 163–71.
11. Elliott, C.M., Tajik, A.J., Giuliani, E.R., and Gordon, H. Idiopathic hypertrophic subaortic stenosis associated with cutaneous neurofibromatosis: report of a case. *Am. Heart J.* **92**: 368–72, 1976.
12. Polany, P.E. and Moynahan, E.J. Progressive cardiomyopathic lentiginosis. *Q. J. Med.* **41**: 205–25, 1972.
13. Somerville, J. and Bonham-Carter, R.E. The heart in lentiginosis. *Br. Heart J.* **34**: 58–66, 1972.
14. St. John Sutton, M.G., Tajik, A.J., Giuliani, E.R., Gordon, H., and Daniel Su, W.P. Hypertrophic obstructive cardiomyopathy and lentiginosis: a little known neural ectodermal syndrome. *Am. J. Cardiol.* **47**: 214–17, 1981.
15. Shub, C., Williamson, M.D., Tajik, A.J., and Eubanks, D.R. Dynamic left ventricular outflow tract obstruction associated with pheochromocytoma. *Am. Heart J.* **102**: 286–90, 1981.
16. Symons, C., Richardson, P.J., and Feizi, O. Hypertrophic cardiomyopathy and hyperthyroidism: a report of three cases. *Thorax* **29**: 713–19, 1974.
17. Bell, R., Barber, P.V., Bray, C.L., and Beton, D.C. Incidence of thyroid disease in cases of hypertrophic cardiomyopathy. *Br. Heart J.* **40**: 1306–9, 1978.
18. Rosenberg, A.M., Haworth, J.C., Degroot, G.W., Trevenen, C.L., and Rechler, M.M. A case of leprechaunism with severe hyperinsulinemia. *Am. J. Dis. Child.* **134**: 170–5, 1980.
19. Goodwin, J.F. Prospects and predictions for the cardiomyopathies. *Circulation* **50**: 210–19, 1974.
20. Pearse, A.G.E. The histochemistry and electron microscopy of obstructive cardiomyopathy. In: Cardiomyopathies, Wolstenholme, G.E.W. and O'Connor, M. (eds.), Ciba Foundation Symposium, Little Brown, Boston, 1964, pp. 132–64.
21. McCallister, B.D. and Brown, A.L. A fine-structure study of idiopathic hypertrophic subaortic stenosis. *Am. J. Cardiol.* **19**: 142, 1967. (abstr.)

22. Van Noorden, S., Olsen, E.G.J., and Pearse, A.G.E. Hypertrophic obstructive cardiomyopathy, a histological, histochemical and ultrastructural study of biopsy material. *Cardiovasc. Res.* **5**: 118–31, 1971.
23. Kawai, C., Yui, Y., Hoshino, T., Sasayama, S., and Matsumori, A. Myocardial catecholamines in hypertrophic and dilated (congestive) cardiomyopathy: a biopsy study. *J. Am. Coll. Cardiol.* **2**: 834–40, 1983.
24. Dargie, H., Boschetti, E., Reid, J., and Goodwin, J.F. Autonomic function in hypertrophic cardiomyopathy. *Circulation* **62** (Suppl.): III-301, 1980. (abstr.)
25. Sugishita, Y., Iida, K., Matsuda, M., Ajisaka, R., Matsumoto, R., Fujita, T., and Ito, I. Plasma norepinephrine concentration during exercise in patients with different types of hypertrophic cardiomyopathy. Annual Report of the Idiopathic Cardiomyopathy Research Committee, The Ministry of Health and Welfare of Japan Publication, 1983, pp. 168–71. (in Japanese)
26. Haneda, T., Miura, Y., Miyazawa, K., Honna, T., Arai, T., Nakajima, T., Miura, T., Yoshinaga, K., and Takishima, T. Plasma norepinephrine concentration in the coronary sinus in cardiomyopathies. *Cath. Cardiovasc. Diag.* **4**: 399–405, 1978.
27. Goldstein, D.S., Lake C.R., Chernow, B., Zeigler, M.G., Coleman, M.D., Taylor, A.A., Mitchell, J.R., Kopin, I.J., and Keiser, H.R. Age-dependence of hypertensive normotensive differences in plasma norepinephrine. *Hypertension* **5**: 100–4, 1983.
28. Koga, Y., Itaya, M., and Toshima, H. Increased cardiovascular response to epinephrine in hypertrophic cardiomyopathy. *Jpn. Heart J.* **26**: 727–40, 1985.
29. Miyazaki, Y. Increased cardiovascular response to norepinephrine in patients with hypertrophic cardiomyopathy. *Junkankika* **22**: 175–84, 1987. (in Japanese)
30. Sagawa, K., Suga, H., Shoukas, A.A., and Bakalar, K.M. End-systolic pressure/volume ratio: A new index of ventricular contractility. *Am. J. Cardiol.* **40**: 748–53, 1977.
31. Iida, K., Sugishita, Y., Matsuda, M., Yamaguchi, T., Ajisaka, R., Matsumoto, R., Fujita, T., Yukisada, K., and Ito, I. Difference in the response to isoproterenol between asymmetric septal hypertrophy and symmetric hypertrophy in patients with hypertrophic cardiomyopathy. *Clin. Cardiol.* **9**: 7–12, 1986.
32. Limas, C.J. Increased number of β-adrenergic receptors in the hypertrophied myocardium. *Biochem. Biophys. Acta* **588**: 174–78, 1979.
33. Tarazi, R.C., Sen, S., Saragoca, M., and Khairallah, P. The multifactorial role of catecholamines in hypertensive cardiac hypertrophy. *Eur. Heart J.* **3** (Suppl. A): 103–10, 1982.
34. Upsher, M.E. and Khairallah, P.A. Beta-adrenergic receptors in rat myocardium during the development and reversal of hypertrophy and following chronic infusions of angiotensin II and epinephrine. *Arch. Int. Pharmacodyn.* **274**: 65–79, 1985.
35. Glaubiger, G., Tsai, B.S., Lefkowitz, R.J., Weiss, B., and Johnson, E.M. Jr. Chronic guanethidine treatment increases cardiac β-adrenergic receptors. *Nature* **273**: 240–42, 1978.
36. Yamada, S., Yamamura, H.I., and Roeske, W.R. Alterations in cardiac autonomic receptors following 6-hydroxydopamine treatment in rats. *Mol. Pharmacol.* **18**: 185–92, 1980.
37. Limas, C. and Limas, C.J. Reduced number of β-adrenergic receptors in the myocardium of spontaneously hypertensive rats. *Biochem. Biophys. Res. Commun.* **83**: 710–4, 1978.
38. Woodcock, E.A., Funder, J.W., and Johnston, C.I. Decreased cardiac β-adrenoceptors in hypertensive rats. *Clin. Exp. Pharmacol. Physiol.* **5**: 545–50, 1978.
39. Robberecht, P., Winand, J., Chatelain, P., Poloczek, P., Camus, J-C., De Neef, P., and Christophe, J. Comparison of β-adrenergic receptors and the adenylate cyclase system with muscarinic receptors and guanylate cyclase activities in the heart of spontaneously hypertensive rats. *Biochem. Pharmacol.* **30**: 385–87, 1981.
40. Hoffman, B.B. and Lefkowitz, R.J. Adrenergic receptors in the heart. *Ann. Rev. Physiol.* **44**: 475–84, 1982.
41. Woodcock, E.A. and Johnston, C.I. Changes in tissue alpha- and beta-adrenergic receptors in renal hypertension in the rat. *Hypertension* **2**: 156–61, 1980.

42. Yamada, S., Ishima, T., Tomita, T., Hayashi, M., Okada, T., and Hayashi, E. Alterations in cardiac alpha and beta adrenoceptors during the development of spontaneous hypertension. *J. Pharmacol. Exp. Ther.* **228**: 454–60, 1984.
43. Golf, S., Myhre, E., Abdelnoor, M., Andersen, D., and Hansson, V. Hypertrophic cardiomyopathy characterised by β-adrenoceptor density, relative amount of β-adrenoceptor subtypes and adenylate cyclase activity. *Cardiovasc. Res.* **19**: 693–99, 1985.
44. Manger, W.M. Catecholamines in Normal and Abnormal Cardiac Function. S. Karger, Basel, 1982.
45. Raum, W.J., Laks, M.M., Garner, P., and Swerdloff, R.S. β-adrenergic receptor and cyclic AMP alterations in the canine ventricular septum during long-term norepinephrine infusion: implications for hypertrophic cardiomyopathy. *Circulation* **68**: 693–99, 1983.
46. Chiba, M., Shida, M., Miyazaki, Y., Inuzuka, S., Nakata, M., Sakai, S., Koga, Y., and Toshima, H. The influence of surgical cardiac denervation and norepinephrine infusion on myocardial hypertrophy in the canine heart. *J. Mol. Cell Cardiol.* **18** (Suppl. 1): 125, 1986. (abstr.)
47. Kajiya, K., Hori, M., Kitabatake, A., Inoue, M., Uchida, S., and Yoshida, H. Cardiac autonomic receptor alterations in cardiomyopathic Syrian hamsters. *Jpn. Circ. J.* **49**: 760, 1985. (abstr.)
48. Sen, S., Tarazi R.C., Khairallah, P.A., and Bumpus, F.M. Cardiac hypertrophy in spontaneously hypertensive rats. *Circ. Res.* **35**: 775–81, 1974.
49. Yamori, Y., Mori, C., Nishio, T., Ooshima, A., Horie, R., Ohtaka, M., Soeda, T., Saito, M., Abe, K., Nara, Y., Nakao, Y., and Kihara, M. Cardiac hypertrophy in early hypertension. *Am. J. Cardiol.* **44**: 964–69, 1979.
50. Toshima, H., Nakata, M., Nohara, M., Chiba, M., and Koga, Y. Increased adrenergic receptor activity and hypertrophic response to norepinephrine in cultured SHR myocardial cell. *Circulation* **76** (suppl. IV): 534, 1987. (abstr.)
51. Simpson, P. Stimulation of hypertrophy of cultured neonatal rat heart cells through an α_1-adrenergic receptor and induction of beating through an α_1- and β_1-adrenergic receptor interaction. *Circ. Res.* **56**: 884–94, 1985.
52. Inuzuka, S. Role of α- or β-adrenergic stimulation in catecholamine induced hypertrophy of the cultured rat myocardial cells. *J. Kurume Med. Assoc.* **49**: 666–74, 1986. (in Japanese)
53. Koga, Y. and Toshima, H. Cardiomyopathy in the elderly. *Jpn. J. Geriat.* **22**: 310 6, 1985. (in Japanese)

Autonomic Nervous Function in Hypertrophic Cardiomyopathy

Yasuro Sugishita, Keiji Iida, and Kimihiko Yukisada

Cardiovascular Division, Department of Internal Medicine, Institute of Clinical Medicine, The University of Tsukuba, Tsukuba, Ibaraki, Japan

ABSTRACT

To investigate the possible role of the autonomic nervous system in hypertrophic cardiomyopathy (HCM), left ventricular and electrocardiographic responses to changes in autonomic nervous function were studied. In HCM, especially asymmetric septal hypertrophy, left ventricular response to isoproterenol was accentuated. Negative T waves in HCM, especially giant negative T waves in apical hypertrophic cardiomyopathy, were highly variable, probably because of changes in β-adrenergic function and others. Parasympathetic function was also abnormal in HCM. In conclusion, characteristic mechanical and electrical responses to autonomic nervous function in HCM might play an important role in the clinical profile of HCM.

INTRODUCTION

Hypertrophic cardiomyopathy (HCM) is an inherited condition that begins in the developing heart before birth. It has been suggested that a disorder of catecholamine function may play a part in the etiology of HCM.[1] The possible role of catecholamine stimulation and excess activity of its two proposed intracellular responses, cyclic AMP and calcium, has been emphasized in animal models of cardiomyopathy.[2] Prolonged infusion with subhypertensive doses of norepinephrine can produce hypertrophy and hemodynamic changes similar to those found in human HCM.[3–5] However, there is no direct resemblance between human HCM and the animal model.

The present paper focuses on the possible role of autonomic nervous function in HCM by describing the responses of left ventricular function and electrocardiogram to changes in autonomic nervous function in patients with HCM.

RESPONSES OF LEFT VENTRICULAR FUNCTION TO ISOPROTERENOL INFUSION IN HCM

The responses of left ventricular function to isoproterenol were studied in 18 patients with HCM.[6] The patients were classified as having asymmetric septal hypertrophy (ASH) or symmetric hypertrophy (SH) on the basis of echocardiogram. ASH was defined by an interventricular septal thickness (IVST) $\geq$ 15 mm and a ratio of IVST to left ventricular wall thickness (PWT) $\geq$ 1.3. SH was defined by a sum of IVST and PWT (IVST + PWT) $\geq$ 26 mm and IVST/PWT $<$ 1.3. Nine male patients with ASH, mean age 53 years (range 42–59 years), nine (seven male and two female) patients with SH, mean age 52 years (range 42–64 years), and nine (seven male and two female) normal controls (NC), mean age 42 years (range 29–55 years), were studied. No patients had heart failure. Left ventricular echograms were recorded before and after five minutes' infusion of isoproterenol (0.02 μg/kg/min). M-mode echograms were digitized by using a digitizing table. Fractional shortening (FS) was obtained as (Dd-Ds)/Dd × 100, where Dd = left ventricular end-diastolic dimension, and Ds = end-systolic dimension, and the normalized peak rate of change of the left ventricular dimension (D) during systole (PVs) was obtained as minimum dD/dt/D.

Figure 1 shows echocardiograms before and during isoproterenol infusion. Echoes of chordae tendineae indicate that these echocardiograms are from the same part of the left ventricle.

The hemodynamic and echocardiographic parameters before and during isoproterenol infusion are listed in Tables 1 and 2. There were no significant differences in FS and pVs between ASH and SH, between SH and NC, before isoproterenol infusion. During

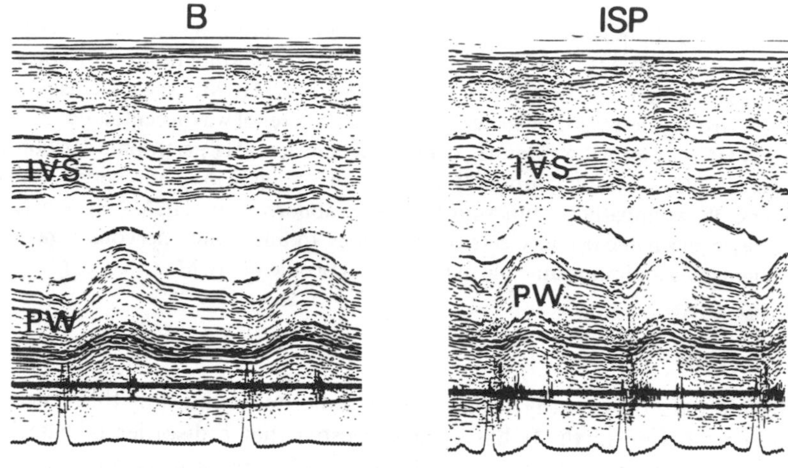

Fig. 1. Left ventricular echocardiograms of symmetric hypertrophy before (B) (left) and during (right) isoproterenol (ISP) infusion. The endocardial echo of the left ventricular posterior wall and left side of the interventricular septum can be seen clearly in both echocardiograms. IVS = interventricular septum; PW = posterior wall of the left ventricle. (From Iida *et al.*,[6] with permission)

TABLE 1. Hemodynamic Data before Isoproterenol Infusion

	HR (beats/min)	SBP (mmHg)	DBP (mmHg)	Dd (mm)	Ds (mm)	FS (%)	pVs (sec)
ASH	58±4	130±19	78±13	45±4	24±2	45±5	3.3±0.7
SH	64±6	147±13	92±10	49±4	29±4	40±6	2.7±0.6
NC	70±6	127±15	80±10	49±3	32±4	36±6	2.3±0.6
ASH-NC	p <0.001	n.s.	n.s.	n.s.	<0.001	<0.01	0.01
ASH-SH	p <0.05	<0.05	n.s.	n.s.	<0.05	n.s.	n.s.
SH-NC	p n.s.	<0.05	n.s.	n.s.	n.s.	n.s.	n.s.

Values are means ± SD.

Abbreviations: HR = heart rate; SBP = systolic blood pressure; DBP = diastolic blood pressure; Dd = left ventricular end-diastolic dimension; Ds = left ventricular end-systolic dimension; FS = fractional shortening; pVs = normalized peak rate of change of left ventricular dimension during systole. (From Iida *et al.*,[6] with permission)

TABLE 2. Hemodynamic Data during Isoproterenol Infusion

	HR (beats/min)	SBP (mmHg)	DBP (mmHg)	Dd (mm)	Ds (mm)	FS (%)	pVs (s)	⊿FS (%)	⊿pVs (sec)
ASH	93±11	147±21	67±9	45±4	18±3	60±6	7.7±1.5	15±4	4.5±1.5
SH	99±18	154±23	81±15	49±4	23±4	53±7	5.2±0.8	12±6	2.5±0.6
NC	100±13	139±20	65±18	48±3	24±4	50±5	4.9±0.8	14±3	2.6±0.8
ASH-NC	n.s.	n.s.	n.s.	n.s.	<0.01	<0.01	<0.001	n.s.	<0.01
ASH-SH	n.s.	n.s.	n.s.	n.s.	<0.01	<0.05	<0.001	n.s.	<0.01
SH-NC	n.s.	n.s.	n.s.	n.s.	n.s.	n.s.	n.s.	n.s.	n.s.

Values are mean ± S1.
Abbreviations: See Table 2; ⊿FS = change in fractional shortening between before and during isoproterenol infusion; ⊿pVs = change in pVs between before and during isoproterenol infusion. (From Iida *et al.*,[6] with permission)

isoproterenol infusion, however, both FS and pVs were significantly greater in ASH tha nSH and NC. The change in pVs (⊿pVs) was significantly higher in ASH than SH and NC, but not ⊿FS, probably due to the difference in sensitivity of the two parameters. (The age of NC was significantly less than that of ASH. However, the inotropic response of catecholamines in the aged myocardium was reported to diminish.[7] Thus the greater response of ASH cannot be attributed to the age difference between the ASH and NC groups.)

From this hyperfunction, hypersensitivity of the β-adrenergic receptor system to isoproterenol can be postulated in ASH.[6] Ejection phase indices, such as fractional shortening and pVs, may be influenced by afterload. When the change in fractional shortening caused by isoproterenol was corrected by the change in afterload (end-systolic wall stress), it was significantly larger in ASH than SH, and was significantly larger in SH than NC.[8]

Safar *et al.*[9] speculated that ASH was probably associated with increased sympathetic tone. It was speculated that the adrenergic system of the ventricular septum was initially different and responded differently to norepinephrine infusion over three months, compared with that of the right and left ventricles before the development of hypertrophy.[5] With norepinephrine infusion, the number of β-receptors increased two or threefold in the septum. The sensitivity of adenylate cyclase to β-agonist stimulation increased in the septum, but remained unchanged in the right and left ventricles, and cyclic AMP concentration decreased in the septum and increased in the right and left ventricles.[5] It has been suggested that the canine ventricular septum might be susceptible to cyclic AMP.[5] The hypersensitivity demonstrated in our study can be proposed to produce the same effect on myocardium as the increased sympathetic tone, and can be expected to play an important role in producing cardiac hypertrophy, septal hypertrophy (ASH) in particular. This hypersensitivity may be one of the causes of the arrhythmia and sudden death often encountered in patients with HCM, especially ASH.

Although it is now apparent that ASH cannot be regarded as a pathognomonic hallmark of HCM, it can be suggested that HCM, especially ASH, is a specific feature of cardiac disease, especially in relation to catecholamines. It has been found that ASH is transmitted as an autosomal dominant genetic abnormality with a high degree of penetrance.[10]

VARIABILITY OF ELECTROCARDIOGRAPHIC FINDINGS, ESPECIALLY NEGATIVE T WAVES, IN HCM

Negative T waves are often seen in HCM.[11,12] Giant negative T waves have been reported in many cases of apical hypertrophic cardiomyopathy, a nonobstructive form of the condition involving concentric hypertrophy of the left ventricular apex, which has been reported from Japan.[13,14] The mechanism of negative T waves or giant negative T waves in HCM has not yet been clarified.

We have tested the hypothesis that negative T waves in HCM, especially giant negative T waves in apical hypertrophic cardiomyopathy, are also sensitive to β-adrenergic function, as is left ventricular function.[15–19]

Thirty-three patients with HCM and negative T waves on a routine electrocardiographic record were studied.[16] Patients in whom systolic anterior movement of the mitral valve was produced or intensified during exercise, as judged by echocardiogram, were excluded. Indeed, changes in loading conditions of the left ventricle evoked by an increase in obstruction during the maneuvers mentioned later may modify the electrocardiographic findings. Twelve standard electrocardiographic leads were recorded. The voltage of the negative T wave was measured from the lower position of the baseline (= T-P segment) to the nadir of the wave, and that of the positive T wave (after the maneuvers, i.e., exercise or isoproterenol infusion, as described later) was measured from the upper position of the baseline to the peak of the wave. The T wave was studied on the electrocardiographic lead in which it was the deepest.

(i) Ambulatory electrocardiographic recording was performed.[17,18] For this test, the patients lay supine on a bed every hour for 10 minutes in the daytime and were observed by nurses to be sleeping in a supine position at night. (ii) Symptom-limited treadmill exercise test was performed.[15–17] (iii) Isoproterenol 0.02 μg/kg/min was infused intravenously for 5 min.[16,17] (iv) Atropine sulfate was administered intravenously in a single dose of 0.01 mg/kg within 30 sec.[18,19] (v) Transesophageal pacing was performed.[19] Electrocardiograms and blood pressure were recorded before and after each of these maneuvers (i–v). (vi) Propranolol was administered orally at a daily dose of 30 mg; this was increased weekly to 60 mg, 90 mg, and finally 120 mg.[16] A treadmill exercise test was performed in these patients at the end of each week of propranolol administration, with the end-point of the test at the same exercise stage as before the administration of propranolol.

Of the 33 patients, hypertrophic obstructive cardiomyopathy was found in seven, in whom giant negative T waves (-1.0 mV or deeper) were seen in only two. In the 26 nonobstructive patients, giant negative T waves were seen in 15 of 16 patients with apical hypertrophic cardiomyopathy (combined with ASH in five patients), in all of the five patients with ASH, and in two of the five patients with SH.

Figure 2 shows ambulatory electrocardiograms in a patient with apical hypertrophic cardiomyopathy.[17] His echocardiograms showed apical hypertrophy. T waves at 12 pm and 3 am (during sleep) were deeper than those at 9 am and 6 pm. In seven of eight patients with apical hypertrophic cardiomyopathy in whom ambulatory electrocardiographic monitoring was performed, negative T wave was deeper at night than during the daytime, except in one who showed no change. Depth of negative T wave was 9.4 ± 3.0 mm at 1, 2, and 3 pm and 12.6 ± 4.5 mm at 1, 2, and 3 am. R-R interval

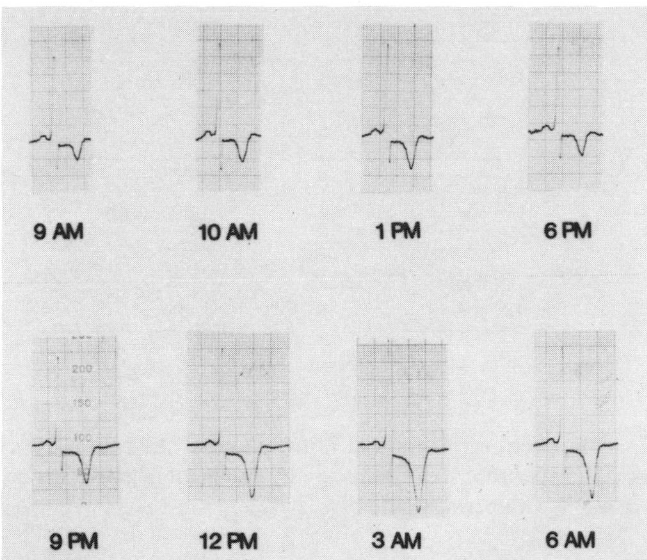

Fig. 2. Ambulatory electrocardiograms in a patient with apical hypertrophic cardiomyopathy with negative T waves. (From Sugishita *et al.*,[17] with permission)

was 793±113 msec at 1, 2, and 3 pm. and 1,055±95 msec at 1, 2, and 3 am. There was a positive correlation between the depth of negative T wave and R-R interval in six patients, but not in two others.[18] Atropine administration caused a significant shortening of R-R interval, but caused no significant change in negative T wave.[19] This suggests the possibility that the change in the depth of T wave observed in ambulatory monitoring was not caused by the change in heart rate.

Figure 3 shows a lead V_5 electrocardiogram before and at the end of exercise in a patient with apical hypertrophic cardiomyopathy and ASH, and giant negative T wave. Heart rate increased from 66 bpm to 129 bpm. The negative T wave became less deep, and the amplitude of the R wave decreased slightly. In all the patients with HCM and negative T wave, heart rate increased during exercise from 70±8 bpm to 128±21 bpm, and systolic blood pressure went from 129±20 mmHg to 164±37 mmHg. (The endpoints of the treadmill exercise test which was performed by increasing 1 stage every 3 min until attaining stage 8 (11.0 METs) were extreme tachycardia (>160 bpm) in eight patients, shortness of breath in seven, 11.0 METs for 3 min in five, leg fatigue in four, significant arrhythmias in two, chest pain in two, and other complaints in five.) In all except four patients, the negative T waves became less deep (no change in three and deeper in one). They became significantly less deep (−1.2±0.5 mV→−0.6±0.5 mV, $P<0.001$), and the change in T wave (ΔT) during exercise averaged +0.6±0.4 mV, ranging from −0.2 mV to +1.6 mV. The ST segment did not change significantly during exercise.

To investigate the determinants of ΔT, the subjects were divided into two groups according to ΔT: group I (21 cases) with a $\Delta T \geq 0.5$ mV, and group II (12 cases) with a $\Delta T < 0.5$ mV (Table 3).[16] Exercise level attained, expressed by METs, heart rate, and the rate pressure product at peak exercise, was related to ΔT. Interventricular septal and posterior left ventricular wall thicknesses at rest, R wave amplitude at rest and at peak exercise, and change in R wave amplitude had no relation to ΔT.

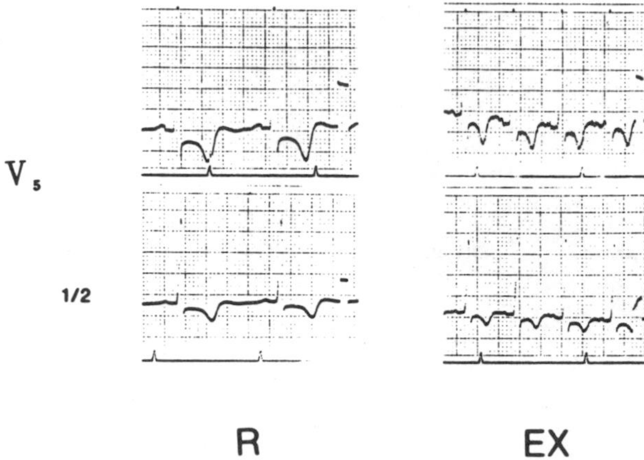

Fig. 3. Lead V_5 electrocardiogram at rest (R) and at the end of exercise (EX) in a patient with hypertrophic cardiomyopathy and giant negative T wave. (From Sugishita *et al.*,[16] with permission)

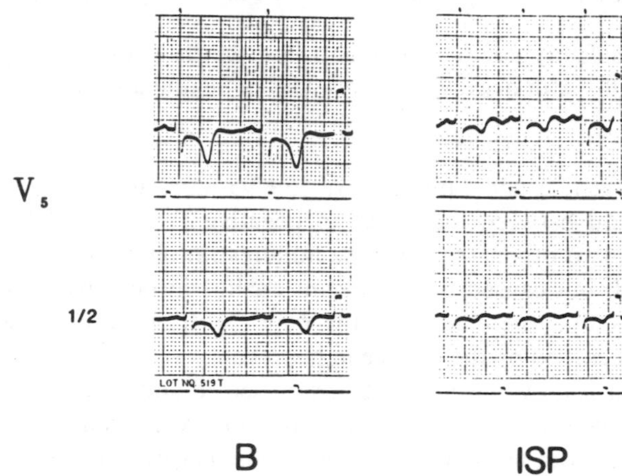

Fig. 4. Lead V_5 electrocardiogram before (B) and at the end of isoproterenol infusion (ISP) in the same case as shown in Fig. 3. (From Sugishita *et al.*,[16] with permission)

Figure 4 shows lead V_5 electrocardiograms before and during isoproterenol infusion test in the same case as shown in Fig. 3. Heart rate increased from 68 bpm to 96 bpm with isoproterenol. The T wave became less deep after five minutes of isoproterenol infusion, but the R wave amplitude did not change. In the 24 patients who performed the isoproterenol infusion test, heart rate increased from 64 ± 11 bpm to 88 ± 15 bpm, and systolic blood pressure, from 134 ± 22 mmHg to 139 ± 23 mmHg. The negative T waves became less deep in all except one patient (no change). The change in depth was significant (-1.2 ± 0.7 mV$\rightarrow -0.4 \pm 0.4$ mV, $P < 0.001$).

Figure 5 shows the depth of the T wave and the rate pressure product during the control period and at the end of exercise or isoproterenol infusion in 24 patients who submitted both to exercise and isoproterenol infusion. The depth of the T wave and the rate pressure product were identical before exercise and isoproterenol infusion. The depth of the T wave was not different after either maneuver: heart rate and the rate

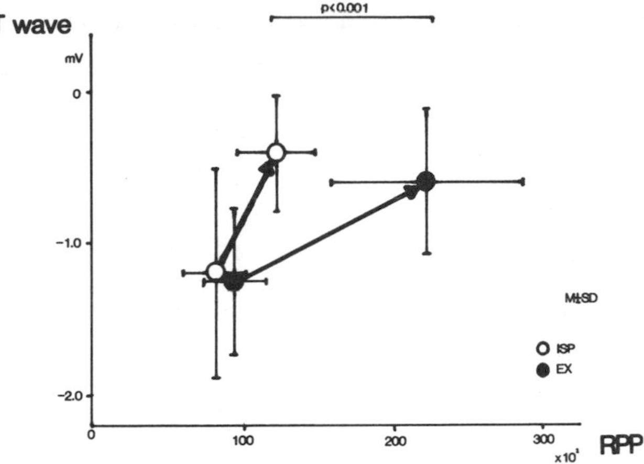

Fig. 5. Relationship between the change in rate pressure product (RPP) and depth of negative T wave during isoproterenol infusion (ISP) and during exercise (EX) in 24 cases. Arrows point from before infusion or at rest to iroproterenol or exercise values. (From Sugishita *et al.*,[16] with permission)

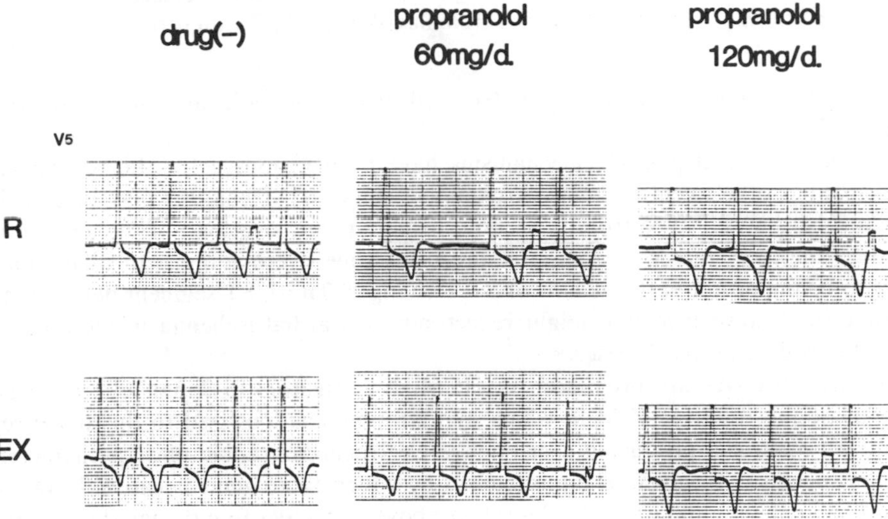

Fig. 6. Influence of propranolol on negative T wave in a case of hypertrophic cardiomyopathy and negative T wave. R: at rest, EX: during exercise. (From Sugishita *et al.*,[16] with permission)

pressure product after exercise were higher than at the end of isoproterenol infusion ($P<0.001$). There was no significant difference in the changes of negative T wave by isoproterenol, between groups I and II, which were divided by ΔT in exercise test, as shown in Table 3.

Figure 6 shows the electrocardiograms at rest and at the end of exercise before propranolol, at 60 mg/d of propranolol, and at 120 mg/d of propranolol in a case of HCM. As shown in Table 4, propranolol made the negative T wave deeper both at rest and during exercise, especially at 120 mg/d. The change in negative T wave caused by

TABLE 3. Hemodynamic Parameters at Rest and during Exercise in Groups I ($\Delta T \geq 0.5$ mV) and II ($\Delta T < 0.5$ mV)

Group	I	II
No. of cases	21	12
Age (years)	54 ± 7	52 ± 14
Sex (male/female)	18/3	12/0
At rest		
IVST (mm)	17 ± 4	19 ± 5
PWT (mm)	15 ± 3	16 ± 4
R Wave amplitude (mV)	3.4 ± 0.9	3.4 ± 1.1
At peak exercise		
Exercise capacity (METs)	7.6 ± 2.7	4.6 ± 2.6*
Heart rate (bpm)	136 ± 19	115 ± 25**
SBP (mmHg)	167 ± 33	158 ± 44
RPP ($\times 10^{-2}$) (mmHg/min)	231 ± 63	182 ± 61*
R wave amplitude (mV)	3.9 ± 0.8	2.9 ± 1.3
ΔR by exercise	−0.5 ± 0.4	−0.4 ± 0.3

Values are mean ± SD
Abbreviations: IVST = interventricular septal thickness, PWT = posterior wall thickness, SBP = systolic blood pressure, RPP = rate pressure product, ΔR = change of R wave amplitude, * $p < 0.02$, ** $p < 0.01$ (modified from Sugishita *et al.*,[16] with permission)

exercise was significant before and at 60 mg/d of propranolol, but not at 120 mg/d of propranolol.

In general, several possible mechanisms have been proposed for the repolarization abnormalities of left ventricular hypertrophy.[20] First, ST-T changes may be associated with myocardial cell hypertrophy. Second, hemodynamic overload of the left ventricle, whether due to increased systolic pressure or volume overloading with dilatation, appears to be important in the genesis of ST-T changes. Third, ST segment depression and asymmetric T wave inversion might reflect subendocardial ischemia in the absence of evident coronary artery disease.

Negative T waves are often seen in HCM. Investigators in Japan[13,14] described a form of nonobstructive HCM in which hypertrophy was localized to the apical region of the left ventricle, producing a distinctive electrocardiographic pattern characterized by giant negative T waves. The mechanism by which these giant negative T waves are provoked remains unknown. As described above, we have found that the negative T waves in HCM are not fixed but are highly variable, especially diurnally and during exercise, or during administration of a β-adrenergic agonist or antagonist.

TABLE 4. Influence of Propranolol on Negative T Wave at Rest and during Exercise

	Depth of negative T wave (mV)	
	at rest	during exercise
Before propranolol	−1.2 ± 0.3	−0.8 ± 0.3†
Propranolol 60 mg/d	−1.4 ± 0.3*	−1.0 ± 0.2†*
Propranolol 120 mg/d	−1.7 ± 0.6*	−1.6 ± 0.5*

Values are mean ± SD
* $p < 0.001$ vs before propranolol (by paired t test)
† $p < 0.001$ vs at rest
(from Sugishita *et al.*,[16] with permission)

Several studies have demonstrated normalization of the negative T wave in various cardiac states (including mild cardiac disorders): by isoproterenol in patients with less advanced heart diseases[21] and by exercise in top-ranking athletes,[22] asymptomatic young men,[23] and those with less advanced coronary artery disease.[24] It has been suggested that the negative T wave in these subjects might be considered "functional"[21,22] or "neurogenic."[22] It was explained by increased sympatho-adrenal activity at rest and enhanced sympatho-adrenal reactivity (plasma norepinephrine concentration) during stresses (mental stress, isometric handgrip, and cold pressor test).[23]

Although remarkable hypertrophy is seen in HCM, the reversal of the abnormal T wave by isoproterenol might not be explainable by morphological changes, but might be related to functional factors. Normalization of the negative T wave might have been related to the increase in heart rate elicited by ambulatory electrocardiographic monitoring and exercise,[15–18] but atropine or transesophageal pacing[19] failed to reverse the abnormal "functional" T wave. Similar changes in the depth of the negative T waves were observed at the end of exercise and isoproterenol infusion. Heart rate and rate pressure product, however, were higher after exercise.[16] This suggests that the plasma level of catecholamines and the activation of the sympatho-adrenergic system rather than heart rate or workload are responsible for the observed changes in the depth of T waves. Propranolol caused a deepening of the negative T wave under control conditions and prevented the reversal of the negative T wave by exercise. In the cases in whom the depth of the negative T wave decreased during exercise by 0.5 mV or more, exercise level attained (METs) and exertional changes of the heart rate and rate pressure product were larger than in those in whom ΔT was smaller. This difference in change in the negative T wave may be related to the higher degree of activation of the sympatho-adrenergic system and the greater rise in the plasma level of catecholamines during the higher level of exercise.

CATECHOLAMINE CONCENTRATION IN HCM

There were some cases of HCM in which the concentration of myocardial norepinephrine was exceptionally high, although its mean value was not significantly higher than that in patients with other types of heart diseases without cardiomyopathy who served as a control group.[25] No significant difference in plasma catecholamines has been reported between normal controls and patients with HCM. There is a large interindividual variability in plasma catecholamines, even if sympatho-adrenergic functions might be abnormal in these patients. It has been reported that the response of blood norepinephrine to postural change and the cold pressor test was abnormal in patients with HCM.[26]

Changes in plasma norepinephrine concentration were studied in eight patients with apical hypertrophic cardiomyopathy (A), 14 with other types of HCM (H), five with hypertensive hypertrophy (HT), nine with mitral valvular regurgitation (V) and 12 normal controls (N) of similar age and sex during symptom-limited supine ergometer exercise.[27] During exercise, M-mode and two-dimensional echocardiograms were recorded, and FS was calculated. There were no significant differences in heart rate among the groups at rest and at the end of exercise. FS was significantly lower in valvular regurgitation than in the others. There were no significant differences in plasma norepinephrine concentration (pg/ml) among the groups (157±54 in N, 103 ±81 in H, 131±21 in A, 245±60 in HT and 218±49 in V). With low-grade exercise plasma concentration norepinephrine (pg/ml) was 284±132 in N, 175±101 in H, 404±147 in A, 460±140 in HT and 539±285 in V, respectively. It was low in H and high in V. In A and HT,

TABLE 5. Coefficient of Variation in Hypertrophic Cardiomyopathy

	Normal control	Hypertrophic cardiomyopathy	NS
At rest	3.24 ± 1.31	2.45 ± 1.56	
At deep breathing	6.07 ± 2.09	3.56 ± 1.53	$p < 0.005$

(from Sugishita *et al.*[31])

it was not low. At the end of exercise, there were no differences between the groups. These results need to be investigated further, as plasma norepinephrine is affected by factors in the sympatho-adrenergic system.

PARASYMPATHETIC NERVOUS SYSTEM IN HCM

The parasympathetic nervous system is another part of the autonomic nervous system. It has, however, not been studied in HCM, possibly because of the lack of appropriate methods to evaluate the function of the parasympathetic nervous system.

It has been shown that beat-to-beat variation in heart rate could be used as a measure of the integrity of the parasympathetic nervous system,[28–30] because the variation was diminished of abolished by blocking the vagus.[28,30]

We measured R-R intervals of 100 consecutive beats at rest and during deep breathing in 14 age-matched normal controls and 14 patients with HCM, and calculated the coefficient of variation (standard deviation/mean $\times 100$) by computer.[31] At rest, the coefficient of variation was not significantly different between the two groups, but during deep breathing, the coefficient of variation of the patients with HCM was significantly lower than that of the normal subjects (Table 5). The patients with HCM were thus suspected to have abnormal functioning of the parasympathetic nervous system.

RELATIONS AMONG CARDIAC HYPERTROPHY, LEFT VENTRICULAR FUNCTION, AND ELECTROCARDIOGRAPHIC FINDINGS IN AUTONOMIC NERVOUS FUNCTION IN HCM

We have shown that isoproterenol infusion causes a significantly greater increase in left ventricular function (FS) in patients with HCM, especially ASH, suggesting hypersensitivity of the β-adrenergic receptor system in the myocardium of HCM, especially ASH.[6,8] We have also shown that negative T waves in HCM, especially giant negative T waves in apical hypertrophic cardiomyopathy, are variable, probably because of changes in β-adrenergic function. These two phenomena may be related, although methodological (e.g., topographical) differences between electrical and echocardiographic techniques can cause discrepancies in results.

We have studied hypertrophied hearts in essential hypertension by left ventricular wall stress and adrenergic response.[32] The patients were divided into three groups: those with subnormal left ventricular end-systolic wall stress (group I); those with normal left ventricular end-systolic wall stress and mild hypertrophy (group IIA), and those with normal left ventricular end-systolic wall stress and severe hypertrophy (group IIB). Plasma norepinephrine concentration was higher in group IIB than in the other groups. Inotropic response to isoproterenol infusion, evaluated by the increase in FS corrected by the decrease in end-systolic left ventricular wall stress, was significantly larger in group I than in group IIA, and was significantly larger in group IIA than in group

IIB.[32] Giant negative T waves were found more often in group I than in group IIB.[33] These results suggest that, in hypertensive hypertrophy with subnormal end-systolic wall stress (inappropriate hypertrophy, e.g., HCM), β-adrenergic response is increased; however, in hypertensive hypertrophy with normal end-systolic wall stress (appropriate hypertrophy), it is normal, or progresses to a depressed state with increased plasma norepinephrine concentration. The results also suggest that the variability in electrocardiographic findings caused by β-adrenergic stimulation might be related to the hypersensitivity to β-adrenergic stimulation in inotropic function.[33]

CONCLUSIONS

The data reviewed here describe the characteristics of left ventricular and electrocardiographic responses to autonomic nervous stimulation in HCM. It is, of course, difficult to determine the etiological role of the autonomic nervous system in HCM from these data, but the autonomic nervous system may, at least, play an important role in modifying clinical profiles, for instance, sudden death during exertion, which is often encountered in HCM.[34]

Acknowledgment

This work was supported by grants from the Japanese Ministry of Health and Welfare for the study of idiopathic cardiomyopathy.

REFERENCES

1. Goodwin, J.F. Mechanisms in cardiomyopathies. *J. Mol. Cell Cardiol.* **17** (Suppl. 2): 5–9, 1985.
2. Opie, L.H., Walpoth, B., and Barsacchi, R. Calcium and catecholamines: Relevance to cardiomyopathies and significance in therapeutic strategies. *J. Mol. Cell Cardiol.* **17** (Suppl. 2): 21–34, 1985.
3. Laks, M.M., Morady, F., and Swan H.J.C. Myocardial hypertrophy produced by chronic infusion of subhypertensive doses of norepinephrine in the dog. *Chest* **64**: 75–78, 1973.
4. Blaufuss, A.H., Laks, M.M., Garner, D., Ishimoto, B.M., and Criley, J.M. Production of ventricular hypertrophy simulating "idiopathic hypertrophic subaortic stenosis" (IHSS) by subhypertensive infusion of norepinephrine in the conscious dog. *Clin. Res.* **23**: 77A, 1975.
5. Raum, W.J., Laks, M.M., Garner, D., and Swerdloff, R.S. Beta-adrenergic receptor and cyclic AMP alterations in the canine ventricular septum during long term norepinephrine infusion: Implications for hypertrophic cardiomyopathy. *Circulation* **68**: 693–699, 1983.
6. Iida, K., Sugishita, Y., Matsuda, M., Yamaguchi, T., Ajisaka, R., Matsumoto, R., Fujita, T., Yukisada, K., and Ito, I. Difference in the response to isoproterenol between asymmetric septal hypertrophy and symmetric hypertrophy in patients with hypertrophic cardiomyopathy. *Clin. Cardiol.* **9**: 7–12, 1986.
7. Lakatta, E.G., Gerstenblith, G., Angell, C.S., Shork, N.W., and Weisfeld, M.C. Diminished inotropic response of aged myocardium to catecholamines. *Circ. Res.* **36**: 262–269, 1975.
8. Sugishita, Y., Iida, K., Matsumoto, R., Fujita, T., Ajisaka, R., Matsuda, M., and Ito, I., Beta-adrenergic responses in clinical cardiac hypertrophy of systemic hypertension and of hypertrophic cardiomyopathy. (abst.) *Jpn. Circ. J.* **49**: 470, 1985.
9. Safar, M.E., Lechner, J.P., Vincent, M.I., Plainfosse, M.T., and Simon, A.C. Echocardiographic dimensions in borderline and sustained hypertension. *Am. J. Cardiol.* **44**: 930–935, 1979.

10. Clark, C.E., Henry, W.I., and Epstein, S.E. Familial prevalence and genetic transmission of idiopathic hypertrophic subaortic stenosis. *N. Engl. J. Med.* **289**: 709–714, 1973.
11. Maron, B.J., Wolfson, J.K., Cirô, E., and Spirito, P. Relation of electrocardiographic abnormalities and pattern of left ventricular hypertrophy identified by 2-dimensional echocardiography in patients with hypertrophic cardiomyopathy. *Am. J. Cardiol.* **51**: 189–194, 1983.
12. McKenna, W., Borggrefe, M., England, D., Deanfield, J., Oakley, C.M., and Goodwin, J.F. The natural history of left ventricular hypertrophy in hypertrophic cardiomyopathy, An electrocardiographic study. *Circulation* **66**: 1233–1240, 1982.
13. Sakamoto, T., Tei, C., Murayama, M., Ichiyasu, H., Hada, Y., Hayashi, T., and Amano, K. Giant T wave invension as a manifestation of asymmetrical septal hypertrophy (ASH) of the left ventricle, echocardiographic and ultrasonocardiotomographic study. *Jpn. Heart J.* **17**: 611–629, 1976.
14. Yamaguchi, H., Ichimura, T., Nishiyama, S., Nagasaki, F., Nakanishi, S. Takatsu, F., Nishijo, T., Umeda, T., and Machii, K. Hypertrophic non-obstructive cardiomyopathy with giant negative T waves (apical hypertrophy): ventriculographic and echocardiographic features in 30 patients. *Am. J. Cardiol.* **44**: 401–412, 1979.
15. Sugishita, Y., Matsuda, M., Iida, K., Ito, I., Yamaguchi, T., and Koseki, S., The influence of exercise on left ventricular outflow tract obstruction, left ventricular performance and electrocardiograms in hypertrophic cardiomyopathy. *Acta Cardiol.* **38**: 455–471, 1983.
16. Sugishita, Y., Yamaguchi, T., Ogawa, T., Iida, K., Matsuda, M., and Ito, I. Variability of negative T wave in hypertrophic cardiomyopathy: Possible role of beta-adrenergic function. *Acta Cardiol.* **42**: 115–133, 1987.
17. Sugishita, Y., Iida, K., Matsuda, M., Ajisaka, R., Ogawa, T., Matsumoto, R., Fujita, T., Ito, I., and Yamaguchi, T. Apical hypertrophy and catecholamine. (abst. in English) *J. Cardiography* **15** (Suppl. IV): 75–83, 1985.
18. Sugishita, Y., Iida, K., and Ito, I. Diurnal change of giant negative T wave in hypertrophic cardiomyopathy. (abst.) *Jpn. Circ. J.* **50**: 301, 1986.
19. Sugishita, Y., Iida, K., Yukisada, K., and Ito, I. Pathophysiology of negative T wave in hypertrophic cardiomyopathy. *Jpn. Circ. J.* (abst. in press)
20. Devereux, R.B. and Reichek, N. Repolarization abnormalities of left ventricular hypertrophy. Clinical, electrocardiographic and hemodynamic correlates. *J. Electrocardiol.* **15**: 47–54, 1982.
21. Daoud, F.S., Surawicz, B., and Gettes, L.S. Effect of isoproterenol on the abnormal T wave. *Am. J. Cardiol.* **30**: 810–819, 1972.
22. Zeppilli, P., Pirrami, M.M., Sussara, M., and Fenici, R. T-wave abnormalities in top-ranking athletes. Effects of isoproterenol, atropine and physical exercise. *Am. Heart J.* **100**: 213–222, 1980.
23. Atterhög, J., Eleassou, K., and Hjemdahl, P. Sympathoadrenal and cardiovascular responses to mental stress, isometric handgrip and cold pressor test in asymptomatic young men with primary T wave abnormalities in the electrocardiogram. *Br. Heart J.* **46**: 311–319, 1981.
24. Sugishita, Y., Koseki, S., Matsuda, M., Ajisaka, R., Iida, K., Ito, I., Ooshima, M., Takeda, T., and Akisada, M. Significance of ST segment and T wave changes in the resting electrocardiograms of patients with exertional angina, studied by exercise radionuclide angiocardiography. *J. Electrocardiol.* **18**: 175–184, 1985.
25. Kawai, C., Yui, T., Hoshino, T., Sasayama, S., and Matsumori, A. Myocardial catecholamines in hypertrophic and dilated (congestive) cardiomyopathy: A biopsy study. *J. Am. Coll. Cardiol.* **2**: 834–840, 1983.
26. Dargie, H., Boshetti, E., Reid, J., and Goodwin, J.F. Autonomic function in hypertrophic cardiomyopathy. *Circulation* **62** (Suppl. III): 301, 1980.
27. Sugishita, Y., Iida, K., Matsuda, M., Ajisaka, R., Matsumoto, R., Fujita, T., and Ito, I.

Plasma norepinephrine concentration at exercise in hypertrophic cardiomyopathy. (abst.) *Jpn. Circ. J.* **47**: 921, 1983.
28. Wheeler, T. and Watkins, P.J. Cardiac denervation in diabetes. *Br. Med. J.* **4**: 584–586, 1973.
29. Sudkvist, G., Almer, L.O., and Lilja, B. Respiratory influence on heart rate in diabetes mellitus. *Br. Med. J.* **1**: 924–925, 1979.
30. Katona, P.G. and Jih, G. Respiratory sinus arrhythmia, non-invasive measurement of parasympathetic cardiac control. *J. Appl. Physiol.* **39**: 801–805, 1975.
31. Sugishita, Y., Yukisada, K., Iida, K., and Ito, I. Assessment of parasympathetic nervous function in patients with hypertrophic cardiomyopathy. *Jpn. Circ. J.* (abst. in press)
32. Sugishita, Y., Iida, K., Yukisada, K., and Ito, I. Classification of hypertrophied hearts in essential hypertension: Evaluation by left ventricular wall stress and adrenergic responses. *Br. Heart J.* **59**: 244–252, 1988.
33. Sugishita, Y. Personal Communication
34. Sugishita, Y., Matsuda, M., Iida, K., Koshinaga, J., and Ueno, M. Sudden cardiac death at exertion. *Jpn. Circ. J.* **47**: 562–572, 1983.

HEREDITY AND ENVIRONMENTAL FACTORS

Patterns of Inheritance and Progression of Left Ventricular Hypertrophy in Hypertrophic Cardiomyopathy

Barry J. Maron

Echocardiography Laboratory, National Heart, Lung, and Blood Institute, National Institutes of Health, Bethesda, Maryland, U.S.A.

Hypertrophic cardiomyopathy (HCM) is unusual among primary cardiac diseases in that it frequently shows a familial pattern of occurrence.[1–17] Indeed, Teare[1] noted in his initial description of the disease in 1958 that HCM could be genetically transmitted. This observation was followed by several reports of single pedigrees and early clinical studies (utilizing history and physical, electrocardiography, chest X-ray and cardiac catheterization) in which clinically overt HCM was identified in consecutive generations in a pattern most consistent with single gene autosomal dominant inheritance.[2–8]

Application of echocardiography to cardiac diagnosis in the early 1970s represented a major advance in the identification of patients with HCM by virtue of permitting the non-invasive recognition of the morphologic marker of the disease, a non-dilated and hypertrophied left ventricle (usually with an asymmetric pattern of wall thickening[18])—in asymptomatic as well as symptomatic patients. Consequently, M-mode and two-dimensional imaging became uniquely applicable to the study and definition of the patterns of inheritance in HCM.

Patterns of Genetic Transmission

Several systematic echocardiographic investigations have been performed in pedigrees with HCM,[11–17] and the findings of these investigations confirmed the initial impressions that HCM is often genetically transmitted as an autosomal dominant trait (Fig. 1). More recent echocardiographic studies, utilizing predominantly two-dimensional imaging, have found the prevalence of the familial form of HCM to be about 50–60% (Fig. 2).[9,15–17] In such studies, only about 15–35% of the first-degree relatives were identified as affected by HCM.[15] In an analyses of 70 pedigrees with HCM, we showed transmission of the morphologic marker of the disease to occur in about 25% of first-degree relatives of the proband (i.e., index case, propositus).[15,16] Although segregation analysis did not support a model of Mendelian autosomal dominant transmission for the overall group of relatives from all families, the vast majority of families with more than one affected relative showed a pattern of inheritance consistent with a dominant single gene trait. However, a substantial minority of probands with HCM (about 45%) were sporadic, having no relative with this disease other than the index case (Fig. 2).

The significance of the sporadic (or non-familial) form of HCM is not known for certain. Some instances of apparent sporadic occurrence could, in fact, be genetic and represent a new mutation or autosomal recessive transmission. Indeed, probands with the familial and sporadic forms of HCM usually have similar clinical or morphologic expressions of their disease. On the other hand, the high frequency with which sporadic cases of HCM occur suggest the possibility of truly non-genetic forms; the identities

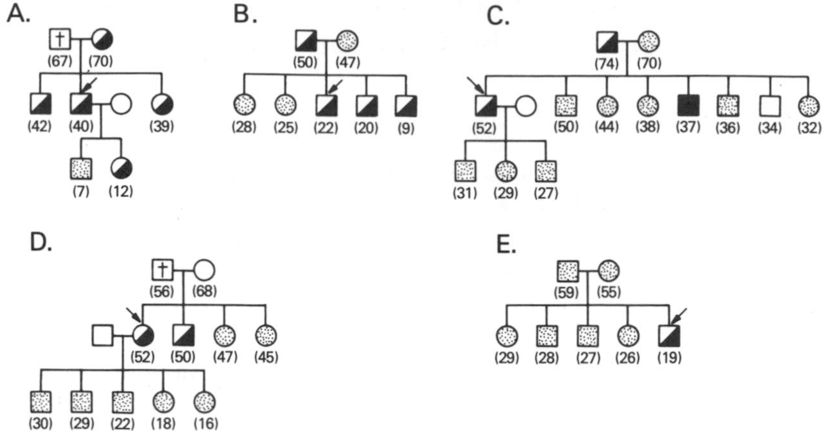

Fig. 1. Five family pedigrees selected as examples of different modes of inheritance. A. most consistent with autosomal dominant inheritance showing 5 affected persons (2 males and 3 females) in 3 consecutive generations; B. probable autosomal dominant transmission with 4 affected men in 2 generations; C. large pedigree showing probable autosomal dominant pattern of transmission, but with a relatively small proportion of affected relatives (*i.e.*, 25%); D. familial transmission of HCM in which only the proband and a brother are affected; this pedigree cannot be classified with regard to a particular Mendelian mode of inheritance; E. sporadic (nonfamilial) occurrence of HCM. Both parents and each sibling of the proband are unaffected by HCM. This pedigree is also compatible with autosomal recessive transmission or a new mutation. Solid symbols indicate death due to HCM; half-filled symbols = alive and HCM was identified by echocardiography; stippled symbols = echocardiographic studies did not show HCM; dagger = noncardiac or nonpremature cardiac death; clear symbols = subject not evaluated by echocardiography; dotted circles = females; dotted squares = males; patient's age (in years) are shown in parentheses below the symbols. Probands are indicated by arrow. Reproduced with permission of American Journal of Cardiology; from Maron *et al.*,[15] *Am. J. Cardiol.*, **53**: 1087, 1984.

of potential non-genetic etiologies are not known at this time. Therefore, it is possible that HCM represents a group of related but etiologically distinct diseases rather than a single disease entity—all with similar phenotypic (morphologic) expression.

Although some investigators have emphasized the possibility that autosomal recessive transmission occurs in HCM, others have found little evidence that this mode of inheritance is common in families with HCM. Only two of the 70 pedigrees we studied suggested autosomal recessive inheritance, i.e., 2 affected siblings born to unaffected parents were identified. Furthermore, a segregation analysis did not support the model of recessive inheritance for the overall group of relatives. Although HCM shows about a 2 to 1 male excess, there is also little evidence for a X-linked pattern of inheritance, as is evidenced by the frequent examples of father-to-son transmission.

Probands and affected relatives within pedigrees appear to differ distinctly with regard to the clinical and morphologic expression of HCM (Fig. 3). This undoubtedly reflects the fact that, in families with HCM screened by echocardiography, probands were referred for cardiologic evaluation (usually because of marked symptoms) while most rela-

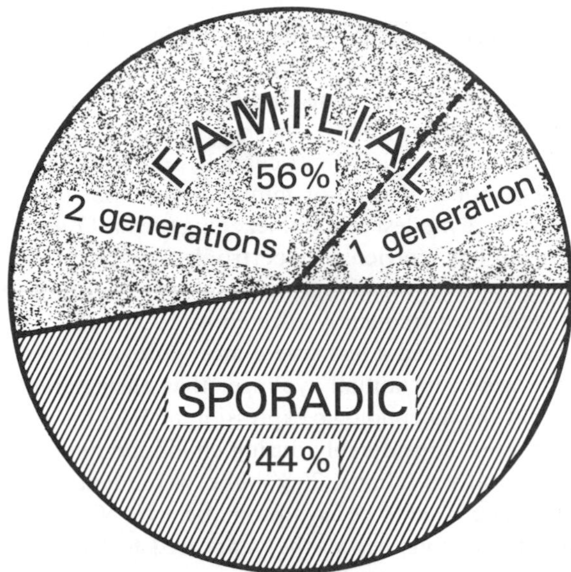

Fig. 2. Prevalence of different modes of inheritance in 70 families with HCM. Reproduced with permission of American Journal of Cardiology; from Maron *et al.*,[15] *Am. J. Cardiol.*, **53**: 1087, 1984.

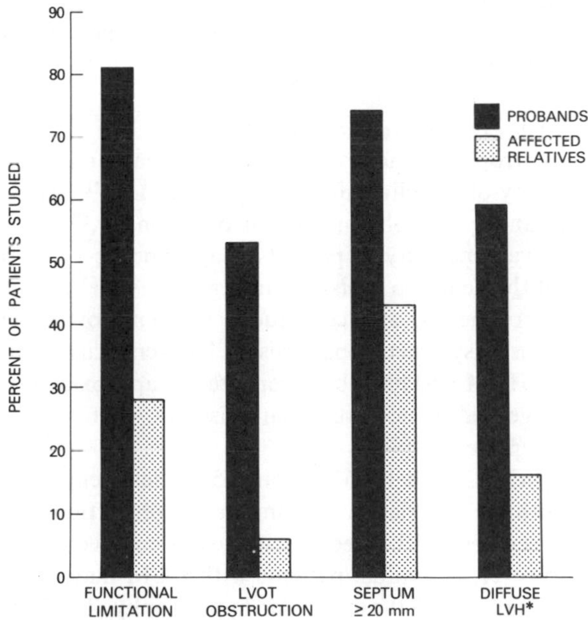

Fig. 3. Comparison of probands and affected relatives from 70 families with HCM with regard to functional limitation, left ventricular outflow tract (LVOT) obstruction, septal thickening and distribution of left ventricular hypertrophy (LVH). Asterisk denotes diffuse hypertrophy involving substantial portions of both ventricular septum and anterolateral free wall. Reproduced with permission of American Journal of Cardiology; from Maron *et al.*,[15] *Am. J. Cardiol.*, **53**: 1087, 1984.

tives were identified as affected for the first time only by virtue of having participated in echocardiographic studies at our initiative. Probands usually showed evidence of clinically significant disease with symptoms and functional limitation (81%), basal obstruction to left ventricular outflow (53%), marked ventricular septal thickening (mean 23 mm) and diffuse distribution of left ventricular hypertrophy (59%). In contrast, affected relatives usually demonstrated no or minimal symptoms (72%), absence of outflow obstruction (94%), more modest septal thickening (mean 17 mm) and more unusual and less diffuse patterns of left ventricular hypertrophy (60%).

When family members were grouped according to their relation to the proband, parents (usually fathers) were most frequently affected by HCM while offspring were much less often affected and also showed a less severe morphologic expression of the disease. Since affected offspring were substantially younger than their parents, this observation supports the concept that the morphologic expression of HCM is not always congenital and may develop or progress considerably during childhood and adolescence.

Many of the affected relatives (almost 20%) who were identified in our echocardiographic survey of pedigrees proved to be asymptomatic, over 50 years of age, and without evidence of subaortic obstruction; hence, they appeared to have a subclinical form in which the sole evidence of HCM was the morphologic expression detectable only with echocardiography. Since this expression of HCM may often constitute a dormant morphologic trait, we do not recommend medical treatment for such individuals. On the other hand, it should be emphasized that some patients with HCM (usually with the obstructive form) achieved advanced ages (over 65 years) before experiencing the onset of symptoms.[19] Indeed, we have observed the initial appearance of symptoms in elderly patients with HCM as late as 80 years of age.

Patterns of Distribution of Left Ventricular Hypertrophy

Left ventricular hypertrophy is the gross anatomical marker and probably the principal determinant of many of the clinical features of HCM.[20,21] Although a symmetric pattern of left ventricular hypertrophy may occur occasionally,[22–24] the distribution of the hypertrophy in the vast majority of patients is asymmetric——with all segments of the left ventricular wall thickened to a dissimilar degree.[20,23–26] Frequently, wall thickening is strikingly heterogeneous, and contiguous segments of the left ventricle may differ greatly in thickness. Asymmetric patterns of left ventricular wall thickening are, however, not unique to HCM and have been reported in approximately 5–10% of adult patients with other congenital or acquired heart diseases, particularly those associated with right ventricular hypertension.[27]

In the majority of patients with HCM (about 55%), left ventricular hypertrophy is diffuse and involves both the ventricular septum and large portions of the anterolateral free wall; the posterior segment of the free wall is least often affected by the hypertrophic process (Fig. 4).[23] However, individual patients with HCM may differ greatly in terms of the pattern and extent of their left ventricular hypertrophy. Thickness of the left ventricular wall is strikingly increased in many patients, including some who have the most severe hypertrophy observed in any cardiac disease.[20,28] For example, not uncommonly we have evaluated patients with maximal wall thickness (usually the ventricular septum) of 35–45 mm with the most extreme dimension observed being 52 mm (Fig. 5A).[28] Such patients with HCM and a "giant heart" exhibit a broad spectrum of clinical manifestations, with the majority having the nonobstructive form of the disease. Although such extreme increases in left ventricular mass might intuitively suggest a unique clinical course for such patients, in our experience their natural history has proven to be rela-

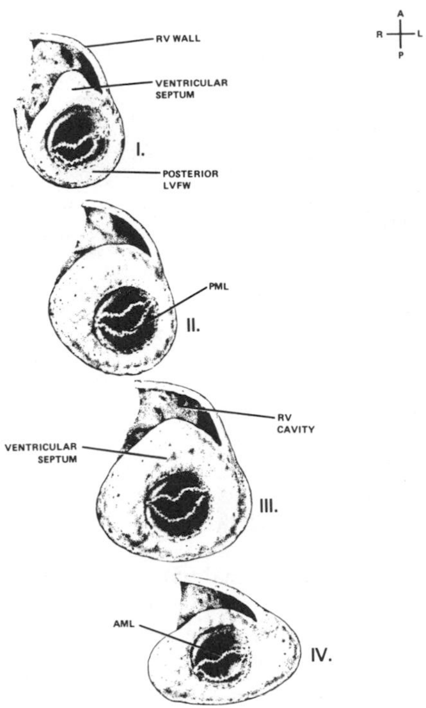

Fig. 4. Four patterns of left ventricular hypertrophy identified by two-dimensional echocardiography in patients with HCM. All patterns are shown in the short-axis cross-sectional plane at the level of the mitral valve. In Type I, the hypertrophy is confined to the anterior segment of the ventricular septum, often involving the basal region alone; the left ventricular free wall and the posterior portion of the septum appear essentially normal. In Type II, the hypertrophy involves substantial portions of the anterior and posterior parts of the septum, but not the free wall. In Type III, the hypertrophy involves substantial portions of both the septum and free wall; often the only segment free of hypertrophy is the posterior portion of the free wall. In Type IV, the hypertrophy involves regions of the left ventricular wall other than the anterior basal ventricular septum—i.e., the posterior septum, the anterolateral free wall, or the apical portion of the left ventricle. AML = anterior mitral leaflet; A = anterior; L = (the patient's) left; LVFW = left ventricular free wall; PML = posterior mitral leaflet; P = posterior; R = (the patient's) right; and RV = right ventricle. Reproduced with permission of American Journal of Cardiology; from Maron *et al.*,[23] *Am. J. Cardiol.*, **48**: 418, 1981.

tively uneventful over an average 6-year period of follow-up; no patient died and two-thirds had no or only mild symptoms at their most recent evaluation.

In contrast, other patients may show wall thickening that is relatively mild and localized to a single segment of myocardium.[29,30] Such mild morphologic expressions of HCM usually selectively involve the anterior and basal portion of ventricular septum. It is important to note that such patterns of left ventricular hypertrophy may represent the patient's native morphologic expression of HCM and that such patients can develop important symptoms and show subaortic obstruction or alternatively may remain asymptomatic for their natural lives. In young athletic individuals, such mild localized

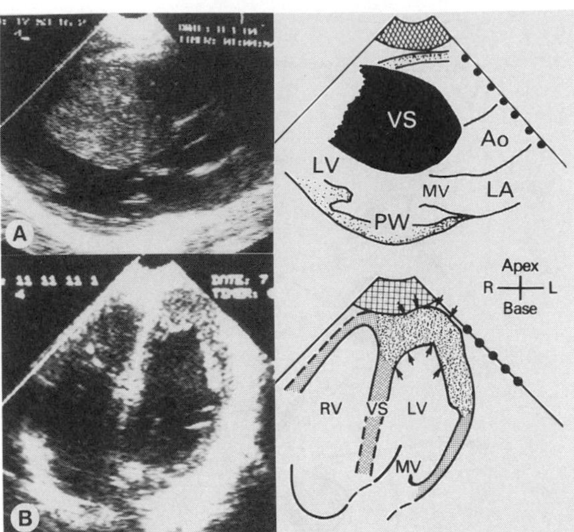

Fig. 5. Stop-frames of two-dimensional echocardiograms in diastole from two patients with HCM showing diverse patterns of left ventricular hypertrophy. Accompanying schematic illustrations are shown to the right. A. Parasternal long-axis plane, showing massive hypertrophy of the ventricular septum (VS), resulting in the appearance of a "lemon drop" protruding into both ventricles. Reproduced with permission of the American College of Cardiology; from Louie and Maron *J. Am. Coll. Cardiol*, **8**:57–65, 1986. B. Modified apical four-chamber view showing relatively mild wall thickening (arrows) which is virtually confined to the true apex of the left ventricle (LV). This morphologic expression of HCM most closely resembles apical hypertrophy of the Japanese type. ALFW = anterolateral free wall; Ao = aorta; LA = left atrium; L = patient's left; MV = mitral valve; PW = posterior free wall; R = patient's right; RV = right ventricle; VS = ventricular septum. Calibration dots are 1 cm apart. Reproduced with permission of the Annals of Internal Medicine; from Louie and Maron,[28] *Ann. Int. Med.*, **106**: 663–670, 1987.

septal hypertrophy (with wall thickness 13–14 mm) may often be difficult to distinguish from the "physiologic" form of left ventricular hypertrophy induced by chronic athletic training.[31] On the other hand, mild left ventricular hypertrophy in HCM may result as a consequence of wall thinning (usually associated with progressive cavity enlargement and impairment in left ventricular systolic function) in certain severely symptomatic patients who had previously demonstrated more typical appearance of the left ventricle for HCM with non-dilated cavity and markedly increased wall thickness.[30,32] In addition, other forms of localized left ventricular hypertrophy may involve the posterior septum, anterolateral free wall, or even the most apical portion of the left ventricle.

The latter form has been most commonly described in Japan. Since 1976, Japanese investigators have reported a subgroup of patients with a form of hypertrophic cardiomyopathy that appeared to differ in several important aspects from the more typical clinical and morphologic expressions of the disease.[33–36] Based primarily on angiographic studies, about 25% of Japanese patients with hypertrophic cardiomyopathy had localized left ventricular hypertrophy that was apparently confined to the true left ventricular apex (below the papillary muscle level). This distribution of hypertrophy characteristically creates the "spade" deformity of the left ventricular cavity on contrast angiocardiogram in diastole, and is also associated with a distinctive electrocardiographic pattern of deep ("giant") T-wave inversion in the precordial leads. Apical hypertrophy in Japanese patients generally appears to be clinically benign and nonfamilial, occurs predominantly in older men and is frequently associated with systemic hypertension.

Apical hypertrophy appears to assume a somewhat different morphologic appearance in patients from "Western" countries (e.g., North America and Europe).[37-39] In the approximately 100 patients who have been reported from outside of Japan to have apical hypertrophy, wall thickening was rarely confined to the true left ventricular apex but appeared to be more diffuse——involving greater portions of the apical one-half of septum and free wall. In addition, patients with the Western variety of apical hypertrophy rarely show marked T wave inversion or the "spade" deformity of the left ventricle, but often incur marked smyptoms and occasionally sudden death. Consequently, these latter patients appear to be part of the "usual" morphologic and clinical spectrum of nonobstructive HCM. For example, of the 965 patients with HCM evaluated by echocardiography at the National Institutes of Health during a 7-year period, 23 (2%) had wall thickening predominantly in the apical (distal) portion of the left ventricle.[38] The patients ranged in age from 15 to 69 years (mean 37) and were predominantly male and white (only 1 was of Oriental descent). Fifteen patients had significant functional limitation, usually exertional dyspnea and fatigue. Several electrocardiographic patterns were identified, but only 4 patients showed "giant" negative T waves. Just 3 patients had the distribution of apical hypertrophy that most closely resembled that described in Japanese patients——i.e., particularly localized hypertrophy confined to the true left ventricular apex (2 of these patients had "giant" negative T waves) (Fig. 5B).

Relationship of Pattern of Hypertrophy to Clinical Presentation

The extent and distribution of left ventricular hypertrophy also appears to be a determinant of clinical features and course in patients with HCM.[20,21] For example, in a population of patients with HCM, marked and diffuse left ventricular hypertrophy confers a predisposition for sudden death (or cardiac arrest),[40] potentially life-threatening arrhythmias such as ventricular tachycardia,[41] and cardiac symptoms and obstruction to left ventricular outflow under basal conditions.[23] However, these relationships of left ventricular mass to clinical findings in HCM are not strong enough to permit prediction of clinical course in individual patients based on the echocardiographic assessment of magnitude of hypertrophy.

The hypertrophied and stiffened left ventricle, characteristic of HCM, results in impaired diastolic relaxation, compliance and filling in about 75% of patients.[42,43] These abnormalities contribute importantly to the congestive symptoms exerienced by many patients with nonobstructive as well as obstructive HCM.[44,45] The early filling phase is prolonged and the rate and volume of rapid filling is decreased. Consequently, there is a compensatory increase in the contribution of atrial systole to overall left ventricular filling.[46] Diastolic dysfunction sufficient to produce symptoms is usually associated with considerable left ventricular hypertrophy, although diastolic abnormalities may also occur in patients with more mild and localized wall thickening.[47]

Finally, the distribution of hypertrophy is an important determinant of whether left ventricular outflow tract obstruction will occur in patients with HCM.[48] In patients with subaortic obstruction, the basal ventricular septum is usually thickened markedly at the level of the mitral valve, the mitral valve is positioned anteriorly within the left ventricular cavity, and the cross-sectional area of the outflow tract (at end-diastole) is considerably reduced. Conversely, in patients with nonobstructive HCM, the outflow tract at mitral valve level is usually larger and maximal septal thickening is evident in more distal portions of the ventricle below the mitral valve.

Morphologic Patterns of HCM within Pedigrees

The morphologic diversity of HCM is underlined by the fact that even closely related first-degree relatives usually show great dissimilarities in the pattern of left ventricular wall thickening (Figs. 6 and 7).[49,50] In fact, variability in the distribution and pattern of left ventricular hypertrophy may be just as great between related members of the same family as between unrelated patients in different families.

In one study[49] left ventricular morphology was compared in pairs of affected first-degree relatives utilizing a detailed echocardiographic analysis of hypertrophy in 10 segments of the left ventricular wall. Only 32 (30%) of 105 pairs with HCM showed phenotypically similar hearts with regard to the pattern of wall thickening (Fig. 6). Morphologic similarities were most common in those relatives who had diffuse hypertrophy involving both the ventricular septum and free wall. Dissimilar morphologic expressions of HCM in closely related relatives probably reflect variation in the expressivity of a single gene; however such phenotypic variability may imply that inheritance is mediated by more than one gene situated in a variety of loci.

Progression, Development and Changing Patterns of Hypertrophy

HCM may occasionally be identified in infants.[51,52] When clinically overt in this age group, the disease is usually associated with severe progressive congestive heart failure and often obstruction to both left and right ventricular outflow. Thus, HCM can represent a congenital heart malformation in which left ventricular wall thickening may begin during fetal development and be evident shortly after birth.

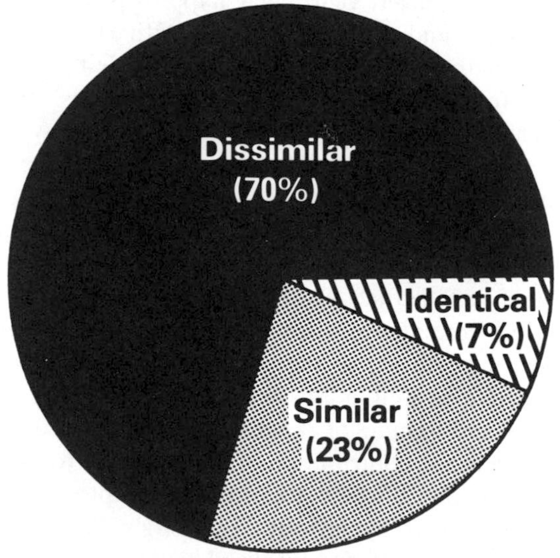

Fig. 6. Proportion of pairs of first-degree relatives with HCM with morphologically identical, similar or dissimilar patterns of left ventricular hypertrophy, based on a two-dimensional echocardiographic segmental wall analysis. From a study of 105 pairs of first-degree relatives (4–74 years old; mean 34) in 40 families with HCM. Reproduced with permission of American Heart Association from Ciro *et al.*,[49] *Circulation* **67**: 1227, 1983.

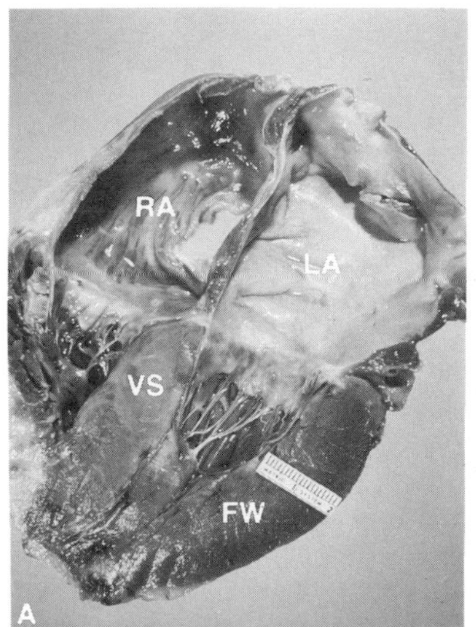

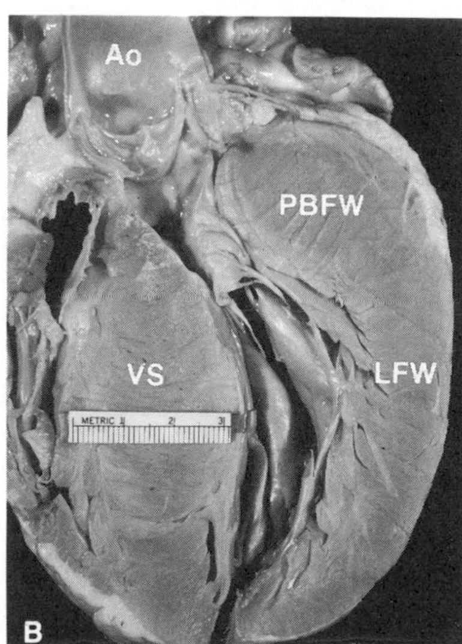

Fig. 7. Hearts of two related patients showing contrasting distribution and magnitude of left ventricular hypertrophy. A. Index patient with symmetric and relatively mild left ventricular wall thickening. Clinical course was characterized by progressive heart failure. Ao = aorta; LA = left atrium; RA = right atrium. B. The 15-year-old niece of the index case; ventricular septum (VS) is markedly hypertrophied (35 mm) and is disproportionately thickened with respect to the left ventricular free wall (FW). Patient was asymptomatic prior to sudden unexpected death. The distribution of hypertrophy in the free wall is also not uniform; posterobasal left ventricular free wall behind the posterior mitral leaflet (arrow) is much thicker (33 mm) than other portions of free wall. Reproduced with permission of American Heart Journal; from Ciro *et al.*,[50] *Am. Heart J.* **104**: 643, 1982.

On the other hand, two-dimensional serial echocardiographic studies in young relatives of patients with HCM have demonstrated that frequently left ventricular hypertrophy is not fully expressed at birth. Wall thicknesses may show substantial changes throughout childhood, but particularly during adolescence when growth development and maturation are most marked. Striking increases in left ventricular wall thickness have been observed in children with pre-existing hypertrophy and also hypertrophy may even develop *de novo* in adolescence (Figs. 8–10). In a recent investigation, 39 children with a family history or morphologic evidence of HCM were studied over a four-year period.[53] Patients were initially investigated at ages 4–15 years (mean 11) and then later at 9–20 years (mean 16). Seventeen of the study patients showed a marked acceleration in the magnitude and extent of established left ventricular hypertrophy, and 5 others demonstrated *de novo* evolution from a morphologically normal-appearing heart to one with substantial, asymmetric wall thickening (Figs. 8 and 9). In these 22 patients, the observed increases in left ventricular wall thickness were striking (6 to 23 mm; 33–250% change, mean 100%), and greatly exceeded that which would have been expected to occur as a consequence of normal growth. The average absolute increase in wall thickness was 12 mm (maximum increase, 23) and was ≥ 10 mm in 14 patients (including 5 with ≥ 15 mm). Of the 22 patients, 45 (or 41%) of 110 left ventricular seg-

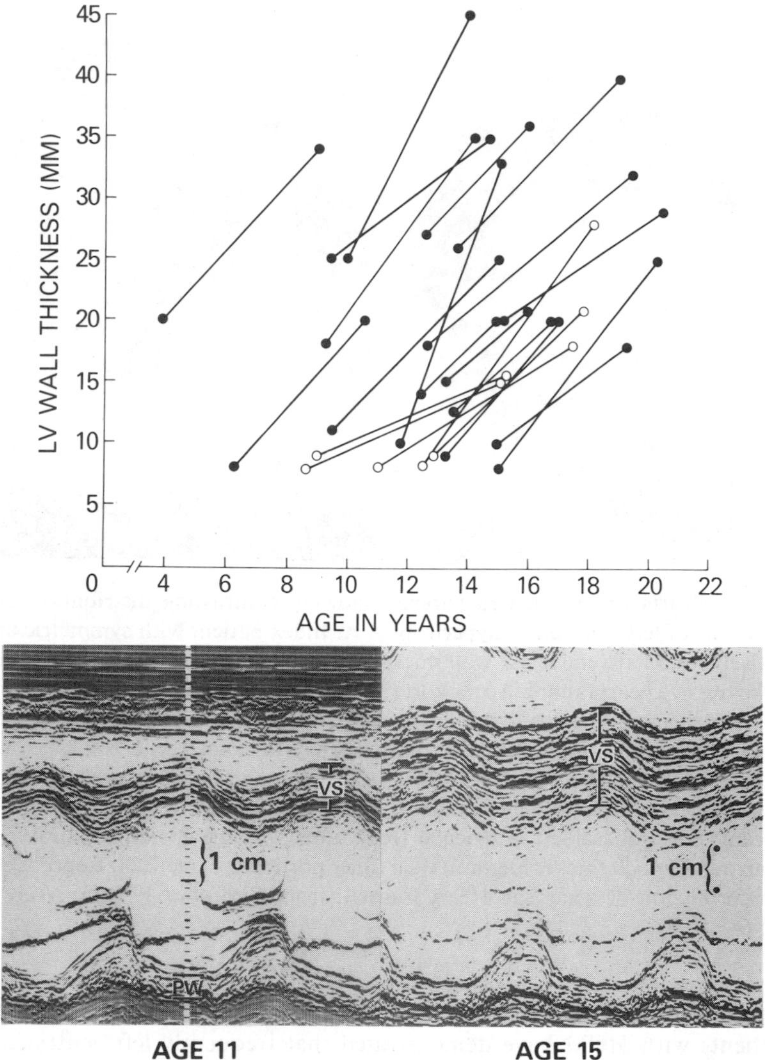

Fig. 8. Development and progression of left ventricular (LV) hypertrophy in children with HCM. *Upper panel.* Dynamic, striking changes in LV wall thickness with age in 22 children with a family history of HCM who were studied with serial two-dimensional echocardiography; each patient is represented by the left ventricular segment that showed the greatest change in wall thickness. Open symbols denote 5 patients who had a family member with HCM, but themselves had no evidence of hypertrophy in any left ventricular segment at the initial evaluation, but subsequently developed wall thickening typical of HCM *de novo. Lower panels.* Development of marked hypertrophy of anterior basal ventricular septum (VS). M-mode echocardiograms were obtained at the same cross-sectional level in a young girl with a family history of HCM. At age 11, anterior ventricular septal thickness was at upper limit of normal (10 mm); at age 15, septal thickness markedly increased (to 33 mm), and the appearance became typical of HCM. PW = posterior free wall. Reproduced with permission of New England Journal of Medicine; from Maron *et al.*,[53] *N. Eng. J. Med.*, **315**: 610, 1986.

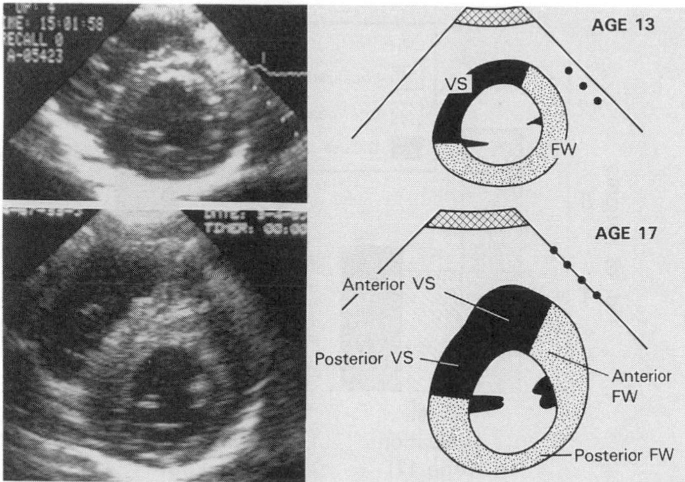

Fig. 9. Development of left ventricular hypertrophy in HCM shown by stop-frame two-dimensional echocardiograms obtained in the short-axis view (at end-diastole) in a boy with a family history of HCM. At age 13, all segments of the left ventricular wall are of normal thickness; at age 17, at the same cross-sectional level, the anterior ventricular septum and contiguous regions of anterior free wall and posterior septum show a marked increase in thickness. FW = free wall; VS = ventricular septum. Reproduced with permission of New England Journal of Medicine; from Maron *et al.*,[53] *N. Eng. J. Med.* **315**: 610, 1986.

ments showed a measurable increase in wall thickness during follow-up; these included 26 segments in which preexisting hypertrophy became greater and 19 previously normal segments in which "new" areas of hypertrophy formed. Therefore, the patterns of hypertrophy become less localized and more diffusely distributed. Ultimately, the region of left ventricular wall most commonly hypertrophied was the anterior ventricular septum, although wall thickening was also frequently identified in the posterior septum and anterior free wall.

These changes in left ventricular mass in children with HCM were generally not associated with symptomatic deterioration, the development of subaortic obstruction, nor changes in electrocardiographic pattern. Although definitive data are not available at this time, it would appear likely that such striking increases in left ventricular wall thickness occur during childhood in the vast majority of patients with HCM and probably represent a morphologic fulfillment of that left ventricular structure genetically predetermined for each patient. Furthermore, in such children with HCM and evolving left ventricular hypertrophy, abnormalities on the 12-lead electrocardiogram may be the initial clinical manifestation of the disease, preceding both the onset of symptoms and the development and appearance of left ventricular hypertrophy on echocardiogram.[54]

In our experience, adult patients with HCM do not experience progression of left ventricular hypertrophy.[55] In one study, none of 65 adult patients (20–50 years of age) with HCM studied by serial two-dimensional echocardiography showed an unequivocal increase in left ventricular wall thickness over a 3 to 6 year follow-up period. Therefore, from these observations we have concluded that the morphologic expression of HCM becomes complete by about age 18 after full physical maturation has been achieved.

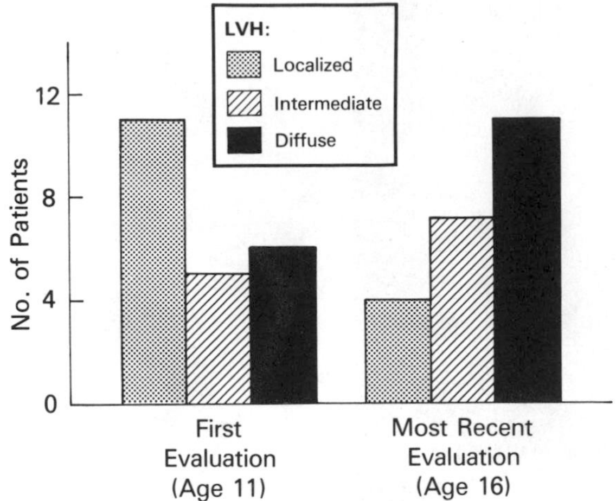

Fig. 10. Changing patterns and extent of left ventricular hypertrophy in 22 patients with HCM. Localized hypertrophy (involving only one left ventricular segment) is common at initial evaluation but later in adolescence more diffuse patterns (involving 3 or more segments) predominate.

Genetic Counseling

Because of the genetic heterogeneity of HCM, no single counseling recommendation can pertain to all families with this disease; rather, counseling should be individualized. For example, if a family shows high gene penetrance with an obvious autosomal dominant inheritance, the risk of transmission of HCM to future offspring may approach 50% and most certainly is greater than 25%. Conversely, in families with only a single (sporadic) occurrence of HCM, the risk of genetic transmission of the disease is probably substantially less than 25%. It is also worth emphasizing that the clinical and morphologic expression of HCM is frequently mild in those affected relatives who are identified solely as a consequence of a systematic echocardiographic survey.[15)]

Furthermore, in formulating genetic counseling recommendations, it is also important to take into consideration the fact that the morphologic expression of HCM may not be complete until adulthood.[53)] Therefore, a single normal echocardiographic examination in a young child with a family history of HCM cannot definitively exclude the disease. If the echocardiogram is initially normal in such children, subsequent echocardiographic studies should be performed at approximately 3-year intervals until the patient attains adult age and mature body size. In addition, after the diagnosis of HCM is made in a patient, it is reasonable to pursue identification of the disease in relatives. This is particularly true for those youthful family members who may contemplate particularly vigorous or competitive athletic activities,[56)] since there appears to be some enhanced risk for premature sudden death in patients with HCM under such conditions.[57)]

REFERENCES

1. Teare, D. Asymmetrical hypertrophy of the heart in young adults. *Br. Heart. J.* **20**: 1–8, 1958.
2. Brent, L.B., Aburano, A., Fisher, D.L., Moran, T.J., Myers, J.D., and Taylor, W.J. Familial muscular subaortic stenosis. An unrecognized form of "idiopathic heart disease", with clinical and autopsy observations. *Circulation* **21**: 167–80, 1960.

3. Hollman, A., Goodwin, J.F., Teare, D., and Renwick, J.W. A family with obstructive cardiomyopathy (asymmetrical hypertrophy). *Br. Heart J.* **22**: 449–56, 1960.
4. Paré, J.A.P., Fraser, R.G., Pirozynski, W.J., Shanks, J.A., and Stubington, D. Hereditary cardiovascular dysplasia. A form of familial cardiomyopathy. *Am. J. Med.* **31**: 37–62, 1961.
5. Wood, R.S., Taylor, W.J., Wheat, M.V., and Schiebler, G.L. Muscular subaortic stenosis in childhood. Report of occurrence in three siblings. *Pediatrics* **30**: 749–58, 1962.
6. Braunwald, E., Lambrew, C.T., Rockoff, S.D., Ross, J., Jr., and Morrow, A.G. Idiopathic hypertrophic subaortic stenosis: I. A description of the disease based upon an analysis of 64 patients. *Circulation* **30** (Suppl IV): 3–119, 1964.
7. Horlick, L., Petkovich, N.J., and Bolton, C.F. Idiopathic hypertrophic subvalvular stenosis. A study of a family involving four generations. Clinical, hemodynamic and pathologic observations. *Am. J. Cardiol.* **17**: 411–8, 1966.
8. Nasser, W.K., Williams, J.F., Mishkin, M.E., *et al.* Familial myocardial disease with and without obstruction to left ventricular outflow. *Circulation* **35**: 638–52, 1967.
9. Branzi, A., Romeo, G., Specchia, S. *et al.* Genetic heterogeneity of hypertrophic cardiomyopathy. *Int. J. Cardiol.* **7**: 129–38, 1985.
10. Emanuel, R., Withers, H., and O'Brien, K. Dominant and recessive modes of inheritance in idiopathic cardiomyopathy. *Lancet* **2**: 1065–7, 1971.
11. Clark, C.E., Henry, W.L., and Epstein, S.E. Familial prevalence and genetic transmission of idiopathic hypertrophic subaortic stenosis. *N. Engl. J. Med.* **289**: 709–14, 1973.
12. van Dorp, W.G., ten Cate, F.J., Vletter, W.B., Dohman, H., and Roelandt, J. Familial prevalence of asymmetric septal hypertrophy. *Eur. J. Cardiol.* **4**: 349–51, 1976.
13. ten Cate, F.J., Hugenholtz, P.G., van Dorp, W.J., and Roelandt, J. Prevalence of diagnostic abnormalities in patients with genetically transmitted asymmetric septal hypertrophy. *Am. J. Cardiol.* **43**: 731–7, 1979.
14. Bjarnason, I., Jonsson, S., and Hardarson, T. Mode of inheritance of hypertrophic cardiomyopathy in Iceland. *Br. Heart J.* **47**: 122–9, 1982.
15. Maron, B.J., Nichols, P.F., Pickle, L.W., Wesley, Y.E., and Mulvihill, J.J. Patterns of inheritance in hypertrophic cardiomyopathy: Assessment by M-mode and two-dimensional echocardiography. *Am. J. Cardiol.* **53**: 1087–94, 1984.
16. Maron, B.J. and Mulvihill, J.J. Genetics of hypertrophic cardiomyopathy. *Ann. Int. Med.* **105**: 610–13, 1986.
17. Greaves, S.C., Roche, A.H.G., Neutze, J.M., and Whitlock, R.M.L. Inheritance of hypertrophic cardiomyopathy: a cross-sectional and M-mode echocardiographic study of 50 families. *Br. Heart J.* **58**: 259–66, 1987.
18. Maron, B.J. and Epstein, S.E. Hypertrophic cardiomyopathy: A discussion of nomenclature. *Am. J. Cardiol.* **43**: 1242–44, 1979.
19. Lewis, J.K. and Maron, B.J. Elderly patients with hypertrophic cardiomyopathy: a subset with distinctive left ventricular morphology and progressive clinical course late in life. *J. Am. Coll. Cardiol.* **13**: 36–45, 1989.
20. Maron, B.J., Bonow, R.O., Cannon, R.O., Leon, M.B., and Epstein, S.E. Hypertrophic cardiomyopathy: Interrelation of clinical manifestations, pathophysiology, and therapy. *N. Engl. J. Med.* **316**: 780–89 and 844–52, 1987.
21. Wigle, E.D., Sasson, Z., and Henderson, M.A., *et al.* Hypertrophic cardiomyopathy. The importance of the site and the extent of hypertrophy. A review. *Prog. Cardiovasc. Dis.* **28**: 1–83, 1985.
22. Shapiro, L.M. and McKenna, W.J. Distribution of left ventricular hypertrophy in hypertrophic cardiomyopathy: a two dimensional echocardiographic study. *J. Am. Coll. Cardiol.* **2**: 437–44, 1983.
23. Maron, B.J., Gottdiener, J.S., and Epstein, S.E. Patterns and significance of distribution of left ventricular hypertrophy in hypertrophic cardiomyopathy. A wide-angle, two-dimensional echocardiographic study of 125 patients. *Am. J. Cardiol.* **48**: 418–28, 1981.

24. Maron, B.J. Asymmetry in hypertrophic cardiomyopathy: the septal to free wall thickness ratio revisited. *Am. J. Cardiol.* **55**: 835–8, 1985.
25. Maron, B.J., Gottdiener, J.S., Bonow, R.O., and Epstein, S.E. Hypertrophic cardiomyopathy with unusual locations of left ventricular hypertrophy undetectable by M-mode echocardiography: Identification by wide-angle, two-dimensional echocardiography. *Circulation* **63**: 409–18, 1981.
26. Maron, B.J., Spirito, P., Chiarella, F., and Vecchio, C. Unusual distribution of left ventricular hypertrophy in obstructive hypertrophic cardiomyopathy: Localized posterobasal free wall thickening in two patients *J. Am. Coll. Cardiol.* **5**: 1474–7, 1985.
27. Maron, B.J. and Epstein, S.E. Hypertrophic cardiomyopathy. Recent observations regarding the specificity of three hallmarks of the disease: asymmetric septal hypertrophy, septal disorganization and systolic anterior motion of the anterior mitral leaflet. *Am. J. Cardiol.* **45**: 141–54, 1980.
28. Louie, E.K. and Maron, B.J. Hypertrophic cardiomyopathy with extreme increase in left ventricular wall thickness: Clinical significance, functional and morphologic features. *J. Am. Coll. Cardiol.* **8**: 57–65, 1986.
29. Spirito, P., Maron, B.J., Bonow, R.O., and Epstein, S.E. Severe functional limitation in patients with hypertrophic cardiomyopathy and only mild localized left ventricular hypertrophy. *J. Am. Coll. Cardiol.* **8**: 537–44, 1986.
30. Spirito, P., Maron, B.J., Bonow, R.O., and Epstein, S.E. Occurrence and significance of progressive left ventricular wall thinning and relative cavity dilatation in patients with hypertrophic cardiomyopathy. *Am. J. Cardiol.* **60**: 123–29, 1987.
31. Maron, B.J. Structural features of the athlete's heart as defined by echocardiography. *J. Am. Coll. Cardiol.* **7**: 190–203, 1986.
32. Maron, B.J., Epstein, S.E., and Roberts, W.C. Hypertrophic cardiomyopathy and transmural myocardial infarction without significant atherosclerosis of the extramural coronary arteries. *Am. J. Cardiol.* **43**: 1086–1102, 1979.
33. Sakamoto, T., Tei, C., Murayama, M., Ichiyasu, H., and Hada, Y. Giant T wave inversion as a manifestation of asymmetrical apical hypertrophy (AAH) of the left ventricle: echocardiographic and ultrasono-cardiotomographic study. *Jpn. Heart J.* **17**: 611–29, 1976.
34. Yamaguchi, H., Ishimura, T., and Nishiyama, S., *et al.* Hypertrophic nonobstructive cardiomyopathy with giant negative T waves (apical hypertrophy): ventriculographic and echocardiographic features in 30 patients. *Am. J. Cardiol.* **44**: 401–12, 1979.
35. Koga, Y., Takahashi, H., Ifuku, M., Itaya, M., Adachi, K., and Toshima, H. Hypertrophic cardiomyopathy with ventricular septal hypertrophy localized to the apical region of the left ventricle (apical ASH). *J. Cardiogr.* **14**: 301–10, 1984.
36. Koga, Y., Itaya, K., and Toshima, H. Prognosis in hypertrophic cardiomyopathy. *Am. Heart J.* **108**: 351–9, 1984.
37. Maron, B.J., Bonow, R.O., Seshagiri, T.N.R., Roberts, W.C., and Epstein, S.E. Hypertrophic cardiomyopathy with ventricular septal hypertrophy localized to the apical region of the left ventricle (apical hypertrophic cardiomyopathy). *Am. J. Cardiol.* **49**: 1838–48, 1982.
38. Louie, E.K. and Maron, B.J. Apical hypertrophic cardiomyopathy: Clinical and two-dimensional echocardiographic assessment. *Ann. Int. Med.* **106**: 663–70, 1987.
39. Keren, G., Belhassen, B., and Sherez, J. *et al.* Apical hypertrophic cardiomyopathy: evaluation by noninvasive and invasive techniques in 23 patients. *Circulation* **71**: 45–56, 1985.
40. Spirito, P. and Maron, B.J. Relation between extent of left ventricular hypertrophy and occurrence of sudden cardiac death in hypertrophic cardiomyopathy. (Submitted for publication).
41. Spirito, P., Watson, R.M., and Maron, B.J. Relation between extent of left ventricular hypertrophy and occurrence of ventricular tachycardia in hypertrophic cardiomyopathy. *Am. J. Cardiol.* **60**: 1137–42, 1987.
42. Bonow, R.O., Rosing, D.R., and Bacharach, S.L., *et al.* Effects of verapamil on left ventricu-

lar systolic function and diastolic filling in patients with hypertrophic cardiomyopathy. *Circulation* **64**: 787–96, 1981.

43. Maron, B.J., Spirito, P., Green, K.J., Wesley, Y.E., Bonow, R.O., and Arce, J. Noninvasive assessment of left ventricular diastolic function by pulsed Doppler echocardiography in patients with hypertrophic cardiomyopathy. *J. Am. Coll. Cardiol.* **10**: 743–7, 1987.
44. St. John Sutton, M.G., Tajik, A.J., and Gibson, D.G., *et al.* Echocardiographic assessment of left ventricular filling and septal and posterior wall dynamics in idiopathic hypertrophic subaortic stenosis. *Circulation* **57**: 512–20, 1978.
45. Sanderson, J.E., Gibson, D.G., and Brown, D.J., *et al.* Left ventricular filling in hypertrophic cardiomyopathy: an angiographic study. *Br. Heart J.* **39**: 661–70, 1978.
46. Bonow, R.O., Frederick, T.M., Bacharach, S.L., *et al.* Atrial systole and left ventricular filling in patients with hypertrophic cardiomyopathy: effect of verapamil. *Am. J. Cardiol.* **51**: 1386–91, 1983.
47. Spirito, P., Maron, B.J., and Chiarella, F., *et al.* Diastolic abnormalities in patients with hypertrophic cardiomyopathy: relation to magnitude of left ventricular hypertrophy. *Circulation* **72**: 310–6, 1985.
48. Spirito, P. and Maron, B.J. Significance of left ventricular outflow tract cross-sectional area in hypertrophic cardiomyopathy: a two-dimensional echocardiographic assessment. *Circulation* **67**: 1100–8, 1983.
49. Ciró, E., Nichols, P.F., and Maron, B.J. Heterogeneous morphologic expression of genetically transmitted hypertrophic cardiomyopathy: two-dimensional echocardiographic analysis. *Circulation* **67**: 1227–33, 1983.
50. Ciró, E., Maron, B.J., and Roberts, W.C. Coexistence of asymmetric and symmetric left ventricular hypertrophy in a family with hypertrophic cardiomyopathy. *Am. Heart J.* **104**: 643–46, 1982.
51. Maron, B.J., Tajik, A.J., Ruttenberg, H.D., Graham, T.P., Atwood, G.F., Victorica, B.E., Lie, J.T., and Roberts, W.C. Hypertrophic cardiomyopathy in infants: clinical features and natural history. *Circulation* **65**: 7–17, 1982.
52. Maron, B.J., Edwards, J.E., Henry, W.L., Clark, C.E., Bingle, G.J., and Epstein, S.E. Asymmetric septal hypertrophy (ASH) in infancy. *Circulation* **50**: 809–20, 1974.
53. Maron, B.J., Spirito, P., Wesley, Y., and Arce, J. Development and progression of left ventricular hypertrophy in children with hypertrophic cardiomyopathy. *N. Eng. J. Med.* **315**: 610–4, 1986.
54. Panza, J.A. and Maron, B.J. Relation of electrocardiographic abnormalities to evolving left ventricular hypertrophy in hypertrophic cardiomyopathy. *Am. J. Cardiol.* (in press).
55. Spirito, P. and Maron, B.J. Absence of progression of left ventricular hypertrophy in adult patients with hypertrophic cardiomyopathy. *J. Am. Coll. Cardiol.* **9**: 1013–17, 1987.
56. Maron, B.J., Gaffney, F.A., Jeresaty, R.M., McKenna, W.J., and Miller, W.W. Task Force III: Hypertrophic cardiomyopathy, other myocardial diseases and mitral valve prolapse. Bethesda Conference No. 16: Cardiovascular Abnormalities in the Athlete: Recommendations Regarding Eligibility for Competition. *J. Am. Coll. Cardiol.* **6**: 1215–17, 1985.
57. Maron, B.J., Roberts, W.C., McAllister, H.A. Rosing, D.R., and Epstein, S.E. Sudden death in young athletes. *Circulation* **62**: 218–29, 1980.

HLA and Hypertrophic Cardiomyopathy

Akira Matsumori and Chuichi Kawai

The Third Division, Department of Internal Medicine, Kyoto University, Kyoto, Japan

ABSTRACT

A close association of certain HLA haplotypes with the occurrence of hypertrophic cardiomyopathy was found in six families. However, these HLA antigens were also found in patients with a sporadic form of the disease. Therefore, HLA-A and HLA-B antigens themselves do not distinguish familial from nonfamilial forms of hypertrophic cardiomyopathy.

Increased frequency of HLA-DR4 was found in patients with hypertrophic obstructive cardiomyopathy, while HLA-DR2 was less frequent in the nonobstructive type of the disease. Although the presence of association suggests that part of the genetic predisposition for hypertrophic cardiomyopathy is associated with the HLA gene complex, it does not necessarily mean that the disease has the HLA-linked single susceptibility gene.

In the majority of family studies on hypertrophic cardiomyopathy, the pattern of transmission is consistent with autosomal inheritance with a high degree of penetrance.[1–3] An autoimmune mechanism may be involved in the pathogenesis of some of these cases of cardiomyopathy,[4] but there is apparently no direct evidence implicating a virus or immunologic mechanisms in the initiation and pathogenesis of the disease. Recent studies have revealed that several HLA antigens are associated with diseases considered to have an immunologic basis and in which a high familial incidence is noted.[5]

We found no significant difference in frequencies of HLA-A, HLA-B, and HLA-C antigens between patients and control subjects. Family studies, however, revealed a close association of the HLA haplotype with the occurrence of hypertrophic cardiomyopathy.[6] We confirmed the HLA haplotype association of hypertrophic cardiomyopathy with familial occurrence in six families.

Family 1 (Fig. 1): The proband was a 41-year-old woman. The diagnosis of hypertrophic cardiomyopathy without obstruction was established by cardiac catheterization. Her mother and younger brother had marked ST-T abnormalities on electrocardiograms, and hypertrophic cardiomyopathy was confirmed by echocardiograms.

Genetic analysis showed that the proband carried the HLA-A9, B7 haplotype. This haplotype was found in her mother and a brother, both of whom were affected. In contrast, her father and elder brother, who did not carry the HLA-A9, B7 haplotype, showed no cardiac abnormality. The proband's child, aged 10 years, had the HLA-A9, B7 haplotype. An inverted T wave through leads V_1 to V_3 was seen on the electrocardiogram, but no echocardiographic abnormalities were evident.

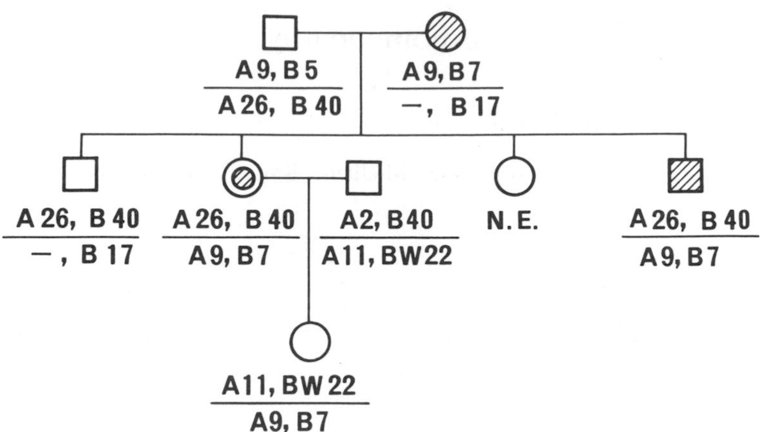

Fig. 1. Family 1 ◉ Proband; □ male; ○ female; ▨◍ affected; N.E.; not examined.
The proband carried the HLA-A9, B7 haplotype. This haplotype was found in her mother and a brother, both affected. Her father and elder brother, not carrying the HLA-A9, B7 haplotype, showed no cardiac abnormality.

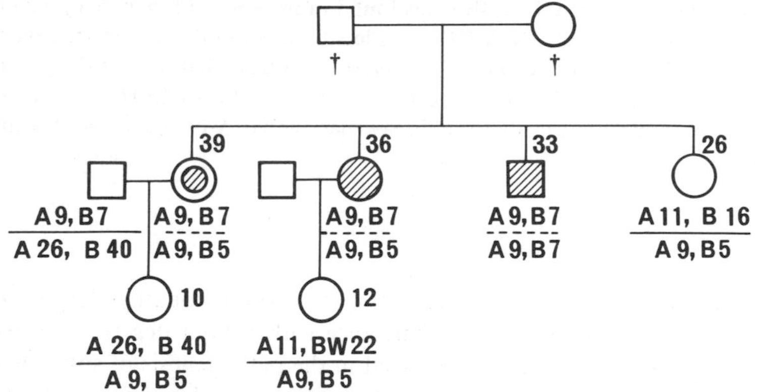

Fig. 2. Family 2 ◉ Proband; □ male; ○ female; ▨◍ affected; † dead.
All the affected members share the HLA-A9, B7 haplotype. In contrast, the youngest sister (26-year-old), the proband's child, and a child of an affected sister, all of whom had no cardiac abnormalities, did not share HLA-B7.

Family 2 (Fig. 2): The proband was a 39-year-old woman whose diagnosis was hypertrophic cardiomyopathy without obstruction. Her mother had "cardiac asthma" and died suddenly at the age of 43. Cardiomyopathy was suspected. The younger sister, 36 years old, also underwent cardiac catheterization in another hospital and was diagnosed as having hypertrophic cardiomyopathy without obstruction. Her brother, 33 years old, had systolic anterior motion of the anterior mitral leaflet (SAM), as determined by echocardiography, and hypertrophic cardiomyopathy with obstruction was confirmed by cardiac catheterization. He gradually developed congestive heart failure; the heart showed dilatation of the left ventricle, and asymmetrical septal hypertrophy and SAM disappeared. Thus, clinical findings were similar to those of dilated cardiomyopathy. He died five years later.

All the affected members shared HLA-A9 and B7. In contrast, the youngest sister (26 years old), the proband's child, and a child of an affected sister, none of whom

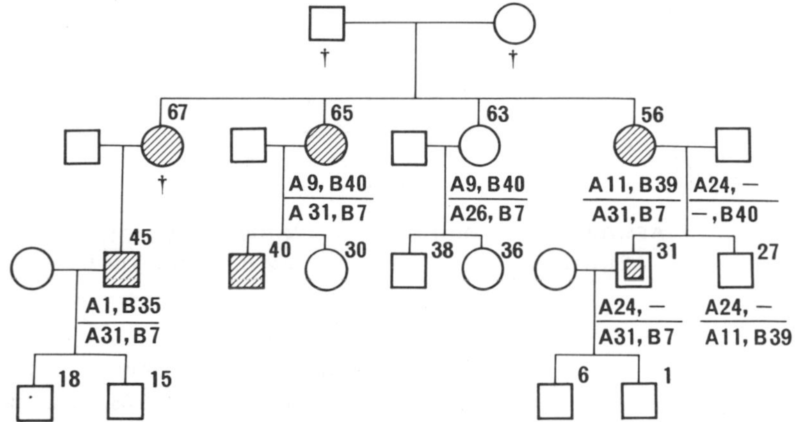

Fig. 3. Family 3 ▣ Proband; □ male; ○ female; ▨● affected; † dead.
All the affected members share the HLA-A31, B7 haplotype. In contrast, the proband's father and 63-year-old maternal aunt, who did not carry the HLA-A31, B7 haplotype, showed no cardiac abnormality.

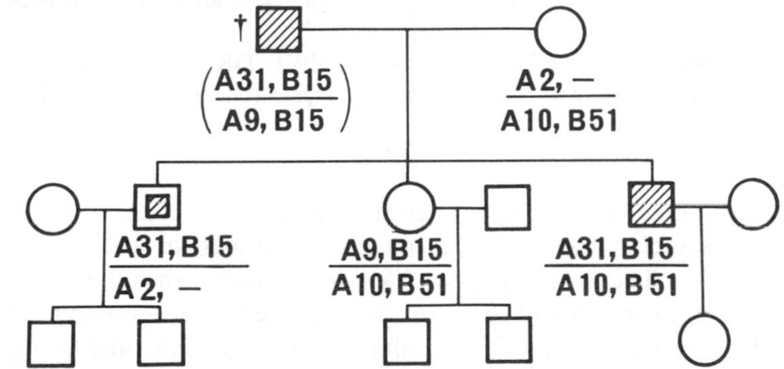

Fig. 4. Family 4 ▣ Proband; □ male; ○ female; ▨● affected; † dead.
Affected members share the HLA-A31, B15 haplotype.

had cardiac abnormalities, did not share HLA-B7. The HLA-A9, B7 haplotype may therefore be associated with the occurrence of the disease in this family. The brother of the proband developed marked cardiomegaly and congestive heart failure, and died five years after the diagnosis. The proband also developed cardiomegaly, and thromboembolism has occurred recently. The clinical manifestations were not similar at the time of diagnosis, but the eventual clinical course of the disease was similar in the two patients.

Family 3 (Fig. 3): The proband was an asymptomatic 31-year-old man. On a routine examination, electrocardiographic abnormalities were noted: left axis deviation, left atrial overload, and abnormal Q waves in leads V_5 and V_6. The diagnosis of hypertrophic cardiomyopathy with obstruction was established by cardiac catheterization and angiocardiography.

A maternal aunt had died suddenly at the age of 67. Another maternal aunt, 65 years old, the proband's cousin, and the proband's mother were found to have hypertrophic cardiomyopathy on the basis of electrocardiographic and echocardiographic abnormalities. All the affected family members shared the HLA-A31, B7 haplotype. In contrast, the proband's father and 63-year-old maternal aunt, who did not carry the

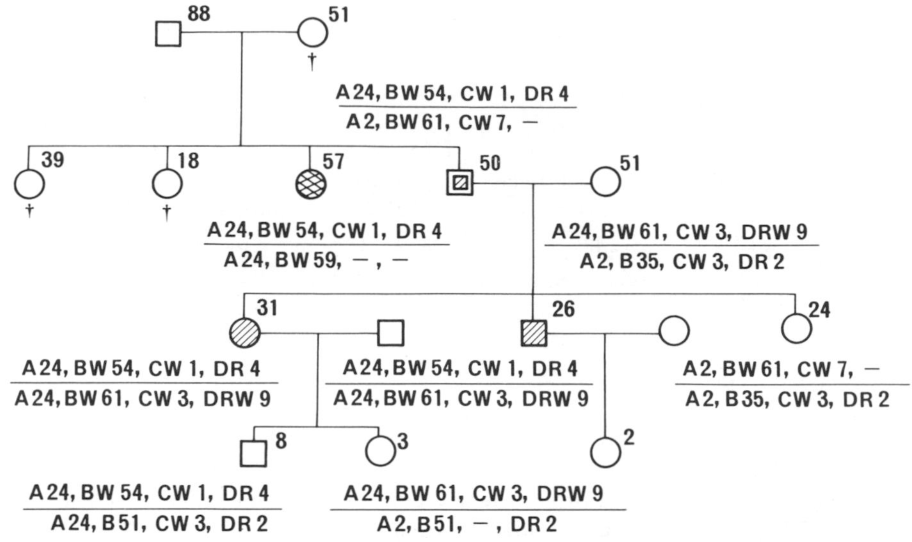

Fig. 5. Family 5 ▩ Proband; □ male; ○ female; ▩● affected; ● suspected; † dead.
Affected members share the HLA-A24, BW54, CW1, DR4 haplotype, whereas a younger daughter, 24 years old, who had no cardiac abnormality, did not share this haplotype.

HLA-A31, B7 haplotype, showed no cardiac abnormality. The HLA-A31, B7 haplotype may, therefore, be associated with the occurrence of the disease in this family.

Family 4 (Fig. 4): The proband was a 37-year-old man with a diagnosis of hypertrophic cardiomyopathy without obstruction. The disease was also found in his brother. His father had died of congestive heart failure, and congestive cardiomyopathy had been diagnosed at necropsy.

The proband's father was suspected of having the HLA-A31, B15 haplotype on the basis of genetic analysis of the rest of the family, because the affected family members shared the HLA-A31, B15 haplotype. Both hypertrophic and congestive cardiomyopathy were seen in this family, so the proband's father might have had hypertrophic cardiomyopathy and developed congestive heart failure in the later years of his life.

Family 5 (Fig. 5): The proband was a 50-year-old man with a diagnosis of hypertrophic cardiomyopathy with obstruction. The proband's mother had died of congestive heart failure; an elder sister had died suddenly at the age of 39. Another elder sister, 57 years old, had echocardiographic evidence of asymmetric septal hypertrophy. The electrocardiogram of the proband's 31-year-old daughter showed inverted T waves in leads II, III, and aVF, and that of his 26-year-old son revealed left ventricular hypertrophy.

All the affected family members shared the HLA-A24, BW54, CW1, DR4 haplotype, whereas a younger daughter, 24 years old, who had no cardiac abnormality, did not share this haplotype. The proband's son and older daughter, whose electrocardiograms were abnormal, may develop typical hypertrophic cardiomyopathy in the future because the proband's electrocardiogram showed only borderline left ventricular hypertrophy 16 years before, when he was 34 years old.

As previously reported, no significant difference was seen in the frequencies of HLA-A, HLA-B, and HLA-C antigens between patients with hypertrophic cardiomyopathy and normal control subjects. However, our family studies revealed a close association of certain HLA haplotypes with the occurrence of hypertrophic cardiomyopathy; however, these HLA antigens were also found in patients with a sporadic form of the disease. Therefore, HLA-A and HLA-B antigens themselves do not distinguish familial from nonfamilial forms of hypertrophic cardiomyopathy. Our previous findings suggested an etiologic heterogeneity of hypertrophic cardiomyopathy. HLA antigen frequencies vary among ethnic groups, and this variance may be important in determining susceptibility to hypertrophic cardiomyopathy.

We found a significant increase in the frequency of HLA-DR4 in patients with hypertrophic cardiomyopathy with obstruction, whereas in the nonobstructive type of this disorder, no significant difference was found. HLA-DR2 was less frequent in the nonobstructive type of the disease, and a decrease in HLA-DR2 may reflect an association that confers resistance.[7,8]

Increased frequency of HLA-DR4 was also found in patients with hypertrophic cardiomyopathy in England, but the increase was not confirmed in those with outflow tract gradient.[9] The difference between Japanese and European studies may be related to different genetic backgrounds of the populations or different criteria for the selection of patients. Hypertrophic cardiomyopathy may also be associated with different HLA-DR antigens in different ethnic groups. None of the disease associations are absolute because not all persons with the genetic determinant have the disease. Several reasons for this phenomenon exist, including environmental factors, other genes, antigen subsets, and disease heterogeneity. In hypertrophic cardiomyopathy, clinical features vary in each patient, and the entity may be heterogenous in its origin. An association of HLA-DRW6 was found with hypertrophic cardiomyopathy in English Caucasian patients,[10] and HLA-DR3 was associated with hypertrophic obstructive cardiomyopathy in Italian patients.[11] In contrast, no significant association of HLA-DR antigens and hypertrophic cardiomyopathy was found in another study performed on European populations.[12] In a recent study using genetic markers of class II MHC (restriction fragment length polymorphism), no significant association was found between HLA genes and the occurrence of hypertrophic cardiomyopathy in familial cases (Kimura, personal communication).

Although the presence of association suggests that part of the genetic predisposition for hypertrophic cardiomyopathy is associated with the HLA gene complex, it does not necessarily mean that the disease has the HLA-linked single susceptibility gene.

Acknowledgment

This work was supported in part by a research grant from the Ministry of Health and Welfare, Japan.

REFERENCES

1. Braunwald, E., Lambrew, C.T., Rockoff, S.D., Ross, J. Jr., and Morrow, A.G. Idiopathic hypertrophic subaortic stenosis. A description of the disease based upon an analysis of 64 patients. *Circulation* **30** (Suppl. IV): 3–119, 1964.
2. Clarke, C.E., Henry, W.L., and Epstein, S.E. Familial prevalence and genetic transmission of idiopathic hypertrophic subaortic stenosis. *N. Engl. J. Med.* **289**: 709–714, 1973.
3. Kawai, C., Sasayama, S., Sakurai, Y., Matsumori, A., and Yui, Y. Recent advances in the study of hypertrophic and dilated (congestive) cardiomyopathy. *Prog. Cardiol.* **12**: 225–248, 1983.

4. Kawai, C. Idiopathic cardiomyopathy: A study on the infectious-immune theory as a cause of the disease. *Jpn. Circ. J.* **35**: 765–770, 1971.
5. Svejgaad, A. and Ryder, L.D. Associations between HLA and disease. In: HLA and Disease, Dausset, J. and Svejgaad, A. (eds.), Munksgaard, Copenhagen, 1977.
6. Matsumori, A., Hirose, K., Wakabayashi, A., Kawai, C., Nabeya, N., Sakurami, T., and Tsuji, K. HLA and hypertrophic cardiomyopathy. *Am. Heart J.* **97**: 428–431, 1979.
7. Matsumori, A., Kawai, C., Wakabayashi, A., Terasaki, P.I., Park, M.S., Sakurami, T., and Ueno, Y. HLA-DRW4 antigen linkage in patients with hypertrophic obstructive cardiomyopathy. *Am. Heart J.* **101**: 14–16, 1981.
8. Matsumori, A., Kawai, C., and Wakabayashi, A. HLA-DR antigen linkage in hypertrophic cardiomyopathy. *Am. Heart J.* **102**: 807, 1981.
9. Zezulka, A., MacKintosh, P., Jobson, S., Lowry, P., and Shapiro, L.M. Human lymphocyte antigens in hypertrophic cardiomyopathy. *Int. J. Cardiol.* **12**: 193–202, 1986.
10. Mourant, A.J., Kafetz, K.M., Bridgen, W.W., Awad, J., D'Amaro, J., Yeatman, N.W.J., and Fastenstein, H. HLA antigen associations in hypertrophic cardiomyopathy. *Tissue Antigens* **20**: 389–393, 1982.
11. Fiorito, S., Autore, C., Fragola, P.V., Purpura, M., Cannata, D., and Sangiorgi, M. HLA-DR3 antigen linkage in patients with hypertrophic obstructive cardiomyopathy. *Am. Heart J.* **111**: 91–94, 1986.
12. Becque, O., Herve P., Bassaud, J.P., Bernard, Y., and Maurat, J.P. HLA-DR antigen linkage in hypertrophic cardiomyopathy. *Am. Heart J.* **102**: 806, 1981.

Genetic and Environmental Factors in Hypertrophic Cardiomyopathy

Masaya Yamaguchi, Komei Matsuyama**, Yoshinori Koga**, Mitsuhiro Tsuruta*, Shuzo Matsuo*, and Hironori Toshima***

* Department of Internal Medicine, Saga Medical School, Saga, Japan
** The 3rd Department of Internal Medicine, Kurume University School of Medicine, Kurume Japan

ABSTRACT

Genetic and environmental factors in 74 families were examined in connection with the pathogenesis of hypertrophic cardiomyopathy (HCM). The segregation ratio was between 0.302 and 0.406, calculated using three kinds of correcting method. However, 27% of the cases were sporadic, lowering the segregation ratio. It is thought that there is some heterogeneity including sporadic type and apical hypertrophy (AH) though the autosomal dominant gene is the main cause for the pathogenesis of HCM. We also performed a case control study to identify the anticipated environmental factors. The result showed that alcohol intake and hypertension made a contribution to this disease.

INTRODUCTION

Hypertrophic cardiomyopathy (HCM) has varied forms of clinical and morphological expression, and numerous nomenclature and classification systems are used based on the presence or absence of left ventricular outflow tract obstruction and differences in distributions of myocardial abnormalities.[1-9] There is broad variation in the degree of hypertrophy, severity, prognosis and clinical onset of symptoms in patients with HCM. In the majority of cases, HCM appears to be a familial disease, with the pattern of inheritance usually most consistent with an autosomal dominant inheritance.[10-15] However, it also appears sporadic (isolated) cases, resulting in a relative decrease in the rate of familial occurrence and the genetic ratio. The rate of familial occurrence is much influenced by factors such as family size, the method and extent of family research, and so on. The sporadic cases also may be a result of mutation or of extreme deviations from probability due to chance.

Are there any essential differences between familial and sporadic cases? At present time, it is very difficult to differentiate them on the basis of clinical symptoms, and we do not know the exact mechanisms of genetic action.

The diversity of clinical findings in patients with HCM could be due to the variation in the expressivity of a dominant gene influenced by genetic background (especially some modifying gene) and enviromental factors, or it could be the result of genetic heterogeneity. These problems might be approachable by study of the extensive family of HCM.

I. PROBLEMS ARISING IN FAMILY STUDY OF HCM

Various types of bias may occur in the process of researching the family of HCM. The method of ascertainment of cases is one of the most important factors, and the results of the study may be influenced by the method of clinical examination and the number of examined relatives of the proband. Furthermore, because of the relatively late onset of this disease, the age structure of the examined family also may influence the result.

Methods of Ascertainment (Selection)

The method of incomplete single ascertainment is usually applied for gathering data on HCM. At first, the pedigree is examined from a proband who has been clinically diagnosed as having HCM. Sometimes double probands are discovered in the same family, in which case we can handle them as a single ascertainment by counting double on the study. In the present study, we applied segregation analysis using *a priori*[16] or *a posteriori* (proband) method,[17] in order to correct for the normal persons who are dropped from the study because of incomplete single ascertainment. Davie's single method is applied in families with dominant inheritance over 2 or 3 generations.[18]

Methodology of Examination of Relatives

Two-dimensional and M-mode echocardiographies are usually performed in the examination of the first-degree relatives of the proband. However, sometimes it is difficult to obtain them from relatives who live in remote places, and only ECG is obtained in some cases.

Examination of the ECG in relatives is quite simple and has the advantage that we can get it by mail from relatives living in remote places. There have been a few reports that ECG has less sensitivity than echocardiography in family research. In Matsuyama *et al.*'s study of 539 relatives of HCM patients, however, ECG was much more sensitive than echocardiography.[19] The discrepancy could result from the use of different criteria for ECG and echocardiography in the study of patients. If we apply mild criteria, the specificity of diagnosis will decrease. Matsuyama *et al.* used a relative mild ECG criterion: an abnormal Q wave or negative T wave in II III aV_F or $V_3 \sim V_6$ for positive evidence. The same thing may happen when the echocardiography criterion of more than 13 mm thickness of the intraventricular septum is used.

There are three patterns of results that can be used for HCM analysis: 1) positive evidence only on ECG, 2) positive evidence only on echocardiography, 3) positive evidence on both ECG and echocardiography. If we examine a family using only echocardiography, we will miss 9.7% of HCM cases. So ECG is preferable for the first screening of relatives. We cannot measure wall thickness on M-mode echocardiography when thickening is located at the anterior base of the ventricular septum or the left ventricular free wall. In that case, M-mode echocardiography is not preferred for the screening.

The percentage of the relatives examined is also an important factor. It is useful to examine all of the first-degree relatives; however, it is sometimes impossible to do this. One of the problems is the prevalence of the small family (nuclear family) in Japan. One of the parents has a high incidence of inheritance in the autosomal dominant trait except for the case of mutation, and siblings tend to resemble the proband in age and environment. So it is important to examine the parents and siblings of the proband in the study of first-degree relatives.

On the other hand, incomplete penetrance is seen in the generation of the children of probands, and it is important to think about this factor in analyzing the data.

Although this criterion cannot be fully applied in a large family, we included a family in the "well-examined" group when we could examine echocardiography in more than four of the first-degree relatives including the proband. We also include diagnosed cases of sudden death, autopsy, and surgery in the sample. More than 15mm of intraventricular septum is considered positive evidence, and apical hypertrophy (AH) having a spade-like left intraventricular cavity is excluded from the study (Chapter III).

II. FAMILIES OF HCM

Familial Occurrence and Sporadic Cases

Three hundred twenty-three family members including 110 probands with HCM were studied by ECG and UCG. Two-dimensional echocardiography was performed in almost all cases (90 %), and some cases were examined at autopsy. Cases of sudden death were included as HCM cases; cases over 70 years and under 16 years of age were excluded.[20] The result showed that 52 of 110 families (47.3 %) had cases of familial occurrence. Similar results were reported by Maron and Greaves *et al.*[14,15] In our study, 74 families were "well examined" (67.3 %); the rate of familial occurrence increased to 70.2 % when we excluded the "poorly examined" families. It appeared that 20 of the 74 "well-examined" families (27.0 %) were sporadic cases. This percentage is difficult to understand even considering the factors of incomplete penetrance (skipping), extreme deviation of probability from the ideal ratio due to contingency, or parental mutation. The mutation rate of the dominant gene in the general population usually seemed to

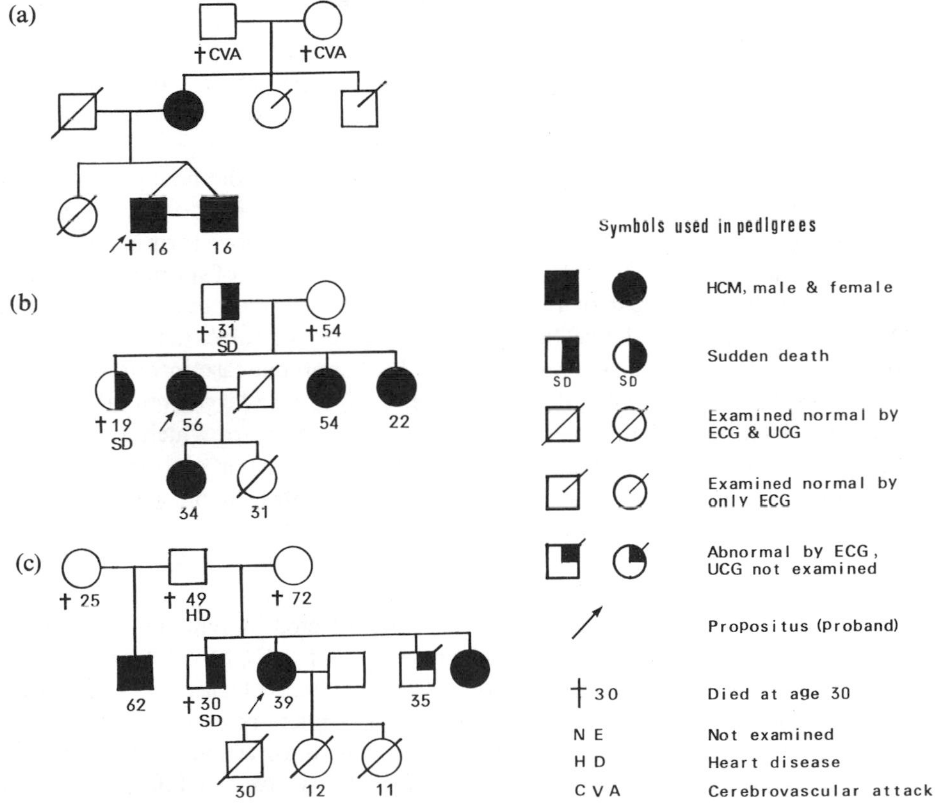

Fig. 1. Typical families of HCM.
(a) Family No. 8: an example of concordant twins
(b) Family No. 4: an example of extreme segregation of HCM
(c) Family No. 45: no segregation in offspring of proband (probability 0.125)

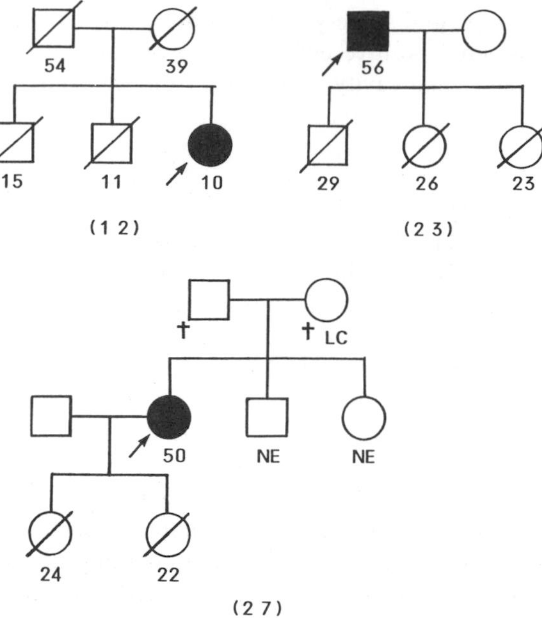

Fig. 2. Sporadic cases of HCM

be small. So the probability of discovering HCM in one parent of a proband or the other is almost equal to penetrance (p). If the parents of a proband are fully examined, the probability of skipping is $(1-p)$. When the proband has two siblings, the probability of normality in both siblings is $(1/2 \cdot p)^2$, as shown in Fig. 2a, and the final probability of negative HCM is $1/4 \cdot (1-p) \cdot p^2 = 1/4 \cdot (p^2 - p^3)$. The P value of the autosomal dominant gene is usually between 0.8 and 0.9. If we put $P = 0.8$ into the above formula, the probability of an sporadic case will be only 3.2%. Many family studies of sporadic cases have difficult problems because most of the parents have already died and their offspring are still relatively young, as shown in Fig. 1 and Fig. 2. We think that more careful examination is necessary in such a case. The 27.0% of sporadic case in our study may have been overestimated; however, the percentage seems to be a large even taking these biases into consideration. That means the existence of HCM cases which are not controlled by the dominant gene, but are caused by a polygenic system and/or by environmental factors. Those cases are described in the following section on a factor of age in segregation.

Segregation in Relatives

The ideal ratio of segregation between normal and affected individuals is 1:1 in the autosomal dominant trait. In such a case, recurrence risk for HCM is 0.5 among first-degree relatives. However, the recurrence risk is often reduced to less than 0.5 by decreased gene penetrance, late onset of the disease, incomplete research on the family, and so on. Another important factor is the segregation ratio, which is often changed by the method of ascertainment used in gathering data.[17] We gathered data on 74 families by the method of incomplete single ascertainment described above. Segregation analysis of autosomal dominant traits is rather more complicated than that of autosomal recessive traits, because one family often has an affected individual in more than one generation. In order to resolve these problems, we corrected the ratios from the pooled

TABLE 1. Segregation Analysis. *A Priori* Method

Size of sibship	No. of sibships	Total No. of children	Observed No. of affected	Expected No. of affected	σ_s^2	σ_s
2	37	74	33	49.32	8.21	
3	32	96	39	54.88	15.68	
4	14	56	26	29.88	10.95	
5	11	55	31	28.39	11.90	
6	7	42	21	21.33	9.65	
sum	101	323	150	183.80	56.39	7.51

data using the *a priori* method, the *a posteriori* method, and the singles method.

(1) Classical method based on an *a priori* expectation

Table 1 shows the observed number of patients and the variance in the size of the sibship. The total number of children in 74 families that can be divided into 101 sibships is 323, and the number of affected individuals is 150 using this method. As the expected number of patients is 183.8 in this case, the difference between the expected and the observed value is 33.8. This is a significant value because the difference is 4 times larger than $\sigma = 7.51$.

(2) *A posteriori* method

There are two methods for the analysis of sibship: one is the analysis of offspring; the other, that of siblings. In the former method, pooling of the data for children born to couples one of whom is a proband and the other normal gives almost complete ascertainment with small loss of specific genotype. These data should be differentiated from those from a siblings sample which needs correction for loss of normal genotype.

In this chapter, we analyzed the pooled data after dividing the sibship into two kinds, which are often found in the same family that carries an autosomal dominant trait. The number of offsping who were born to proband-normal spouse couples is 119 in 52 groups. There were 36 patients with HCM among them, and the segregation ratio was 0.302. Twenty-nine sporadic cases in 13 families indicates a different entity of disease from the usual HCM. If we exclude these sporadic cases from our data, the segregation ratio increases to 0.396. However, both segregation ratios are quite different from the expected value of 0.5. On the other hand, 129 affected patients (56.8%) out of 227 sibships in 62 groups were identified by analyzing the siblings of the probands. If we exclude the probands from these data in order to compensate for error, the final segregation ratio becomes 0.406. This ratio significantly differs by 5.82 of χ^2 from the expected values.[17] If we exclude 13 sporadic families which are supposed to be different entities, the ratio and value of χ^2 become 0.463 and 0.06, respectively. These data are compatible with the expectation of dominant inheritance. As described above, the segregation ratio of HCM shows relatively great differences between the analysis of siblings and that of offspring of the proband. This could be due to the factor of age in penetrance of the HCM gene.

The age of onset of HCM has a wide variation ranging from puberty to middle age. The segregation ratios differ significantly, by 5%, between the group under 30 years and that over 30 years of age.[20] Although the analysis of offspring of probands is thought to be a good method, the difference in average age between offspring and siblings (20 $\pm$ 7.8 years and 41 $\pm$ 14.6 years) seemed to decrease the penetrance of this disease.

(3) The singles method

In the *a posteriori* method, we tested the data by dividing the cases into different types of sibship in the same family. However, we can also analyze the data without dividing each pedigree, using the singles method.[18]

In this method, the number of affected individuals, normal individuals, single pedigrees, and double pedigrees are 161, 182, 56, and 2, respectively; thus, the ratio and σ are 0.366 and 0.0288, respectively. If we exclude the sporadic cases, as we did in the *a posteriori* method, the ratio and σ become 0.451 and 0.0325, respectively, which is somewhat different from the expected value.

Analyzed by these three methods, the segregation ratio is between 0.302 and 0.406 in all families with HCM. This value is less than the ideal ratio in the autosomal dominant case. The following factors are thought to account for the paucity of the ratio: (1) the relatively large number of sporadic cases, (2) the low penetrance of the HCM-gene, especially in younger family members for whom the penetrance is less than 1.0, and (3) insufficient follow-up in family research. If we exclude the sporadic cases as cases of a different entity, as discussed above, the segregation ratio approaches 0.5. The segregation ratio for siblings of the proband becomes especially close to 0.5. That means that HCM is a complex entity including sporadic cases and heterogenous type such as apical hypertrophy, although most cases are considered to be controlled by the autosomal dominant gene.

III. APICAL HYPERTROPHY

Apical hypertrophy (AH) is a type of HCM that is characterized by disproportionate hypertrophy of the left ventricular apical region and that shows the "ace of spades configuration" on left ventriculograms.[4,5] This type is relatively frequently reported in Japan. AH should be differentiated from apical ASH[9] or apical hypertrophic cardio-

TABLE 2. Comparison of Apical Hypertrophy (AH) and Apical Asymmetric Septal Hypertrophy (ASH)[9,22]

	Apical hypertrophy ($N=29$)	Apical ASH ($N=26$)	P
Age	53 ± 7	32 ± 13	<0.001
Sex (Male: Female)	26 : 3	8 : 5	<0.05
Rate of familial occurrence	10%	56% – 74%	-
Blood pressure			
systoric	131 ± 20	116 ± 11	<0.01
diastoric	81 ± 14	67 ± 12	<0.001
NYHA (III, IV) %	0	31	<0.01
ECG			
RV1 (mm)	3 ± 2	11 ± 11	<0.001
RV5 (mm)	41 ± 10	29 ± 13	<0.001
T (mm)	−16 ± 6	−3 ± 5	<0.001
UCG			
LVDs (mm)	26 ± 4	30 ± 6	<0.01
LVDd(mm)	45 ± 5	46 ± 5	NS
FS (%)	44 ± 6	34 ± 9	<0.001

NYHA: New York Heart Association, ECG: Electrocadiogram, UCG: Echocardiography, LVDs: Left ventricular systoric dimension, LVDd: Left ventricular diastoric dimension, FS: Fractional shortening

myopathy (AHCM),[8] which has abnormal hypertrophic septum near the apex. AH has less frequent familial occurrence and relatively high incidence in older men compared with apical ASH.[21] The difference between apical ASH and AH has been clarified recently.[9,22] The typical AH patient has a tendency to hypertension in his background and has a good clinical prognosis compared with the apical ASH patient, who often has the problem of congestive heart failure in the clinical course (Table 2). The relatives of the AH patient show less clear findings of abnormal ECG and 2-D echocardiography, and almost none of them has apical ASH or typical HCM. Mild hypertension and aging are thought to be acceralating factors of this disease. Though not major, a genetic factor may be involved because of the recurrence risk of about 10% in relatives. Apical ASH and AHCM are usually thought to be a part of the wide spectrum of HCM. These data suggest that the AH which is seen in Japan is a different entity of disease from apical ASH or AHCM. However, the non-familial case of HCM in an older man who has a history of mild hypertension may have the same pathogenecity as AH.

IV. FACTORS INFLUENCING GENE EXPRESSION

The gene penetrance in the dominant type of HCM is smaller than 100%, as is frequently seen in dominant genes. We have already demonstrated that aging is one of the important factors. Males are significantly more often affected than females, with a 96:65 ($\chi^2 = 5.97$) advantage in the sex ratio. It is of interest to know whether this different incidence is caused by internal environmental factors such as testosterone or external environmental factors such as smoking, drinking, physical exercise, and so on. In this point of view, we performed a case control study focusing on several environmental factors that were anticipated to influence gene expressivity.

We selected the following four groups for the case control study: 84 patients with definite HCM (55 males, 29 females) (Group 1), 84 normal relatives (Group 2), 59 abnormal relatives with HCM (Group 3), and 168 patients in our out-patient clinics (110 males, 58 females) (Group 4). The anticipated factors were examined and compared in each paired group as shown in Table 3. If an sporadic case is one with a non-genetic type of disease, external environmental factors may be more important factors. Therefore, we also did a study comparing 22 sporadic cases with familial cases.

In this study, the out-patient group (Group 4) is a group of patients without HCM who are treated in our out-patient cardiology clinics; it is not a group of normal control subjects. First-degree relatives who have normal ECG and UCG are more likely to be controls in the strict sense, because their environmental conditions are likely to bear a relatively close resemblance to their index cases. There is no significant difference in average age between Group I (46.2 ± 14.1) and Group 4 (46.1 ± 14.0). Relative risk (RR) was calculated for the comparison of each paired group, and the χ^2 test was used to examine the significance of the RR value.

As shown in Table 3, alcohol intake in cases with HCM significantly increased RR in the three comparative studies. A history of drinking to a moderate degree or more is certainly found in many patients with HCM, giving a RR of 3.22 to 6.67. Hypertension had a RR of 3.17 in the comparative study between the HCM cases (Group 1) and normal relatives (Group 2), and a RR of 2.43 (not significant) between sporadic cases and normal relatives. It is natural that many patients in the out-patient group (Group 4) had histories of illness and of medication. Sporadic cases had a significantly higher alcohol intake than normal relatives, but had no other significantly increased factors.

TABLE 3. Environmental Factors in HCM

Factor	Relative risk				
	all HCM: out-pt*	Case: Normal relatives	Case: Abnormal relatives	Sporadic: Familial	Sporadic: Normal relatives
School career (college or above)	0.46*	1.02	0.55	2.36	1.71
Susceptibility to common cold	0.65	0.61	0.82	2.12	1.01
Past history of illness	0.17***	1.89	2.00	2.17	3.00
Smoking	0.89	1.83	1.16	1.16	2.01
Alcohol intake	1.91	5.95***	3.22*	1.19	6.67***
Sports	2.26	1.36	0.86	2.54	2.45
Labor (physical)	1.62	1.26	1.62	0.51	0.77
Weight gain	1.18	0.49	1.91	1.85	0.73
Hypertension	0.84	3.17*	0.83	0.68	2.43
History of medication	0.25***	0.59	0.44	1.27	0.70

*** $P < 0.005$ ** $P < 0.01$ * $P < 0.05$ all HCM: case and relatives with HCM. out-pt: group of out-patients

In summary, though alcohol intake may be a promoting factor for HCM, it was not so great a factor in terms of its RR value of 3 to 6. Hypertension was found to be significant only in the comparison between the HCM cases and normal relatives, but it seemed to be less important than apical hypertrophy. There may be other promoting factors for HCM, such as hormonal and metabolic error, infection, intrauterine environment, and other unknown factors. However, there has been no detailed study of them. Considering these conditions, at the present time there is no clear explanation for the wide clinical manifestation of HCM even in the same family. Furthermore, the probable existence of a hypostatic modifying gene (accelerating or resistent) is conceibable.

Further extensive studies about primary genic function of the dominant gene, genetic or environmental modifying factors, and mutation rate will be needed in future.

REFERENCES

1. Frank, S. and Braunwald, E. Idiopathic subaortic stenosis. Clinical analysis of 126 patients with emphasis on the natural history. *Circulation* **37**: 759–788, 1968.
2. Abbasi, A.S., MacAlpin, R.N., Eber, L.M. and Pearce, M.L. Echocardiographic diagnosis of idiopathic hypertrophic cardiomyopathy without outflow obstruction. *Circulation* **46**: 897–904, 1972.
3. Henry, W.L., Clark, C.E., and Epstein, S.E. Echocardiographic identification of the pathognomonic anatomic abnormality of IHSS. *Circulation* **47**: 225–233, 1973.
4. Sakamoto, T., Tei, C., Murayama, M., Ichiyasu, H., Hada, Y., Hayashi, T., and Amano, K. Giant T wave inversion as a manifestation of asymmetrical apical hypertrophy (AAH) of the left ventricle. Echocardiographic and ultrasonocardiotomographic study. *Jpn. Heart J.* **17**: 611–629, 1976.
5. Yamaguchi, H., Ishimura, T., Nishiyama, S., Nagasaki, F., Nakanishi, S., Takatsu, F., Nishijo, T., Umeda, T., and Machii, K. Hypertrophic nonobstructive cadiomyopathy with

giant negative T waves (apical hypertrophy): Ventriculographic and echocardiographic features in 30 patients. *Am. J. Cardiol.* **44**: 401–412, 1979.

6. Maron, B.J. and Epstein, E.S. Hypertrophic cardiomyopathy: a discussion of nomenclature. *Am. J. Cardiol.* **43**: 1242–1244, 1979.
7. Maron, B.J., Gottdiener, J.S., and Epstein, S.E. Patterns and significans of distribution of left ventricular hypertrophy in hypertrophic cardiomyopathy. A wide angle, two dimensional echocardiographic study of 125 patients. *Am. J. Cardiol.* **48**: 418–428, 1981.
8. Maron, B.J., Bonow, R.O., Seshagiri, T.N.R., Roberts, W.C., and Epstein, S.E. Hypertrophic cardiomyopathy with ventricular septal hypertrophy localized to the apical region of the left ventricle (Apical hypertrophic cardiomyopathy). *Am. J. Cardiol.* **49**: 1838–1848, 1982.
9. Koga, Y., Takahashi, H., Ifuku, M., Itaya, M., Adachi, K., and Toshima, H. Hypertrophic cardiomyopathy with ventricular septal hypertrophy localized to the apical region of the left ventricle (apical ASH). *J. Cardiol.* **14**: 301–310, 1984. (in Japanese)
10. Emanuel, R., Withers, R., and O'Brien, K. Dominant and recessive modes of inheritance in idiopathic cardiomyopathy. *Lancet* **2**: 1065–1067, 1971.
11. Clark, C.E., Henry, W.L., and Epstein, S.E. Familial prevalence and genetic transmission of idiopathic hypertrophic subaortic stenosis. *N. Eng. J. Med.* **289**: 709–714, 1973.
12. Yamaguchi, M., Toshima, H., Yanase, T., Ikeda, H., Koga, Y., Yoshioka, H., Ito, M., Fujino, T., and Yasuda, H. A family study of idiopathic cardiomyopathy. *Proc. Jpn. Acad.* **53** (Series B) 209–214, 1977.
13. ten Cate, F.J., Hugenholtz, P.G., Dorp, W.G., and Roelandt, J. Prevalence of diagnostic abnormalities in patient with genetically transmitted asymmetric septal hypertrophy. *Am. J. Cardiol.* **43**: 731–737, 1979.
14. Maron, B.J., Nichols, III., P.F., Pickle, L.W., Wisley, Y.E., and Mulvihill, J.J. Patterns of inheritance in hypertrophic cardiomyopathy: Assessment by M-mode and two-dimensional echocardiography. *Am. J. Cardiol.* **53**: 1087–1094, 1984.
15. Greaves, S.C., Roche, A.H.G., Neutze, J.M., and Whitlock, R.M.L. Inheritance of hypertrophic cardiomyopathy: a cross sectional and M mode echocardiographic study of 50 families. Br. *Heart J.* **58**: 259–266, 1987.
16. Hogben, L. An Introduction to Mathematical Genetics. W.W. Norton & Co. Inc., N.Y., 1946.
17. Stern, C. Principles of Human Genetics. Freeman Co., Sanfrancisco, 1973, pp195–200.
18. Davie A: Segregation Analysis. In: Principles and Practice of Medical Genetics, Emery A.E.H., and Rimoin, D.L. (eds.), Churchill Livingstone, N.Y., 1983, pp75–79.
19. Matsuyama, K., Ogata, M., Shida, M., Miyazaki, Y., Koga, Y., Utsu, F., and Toshima, H. Usefulness of ECG and 2-D ECHO in family survey of hypertrophic cardiomyopathy. *Jpn. Circ. J.* **46**: 803–804, 1985 (Abst).
20. Matsuyama, K., Nishi, H., Shida, M., Miyazaki, Y., Toshima, H., Koga, Y., and Yamaguchi, M. The mode of inheritance of hypertrophic cardiomyopathy determined by two-dimensional echocardiography. Presented at the 52nd annual scientific meeting of Japanese Circulation Society, Akita, 1988.
21. Yamaguchi, M., Setoguchi, Y., Toshima, H., and Koga, Y. Genetic study of hypertrophic cardiomyopathy: with special reference to apical hypertrophy. *Jpn. Circ. J.* **46**: 735, 1982 (Abst.).
22. Miyazaki, Y., Shida, M., Matsuyama, K., Chiba, M., Nakata, M., Sakai, S., Inuzuka, S., Nohara, M., Toshima, H., and Koga, Y. Japanese apical hypertrophy is distinct from apical hypertrophic cardiomyopathy (Maron). *Heart* **19**: 554–568, 1987 (in Japanese).
23. Yamaguchi, M., Setoguchi, Y., Matsuo, S., Koga, Y., Hayano, M., Tsuruta, M., and Inoue, J. Further study of environmental factors in patient with hypertrophic cardiomyopathy. *Jpn. Circ. J.* **50**: 296–297, 1986 (Abst).

A Possible Role of Systemic Hypertension in the Pathogenesis of Hypertrophic Cardiomyopathy

Yoshinori Koga and Hironori Toshima

The Third Department of Medicine, Kurume University School of Medicine, Kurume, Japan

ABSTRACT

Asymmetric septal hypertrophy, although initially considered to be a pathognomonic sign of hypertrophic cardiomyopathy (HCM), is now recognized to occur in various other conditions, including systemic hypertension. The advent of echocardiography has also revealed that HCM is not at all unusual in elderly people, and is often associated with hypertension. These observations have raised the important question as to whether an association of hypertension in patients with HCM is purely coincidental or represents some etiological relationship. We therefore performed a case-control study and found that the association is statistically significant, suggesting an etiological relationship. When our patients with HCM were subdivided into several groups according to the presence or absence of familial occurrence of HCM and history of hypertension, we found that the hypertensive group consisted predominantly of elderly males and presented a milder form of the disease with less impaired cardiac function and infrequent sudden death. Apical hypertrophy of Japanese form also appeared to suggest an association of abnormal hypertrophy and hypertension.

From these observations, we propose that HCM represents a group of related but etiologically distinct diseases rather than a single disease entity. Particularly in elderly patients, there may exist an etiologically distinct form of the disease that may be related to hypertension and in which the morphologic expression of HCM nevertheless appears to be similar to that of the classical genetic form of the disease.

ASYMMETRIC HYPERTROPHY IN PATIENTS WITH SYSTEMIC HYPERTENSION

The clinical diagnosis of hypertrophic cardiomyopathy (HCM) relies upon a demonstration of unexplained left ventricular hypertrophy. The distribution of hypertrophy is most often asymmetrical, predominantly involving the ventricular septum and occasionally the distal ventricle, while symmetrical hypertrophy may also be found.[1,2] Outflow obstruction of the ventricle, another feature characteristic of HCM, is observed in about one-third of patients under basal condition. These hallmarks of HCM, asymmetric ventricular hypertrophy and outflow obstruction, can reliably be assessed noninvasively with echocardiography and were initially considered to be the pathognomonic signs of HCM.[3–5] Subsequent studies,[6,7] however, have shown that these findings are neither characteristic nor highly specific to HCM but can also occur in other cardiac diseases such as congenital anomalies with long-standing right ventricular pressure overload, congenital or acquired aortic valvular diseases, and systemic hypertension. Accordingly, the term "disproportionate septal thickening (DST)" has been proposed by Maron *et al.*[6,7] to describe the secondary form of abnormal ventricular septal thickening, since the term "asymmetric septal hypertrophy (ASH)" implies the existence of a primary cardiomyopathy.

A possible association of asymmetric septal hypertrophy in patients with systemic hypertension has been given considerable attention, often resulting in a diagnostic dilemma, as hypertension is the most common condition in the general population and such an association is not rare in clinical practice. In 1975, we[8] demonstrated with echocardiography that asymmetric septal hypertrophy could occur in patients with borderline hypertension, some of them being associated with left ventricular outflow obstruction. Subsequent studies[7,9–20] have confirmed our observation, though the reported prevalence of asymmetric septal hypertrophy in hypertensives has varied considerably (4–30%), possibly depending on the study population. These studies have raised the important question of whether the presence of asymmetric septal hypertrophy in patients with hypertension represents an etiological relationship or is a purely coincidental occurrence.

Figure 1 shows our recent observations on left ventricular wall thickness (as expressed by adding ventricular septal and posterial wall thickness) determined by echocardiography in patients with systemic hypertension. Patients with sustained hypertension and severe retinal changes (Scheie grade III) showed left ventricular wall thickness of around 30 mm to 40 mm. In contrast, left ventricular wall thickness was quite variable in patients with mild hypertension and less severe retinal damage. Some of them manifested asymmetric septal hypertrophy or apical hypertrophy showing a spade-shaped configuration on the left ventriculogram. These observations were con-

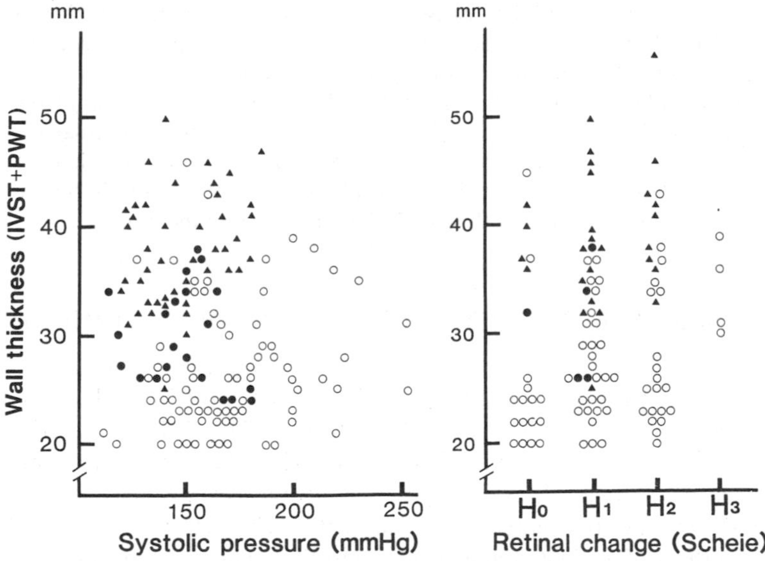

Fig. 1. Relationship of left ventricular wall thickness (ventricular septum + posterior wall) to systolic blood presure during admission (left) or retinal change on Scheie's classification (right). Note the greater variation in wall thickness in those with borderline elevation in systolic blood presure and milder retinal change. Asymmetric septal hypertrophy or apical hypertrophy is observed in those with a systolic pressure of 180 mmHg or less, or in those with Scheie grade II or less. Closed circles represent patients with asymmetric septal hypertrophy, closed triangles those with apical hypertrophy, and open circles those with symmetric hypertrophy.

sistent with findings in previous reports by others[11,17,18,20] as well as ourselves[8] that asymmetric hypertrophy is more prevalent in patients with borderline hypertension than in those with sustained hypertension. Since asymmetric hypertrophy cannot thus be ascribed solely to increased afterload, Safer *et al.*[11] and Corea *et al.*[18] have suggested that augmented sympathetic activity might be related to the abnormality. We[8] alternatively postulated that these patients might have developed excessive hypertrophy based on some genetic predisposition, the expression of which is evoked by hypertension. Savage *et al.*[21] performed an echocardiographic study on the first-degree relatives of patients with hypertension and disproportionate septal thickening. They found that disproportionate septal thickening occurred in four of seven hypertensive relatives, but in only one of 16 normotensive relatives. From these results, they also suggested that hypertensives with disproportionate septal thickening have a heritable predisposition that is expressed only in the presence of hypertension.

HYPERTENSION IN PATIENTS WITH HYPERTROPHIC CARDIOMYOPATHY

In patients with HCM, an association with hypertension[22–26] has long been noted since the first report by Brock,[22] who implied that the condition might be an acquired entity, secondary to hypertension. Later reports[27–30] on larger series of patients with HCM have focused upon the high incidence of familial occurrence of the disease and have paid less attention to its association with hypertension. Clark *et al.*,[31] who performed a familial survey using M-mode echocardiography, further emphasized the genetic aspect of the disease, describing that familial occurrence is demonstrable in the majority of patients with HCM. It is noteworthy, however, that these studies were performed at large referral centers where young or middle-aged symptomatic patients are more likely to be sent. Exclusion of elderly patients could thus be a possible explanation for the low prevalence of hypertension in these studies. With the advent of echocardiography, however, HCM has been increasingly recognized to be not at all unusual in elderly patients.[32–41] Approximately half of these elderly HCM patients have been reported to show associated hypertension[33,34,36–38,40,41] and less frequent familial occurrence.[33,34,37,38,40] Recent re-evaluations[42–45] of familial occurrence using two-dimensional echocardiography have revealed that the prevalence of the familial form of HCM was only about 50% to 60%, substantially less frequent than those found in previous M-mode echocardiographic studies.[31] Some sporadic cases could be genetic and represent new mutations or autosomal recessive transmission. In contrast, Maron[2,45] has suggested that the high frequency with which the sporadic variety of HCM occurs indicates that

TABLE 1. Sex Incidence, Familial Occurrence, and History of Hypertension in Three Age-groups of Patients with Hypertrophic Cardiomyopathy

	Obstructive			Nonobstructive (ASH)		
Age (years)	≤29	30–49	≥50	≤29	30–49	≥50
No. of patients	10	17	11	25	50	32
Sex (% male)	50	76	82	60	64	78
Family Hx (%)	80	47	25[a]	72	60	50
Hx of hypertension (%)	0	35	64[b,d]	4	24	63[c,f]

[a]P<0.05, [b]P<0.01, [c]P<0.001 as compared with the young group; [d]P<0.05, [e]P<0.01, [f]P<0.001 as compared with the middle-aged group. ASH = Asymmetric septal hypertrophy, Hx = history.

other nongenetic causes may exist and that these produce phenotypically similar expressions of the disease. Hence, it appears possible that HCM represents a group of related but etiologically distinct diseases rather than a single disease entity.

Table 1 shows the sex incidence, frequency of familial occurrence, and history of hypertension correlated with age in our patients with HCM. Although sustained hypertension could occur in patients with HCM, the majority of them manifest mild and labile hypertension. Our primary interest was then focused on the association of mild or labile hypertension and HCM, and patients who showed high blood pressure exceeding 160/95 mmHg were excluded from the analysis. In younger patients with HCM (less than 30 years old), there was a nearly equal sex incidence with frequent familial occurrence, suggesting autosomal dominant inheritance. On the other hand, elderly patients of 50 years of age or older were predominantly males, had a frequent association with a history of hypertension, and showed less common familial occurrence. The middle-aged patients (30 to 49 years old) manifested a profile intermediate between those of the younger and older patients. These observations may further support the concept that there are etiologically distinct forms of the disease, particularly in elderly patients, that are possibly related to hypertension and in which the morphologic expression of HCM nevertheless appears to be similar to that in the classical genetic from of the disease.

CASE-CONTROL STUDY ON THE ASSOCIATION OF HYPERTENSION WITH HCM

The issue that is therefore important is whether hypertension and HCM are significantly related or are purely coincidental. The most desirable way to address this question would be to perform a cohort study, comparing the eventual outcomes of groups of subjects with or without systemic hypertension. The relative occurrence of abnormal hypertrophy indicating HCM noted when each group was followed forward in time would provide the controlled measure of risk. Although such an investigative method is logically appealing, it cannot readily be used to study uncommon diseases, such as HCM, because extremely large groups of people would have to be followed for long periods to obtain statistically meaningful estimates of risk. Because of these logistic problems, the case-control study has become a popular activity with widespread acceptance as an alternative approach which allows statistically meaningful results to be obtained with a manageable sample size. The approach ascertains the relative frequencies of the risk of interest in two groups, a case group of patients who have the disease and a control group who have not, and provides a controlled estimate of risk.

We then performed the case-control study to investigate whether hypertension and HCM are significantly associated or not. The study subject included 102 consecutive patients with HCM, aged 35 years or more, who were admitted to our hospital. Patients who presented hypertension exceeding 160/95 mmHg during admission were excluded from the study. The subjects were divided into two groups: one consisted of 65 patients with asymmetric septal hypertrophy (50 males and 15 females with an average age of 51 ± 9 years), and the other of 37 patients with apical hypertrophy (34 males and 3 females with an average age of 52 ± 9 years). Patients with asymmetric septal hypertrophy included 18 patients with outflow obstruction in the resting condition and 47 with no obstruction while resting. Those with apical hypertrophy showed a spade-shaped configuration on the left ventriculogram, and neither outflow obstruction nor asymmetric septal hypertrophy was noted. For each case of HCM, two controls, matched for age and sex,

TABLE 2. History of High Blood Pressure and Use of Antihypertensive Medication among Cases and Controls

	Asymmetric septal hypertrophy			Apical hypertrophy		
	Case	Control	Relative risk (CI)	Case	Control	Relative risk (CI)
History of high blood pressure						
	51%	27%	2.9 (1.5–5.4)[b]	54%	25%	3.5 (1.5–8.1)[b]
Frequency of high blood pressure documentation						
Occasional	16%	20%	1.2 (0.5–2.8)	24%	19%	2.0 (0.7–5.6)
Often	35%	7%	7.5 (3.0–18.4)[c]	30%	6%	8.1 (2.3–28.8)[c]
Use of antihypertensive medication						
	31%	18%	2.1 (1.0–4.2)[a]	22%	19%	1.1 (0.4–3.1)

[a] $P<0.05$, [b] $P<0.01$, [c] $P<0.001$.
CI = 95% confidence interval.

were selected randomly from the population register of the suburban town of Kurume, where our hospital is located. Trained interviewers successfully carried out telephone interviews in all patients with HCM and 93% of 204 control subjects. The interview schedule involved ascertaining the number of previous blood pressure measurements, history of high blood pressure, and use of antihypertensive medications. We also obtained histories related to incidences of common cold, diabetes, recent weight changes, smoking, alcohol intake, regularity of exercise, and the usual demographic information with regard to such factors as education and occupation. Points estimates of relative risk were calculated by the odds ratio. Confidence intervals were computed by the method of Miettinen.[46] Statistical significance was determined at a level of $p < 0.05$ by Chi-square test for two-by-two tables or by Bartholomew's test[47] for dose-response relationships.

Table 2 presents the histories of high blood pressure and use of antihypertensive medications among patients with asymmetric septal hypertrophy or apical hypertrophy, and among the control subjects. High blood pressure was reported to be mentioned by family physicians or at the time of regular medical screening in 51% of patients with asymmetric septal hypertrophy and in only 27% of the controls. The relative risk estimate of HCM was significantly increased to 2.9 for those with a history of hypertension. Use of antihypertensive medications was again higher in patients with asymmetric septal hypertrophy than in controls (31% vs 18%), with a relative risk estimate of 2.1. Patients with apical hypertrophy of Japanese form reported a history of high blood pressure significantly more frequently than did controls with a relative risk estimate of 3.5. The relative risk estimates of both asymmetric septal hypertrophy and apical hypertrophy increased with an increasing frequency of reports of high blood pressure. In contrast, there were no differences among the HCM patients and controls in the number of blood pressure determinations, history of diabetes, recent weight gain, smoking, or alcohol intake.

Thus the case-control study clearly indicated that the association of hypertension and HCM is not a coincidental occurrence, but is significantly and possibly etiologically related. Although excessive hypertrophy in these patients can apparently not be ascribed solely to increased afterload, it is likely that hypertension provoked or promoted abnormal hypertrophy in association with some other predisposition, possibly genetic. An alternative possibility might be that a common but unknown abnormality is related to both excessive hypertrophy and hypertension.

DIFFERENCES IN CLINICAL PROFILES BETWEEN HCM PATIENTS WITH FAMILIAL OCCURRENCE AND THOSE WITH A HISTORY OF HYPERTENSION

The significant association of hypertension with HCM may raise the further question of whether or not these hypertensive patients present clinical features similar to those with the classical familial form (familial group) of the disease. We therefore subdivided patients with HCM into several groups according to familial occurrence and history of hypertension, and compared their clinical features (Tables 3–5). In nonobstructive patients with asymmetric septal hypertrophy, the hypertensive group who showed a history of hypertension but no familial occurrence was significantly older than the familial group. Eighty-two percent of the hypertensive group were males. In addition to higher systolic and diastolic blood pressures, the hypertensive group presented greater ventricular septal thickening. This could be explained by the inclusion of those with atypical septal hypertrophy mainly involving the distal or postero-basal septum in the familial group. The significantly thicker posterior wall in the hypertensive group might be related to increased afterload. On the other hand, left ventricular end-diastolic pressure was less elevated and myocardial fibrosis in the endomyocardial biopsy samples was less extensive in the hypertensive group. Patients who presented both familial occurrence and a history of hypertension showed a clinical profile comparable to that of the hypertensive group. This similarity may offer further evidence that hypertension is related to the morphologic expression of the disease in these patients. Patients who showed neither history of hypertension nor familial occurrence demonstrated clinical features comparable to those of the familial group. The incomplete family survey in these patients could explain the similarities, although we examined at least three first-degree relatives using either electrocardiography or echocardiography (or both).

In patients with obstructive HCM (Table 4), the resting pressure gradient within the left ventricle was even greater in the hypertensive group. Patients in this group were older and presented higher QRS amplitude and greater posterior wall thickening in

TABLE 3. Clinical Profiles of Hypertrophic Nonobstructive Cardiomyopathy with Asymmetric Septal Hypertrophy in Relation to Familial Occurrence and History of Hypertension

	HT (+) FH (−)	HT (+) FH (+)	HT (−) FH (−)	HT (−) FH (+)
No. of patients	22	11	32	42
Age (years)	53±11[c]	53±12[c]	41±12[a]	34±14
Sex (% male)	82%	73%	47%	71%
Blood pressure (mmHg)				
Systolic	148±20[c]	130±14[b]	117±14	117±11
Diastolic	85±9[c]	78±9[b]	67±10	66±12
SV_1 + RV_5 (mm)	50±14	45±14	39±19	45±16
T in V_5 (mm)	−9±8[b]	−6±9	−4±6	−3±6
Wall thickness (mm)				
Septum	24±4[b]	23±4	22±6	19±7
Posterior wall	15±3[b]	13±1	13±2	12±3
LVEDP (mmHg)	11±5[b]	11±2[a]	17±7	17±7
% Fibrosis (%)	15±11	19±14	24±10	22±9

[a] $P<0.05$, [b] $P<0.01$, [c] $P<0.001$ compared with those of HT(−) and FH(+). HT = history of hypertension, FH = family history, LVEDP = left ventricular end-diastolic pressure

TABLE 4. Clinical Profiles of Hypertrophic Obstructive Cardiomyopathy in Relation to Familial Occurrence and History of Hypertension

	HT (+) FH (−)	HT (−) FH (−)	HT (−) FH (+)
No. of patients	12	8	17
Age (years)	$53\pm9^{c)}$	41 ± 18	30 ± 13
Sex (% male)	75%	75%	65%
Blood pressure (mmHg)			
Systolic	$134\pm19^{a)}$	108 ± 10	117 ± 12
Diastolic	$80\pm16^{b)}$	56 ± 15	62 ± 13
SV_1+RV_5(mm)	$60\pm22^{a)}$	41 ± 14	42 ± 20
T in V_5 (mm)	-3 ± 9	-3 ± 6	0 ± 6
Wall thickness (mm)			
Septum	$22\pm5^{b)}$	24 ± 5	28 ± 6
Posterior wall	$19\pm4^{b)}$	14 ± 3	14 ± 3
Pressure gradient (mmHg)	72 ± 49	40 ± 18	59 ± 30
LVEDP (mmHg)	21 ± 5	$16\pm5^{a)}$	22 ± 6
FAI (%)	$38\pm19^{a)}$	$29\pm12^{b)}$	51 ± 11

$^{a)}P<0.05$, $^{b)}P<0.01$, $^{c)}P<0.001$ compared with those of HT (−) and FH (+). HT = history of hypertension, FH = family history, LVEDP = left ventricular end-diastolic pressure, FAI = functional aerobic impairment

addition to elevated blood pressure, as compared with the familial group. On exercise stress test, however, functional aerobic impairment was significantly lower in the hypertensive group, while left ventricular end-diastolic pressure was comparable.

HCM patients in the hypertensive group thus presented similar or even greater morphologic expression of asymmetric septal hypertrophy as well as hemodynamic manifestation of left ventricular outflow obstruction. Nevertheless, these patients in the hypertensive group showed trends toward lower left ventricular end-diastolic pressure, less extensive myocardial fibrosis, and milder limitation in exercise capacity. The long-term prognosis is usually favorable and sudden death is rare in these patients.[48] The hypertensive group of HCM thus appeared to have a milder form of the disease despite their advanced age. We would therefore suggest that the hypertensive group may present a disease that is etiologically distinct from the classical genetic form of HCM which is compatible with autosomal dominant inheritance. Although this postulation has not been substantiated by pathological studies, Maron *et al.*[49] failed to find extensive disarray of myocardial cells consistent with classical HCM in two hypertensive patients with disproportionate ventricular septal thickening.

These different clinical manifestations in hypertensive and familial forms of HCM have not been fully described previously, but it has been well recognized that elderly patients, frequently associated with hypertension, are often minimally symptomatic and may be unexpectedly diagnosed by routine echocardiographic examination.[33,34,37,40] Some elderly patients are able to live a long life and are incidentally found to have HCM at the time of autopsy for noncardiac diseases. Accordingly, Davies *et al.*[33] suggested that, at one end of the spectrum of HCM, there are young patients, often familial, who usually show the classical form of the disease with severe functional limitations and frequent sudden death, while at the other end there are elderly patients with similar morphological appearance but who have no or minimal symptoms of cardiac disease. Their suggestion appears to be consistent with our experience.[40]

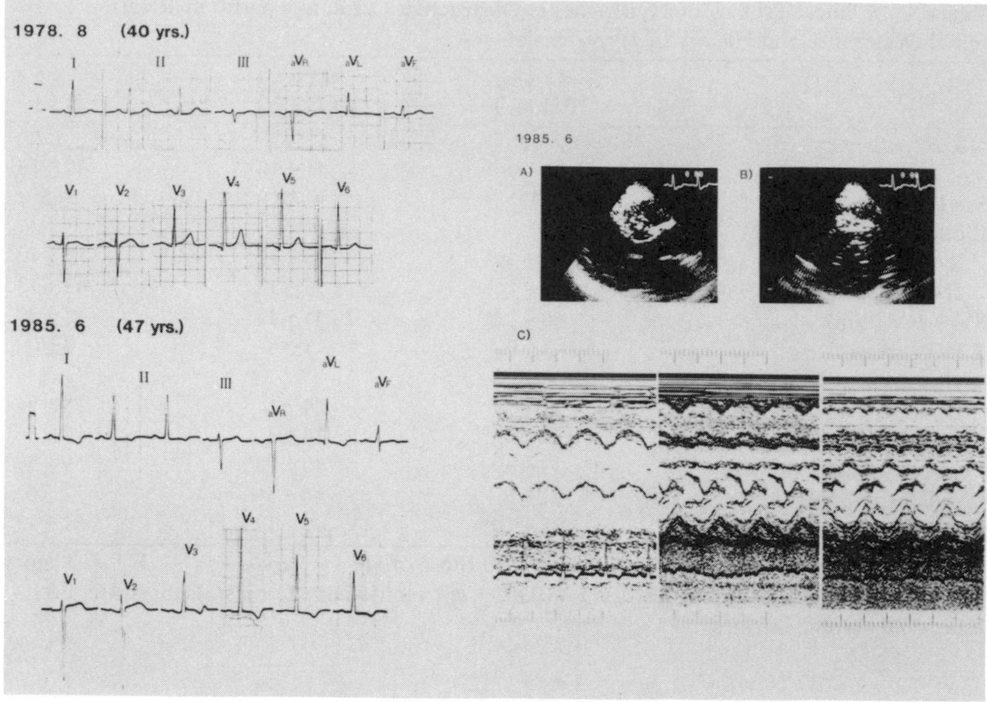

Fig. 2. A representative patient suggesting that hypertension has provoked asymmetric septal hypertrophy. She presented a nealy normal electrocardiogram (left upper) at age 40, when she was diagnosed as being hypertensive (190/100 mmHg). During the following years, she developed left ventricular hypertrophy with negative T waves (left lower). Echocardiograms at age 47 demonstrate asymmetric septal hypertrophy and systolic anterior motion of the mitral valve (right). Cardiac catheterization revealed a pressure gradient of 50 mmHg in the left ventricle and confirmed a diagnosis of hypertrophic obstructive cardiomyopathy.

The explanation for this more benign and milder form of the disease in elderly hypertensive patients is not clear. Figure 2 presents an interesting patient in this regard who suggested a mode of expression of abnormal hypertrophy. Although the initial echocardiogram was not available, she presented a nearly normal electrocardiogram at the age of 40 years, when she was diagnosed as hypertensive (190/100 mmHg). During the following seven years, she developed T wave inversion in the left precordial leads and presented asymmetric septal hypertrophy and left ventricular outflow obstruction of 50 mmHg. Several investigators[24,25] have also reported patients with hypertension in whom clinical and hemodynamic features of HCM later developed. It is therefore likely that such elderly hypertensive patients express abnormal hypertrophy later in life in the presence of coexistent hypertension and accordingly present a relatively milder form of the disease.

The greater thickening of the posterior wall in the hypertensive group was again in agreement with previous autopsy studies[33,34] which have noted more uniform left ventricular hypertrophy in elderly patients with HCM. Although they attributed this morphological difference to long-standing outflow obstruction in elderly patients, the tendency was also observed in nonobstructive patients in our series. We therefore suppose

TABLE 5. Clinical Profiles of Apical Hypertrophy in Relation to History of Hypertension

	History of hypertension	
	(+)	(−)
No. of patients	23	25
Age (years)	52±10	50±6
Sex (% male)	97%	89%
Blood pressure (mmHg)		
Systolic	148±20[b]	124±14
Diastolic	88±13[a]	77±11
SV_1+RV_5 (mm)	59±12	56±16
T in V_5 (mm)	−16±5	−16±7
Wall thickess (mm)		
Septum	15±3	15±3
Posterior wall	14±2	14±3
LVEDP (mmHg)	14±5	15±6
FAI (%)	24±17	27±18

[a] $P<0.01$, [b] $P<0.001$. LVEDP = left ventricular end-diastolic pressure, FAI = functional aerobic impairment

that hypertension may have also contributed to the posterior wall thickening. An interesting difference has emerged in the sex predilection between Japanese and Western elderly hypertensive patients with HCM. Among our Japanese patients, males predominated, while a majority of reports from Western countries[32,35–39,41] have described the preponderance of female patients. The discrepancy is difficult to explain, but may be related to different racial, socioeconomic, or nutritional factors between the countries. The much higher incidence of coronary artery diseases in Western males could alternatively have masked the occurrence of HCM. Whatever the reason, the sex difference may provide a clue to investigate the role of environmental or acquired factors in the development of excess hypertrophy in elderly HCM.

Apical hypertrophy of Japanese form,[51,52] which manifests as a spade-shaped deformity of the left ventricle, is another example that suggests an association of hypertension with abnormal hypertrophy. As described in detail elsewhere in this monograph, the condition occurs exclusively in middle-aged or elderly males.[53,54] Around half of them present a history of hypertension, though few patients demonstrate familial occurrence. Our case-control study revealed a significant association of hypertension with apical hypertrophy, as previously described. The majority of these patients are asymptomatic or minimally symptomatic, and are incidentally identified by a characteristic electrocardiographic finding (giant negative T waves) at the time of routine health checks, either at home or at the workplace. They show mildly elevated left ventricular end-diastolic pressure and minimal impairment of exercise capacity, with no reported sudden death until recently. Apical hypertrophy thus again appears to be distinct from the classical familial form of HCM. When these patients were subdivided into those with and without a history of hypertension, the two groups did not differ in their clinical features except for higher blood pressure in the hypertensive group (Table 5). Both groups, irrespective of a history of hypertension, demonstrated an increased response of systolic pressure elevation during exercise compared with age- and sex-matched control subjects who had comparable resting blood pressures. It is not uncommon to obtain a nearly normal electrocardiogram taken several years earlier in these patients. We[53] thus

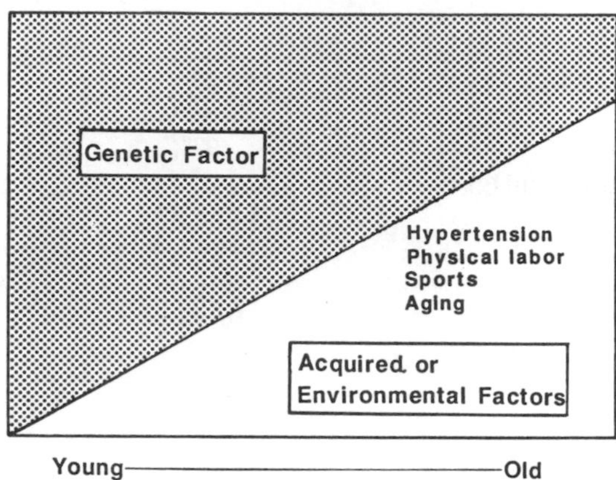

Fig. 3. A diagram illustrating the proposed disease spectrum of hypertrophic cardiomyopathy. See text for details.

suggested that these patients with apical hypertrophy developed the abnormality through provocation by increased afterload, although hypertension is apparently not the sole factor.

Figure 3 depicts our current hypothesis on the disease spectrum of HCM. It is possible that HCM represents a group of related but etiologically distinct diseases rather than a single disease entity. At one end of the spectrum are young patients who develop the disease based on a genetic defect inherited as an autosomal dominant trait, while at the other end are elderly patients who express excessive hypertrophy in association with coexisting acquired or environmental factors related to hypertension, physical labor, sports, or aging. Since these acquired factors do not fully explain the abnormal hypertrophy in the latter group, we have also postulated the contribution of some genetic predisposition different from the autosomal dominant trait. In conclusion, there may be etiologically distinct forms of the disease that are related to acquired factors such as hypertension and in which the morphologic expression of hypertrophic cardiomyopathy nevertheless appears to be similar to that in the classical genetic form of the disease.

Acknowledgment

This study was supported in part by the Research Grant for Intractable Diseases from the Ministry of Health and Welfare of Japan.

REFERENCES

1. Wigle, E.D., Sasson, Z., Henderson, M.A., Ruddy, T.D., Fulop, J., Rakowski, H., and Williams, W.G. Hypertrophic cardiomyopathy. The importance of the site and the extent of hypertrophy. A review. *Progr. Cardiovas. Dis.* **28**: 1–83, 1985.
2. Maron, B.J., Bonow, R.O., Cannon, R.O. III, Leon, M.B., and Epstein, S.E. Hypertrophic cardiomyopathy. Interrelations of clinical manifestations, pathophysiology, and therapy. *N. Engl. J. Med.* **361**: 780–89, 1987.
3. Shah, P.M., Gramiak, R., Adelman, A.G., and Wigle, E.D. Role of echocardiography in diagnostic and hemodynamic assessment of hypertrophic subaortic stenosis. *Circulation* **44**: 891–8, 1971.

4. Henry, W.L., Clark, C.E., and Epstein, S.E. Asymmetric septal hypertrophy. Echocardiographic identification of the pathognomonic anatomic abnormality of IHSS. *Circulation* **47**: 225–33, 1973.
5. Epstein, S.E., Henry, W.L., Clark, C.E., Roberts, W.C., Maron, B.J., Ferrans, V.J., Redwood, D.R., and Morrow, A.G. Asymmetric septal hypertrophy. *Ann. Intern. Med.* **81**: 650–80, 1974.
6. Maron, B.J., Edwards, J.E., Ferrans, V.J., Clark, C.E., Lebowitz, E.A., Henry, W.L., and Epstein, S.E. Congenital heart malformations associated with disproportionate ventricular septal thickening. *Circulation* **52**: 926–32, 1975.
7. Maron, B.J. and Epstein, S.E. Hypertrophic cardiomyopathy. Recent observations regarding the specificity of three hallmarks of the disease: Asymmetric septal hypertrophy, septal disorganization and systolic anterior motion of the anterior mitral leaflet. *Am. J. Cardiol.* **45**: 141–54, 1980.
8. Toshima, H., Koga, Y., Yoshioka, H., Akiyoshi, T., and Kimura, N. Echocardiographic classification of hypertensive heart disease: A correlative study with clinical features. *Jpn. Heart J.* **16**: 377–93, 1975.
9. Criley, J.M., Blaufuss, A.H., and Abbasi, A.S. Nonobstructive IHSS. *Circulation* **52**: 963, 1975.
10. Dunn, F.G., Chandraratna, P., de Carvalho, J.G.R., Basta, L.L., and Frohlich, E.D. Pathophysiologic assessment of hypertensive heart disease with echocardiography. *Am. J. Cardiol.* **39**: 789–95, 1977.
11. Safar, M.E., Lehner, J.P., Vincent, M.I., Plainfosse, M.T., and Simon, A.Ch. Echocardiographic dimensions in borderline and sustained hypertension. *Am. J. Cardiol.* **44**: 930–35, 1979.
12. Savage, D.D., Drayer, J.I.M., Henry, W.L., Mathews, E.C. Jr., Ware, J.H., Gardin, J.M., Cohen, E.R., Epstein, S.E., and Laragh, J.H. Echocardiographic assessment of cardiac anatomy and function in hypertensive subjects. *Circulation* **59**: 623–32, 1979.
13. Kansal, S., Roitman, D., and Sheffield, L.T. Interventricular septal thickness and left ventricular hypertrophy. An echocardiographic study. *Circulation* **60**: 1058–65, 1979.
14. Gibson, D.G., Traill, T.A., Hall, R.J.C., and Brown, D.J. Echocardiographic features of secondary left ventricular hypertrophy. *Br. Heart J.* **41**: 54–9, 1979.
15. Doi, Y.L., Deanfield, J.E., McKenan, W.J., Dargie, H.J., Oakley, C.M., and Goodwin, J.F. Echocardiographic differentiation of hypertensive heart disease and hypertrophic cardiomyopathy. *Br. Heart J.* **44**: 395–400, 1980.
16. Cohen, A., Hagan, A.D., Watkins, J., Mitas, J., Schvartzman, M., Mazzoleni, A., Cohen, I.M., Warren, S.E., and Vieweg, W.V.R. Clinical correlates in hypertensive patients with left ventricular hypertrophy diagnosed with echocardiography. *Am. J. Cardiol.* **47**: 335–41, 1981.
17. Niederle, P., Widimsk'y, J., Jandova', R., Ressel, J., and Grospic, A. Echocardiographic assessment of the left ventricle in juvenile hypertension. *Int. J. Cardiol.* **2**: 91–101, 1982.
18. Corea, L., Bentivoglio, M., Verdecchia, P., and Motolese, M. Left ventricular wall thickness and plasma catecholamines in borderline and stable essential hypertension. *Eur. Heart J.* **3**: 164–70, 1982.
19. Shapiro, L.M., Kleinebenne, A., and McKenna, W.J. The distribution of left ventricular hypertrophy in hypertrophic cardiomyopathy: comparison to athletes and hypertensives. *Eur. Heart J.* **6**: 967–74, 1985.
20. Hammond, I.W., Devereux, R.B., Alderman, M.H., Lutas, E.M., Spitzer, M.C., Crowley, J.S., and Laragh, J.H. The prevalence and correlates of echocardiographic left ventricular hypertrophy among employed patients with uncomplicated hypertension. *J. Am. Coll. Cardiol.* **7**: 639–50, 1986.
21. Savage, D.D., Devereux, R.B., Sachs, I., and Laragh, J.H. Disproportionate ventricular septal thickness in hypertensive patients. *J. Cardiovasc. Ultrasonography* **1**: 79–85, 1982.
22. Brock, R. Functional obstruction of the left ventricle (acquired aortic subvalvular stenosis)

Guys Hosp. Rep. **106**: 221–38, 1957.
23. Ewy, G.A., Marcus, F.I., Bohajalian, O., Burke, H.L., and Roberts, W.C. Muscular subaortic stenosis. Clinical and pathologic observations in an elderly patient. *Am. J. Cardiol.* **22**: 126–32, 1968.
24. Moreyra, E., Knibbe, P., and Brest, A.N. Hypertension and muscular subaortic stenosis. *Chest* **57**: 87–90, 1970.
25. Hamby, R.I., Roberts, G.S., and Meron, J.M. Hypertension and hypertrophic subaortic stenosis. *Am. J. Med.* **51**: 474–80, 1971.
26. Alday, L.E., Wagner, H.R., and Vlad, P. Severe systemic hypertension and muscular subaortic stenosis. *Am. Heart J.* **83**: 395–400, 1972.
27. Frank, S., and Braundwald, E. Idiopathic hypertrophic subaortic stenosis: Clinical analysis of 126 patients with emphasis on the natural history. *Circulation* **37**: 759–88, 1968.
28. Adelman, A.G., Wigle, E.D., Ranganathan, N., Webb, G.D., Kidd, B.S.L., Bigelow, W.G., and Silver, M.D. The clinical course in muscular subaortic stenosis. *Ann. Intern. Med.* **77**: 515–25, 1972.
29. Hardarson, T., de la Calzada, C.S., Curiel, R., and Goodwin, J.F. Prognosis and mortality of hypertrophic obstructive cardiomyopathy. *Lancet* ii: 1462–67, 1973.
30. Shah, P.M., Adelman, A.G., Wigle, E.D., Gobel, F.L., Burchell, H.B., Hardarson, T., Curiel, R., de la Calzada, C., Oakley, C.M., and Goodwin, J.F. The natural (and unnatural) history of hypertrophic obstructive cardiomyopathy. *Circ. Res.* **35** (Suppl. 2): 179–95, 1974.
31. Clark, C.E., Henry, W.L., and Epstein S.E. Familial prevalence and genetic transmission of idiopathic hypertrophic subaortic stenosis. *N. Engl. J. Med.* **289**: 709–14, 1973.
32. Whiting, R.B., Powell, W.J. Jr., Dinsmore R.E., and Sanders, C.A. Idiopathic hypertrophic subaortic stenosis in the elderly. *N. Engl. J. Med.* **285**: 196–200, 1971.
33. Davies, M.J., Pomerance, A., and Teare, R.D. Pathological features of hypertrophic obstructive cardiomyopathy. *J. Clin. Path.* **27**: 529–35, 1974.
34. Pomerance, A. and Davies, M.J. Pathological features of hypertrophic obstructive cardiomyopathy (HOCM) in the elderly. *Br. Heart J.* **37**: 305–12, 1975.
35. Hamby, R.I. and Aintablian, A. Hypertrophic subaortic stenosis is not rare in the eighth decade. *Geriatrics* **32**: 71–4, 1976.
36. Battle, W.E., Siegel, F.A., and Fox, L.M. The older patient with idiopathic hypertrophic subaortic stenosis. *Geriatrics* **32**: 61–69, 1977.
37. Krasnow, N. and Stein, R.A. Hypertrophic cardiomyopathy in the aged. *Am. Heart J.* **96**: 326–36, 1978.
38. Petrin, T.J. and Tavel, M.E. Idiopathic hypertrophic subaortic stenosis as observed in a large community hospital: Relation to age and history of hypertension. *J. Am. Geriat. Soc.* **27**: 43–46, 1979.
39. Berger, M., Rethy, C., and Goldberg, E. Unsuspected hypertrophic subaortic stenosis in the elderly diagnosed by echocardiography *J. Am. Geriat. Soc.* **27**: 178–82, 1979.
40. Koga, Y. and Toshima, H. Cardiomyopathy in the elderly. *Jpn. J. Geriat.* **22**: 310–16, 1985. (in Japanese)
41. Shenoy, M.M., Khanna, A., Nejat, M., Greif, E., and Friedman, S.A. Hypertrophic cardiomyopathy in the elderly. A frequently misdiagnosed disease. *Arch. Intern. Med.* **146**: 658–61, 1986.
42. Maron, B.J., Nichols, P.F. III, Pickle, L.W., Wesley, Y.E., and Mulvihill, J.J. Patterns of inheritance in hypertrophic cardiomyopathy: Assessment by M-mode and two-dimensional echocardiography. *Am. J. Cardiol.* **53**: 1087–94, 1984.
43. Branzi, A., Romeo, G., Specchia, S., Lolli, C., Binetti, G., Devoto, M., Bacchi, M., and Magnani, B. Genetic heterogeneity of hypertrophic cardiomyopathy. *Int. J. Cardiol.* **7**: 129–33, 1985.
44. Greaves S.C., Roche, A.H.G., Neutze, J.M., and Whitlock, R.M.L. Inheritance of hypertrophic cardiomyopathy: A cross sectional and M mode echocardiographic study of 50

families. *Br. Heart J.* **58**: 259–66, 1987.

45. Maron, B.J. and Mulvihill, J.J. The genetics of hypertrophic cardiomyopathy. *Ann. Intern. Med.* **105**: 610–13, 1986.
46. Miettinen, O.S. Estimability and estimation in case-referent studies. *Am. J. Epidemiol.* **103**: 226–35, 1976.
47. Barlow, R.E., Bartholomew, D.J., Bremner, J.M., and Brunck, H.D. Statistical inference under order restrictions. New York, Wiley, 1972.
48. Koga, Y., Itaya, K., and Toshima, H. Prognosis in hypertrophic cardiomyopathy. *Am. Heart J.* **108**: 351–59, 1984.
49. Maron, B.J., Edwards, J.E., and Epstein, S.E. Disproportionate ventricular septal thickening in patients with systemic hypertension. *Chest* **73**: 466–70, 1978.
50. Miller, R.A., Flowers, N.C., Berndt, T.B., *et al.* Polycystic kidney disease, hypertension and subaortic stenosis. *South Med. J.* **67**: 354, 1974.
51. Sakamoto, T., Tei, C., Murayama, M., Ichiyasu, H., Hada, Y., Hayashi, T., and Amano, K. Giant T wave inversion as a manifestation of asymmetrical apical hypertrophy (AAH) of the left ventricle. Echocardiographic and ultrasono-cardiotomographic study. *Jpn. Heart J.* **17**: 611–29, 1976.
52. Yamaguchi, H., Ishimura, T., Nishiyama, S., Nagasaki, F., Nakanishi, S., Takatsu, F., Nishijo, T., Umeda, T., and Machii, K. Hypertrophic nonobstructive cardiomyopathy with giant negative T wave (apical hypertrophy): Ventriculographic and echocardiographic features in 30 patients. *Am. J. Cardiol.* **44**: 401–12, 1979.
53. Koga, Y., Itaya, M., Takahashi, H., Koga, M., Ikeda, H., Itaya, K., and Toshima, H. Apical hypertrophy and its genetic and acquired factors. *J. Cardiography* **15** (Suppl. VI): 65–74, 1985. (in Japanese)
54. Miyazaki, Y., Shida, M., Matsuyama, K., Chiba, M., Nakata, M., Sakai, S., Inuzuka, S., Nohara, M., Toshima, H., and Koga, Y. Japanese apical hypertrophy is distinct from apical hypertrophic cardiomyopathy. *Shinzo* **19**: 559–68, 1987. (in Japanese)

PATHOPHYSIOLOGICAL AND CLINICAL ASPECTS

Myocardial Ischemia in Hypertrophic Cardiomyopathy

Richard O. Cannon, III

Cardiovascular Diagnosis Section, Cardiology Branch, NHLBI, National Institutes of Health, Bethesda, Maryland, U.S.A.

ABSTRACT

Patients with hypertrophic cardiomyopathy, especially those symptomatic with angina pectoris, are commonly found to have myocardial ischemia during stress. The most likely mechanisms responsible for ischemia relate to imbalances between myocardial oxygen demands and appropriate coronary flow delivery. Patients with obstruction to left ventricular outflow may have high metabolic demands during stress with rapid exhaustion of coronary flow reserve. Patients without obstruction may have greater impairment in coronary flow delivery with rapid exhaustion of a more limited flow reserve compared with patients with obstruction. In both groups, multiple considerations including factors relating to myocardial oxygen demand (muscle mass, systolic and diastolic wall stress) and appropriate coronary flow delivery (abnormal myocellular architecture and capillary/myocyte relationships, effects of abnormal diastolic filling on coronary flow, septal perforator compression, coexisting coronary artery disease) may impact to varying degrees on the pathogenesis of myocardial ischemia.

INTRODUCTION

The majority of patients with hypertrophic cardiomyopathy come to medical attention because of symptoms such as exertional dyspnea, chest pain, fatigue, and sudden alterations in consciousness. In patients with coronary artery disease, these symptoms may be consequences of myocardial ischemia due to limitation to appropriate blood flow delivery because of atherosclerotic disease of epicardial coronary arteries. However, in hypertrophic cardiomyopathy, symptoms commonly occur in the presence of angiographically normal epicardial coronary arteries and hyperdynamic left ventricles. Thus, if myocardial ischemia does occur in hypertrophic cardiomyopathy and is responsible for symptoms, the pathophysiology must differ considerably from patients with coronary artery disease.

METABOLIC EVIDENCE FOR ISCHEMIA IN HYPERTROPHIC CARDIOMYOPATHY

The most convincing evidence for ischemia in hypertrophic cardiomyopathy is metabolic evidence for anerobic metabolism, especially during stress. This might result from an imbalance between myocardial oxygen demands and appropriate oxygen delivery via coronary blood flow, although a primary cellular abnormality involving energy substrate utilization or oxidative metabolism unrelated to supply-demand considerations is possible. Classically, the biochemical marker for ischemia most commonly sought in experimental and clinical studies is myocardial production of lactate. Lactate is extracted from the coronary circulation by myocytes and enters the mitochondria after conversion to pyruvate, and subsequently acetyl CoA. However, conversion to pyruvate can only occur if NAD^+ (nicotinamide adenine dinucleotide) is available in the cytosol, which in turn is dependent upon appropriate delivery of oxygen to the mitochondria to act as a hydrogen receptor. Thus, the venous drainage from normally perfused and oxygenated myocardium contains less lactate than coronary arterial inflow. However, during situations of oxygen deprivation, NAD^+ is less available, or unavailable, and lactate metabolism is interrupted. Increases in myocardial cytosol lactate result in lactate spillover into the venous drainage, and lactate concentration exceeds that of the arterial inflow (lactate production). Actual demonstration of lactate production during suspected ischemia is hampered by the necessity in humans to collect venous drainage from all layers of the myocardium, not just the subendocardium, where ischemia is most likely to occur earliest during stress because of the greater metabolic requirements of the subendocardium and greater vulnerability to flow delivery, as will be discussed later. Thus, early ischemia will result in confluence of increased lactate content of venous blood drained from the subendocardium with venous blood containing a more normal concentration of lactate from the mid and epicardial regions of the myocardium. The net sum of the lactate concentrations from these regions may result in an overall decrease in lactate extraction, because of an increase in coronary venous lactate content (or, if multiplied by coronary flow, a decrease in lactate consumption) compared with basal measurements. If myocardial ischemia is more severe, or if ischemia is more transmural, then net lactate production would be demonstrable. Thus, although lactate production as demonstrated in coronary venous blood is specific for myocardial ischemia, the sensitivity for demonstration of ischemia is relatively low, but to an unknown degree.[1-3]

Several studies have demonstrated abnormal lactate metabolism during stress in symptomatic patients with hypertrophic cardiomyopathy and angiographically normal coronary arteries. Thompson *et al.*[4] performed pacing studies in 13 patients (hypertrophic cardiomyopathy diagnosed by biventricular angiography), and noted a decrease in lactate extraction in five, with lactate production in this group of five as a whole at a heart rate of approximately 150. This metabolic response to pacing was improved in only one of the five patients during repeat pacing following propranolol 0.2 mg/kg intravenously. Pasternac *et al.*[5] reported lactate metabolism in four symptomatic patients with obstructive hypertrophic cardiomyopathy based on angiographic demonstration of increased left ventricular mass with the ejection fraction of greater than 50%, and echocardiographic demonstration of asymmetric septal hypertrophy. During pacing tachycardia, all four patients experienced chest pain, and an increase in coronary sinus lactate was found in all four compared with basal values, although in no patient was coronary sinus lactate concentration higher than the arterial concentration.

We reported lactate metabolism in 50 symptomatic patients with echocardiographic diagnosis of hypertrophic cardiomyopathy, 23 with basal left ventricular outflow gradients equal to or greater than 30 mmHg and 27 without basal gradients.[6] During atrial pacing to a heart rate of 130, 41 of 50 patients experienced chest pain, while 46 of 48 patients paced to a heart rate of 150 experienced chest pain. At this highest paced heart rate, great cardiac vein and arterial blood sampling demonstrated lactate production in 14 of 22 patients with basal obstruction and 11 of 26 patients without basal obstruction. In four additional patients with basal obstruction and eight without obstruction, a decrease in lactate consumption was noted at a heart rate of 150. Overall, 39 of 50 patients demonstrated either lactate production or decrease in consumption compared with basal measurements. Although patients with basal left ventricular outflow obstruction had more severe metabolic evidence of ischemia in terms of absolute measurements of lactate production during pacing stress, the difference from patients without obstruction was not statistically significant. Isoproterenol stress not only produced chest pain in 13 patients with obstructive hypertrophic cardiomyopathy, but also metabolic evidence of more severe myocardial ischemia at a heart rate of 130, compared with pacing stress at the same heart rate.[7]

Ogata *et al.*[8] reported results of pacing stress in 18 patients with hypertrophic cardiomyopathy (17 without basal obstruction), seven of whom had a history of chest pain. At a heart rate of approximately 150, the eight patients complaining of chest pain showed a marked decrease in lactate extraction or actual production, as did three additional patients without chest pain during pacing. In contrast, the seven patients with lesser decreases in lactate extraction during pacing were all pain free during pacing. Cuccurullo *et al.*[9] measured lactate metabolism during isoproterenol infusion in 14 patients with obstructive hypertrophic cardiomyopathy, eight of whom had a history of angina and six of whom did not. All eight of the chest pain group demonstrated lactate production by coronary sinus sampling during isoproterenol infusion to a heart rate of approximately 120. In contrast, lactate extraction increased in the asymptomatic group.

Thus, multiple studies of symptomatic patients with hypertrophic cardiomyopathy have demonstrated unequivocal metabolic evidence of myocardial ischemia, often to a severe degree, during pacing and β-agonist catecholamine stress. Further, ischemia has been convincingly demonstrated in patients with and without obstruction to left ventricular outflow. Patients with hypertrophic cardiomyopathy but asymptomatic for chest pain do not appear to have the same ischemic metabolic response to these stresses.

POTENTIAL MECHANISMS OF MYOCARDIAL ISCHEMIA

Classically, myocardial ischemia results from inappropriate matching of myocardial demands for oxygen utilization and myocardial oxygen delivery via coronary blood flow. As has been discussed elsewhere in this monograph, hypertrophic cardiomyopathy is a disease with multiple pathophysiologic and hemodynamic features, including hypertrophy, obstruction to the left ventricular outflow in some patients, morphologically

TABLE 1. Potential Mechanisms of Myocardial Ischemia

Myocardial oxygen demand considerations
- –increased muscle mass
- –increased left ventricular diastolic pressures
- –increased left ventricular systolic pressures in patients with obstruction to outflow

Myocardial oxygen supply considerations
- –increased oxygen diffusion distances from capillary to center of hypertrophied myocyte
- –abnormal myocellular/capillary relationships
- –fibrous replacement of capillaries
- –abnormal intramural small arteries, with luminal narrowing
- –systolic compression of septal perforators and epicardial artery segments
- –effects of abnormal diastolic filling on myocardial perfusion
- –coexisting coronary artery disease

abnormal myocellular architecture and intramural coronary arteries, and abnormal diastolic filling, all of which could influence myocardial oxygen supply and demand relationships, even in the presence of normal epicardial coronary arteries. As shown in Table 1, myocardial oxygen demand considerations include increased muscle mass, a hallmark of this disease. Hypertrophied tissue generally requires greater absolute basal and stress coronary flow because of greater muscle mass and contractile protein content, which require greater rates of oxidative metabolism for providing high energy phosphates. Even though the coronary flow per unit mass may be normal, the higher absolute flow at rest and during stress necessitates greater vasodilatation of autoregulatory arterioles, thus partially exhausting further dilatory capacity and coronary flow reserve. The necessity for greater absolute flow to satisfy the energy requirements of greater myocardial mass is partially offset by decreased regional wall stress, which is inversely related to wall thickness by Laplace's law. Thus, for any diastolic or systolic left ventricular chamber pressure, the wall stress, especially in the mid and outer walls of the hypertrophied myocardium, may be lower than normal. However, wall tension in the subendocardium would still be higher than normal in the presence of increased left ventricular systolic and diastolic pressures.

POTENTIAL MECHANISMS OF MYOCARDIAL ISCHEMIA AND HYPERTROPHIC CARDIOMYOPATHY: SUPPLY CONSIDERATIONS

Several features of hypertrophic cardiomyopathy might affect appropriate blood flow and oxygen delivery to the myocardium. Even if the coronary microcirculation remained normal in absolute numbers and maximum cross-sectional area, the diffusion distance from capillaries to the center of hypertrophied myocytes might impair appropriate oxygen delivery, especially during stress when oxygen requirements are high. Although new capillary formation that has been demonstrated in some chronic hypertensive animal models might alleviate this concern somewhat by bringing more capillaries in contact with hypertrophied myocytes, diffusion distances might still be greater than normal for the most hypertrophied cells. Whether neovascularization occurs in hypertrophic cardiomyopathy in response to the hypertrophic process is unknown. Indeed, fibrous tissue formation and the bizarre myocellular architecture, which are morphologic features in hypertrophic cardiomyopathy, might actually reduce the absolute numbers of small vessels and result in both increased diffusion distances from capillaries to myocytes and impaired peak flow capacity of the microcirculation during stress, thus compromising peak vasodilator reserve.

Another morphologic feature which might compromise appropriate blood flow delivery is "small vessel disease," described in detail elsewhere in this monograph. Intimal proliferation and muscular hyperplasia in small intramural arteries appear capable of compromising the lumen of these vessels, and since resistance is inversely proportional to the radius to the fourth power, small reductions in the radius of a small vessel can have marked effects on flow resistance in the microcirculation. Abnormal small vessels have been seen at necropsy in patients with and without obstruction to left ventricular outflow.[10,11]

Two hemodynamic features might also compromise coronary flow delivery. First, systolic compression of epicardial and septal perforator vessels is often noted in patients with hypertrophic cardiomyopathy during angiography.[12,13] Although approximately 85% of transmural coronary blood flow occurs in diastole, there is a small systolic flow component which might be of considerable importance given the concerns of supply and demand discussed in this section, thus limiting peak flow capacity during stress. Further, if there is protracted compression lasting into early diastole when intramyocardial blood flow normally occurs, the impact of systolic compression might even be more important with regard to compromising myocardial oxygen delivery during stress. Systolic compression of septal vessels is probably responsible for the "stop and go," or stuttering appearance of contrast dye transit down the left anterior descending artery frequently noted during angiography of patients with hypertrophic cardiomyopathy, especially those with obstruction, due to cessation of flow during systole, followed by rapid dye transit during diastole.

Even in the absence of systolic compression of septal perforating vessels, abnormal diastolic properties of the myocardium, common to most hypertrophic cardiomyopathic ventricles, might impair early diastolic filling of the microcirculation, when coronary flow is normally maximal because of the normal rapid fall in left ventricular tissue pressure.[14]

All of the above considerations regarding coronary flow delivery would be expected to be of greatest impact in the subendocardium because of the greater oxygen requirements of the inner regions of the myocardium proximate to high ventricular chamber pressures, compared with the mid and outer walls of the myocardium. Thus the subendocardium is more vulnerable to developing ischemia if appropriate blood flow cannot meet myocardial oxygen demands.

CLINICAL STUDIES ELUCIDATING MECHANISMS OF MYOCARDIAL ISCHEMIA

Most clinical studies which offer insight as to mechanisms of myocardial ischemia involve noninvasive and invasive measurements of coronary blood flow or myocardial perfusion in symptomatic patients. Several studies have employed thallium scintigraphy during treadmill exercise stress to assess the presence and severity of regional abnormalities in myocardial perfusion. Rubin *et al.*[15] studied 10 patients, all symptomatic with angina pectoris, with echocardiographic evidence of asymmetric septal hypertrophy. Nine had systolic anterior motion on echo and four had basal gradients greater than 30 mmHg at catheterization. No patient had angiographic evidence of septal perforator artery compression, and all had angiographically normal coronary arteries. Seven of 10 had resting ST-T abnormalities secondary to left ventricular hypertrophy, thus precluding analysis of ST segment shifts during exercise. During exercise stress using a graded treadmill exercise protocol, five of 10 stopped because of chest pain while the other five stopped after achieving 85% of their predicted maximum heart rate. In one of three patients with normal baseline ST segments, significant ST segment depression was noted. Only one patient was found to have a perfusion defect on exercise not present at rest. The authors suggested that ischemia might be due to homogenously diminished perfusion or a metabolic abnormality, but regional perfusion abnormalities during stress comparable to patients with coronary artery disease were uncommon in hypertrophic cardiomyopathy.

In contrast, Pitcher *et al.*[16] found a high incidence of thallium perfusion defects during exercise in 23 patients with hypertrophic cardiomyopathy, 11 of whom had a history of recurrent chest pain. Twenty underwent cardiac catheterization, and 10 had basal left ventricular outflow gradients. Coronary arteriography was performed in 17 patients: 16 had angiographically normal arteries and an additional patient had minor luminal irregularities. Fifteen patients had thallium perfusion defects; 12 had defects on exercise which reperfused after rest or were fixed, and three had septal defects visible only on delayed images after rest. Eight of 11 patients with the history of recurrent chest pain had reperfusion defects suggestive of ischemia; three additional patients with recurrent angina had normal scintigrams. In contrast, only three of 13 patients without reperfusion defects had a history of persistent angina. Seventeen of the 23 patients had resting ST-T wave abnormalities on ECG. Only two of 23 patients had at least 2 mm ST segment depression during exercise, both patients with perfusion defects.

In 14 patients with hypertrophic cardiomyopathy, Hanrath *et al.*[17] performed studies of lactate metabolism via great cardiac vein sampling during atrial pacing (heart rate approximately 150) and thallium scintigraphy during graded exercise testing approximately one week later. Ten of 14 patients had basal left ventricular outflow gradients. During pacing study, seven of 14 patients produced lactate; of this group, three had fixed and reversible thallium perfusion defects and two had fixed defects only during exercise and subsequent rest. Of the other seven patients who did not produce lactate during pacing, one had fixed and reversible defects and four had fixed defects only. They concluded that hypertrophic cardiomyopathy is commonly associated with ischemia or fibrosis.

O'Gara *et al.* from the Cardiology Branch, NHLBI, National Institutes of Health,[18] recently reported perfusion studies in 72 patients with hypertrophic cardiomyopathy using ^{201}Tl emission computed tomography. Thirty-six of the 72 patients had a history of chest pain and 45 had a history of exertional dyspnea. Twenty-three patients were judged to have basal outflow gradients by catheterization and/or echocardiographic demonstration of systolic anterior motion of the mitral valve. Left ventricular ejection fractions were calculated by gated blood pool radionuclide angiography. Regional perfusion defects were detected in 41 of 72 patients (57%) and were noted in all regions of the left ventricle. In 26 patients, tomographic images showed apparent left ventricular cavity dilatation immediately after exercise, not noted on delayed images. Radionuclide angiograms in five of these patients showed no left ventricular enlargement during exercise, suggesting that the apparent cavity enlargement on thallium tomograms was probably due to subendocardial hypoperfusion. In the 17 patients with fixed or only partially reversible defects, 14 had rest ejection fractions $<50\%$, suggesting extensive scarring. In contrast, the 24 patients with exercise-induced perfusion defects that reperfused at rest all had ejection fractions of $>50\%$. Neither a history of chest pain nor its precipitation during treadmill exercise was predictive of an abnormal study; defects were present in 10 of 18 asymptomatic patients and 31 of 54 symptomatic patients.

Thus, thallium perfusion defects can commonly be demonstrated in patients with hypertrophic cardiomyopathy, both with and without symptoms of chest pain and with and without obstruction to the left ventricular outflow. Whether reversible thallium defects in hypertrophic cardiomyopathy are actually representative of impaired regional blood flow delivery during stress, as is considered to be the case in patients with coronary artery disease, is unknown. Fixed thallium defects probably correspond to regions of scarring and are common in patients with impaired left ventricular function. Whether patients with reversible defects are more likely to progress over time to scarred ventricles with poor left ventricular systolic function is unknown.

VENTRICULOGRAPHIC STUDIES

St. John Sutton *et al.*[19] performed videometric analyses of RAO ventriculograms in

18 patients with echocardiographic diagnosis of hypertrophic cardiomyopathy (14 patients on propranolol up to 12 hr prior to catheterization), calculating peak rates of systolic thickening and diastolic thinning of the mid-anterior left ventricular wall. Fourteen of 18 patients had basal left ventricular outflow gradients (mean 32 mmHg). Compared with identical studies in 20 patients with normal coronary arteries and left ventricles with atypical chest pain syndromes, the peak rates of systolic thickening and diastolic thinning were not significantly different between the two groups. However, the seven patients with hypertrophic cardiomyopathy and a history of angina did have significantly lesser peak rates of systolic wall thickening and diastolic wall thinning compared with the 11 patients with hypertrophic cardiomyopathy without a history of angina, and the control subjects. Although the ratio of diastolic pressure-time index (DPTI) to systolic pressure-time index (SPTI) was reduced in patients with hypertrophic cardiomyopathy compared with controls, there was no difference in the DPTI/SPTI ratio between patients with hypertrophic cardiomyopathy with angina and patients with hypertrophic cardiomyopathy without angina. Thus, patients with hypertrophic cardiomyopathy and angina commonly had impaired systolic and diastolic wall dynamics, but whether this was a cause or consequence of ischemia could not be determined from this study.

ANGIOGRAPHIC STUDIES

Typically, the coronary arteries in patients with hypertrophic cardiomyopathy are larger than normal, often with rapid dye transit, particularly in those patients with outflow obstruction. Systolic compression of septal perforator branches was described by Pichard *et al.*[12] in 13 patients with hypertrophic cardiomyopathy, eight of whom were symptomatic with chest pain and seven of whom were symptomatic with effort dyspnea; only two were asymptomatic. Although all 13 patients had some degree of septal perforator compression during systole, those patients with the most marked degree of compression were those with basal left ventricular outflow gradients. Two patients also had dynamic systolic compression of the mid left anterior descending artery. In comparison, none of 10 patients with normal left ventricles or 10 patients with left ventricular hypertrophy due to aortic stenosis (5) or "idiopathic" hypertrophy (5) had evidence of septal perforation compression. Ruddy *et al.*[13] studied 47 patients with hypertrophic cardiomyopathy, 21 with basal left ventricular outflow obstruction. Thirty patients had septal perforator compression during systole, the presence and severity of which correlated with the extent of septal hypertrophy and the presence of basal obstruction. Of note, a history of angina was present in 76% of patients with septal perforation compression and only 13% of patients without compression. Only 15% of patients had systolic compression of epicardial coronary artery segments. In our series of 50 consecutive patients with hypertrophic cardiomyopathy who underwent angiographic and coronary hemodynamic study, all of whom were symptomatic with chest pain, systolic compression of septal perforator vessels was noted in 86% of patients with obstruction and 64% of patients without obstruction.[6] Thus, septal perforator artery compression is frequently noted in symptomatic patients with hypertrophic cardiomyopathy, especially in those with basal left ventricular outflow obstruction. In no study could the relative contribution of septal perforator artery compression to impaired blood flowd elivery be determined.

INVASIVE STUDIES OF CORONARY BLOOD FLOW IN HYPERTROPHIC CARDIOMYOPATHY

Early studies by Gorlin *et al.*[20] and Brink *et al.*[21] utilizing inert gas washout methods for measurement of coronary blood flow were performed in six patients with obstructive hypertrophic cardiomyopathy. These studies found that basal left ventricular flow and myocardial oxygen consumption, normalized for mass, were similar to those in patients with nonhypertrophied ventricles, although in absolute terms they were higher than normal. Weiss *et al.*[22] utilizing scintillation detection of ^{133}Xe washout for estimating left coronary artery blood flow, reported that in five patients with ventriculographic determination of hypertrophic cardiomyopathy (three with basal left ventricular outflow gradients), coronary flow per unit mass was lower than normal. However, the absolute basal flows were higher than normal when calculated perfusion was multiplied by angiographically determined left ventricular mass. Thompson *et al.*[4] measured coronary sinus blood flow by thermodilution in 13 symptomatic patients with hypertrophic cardiomyopathy, 11 of whom had significant basal left ventricular outflow gradients. Coronary sinus flow increased from 216±38 ml/min to 374±74 ml/min (mean±SD) during pacing to a heart rate of 150. During pacing, the eight patients with normal lactate extraction had increases in coronary sinus flow with each increment in heart rate. In contrast, four out of five patients with lactate production had little or no increase in coronary sinus flow with each pacing increment. Four of five in this group with pacing-induced ischemia also had the highest oxygen consumption at rest and during low paced heart rates. These authors concluded that ischemia in obstructive hypertrophic cardiomyopathy is due to high myocardial oxygen demand or inability of coronary flow to increase with increases in heart rate.

Pasternac *et al.*[5] measured coronary sinus flow by thermodilution in four symptomatic patients with obstructive hypertrophic cardiomyopathy at rest and during pacing, comparing these findings with those of five control subjects. Coronary sinus flow was significantly higher in patients than control at rest (177±50 vs 116±24 ml/min, mean± S.D.), as well as during pacing to a heart rate of 150. However, when flows were divided by mass estimates determined from the RAO ventriculogram, the basal and pacing-induced flows per unit at mass were lower in patients than controls. Likewise, the absolute, but not mass-corrected myocardial oxygen consumption was higher at rest and during pacing in patients with hypertrophic cardiomyopathy compared with controls. All four patients experienced chest pain, associated with an increase in coronary sinus venous lactate concentration. During pacing, the DPTI/SPTI ratio was significantly lower in patients than controls, which the authors interpreted as causing subendocardial ischemia.

Cuccurulo *et al.*[9] performed measurements of coronary sinus flow in the basal state and during isoproterenol infusion (2 to 4 mcg/min) in 14 patients with obstructive hypertrophic cardiomyopathy and angiographically normal coronary arteries, eight of whom had a history of angina and six of whom did not. Patients with angina developed a greater systolic outflow tract gradient (102±8 vs 52±8 mmHg, $P<.0001$), higher left ventricular end-diastolic pressure (33±4 vs 20±6 mmHg, $P<.001$), and smaller increase in coronary sinus flow (176±9 vs 262±34 ml/min, $P<.001$), all with lactate production, compared with the six patients without a history of angina. Shimamatsu and Toshima administered dipyridamole 0.56 mg/kg to 19 patients with nonobstructive hypertrophic cardiomyopathy and seven control subjects.[23] They found that the maximum coronary sinus flow was significantly lower in patients with hypertrophic cardiomyopathy compared with control subjects. These investigators found a significant correlation between the minimum coronary vascular resistance after dipyridamole and left ventricular muscle mass, but no correlation with left ventricular end-diastolic pressure and the severity of septal perforator compression.

In our initial series of 20 symptomatic patients with echocardiographically determined hypertrophic cardiomyopathy, nine of whom had resting left ventricular outflow tract gradients equal to or greater than 30 mmHg, basal great cardiac vein flow was significantly higher (91 ± 27 vs 66 ± 17 ml/min) and coronary resistance lower ($1.13 \pm .38$ vs $1.55 \pm .45$ mm × Hg/ml/min) compared with 28 control subjects without hypertrophic cardiomyopathy (Fig. 1).[24] During pacing, coronary flow rose in both groups, although patients with hypertrophic cardiomyopathy as a group demonstrated an initial rise in flow to 130 beats/min, at which point 12 of 20 patients developed their typical chest pain (Fig. 2). With continued pacing to a heart rate of 150 beats/min, the mean coronary flow actually fell to 114 ± 29 ml/min, with 18 of 20 patients experiencing their typical chest pain and metabolic evidence of myocardial ischemia. This fall in coronary flow was associated with a substantial rise in left venticular end-diastolic pressure (30 ± 9 mmHg immediately after peak pacing) (Fig. 3). In the 14 patients whose great cardiac vein flow actually fell from intermediate to peak pacing, the rise in left ventricular end-diastolic pressure was greater than in the six whose flow remained unchanged or increased (11 ± 8 vs 2 ± 10 mmHg, $P < .01$). In our recently reported series of 50 patients with hypertrophic cardiomyopathy, 23 of whom had basal obstruction to left ventricular outflow, patients with obstruction had significantly greater basal great cardiac vein

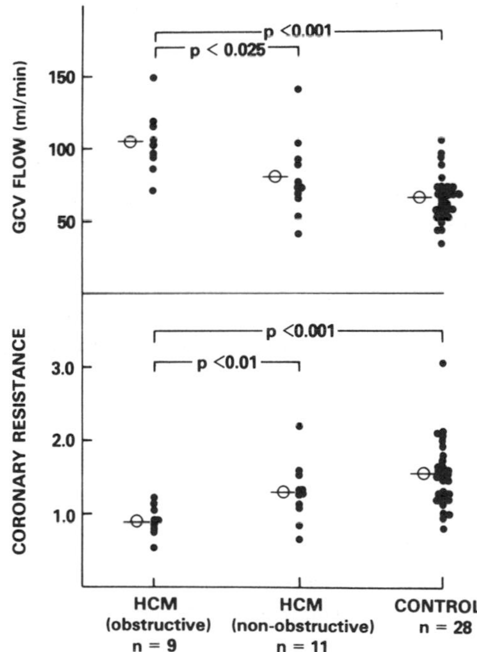

Fig. 1. Great cardiac vein (GCV) flow and resistance at rest in 20 patients with hypertrophic cardiomyopathy (HCM) and 28 control subjects. Nine patients with hypertrophic cardiomyopathy had resting left ventricular outflow tract gradients of 30 mmHg or more. Circle with bar represents mean value. (Reprinted from reference 24 by permission of the American Heart Association, Inc.)

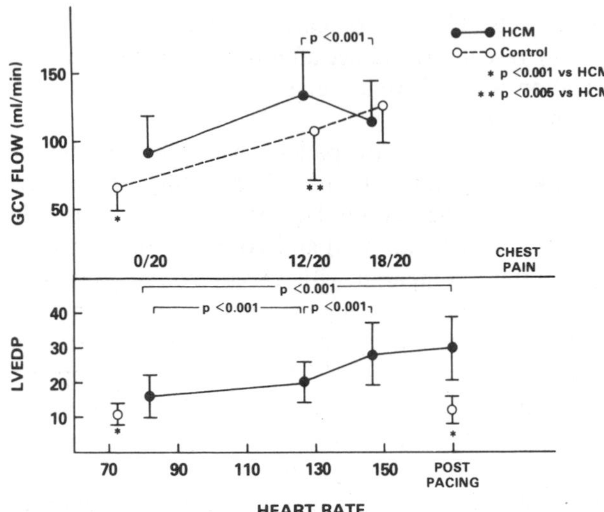

Fig. 2. Top: Great cardiac flow at rest, intermediate pacing, and peak pacing in patients with hypertrophic cardiomyopathy (HCM) and control subjects. Number at bottom represents number of patients with hypertrophic cardiomyopathy experiencing chest pain at each heart rate. Bottom: Corresponding LVEDP for the heart rates above. Circles represent mean values with standard deviation bars. (Reprinted from reference 24 by permission of the American Heart Association, Inc.)

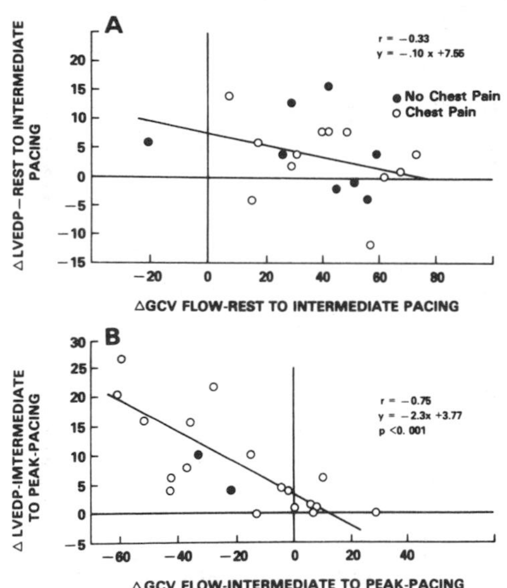

Fig. 3. A: Absence of relationship between the change in great cardiac vein (GCV) flow and change in LVEDP from rest to intermediate pacing in patients with hypertrophic cardiomyopathy. B: Significant relationship between change in great cardiac vein flow and change in LVEDP from intermediate to peak pacing. (Reprinted from reference 24 by permission of the American Heart Association, Inc.)

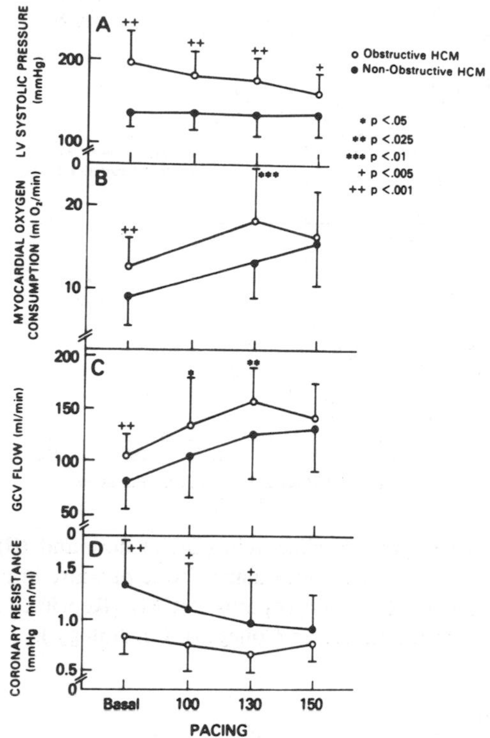

Fig. 4. A: Left ventricular (LV) systolic pressure; B: myocardial oxygen consumption in the anterior coronary circulation; C: great cardiac vein (GCV) flow; and D: coronary resistance in the anterior circulation for patients with hypertrophic cardiomyopathy. With (open circles) and without (closed circles) obstruction to left ventricular outflow. Mean values with 1 SD are plotted in the basal state and during pacing. $*P<0.05$, $**P<0.025$, $***P<0.01$, $++P<0.001$ vs patients without obstruction to left ventricular outflow. (Reprinted from reference 6 with permission from the American College of Cardiology.)

flow and myocardial oxygen consumption of the anterior left ventricle compared with the 27 patients without basal obstruction (Figs. 4 and 5).[6] Myocardial oxygen consumption in great cardiac vein flow was also significantly higher at a paced heart rate of 100 and 130 beats/min (the anginal threshold for 41 of the 50 patients). In patients with obstruction, transmural coronary flow reserve was exhausted at a peak rate of 130 beats/min; higher heart rates resulted in more severe metabolic evidence of ischemia, with all patients experiencing chest pain and with an actual increase in coronary resistance (Fig. 4). Patients without obstruction also demonstrated evidence of ischemia at heart rates of 130 and 150 beats/min with 25 of 27 patients experiencing chest pain. In this group, myocardial ischemia occurred at significantly lower coronary flow, higher coronary resistance, and lower myocardial oxygen consumption, suggesting more severely impaired flow delivery in this group compared with those with obstruction. Of interest, despite metabolic evidence of severe ischemia (Fig. 6), there was no net increase in myocardial oxygen extraction in patients with hypertrophic cardiomyopathy regardless of whether or not they had basal left ventricular outflow obstruction (Fig. 7).

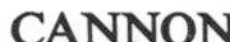

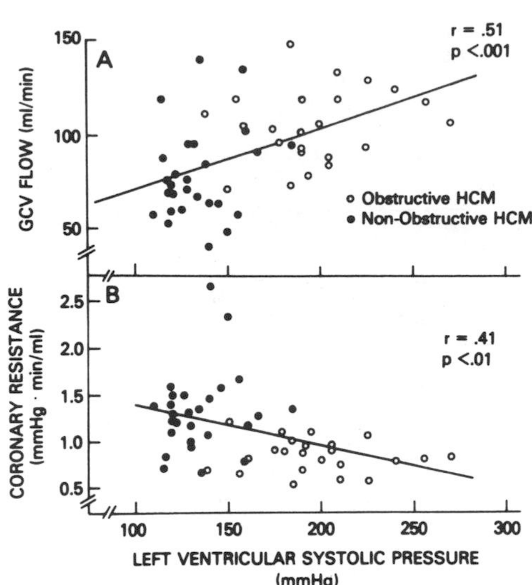

Fig. 5. Relation of (A) great cardiac vein (GCV) flow and (B) coronary resistance in the basal state of left ventricular systolic pressure in obstructive and nonobstructive hypertrophic cardiomyopathy (HCM). (Reprinted from reference 6 with permission from the American College of Cardiology.)

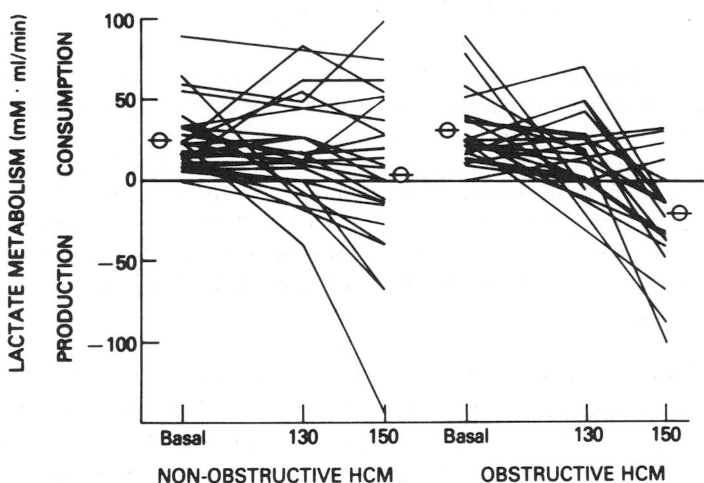

Fig. 6. Lactate consumption in the basal state and during pacing at rates of 130 and 150 beats/min in patients with hypertrophic cardiomyopathy (HCM) with and without obstruction to left ventriuclar outflow. Lactate consumption <0 indicates production of lactate by the myocardium. (Reprinted from reference 6 with permission from the American College of Cardiology.)

Figure 8 outlines the pathophysiology of ischemia in patients with and without obstruction supported by our studies. Although the basal flow and myocardial oxygen consumption per unit mass may be normal, as suggested by previous studies, patients with obstruction to left ventricular outflow have high absolute basal coronary flow and oxygen consumption and rapidly exhaust their coronary flow reserve during stress.

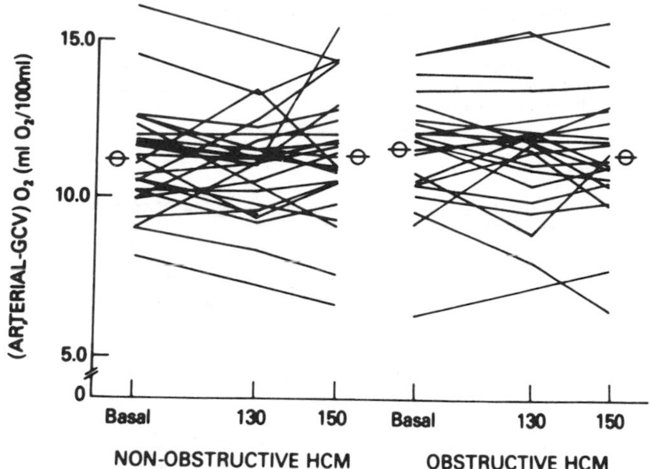

Fig. 7. Arterial minus great cardiac vein (GCV) oxygen content in the basal state and during pacing in patients with and without obstruction to left ventricular outflow. (Reprinted from reference 6 with permission from the American College of Cardiology.)

These high flows appear to be particularly vulnerable to increases in left ventricular filling pressures, with an actual drop in flow and increase in coronary resistance with higher paced heart rates. In contrast, patients without obstruction appear to have more severe impairment in coronary flow delivery, with metabolic evidence of severe ischemia precipitating chest pain at lower peak coronary flows. Preliminary studies in six patients with obstructive hypertrophic cardiomyopathy that underwent left ventricular myotomy/myectomy indicate in postoperative studies a decrease in basal and pacing-induced great cardiac vein flows and myocardial oxygen consumption, improved indices of myocardial ischemia by lactate metabolism, and an improvement in pacing anginal threshold.[25] Undoubtedly, other considerations outlined in Table 1 with regard to potential mechanisms of altering myocardial oxygen supply and demand relationships are operative to varying degrees in patients with hypertrophic cardiomyopathy. Unfortunately, because of the multiplicity of factors and complex inter-relationships amongst them, their relative contribution cannot be ascertained from any one study.

CORONARY ARTERY DISEASE IN PATIENTS WITH HYPERTROPHIC CARDIOMYOPATHY

Of course, patients with hypertrophic cardiomyopathy may have coexisting heart disease unrelated to the hypertrophic process. Several studies have reported coronary artery disease in patients with hypertrophic cardiomyopathy presenting with anginal symptoms,[26–29] and improvement in symptom status after surgical revascularization.[29] As is evident in the discussion of studies demonstrating myocardial ischemia and attempting to elucidate mechanisms of ischemia presented in this chapter, noninvasive testing is not helpful in separating those patients with coexisting coronary artery disease and thus coronary angiography is the only means of detecting coexisting coronary disease in symptomatic patients.

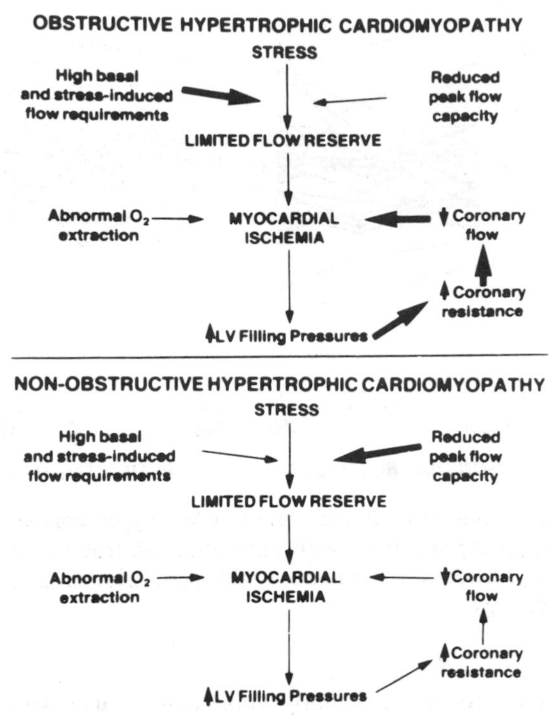

Fig. 8. Proposed mechanisms of myocardial ischemia in hypertrophic cardiomyopathy (large arrows indicate mechanisms of greater importance than those indicated by small arrows). Top panel: Patients with significant basal left ventricular (LV) outflow obstruction have high basal flow requirements primarily because of high left ventricular systolic pressure and wall stress. Flow requirements increase further with stress, rapidly exhausting peak flow capacity, which in absolute terms may be relatively normal. Abnormal oxygen extraction capacity may also contribute to or aggravate ischemia. Elevated filling pressures resulting from ischemia have a deleterious compressive effect on the maximally vasodilated transmural coronary bed, resulting in increased coronary resistance and a decrease in flow. Lower panel: Patients with little or no obstruction and lower left ventricular systolic pressure have lower basal flow requirements (although higher than those of patients without structural heart disease). During stress, flow reserve may be compromised by greater impairment in the capacity for augmenting coronary flow delivery, resulting in ischemia at lower coronary flow and myocardial oxygen consumption than in patients with obstruction. Abnormal oxygen extraction capacity may contribute to or aggravate ischemia. Elevation of filling pressures related to ischemia appears to have a less deleterious effect on coronary flow than that in patients with obstruction. (Reprinted from reference 6 with permission from the American College of Cardiology.)

SUMMARY

Patients with hypertrophic cardiomyopathy, especially those symptomatic with angina pectoris, clearly have inducible myocardial ischemia, most likely related to imbalances between myocardial oxygen demands and appropriate coronary flow delivery.

Patients with obstruction to left ventricular outflow may have greater metabolic demands during stress, with more rapid exhaustion of coronary flow reserve. Patients without obstruction may have greater impairment in coronary flow delivery, with rapid exhaustion of a more limited flow reserve compared with patients with obstruction. However, in both groups, multiple considerations including factors relating to myocardial oxygen requirements (muscle mass and distribution, systolic and diastolic wall stress) and appropriate coronary flow delivery (abnormal myocellular architecture and capillary/myocyte relationships, effects of abnormal diastolic filling on coronary flow, septal perforator compression, coexisting coronary artery disease) may impact to varying degrees on the pathogenesis of myocardial ischemia. Unfortunately, at present it is impossible to separate accurately the most important influences on the induction of myocardial ischemia in a given patient. Also unknown is whether myocardial ischemia may result in the extensive regional and global scarring seen in some patients with hypertrophic cardiomyopathy resulting in either wall motion abnormalities or progression to a dilated, hypocontractile ventricle,[30–32] or whether these processes are independent of myocardial ischemia. If myocardial ischemia does contribute to myocardial scarring, it is further unknown whether medication or operative relief of outflow obstruction alters this process. Also unknown at present is whether metabolic abnormalities in substrate utilization and oxidative metabolism may contribute to myocardial ischemia in some patients with hypertrophic cardiomyopathy.

REFERENCES

1. Neil, W.A. Myocardial hypoxia and anaerobic metabolism in coronary heart disease. *Am. J. Cardiol.* **22**: 507–515, 1968.
2. Case R.B., Nasser, M.G., and Crampton, R.S. Biochemical aspects of early myocardial ischemia. *Am. J. Cardiol.* **24**: 766–775, 1969.
3. Gorlin, R. Evaluation of myocardial metabolism in ischemic heart disease. *Circulation* 1969: 39–40 (Suppl IV): 155–163.
4. Thompson, D.S., Naqvi, N., Juul, S.M., Swanton, R.H., Coltart, D.J., Jenkins, B.S., and Webb-Peploe, M.M. Effects of propranolol on myocardial oxygen consumption, substrate extraction and haemodynamics in hypertrophic cardiomyopathy. *Br. Heart J.* **44**: 488–498, 1980.
5. Pasternac, A., Noble, J., Streulens, Y, Elie, R., Henschke, C., and Bourassa, M.G. Pathophysiology of chest pain in patients with cardiomyopathies and normal coronary arteries. *Circulation* **65**: 778–789, 1982.
6. Cannon, R.O., Schenke, W.H., Maron, B.J., Tracy, C.M., Leon, M.B., Brush, J.E., Rosing, D.R., and Epstein, S.E. Differences in coronary flow and myocardial metabolism at rest and during pacing between patients with obstructive and patients with nonobstructive hypertrophic cardiomyopathy. *J. Am. Coll. Cardiol.* **10**: 53–62, 1987.
7. Cannon, R.O., Brush, J., and Tracy, C.M. Contribution of left ventricular contractility and outflow gradient to ischemia in hypertrophic cardiomyopathy (abstr). *J. Am. Coll. Cardiol.* **9**: 230A, 1987.
8. Ogata, Y., Hiyamuta, K., Terasawa, M., Ohkita, Y., Bekki, H., Koga, Y., and Toshima, H. Relationship of exercise or pacing induced ST segment depression and myocardial lactate metabolism in patients with hypertrophic cardiomyopathy. *Jpn. Heart J.* **27**: 145–158, 1986.
9. Cuccurullo, F., Mezzetti, A., Lapenna, D., *et al.* Mechanism of isoproterenol-induced angina pectoris in patients with obstructive hypertrophic cardiomyopathy and normal coronary arteries. *Am. J. Cardiol.* **60**: 667–673, 1987.
10. Maron, B.J., Wolfson, J.K., Epstein, S.E., and Roberts, W.C. Intramural ("small vessel")

coronary artery disease in hypertrophic cardiomyopathy. *J. Am. Coll. Cardiol.* **8**: 545–557, 1986.

11. Tanaka, M., Fujiwara, H., Onodera, T., Wu, D-J., Matsuda, M., Hamashima, Y., and Kawai, C. Quantitative analysis of narrowings of intramyocardial small arteries in normal hearts, hypertensive hearts, and hearts with hypertrophic cardiomyopathy. *Circulation* **75**: 1130–1139, 1987.
12. Pichard, A.D., Meller, J., Teichholz, L.E., Lipnick, S., Gorlin, R., and Hermon, M.V. Septal perforator compression (narrowing) in idiopathic hypertrophic subaortic stenosis. *Am. J. Cardiol.* **40**: 310–314, 1977.
13. Ruddy, T.D., Henderson, M.A., Rakowski, H., and Wigle, E.D. Systolic constriction of the coronary arteries in hypertrophic cardiomyopathy (abstr). *Circulation* **54**: IV-239, 1981.
14. Brutsaert, D.L., Housmans, P.R., and Goethals, M.A. Dual control of relaxation: Its role in the ventricular function in the mammalian heart. *Circ. Res.* **47**: 637–652, 1980.
15. Rubin, K.A., Morrison, J., Padnick, M.B., Binder, A.J., Chiaramida, S., Margouleff, D., Padmanabhan, V.T., and Gulotta, S.J. Idiopathic hypertrophic subaortic stenosis: Evaluation of anginal symptoms with thallium-201 myocardial imaging. *Am. J. Cardiol.* **44**: 1040–1045, 1979.
16. Pitcher, D., Wainwright, R., Maisey, M., Curry, P., and Sowton, E. Assessment of chest pain in hypertrophic cardiomyopathy using exercise thallium-201 myocardial scintigraphy. *Br. Heart J.* **44**: 650–656, 1980.
17. Hanrath, P., Mathey, D., Montz, R., Thiel, G., Vorbringer, H., Kupper, W., Schneider, C., and Bleifeld, W. Myocardial thallium-201 imaging in hypertrophic obstructive cardiomyopathy. *Eur. Heart J.* **2**: 177–185, 1981.
18. O'Gara, P.T., Bonow, R.O., Maron, B.J., Damske, B.A., Van Lingen, A., Bacharach, S.L., Larson, S.M., and Epstein, S.E. Myocardial perfusion abnormalities in patients with hypertrophic cardiomyopathy: assessment with thallium-201 emission computed tomography. *Circulation* **76**: 1214–1223, 1987.
19. St. John Sutton, M.G., Tajik, A.J., Smith, H.C., and Ritman, E.L. Angina in idiopathic hypertrophic subaortic stenosis. A clinical correlate of regional left ventricular dysfunction: A videometric and echocardiographic study. *Circulation* **61**: 561–568, 1980.
20. Gorlin, R., Cohen, L.S., Elliott, W.C., Klein, M.D., and Lane, F.J. Hemodynamics of muscular subaortic stenosis (obstructive cardiomyopathy). In: Ciba Foundation Symposium: Cardiomyopathies, Wolstenholme, G.E.W. and O'Connor, M. (eds.), London 1964, p. 76.
21. Brink, A.J., Lewis, C.M., and Van Heerden, P.D.R. Coronary blood flow and myocardial metabolism in obstructive cardiomyopathy: Observations before and after treatment with a beta adrenergic blocking agent. *Am. J. Cardiol.* **19**: 548–555, 1967.
22. Weiss, M.B., Ellis, K., Sciacca, R.R., Johnson, L.L., Schmidt, D.H., and Cannon, P.J. Myocardial blood flow in congestive and hypertrophic cardiomyopathy. *Circulation* **54**: 484–493, 1976.
23. Shimamatsu, M. and Toshima, H. Impaired coronary vasodilatory capacity after dipyridamole administration in hypertrophic cardiomyopathy. *Jpn. Heart J.* **28**: 387–401, 1987.
24. Cannon, R.O., Rosing, D.R., Maron, B.J., Leon, M.B., Bonow, R.O., Watson, R.M., and Epstein, S.E. Myocardial ischemia in patients with hypertrophic cardiomyopathy: Contribution of inadequate vasodilator reserve and elevated left ventricular filling pressures. *Circulation* **71**: 234–243, 1985.
25. Cannon, R.O., Rosing, D.R., McIntosh, C.L., and Epstein, S.E. Hypertrophic cardiomyopathy: Improved hemodynamics, metabolism, and anginal threshold following surgical relief of outflow obstruction (abstr). *Circulation* **75**: III-447, 1985.
26. Gulotta, S.J., Hamby, R.I., Aronson, A.L., and Ewing, K. Coexistent idiopathic hypertrophic subaortic stenosis and coronary artery disease. *Circulation* **46**: 890–896, 1972.
27. Oran, E., Gupta, S., Yeo, B., *et al.* Idiopathic hypertrophic subaortic stenosis in patients

with coronary artery disease. Importance of recognition and principles of management. *Angiology* **24**: 538–547, 1973.

28. Marcus, G.B., Popp, R.L., and Stinson, E.B. Coronary artery disease with idiopathic hypertrophic subaortic stenosis. *Lancet* **i**: 901–903, 1974.
29. Cokkinos, D.V., Krajcer, Z., and Leachman, R.D. Coronary artery disease in hypertrophic cardiomyopathy. *Am. J. Cardiol.* **55**: 1437–1438, 1985.
30. Maron, B.J., Epstein, S.E., and Roberts, W.C. Hypertrophic cardiomyopathy and transmural myocardial infarction without significant atherosclerosis of the extramural coronary arteries. *Am. J. Cardiol.* **43**: 1086–1102, 1979.
31. Waller, B.F., Maron, B.J., Epstein, S.E., and Roberts, W.C. Transmural myocardial infarction in hypertrophic cardiomyopathy. A cause of conversion from left ventricular asymmetry to symmetry and from normal-size to dilated left ventricular cavity. *Chest* **79**: 461–465, 1981.
32. Nagata, S., Park, Y., Minamikawa, T., Yutani, C., Kamiya, T., Nishimura, T., Kozuka, T., Sakakibara, H., and Nimura, Y. Thallium perfusion and cardiac enzyme abnormalities in patients with familial hypertrophic cardiomyopathy. *Am. Heart J.* **109**: 1317–1322, 1985.

Regional Myocardial Blood Flow and Metabolism at Rest and during Exercise in Hypertrophic Cardiomyopathy

Maleah Grover-McKay, Heinrich R. Schelbert,** Joseph K. Perloff,*** and Janine Krivokapich*****

* Division of Nuclear Medicine and Biophysics, Department of Radiological Science, UCLA School of Medicine, University of California, Los Angeles, California, U.S.A.
** Division of Nuclear Medicine and Biophysics, Department of Medicine, UCLA School of Medicine, University of California, Los Angeles, California, U.S.A.
*** Division of Cardiology, University of California, Los Angeles, California, U.S.A.
**** Laboratory of Nuclear Medicine and Non-Invasive Laboratory, University of California, Los Angeles, California, U.S.A.

INTRODUCTION

It has been postulated that the the genetic marker for classic genetic hypertrophic cardiomyopathy[1,2] may result in regional metabolic abnormalities in the disproportionately thick ventricular septum.[3] Increased septal glycogen observed in these patients may be evidence for regional metabolic differences.[4–6]

Angina in patients with classic hypertrophic cardiomyopathy has been assumed to reflect myocardial ischemia, most likely originating in the disproportionately thick ventricular septum.[7–14] Using positron emission tomography (PET) and radiolabeled compounds which trace blood flow and biochemical pathways in a known manner, it is possible to investigate regional myocardial blood flow and metabolism and to assess whether or not ischemia is present.[15,16] Accordingly, we studied 13 patients with hypertrophic cardiomyopathy using PET and tracers of blood flow and metabolism in order to examine whether regional myocardial differences are present and whether these differences are consistent with the hypothesis of septal ischemia.[17]

METHODS

Patient Population

Ninc malcs and four fcmalcs with a mcan agc of 44 ycars wcrc studicd. Clinical, ccho-cardiographic, and angiographic criteria were used to establish the diagnosis of hypertrophic cardiomyopathy with asymmetric septal hypertrophy.[18,19] In five patients there was evidence of genetic transmission. Diseases believed to have an association with hypertrophic cardiomyopathy, such as hyperthyroidism[20] or systemic hypertension,[21] were remote in the histories of four patients. The majority of patients had good exercise capacities and only occasional dyspnea or chest discomfort, which was not convincingly angina. Two patients were on no medications, 11 were taking either verapamil or beta-

* Operated for the U.S. Department of Energy by the University of California under Contract DE-AC03-76-SF00012. This work was supported in part by the Director of the Office of Energy Research, Offices of Health and Environmental Research, by NIH Grant ♯ HL 29845, and by an Investigative Group Award by the Greater Los Angeles Affiliate of the American Heart Association.

blockers. Two patients had normal planar ^{201}Tl exercise tests. Of the five who underwent cardiac catheterization, four patients had a resting left ventricular to aortic pressure gradient and one had a provokable gradient. Two patients had minimal to moderate disease of the left anterior descending coronary artery (40% and 60% diameter narrowing).

Study Protocol

Eleven patients fasted overnight. Seven who were on medications discontinued them overnight, but two continued to take verapamil and four were taking β-blockers. Immediately prior to the PET study, the following data were obtained: heart rate and blood pressure to estimate cardiac workload, a 12-lead electrocardiogram to evaluate electrocardiographic evidence of left ventricular hypertrophy, and two-dimensional and M-mode echocardiograms to determine the extent of hypertrophy and the degree of systolic anterior motion of the anterior mitral leaflet.[18] The patients were then placed into the UCLA whole body positron emission tomograph (ECAT II; CTI, Knoxville, TN).[22] In order to correct the emission images for photon attenuation, transmission images at five to six contiguous myocardial cross-sectional levels 1.0 to 1.5 cm apart were obtained.

Seven patients were studied only in the resting state using the blood flow tracer ^{13}N ammonia, the tracer of fatty acid metabolism ^{11}C palmitate, and the tracer of exogenous glucose uptake ^{18}F deoxyglucose. In the six other patients, ^{13}N ammonia or the blood flow tracer ^{82}Rb was administered in the resting state and ^{18}F deoxyglucose injected during maximum exercise. In three of these six patients, injection of both ^{13}N ammonia or ^{82}Rb and ^{18}F deoxyglucose was repeated at rest on separate days. In one of these six patients, ^{13}N ammonia was injected at rest and during maximum exercise, and ^{18}F deoxyglucose imaging was accomplished after tracer injection during a second, identical exercise test on the same day. In another patient, ^{13}N ammonia was injected at rest and also during maximum exercise. The following number of studies were therefore obtained: 17 studies of myocardial blood flow at rest and two at maximum exercise, seven studies of ^{11}C palmitate at rest, and 10 studies of ^{18}F deoxyglucose uptake at rest and six during maximum exercise.

Regional myocardial blood flow images were obtained after 15 to 20 mCi ^{13}N ammonia were given intravenously.[23,24] In two patients ^{13}N ammonia was not available and the blood flow tracer ^{82}Rb (30 to 40 mCi iv per injection[25,26]) was used. Because of the short physical half-life of ^{82}Rb (75 seconds), three to four separate injections were necessary, one for each image. When myocardial blood flow was evaluated during exercise, ^{13}N ammonia was injected one minute prior to cessation of maximum exercise, the patient was repositioned in the tomograph, and imaging commenced approximately three minutes after injection.

Myocardial fatty acid metabolism was evaluated with 15 to 20 mCi intravenous ^{11}C palmitate by recording serial images at a single mid-left ventricular level for 60 min.[27-31]

Regional myocardial utilization of exogenous glucose was evaluated with 10 mCi of ^{18}F deoxyglucose,[32,33] which was injected intravenously either at rest or one minute prior to stopping maximum treadmill[34] or semisupine bicycle exercise. Forty minutes after tracer injection, five to six contiguous cross-sectional images were recorded.

Production of ^{13}N ammonia, ^{11}C palmitate, and ^{18}F deoxyglucose have been described previously.[35-37] Images were acquired using the medium spatial resolution mode (18 mm at full-width half-maximum of a line source). For ^{13}N ammonia the acquisition time per image increased as ^{13}N decayed so that approximately one million counts were collected for each image. ^{82}Rb images were acquired from 1.5 to 6 min following tracer injection. Serial ^{11}C palmitate images were acquired for successively longer times (e.g., 90, 180, or 300 seconds); at least 400,000 counts were collected per image (maximum counts were as high as 2,400,000). ^{18}F deoxyglucose images were acquired for 10 to 12 min. All images were corrected for isotope decay.

Positron Emission Tomography Image Analysis and Statistics

Myocardial uptake of ^{13}N ammonia, ^{82}Rb, and ^{18}F deoxyglucose, and myocardial uptake and clearance of ^{11}C palmitate were analyzed by assigning six circular regions of interest to PET images of the left ventricular myocardium, three each in the septum and the lateral wall.[31] Only cross-sectional images that included the hypertrophied septum were analyzed.

Average myocardial tracer concentration in the septum and lateral wall were determined by averaging counts for the three regions of interest assigned to each area. In order to compare regional myocardial blood flow in the disproportionately thick septum with that in the normal lateral wall, a ratio of septal counts divided by lateral wall counts was calculated. The ratios of counts recovered from the septum and lateral wall in patients were compared with those obtained for ten normal volunteers.

Regional myocardial uptake of ^{11}C palmitate was determined at 6–8 min when tissue ^{11}C concentrations were highest.[31] From the tissue clearance curve of ^{11}C palmitate, two variables were derived: (1) the half-time of the early rapid clearance phase ($t_{1/2}$) and (2) the fraction of maximum myocardial ^{11}C activity at the end of the early rapid phase (the residual fraction).

In order to detect the presence of areas of increased ^{18}F deoxyglucose uptake relative to ^{13}N ammonia uptake, circumferential profile analysis[38] was performed on the ^{13}N ammonia and ^{18}F deoxyglucose images. Data for the one patient with this finding and a 60% stenosis in the left anterior descending coronary artery are not included in summed data from patients without this finding.

Mean values are given with standard deviations. All data were analyzed with paired or unpaired Student's *t*-test. Statistical significance was defined as P values of less than or equal to 0.05.

RESULTS

Clinical, Hemodynamic, and Laboratory Data

Three patients experienced transient chest discomfort on the study day, two at the beginning of the day and one during acquisition of the ^{18}F deoxyglucose images.

Resting heart rates averaged 66 $\pm$ 12 bpm, systolic blood pressure 126 $\pm$ 9 mmHg, and diastolic blood pressure 80 $\pm$ 8 mmHg. The resting heart rate-systolic blood pressure product was 8,402 $\pm$ 1,701.

As determined by venous blood samples in five patients with studies performed at rest and in three patients in whom blood was drawn before and following maximum exercise, neither venous glucose or neutral fatty acids rose significantly either during the rest studies or following exercise.

Electrocardiograms met standard criteria for left ventricular hypertrophy in 10 patients. The patient with a 60% left anterior descending coronary artery stenosis had first-degree atrioventricular block and right bundle branch block.

The echocardiographic septal to posterior wall thickness ratio averaged 1.8 $\pm$ 0.3.

Systolic septal thickening appeared normal in 10 patients. The echocardiographic hypertrophy score[18] was equal to or less than 3 in four patients, between 4 and 6 in five, and equal to or greater than 7 in four. Systolic anterior motion of the anterior mitral leaflet was mild in four patients, moderate in two, and severe in six.

Exercise

Six of seven patients reached at least 75% of the maximum predicted heart rate during exercise. In these six patients. the maximal heart rate averaged 156 ± 12 bpm and the maximal systolic and diastolic blood pressure were 176 ± 13 and 86 ± 5 mmHg, respectively. The heart rate-systolic blood pressure product averaged 27,561 ± 3,904. The mean time of treadmill exercise was 15 ± 3 min (i.e., 6 to 8 metabolic equivalents). No patient experienced chest pain or an abnormal blood pressure response. Left ventricular hypertrophy precluded evaluation of ischemic changes during exercise.

Positron Emission Tomography Images

Segmental analysis of ^{13}N ammonia or ^{82}Rb and ^{18}F deoxyglucose uptake

Images in the patient with 60% diameter narrowing of the left anterior descending coronary artery demonstrated in the distal septal and anterior walls a relative increase in ^{18}F deoxyglucose uptake compared to ^{13}N ammonia uptake, a pattern that has been described as evidence of ischemia.[38–40] This patient did not have chest pain on the study day. His findings are presented but excluded from further statistical analysis. Accordingly, the summed data for resting studies will be at least one less than the total number of studies performed.

^{13}N ammonia or ^{82}Rb uptake (n = *16 studies at rest) (Fig. 1)*

Observed myocardial counts for ^{13}N ammonia or ^{82}Rb uptake were similar for the

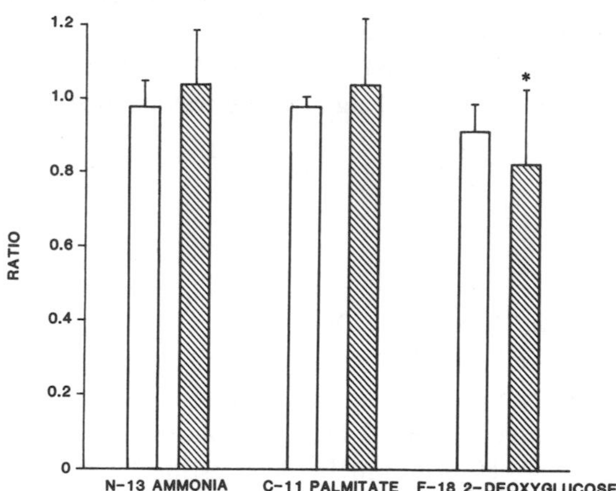

Fig. 1. Ratios of observed septal to lateral wall counts in normals (open bars) and patients with hypertrophic cardiomyopathy (hatched bars) for ^{13}N ammonia (on left), ^{11}C palmitate (in middle), and ^{18}F deoxyglucose (on right). The ratios of observed counts are similar for all three tracers although the ratio for ^{18}F deoxyglucose in patients with hypertrophic cardiomyopathy is lower than the ratio in normals, whereas the ratios for the two other tracers are slightly higher in patients than in normals. In patients, the ratio for ^{18}F deoxyglucose is significantly lower than the ratio for ^{13}N ammonia. *$p \leq 0.05$ vs ^{13}N ammonia for normals.

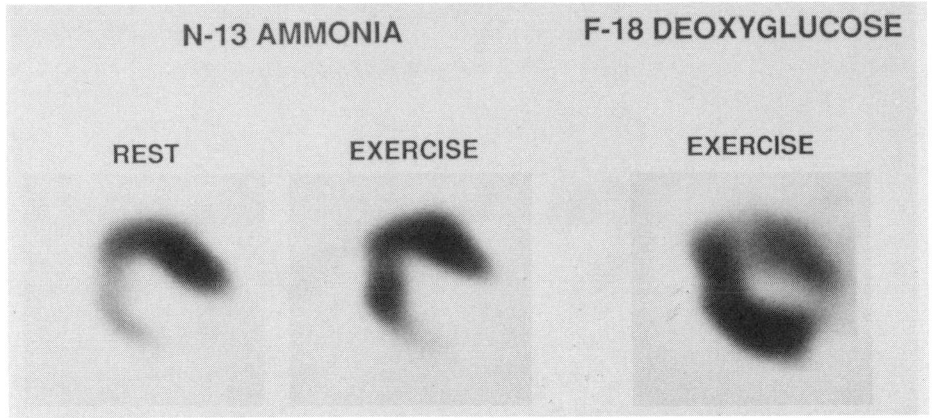

Fig. 2. ^{13}N ammonia images obtained at rest (left) and ^{13}N ammonia (middle) and ^{18}F deoxyglucose (right) images acquired at maximum exercise. The patient performed two identical exercise tests on the same day. Although observed ^{13}N ammonia uptake appears less in the lateral wall (lower left) than the septum (upper right), after observed counts were corrected for the partial volume effect, ^{13}N ammonia uptake in the septum was 33% lower than uptake in the lateral wall at rest, and 44% lower at maximal exercise. Corrected ^{18}F deoxyglucose uptake at maximal exercise was 43% lower in the septum than in the lateral wall.

septal and lateral wall (20,131 ± 4,114 and 19,348 ± 4,336; NS). The ratio for observed septal to lateral wall counts was 1.04 ± 0.12, similar to the ratio of 0.98 ± 0.07 in 10 normal volunteers.

Myocardial ^{13}N ammonia or ^{82}Rb uptake was evaluated on two separate days in four patients and yielded similar values (0.95 vs 0.96, 1.10 vs 1.00, 1.17 vs 1.31, and 1.02 vs 0.82).

Myocardial blood flow studies were acquired on the same day at rest and during exercise in two patients. In the images seen in Fig. 2, the ratio of observed septal to lateral wall counts was lower during exercise than at rest (1.07 vs 1.31).

^{11}C palmitate uptake and clearance (summed data, n=6) (Fig. 1)

The observed myocardial counts at the time of maximum ^{11}C palmitate uptake for the septal and lateral walls were also similar (17.912±2,566 and 17,708±4,348; NS). The ratio of observed septal to lateral wall counts was 1.04. .0.18, similar to the ratio of 0.98±0.03 in seven normal volunteers.

The half-time of the early rapid phase (septum: 21.0±4.7 min; lateral wall: 20.2±4.2 min) and the residual fractions (septum: 57.3±3.0 minutes; lateral wall: 58.5±5.2 min) were similar in the septal and lateral walls. In the patient with PET evidence of ischemia and a 60% diameter narrowing in the left anterior descending coronary artery, the half-time of the early rapid phase was longer in the septum than in the lateral wall (33.8 vs 22.5 min). Although data for the patient with a 40% diameter narrowing in the left anterior descending coronary artery were included in the summed data, it is of interest that the half-time of the early rapid phase in the disproportionately thick septum supplied by this minimally stenotic artery was longer than in the lateral wall (27.5 vs 19.3 min).

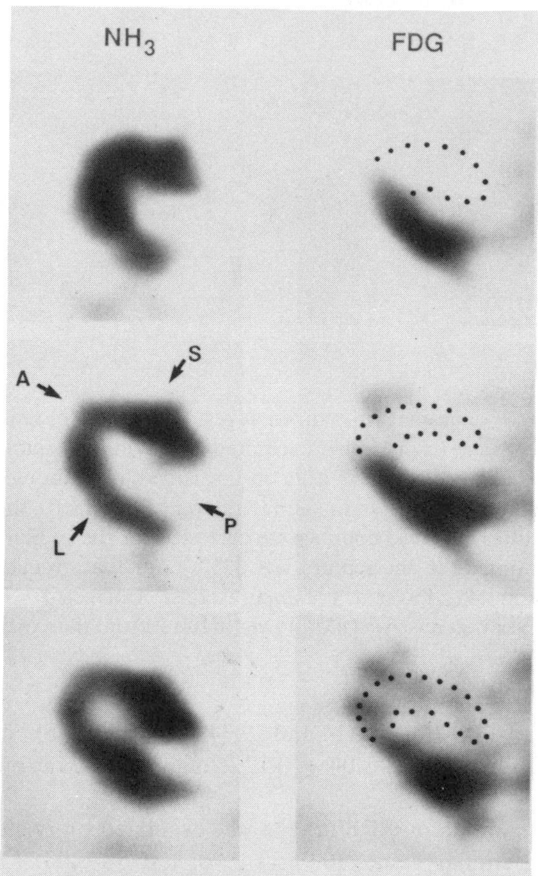

Fig. 3. ^{13}N ammonia images (left) and ^{18}F deoxyglucose (FDG) images (right) acquired at rest. Three contiguous myocardial levels are shown from the base of the heart, on the top, toward the apex, and on the bottom. The septum (S) is at the upper right, the anterior wall (A) at the upper left, the lateral wall (L) at the lower left, and the posterior (P) mitral valve at the right. Prior to correction for the partial volume effect, ^{13}N ammonia uptake in the septum appears similar to uptake in the lateral wall. Observed ^{13}N ammonia septal and lateral wall counts were 22,718 and 36,121, whereas corrected counts were 20,560 and 19,836, respectively. Septal uptake of ^{13}F deoxyglucose (within dotted lines) is severely reduced compared with uptake in the lateral wall. This reduction can be detected visually. Observed ^{18}F deoxyglucose septal and lateral wall counts were 10,464 and 25,791, whereas corrected counts were 11,562 and 46,964, respectively. Thus, septal ^{18}F deoxyglucose uptake is decreased compared with ^{13}N ammonia uptake in this study acquired at rest. This pattern is the opposite of the pattern indicative of ischemia.

^{18}F deoxyglucose uptake (Fig. 1)

Because in two patients myocardial ^{18}F deoxyglucose uptake at rest was not adequate for analysis, uptake values are presented for only seven patients. Unlike uptake of ^{13}N

ammonia and ^{11}C palmitate, uptake of ^{18}F deoxyglucose at rest in the septum was decreased relative to the lateral wall (15,768±4,314 vs 19,818±5,234; NS; Fig. 3). The ratio of observed septal to lateral wall counts was 0.83±0.22, lower than the ratio in 10 volunteers (0.98±0.07; $P \leq 0.05$). In addition, this ratio was significantly lower than the ratio for ^{13}N ammonia at rest ($P \leq 0.03$).

In two of the six patients studied at maximal exercise, one of whom fasted and one of whom had eaten, myocardial ^{18}F deoxyglucose uptake was not adequate for analysis ($n=4$). The patient who had eaten did not achieve 75% of her maximum predicted heart rate during bicycle exercise. The ratio at maximal exercise (0.81±0.23) was not significantly different from the ratio obtained at rest.

Patients with chest pain on the study day

The septal to lateral wall ratio for blood flow in the three patients with chest pain on the day of the study was slightly but not significantly lower than the ratio in patients without chest pain (0.97±0.07 vs 1.06±0.17; NS). Myocardial ^{18}F deoxyglucose uptake was not adequate for analysis in two of the three patients with chest pain. In the third patient, who had pain during acquisition of the ^{18}F deoxyglucose image, the observed septal to lateral wall ratio was 0.81.

DISCUSSION

Without correcting observed counts for wall thickness, the uptake of blood flow tracers—^{13}N ammonia and ^{82}Rb—appeared similar in the septum relative to the lateral wall, suggesting that blood flow was similar in these two myocardial regions. For ^{11}C palmitate, the uptake, clearance half-time of the early rapid clearance phase, and residual fraction were similar in the septum and the lateral wall except for two patients with minimal to moderate left anterior descending coronary artery disease. These findings suggest that fatty acid metabolism was similar in these two myocardial regions. However, in the interventricular septum, uptake of the tracer of exogenous glucose utilization—^{18}F deoxyglucose—was significantly more depressed than uptake of tracers of blood flow. Although the number of patients studied during maximum exercise was small, the tracer of myocardial blood flow decreased in the septum relative to the lateral wall during exercise compared with rest. This finding suggests a decrease in septal blood flow relative to the lateral wall during maximum exercise. The ratio of septal to lateral wall exogenous glucose utilization was slightly less during maximum exercise compared with the ratio obtained at rest. The reduction of ^{18}F deoxyglucose uptake in the interventricular septum both at rest and during maximum exercise, together with normal ^{11}C palmitate kinetics (i.e., fatty acid metabolism) at rest, argue against the presence of ischemia and raise the question of a primary metabolic abnormality in the disproportionately thickened septum of patients with hypertrophic cardiomyopathy.

Myocardial Blood Flow

Using alternative markers of blood flow (e.g., ^{201}Tl and ^{133}Xe), some investigators have reported normal blood flow to the interventricular septum, while others have reported stress-induced perfusion abnormalities which normalized on delayed ^{201}Tl scintigraphy.[7,8,10,14,41] One report described reduced blood flow to the interventricular septum even at rest.[42] Visual observation of homogenous distribution of ^{13}N ammonia on images acquired in our 13 patients suggest that blood flow to the interventricular

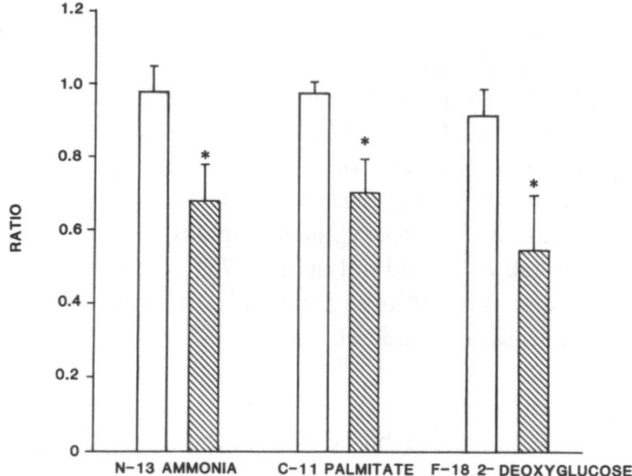

Fig. 4. Septum to lateral wall activity ratios for counts corrected for the thickness of the septum and lateral wall, as measured by echocardiography, in patients with hypertrophic cardiomyopathy. The data for normals are shown by open bars and for patients with hypertrophic cardiomyopathy by hatched bars for ^{13}N ammonia (on left), ^{11}C palmitate (in middle), and ^{18}F 2-deoxyglucose (on right). The corrected activity ratios are significantly lower in patients with hypertrophic cardiomyopathy than in normals for all three tracers. $*p \leq 0.001$ vs normals.

septum was normal. In these patients, the average ratio of septal to lateral wall counts approached unity (1.04 ± 0.12), a value similar to that obtained in normal subjects.

However, myocardial counts as seen and determined from cross-sectional images do not necessarily represent true tracer tissue concentrations. The partial volume effect, common to all imaging techniques, causes an underestimation of true tissue tracer counts when the size of the imaged object (in our study, the thickness of the myocardial wall) is less than twice the spatial resolution of the imaging device.[42] Therefore, the marked regional differences in myocardial wall thickness in our patients with hypertrophic cardiomyopathy and a disproportionately thick septum would lead to heterogeneity of observed tracer concentrations on the cross-sectional images. For example, if blood flow or glucose utilization in units per gram myocardium were identical, ^{13}N ammonia and ^{18}F deoxyglucose concentrations should be larger in the septum than in the lateral wall. True tissue concentrations can be calculated from the images by correcting observed counts for this underestimation by using the known relationship between wall thickness and the degree of underestimation. Assuming that the echocardiographically measured thickness of the posterior wall equaled that of the posterolateral wall imaged with PET (an assumption which magnetic resonance images confirmed as accurate in three of our patients), correction of the regional tissue concentrations for regional partial volume effect altered the septal to lateral wall activity ratio (Fig. 4). The septal to lateral wall ratio for uptake of the blood flow tracer declined to 0.72 ± 0.09, indicating an average 28% reduction of blood flow in the interventricular septum relative to the lateral wall. Thus, all patients analyzed in this manner revealed a relative decrease in blood flow to the disproportionately thick septum. Reports of abnormal intramural septal coronary arteries,[44,45] decreased septal ^{201}Tl uptake,[10,46] and abnormal coronary vasodilator reserve[12] provide additional evidence for impaired septal blood flow. The corrected septal to lateral wall ratio for ^{13}N ammonia uptake declined from the value obtained at rest in two patients studied at maximal exercise (0.83 vs 0.68 and 0.66 vs 0.56), findings which raise the possibility of an attenuated flow response to exercise in the disproportionately hypertrophied septum.

Fatty Acid Metabolism and Exogenous Glucose Utilization

Myocardial uptake of ^{11}C palmitate also appeared to be homogenous on the PET images in our patients. This observation was confirmed by the average septal to lateral wall activity ratio of 1.04 ± 0.18, which approached unity and was similar to the average ratio in the seven normal volunteers. However, after correction for partial volume effect, the septal to lateral wall activity ratio declined to 0.68 ± 0.10. Thus, relative to the lateral wall, ^{11}C palmitate uptake was decreased by 32% in the septum and, therefore, paralleled the reduction in blood flow. Rather than reflecting an abnormality of fatty acid metabolism, this decrease in the interventricular septum was most likely a function of decreased blood flow, as previously demonstrated in animal experiments.[27] The normal half-time of the early rapid phase and residual fraction in the septum are also consistent with normal fatty acid metabolism and a flow-dependent decrease in ^{11}C palmitate uptake, arguing against the presence of ischemia.

While the reduction of blood flow and ^{11}C palmitate uptake in the thickened septum is consistent with decreased blood flow and fatty acid uptake, the myocardial clearance kinetics of ^{11}C palmitate do not favor ischemia. First, no significant difference existed in clearance half-times of the early rapid clearance phase and in residual fractions between the septal and lateral wall in patients with hypertrophic cardiomyopathy without coronary artery disease. Second, the average clearance half-times and residual fractions observed in the septum of our patients were virtually identical with those previously reported in normal human myocardium.[31] It is of interest that even minimal obstructive disease of a coronary artery supplying the disproportionately thick ventricular septum resulted in altered clearance half-times of the early rapid phase, a finding which differs from patients with more severe coronary artery disease but normal myocardial wall thickness.[31] In the presence of increased septal thickness and inadequate vasodilator reserve,[12] even a minimal coronary artery stenosis may be physiologically significant.

The relative decrease in the septal to lateral wall ratio for ^{18}F deoxyglucose argues further against the presence of ischemia at rest in the interventricular septum. After regional tracer tissue concentrations were corrected for partial volume effect, the average septal to lateral wall activity ratio declined even more to 0.55 ± 0.14.

If the metabolic abnormality in the disproportionately thick interventricular septum at rest had been caused by ischemia, we would have anticipated a delay in septal ^{11}C palmitate clearance as well as a relative or absolute increase in septal ^{18}F deoxyglucose uptake. Such ischemia-related abnormalities had previously been observed in animal experimental studies and in patients with ischemic heart disease.[38-40,47] Our findings with PET are at variance with reports of decreased extraction or even release of lactate in patients with hypertrophic cardiomyopathy as a sign of ischemia, although the majority of these reported abnormalities in lactate metabolism were observed only during exercise or atrial pacing.[9,11,12] In light of the previously reported vascular abnormalities and limited coronary flow reserve in patients with hypertrophic cardiomyopathy, it is possible that exercise or atrial pacing in a large number of symptomatic patients would induce an ischemia metabolic pattern on PET. In our study, exercise was performed in a small number of patients with relatively good physical tolerance, so the results only reflect trends. It is of note that even the patient who experienced chest pain during the PET study did not have PET evidence of ischemia, suggesting that the pain was either of nonischemic origin or that the ischemia did not evoke metabolic abnormalities sufficient to be imaged.

A possible explanation for the relative decrease in septal glucose utilization is inhibition at the level of glucose uptake either due to insulin[48,49] or its effects on the ATP-dependent translocation of glucose transporters from the Golgi complex to the plasma membrane.[50–52] Alternatively, the increased septal glycogen content observed in hypertrophic cardiomyopathy[4–6] might indicate impairment of glucose utilization rather than of glucose transport.

Our data suggest that patients with hypertrophic cardiomyopathy might have a nonischemic metabolic abnormality in the disproportionately thick ventricular septum. It is not known whether the presumed metabolic defect is primary or secondary. A primary genetic biochemical fault may affect the ventricular septum and initiate the subsequent pathogenetic mechanism(s).[3]

REFERENCES

1. Clark, C.E., Henry, W.L., and Epstein, S.E. Familial prevalence and genetic transmission of hypertrophic subaortic stenosis. *N. Engl. J. Med.* **289**: 709–714, 1973.
2. Maron, B.J. and Mulvihill, J.J. The genetics of hypertrophic cardiomyopathy. *Ann. Int. Med.* **105**: 610–613, 1986.
3. Perloff, J.K. Pathogenesis of hypertrophic cardiomyopathy. In: Heart Muscle Disease, Goodwin, J.F. (ed.), MTP Press Limited, Boston, 1985, pp. 7–22.
4. Snijder, J., Dejong, J., and Meijr, A.E.F.H. Light microscopical, ultrastructural and histochemical aspects of hypertrophic obstructive cardiomyopathy (subaortic stenosis). *J. Molec. Cell. Cardiol.* **3**: 81–92, 1971.
5. Van Noorden, S., Olsen, E.G.J., and Pearse, A.G.E. Hypertrophic obstructive cardiomyopathy, a histological, histochemical, and ultrastructural study of biopsy material. *Cardiovasc. Res.* **5**: 118–131, 1971.
6. Emeriau, J.P., Le Menn, R., Besse, P., and Bricaud, H. Etude ultrastructurale de 11 cas de myocardiopathie obstructive du ventricule gauche. *Arch. Mal. Coeur* **5**: 475–483, 1976.
7. Rubin, K.A., Morrison, J., Padnck, M.B., Binder, A.J., Chiaramida, S., Margouleff, D., Padmanabhan, V.T., and Gulotta, S.J. Idiopathic hypertrophic subaortic stenosis: Evaluation of anginal symptoms with thallium-201 myocardial imaging. *Am. J. Cardiol.* **44**: 1040, 1979.
8. Pitcher, D., Wainwright, R., Maisey, M., Curry, P., and Sowton, E. Assessment of chest pain in hypertrophic cardiomyopathy using exercise thallium-201 myocardial scintigraphy. *Br. Heart J.* **44**: 650, 1980.
9. Thompson, D.S., Naqvi, N., Juul, S.M., Swanton, R.H., Coltart, D.J., Jenkins, B.S., and Webb-Peploe, M.M. Effects of propanolol on myocardial oxygen consumption, substrate extraction, and hemodynamics in obstructive cardiomyopathy. *Br. Heart J.* **44**: 488–498, 1980.
10. Hanrath, P., Mathey, D., Montz, R., Thiel, U., Vorbringer, H., Kupper, W., Schneider, C., and Bleifeld, W. Myocardial thallium 201 imaging in hypertrophic obstructive cardiomyopathy. *Eur. Heart J.* **2**: 177–185, 1981.
11. Pasternac, A., Wagniart, P., Olivenstein, R., Petitclerc, R., Krol, R., Andermann, E., Melancon, S., Geoffroy, G., de Champlain, J., and Barbeau, A. Increased plasma catecholamines in patients with Friedreich's ataxia. *Can. J. Neurol. Sci.* **9**: 195, 1982.
12. Cannon, R.O. III, Rosing, D.R., Maron, B.J., Leon, M.B., Bonow, R.O., Watson, R.M., and Epstein, S.E. Myocardial ischemia in patients with hypertrophic cardiomyopathy: Contribution of inadequate vasodilator reserve and elevated left ventricular filling pressures. *Circulation* **71**: 234–243, 1985.

13. Maron, B.J., Bonow, R.O., Cannon, R.O., Leon, M.B., and Epstein, S.E. Hypertrophic cardiomyopathy: Interrelations of clinical manifestations, pathophysiology, and therapy. *N. Engl. J. Med.* **316**: 780–789, 884–852, 1987.
14. O'Gara, P.T., Bonow, R.O., Maron, B.J., Damske, B.A., Van Lingen, A., Bachrach, S.L., Larson, S.M., and Epstein, S.E. Myocardial perfusion abnormalities in patients with hypertrophic cardiomyopathy: Assessment with thallium-201 emission computed tomography. *Circulation* **76**: 1214–1223, 1987.
15. Grover, M. and Schelbert, H.R. Positron emission computed tomography. In: Digital Cardiac Imaging, G.K. Hall Medical Publishers, Boston, 1985, pp. 158–182.
16. Schelbert, H.R. and Schwaiger, M. PET studies of the heart. In: Positron Emission Tomography and Autoradiography, Phelps, M., Mazziotta, J., and Schelbert, H. (eds.), Raven Press, New York, 1986, pp. 581–661.
17. Grover-McKay, M., Schwaiger, M., Krivokapich, J., Perloff, J.K., Phelps, M.E., and Schelbert, H.R. Regional myocardial blood flow and metabolism in mildly symptomatic patients with hypertrophic cardiomyopathy. *J. Am. Coll. Cardiol.* (in press)
18. Wigle, E.D., Sasson, Z., Henderson, M.A., Ruddy, T.D., Fulop, J., Rakowski, H., and Williams, W.G. Hypertrophic cardiomyopathy. The importance of the site and the extent of hypertrophy. A review. *Prog. Cardiovasc. Dis.* **28**: 1–83, 1985.
19. Wigle, E.D. Hypertrophic cardiomyopathy: A 1987 viewpoint. *Circulation* **75**: 311–322, 1987.
20. Bell, R., Barber, P.V., Bray, C.L., and Beton, D.C. Incidence of thyroid disease in cases of hypertrophic cardiomyopathy. *Br. Heart J.* **40**: 1306–1309, 1978.
21. Topol, E.J., Traill, T.A., and Fortuin, N.J. Hypertensive hypertrophic cardiomyopathy of the elderly. *N. Engl. J. Med.* **312**: 277–283, 1985.
22. Phelps, M.E., Hoffman, E.J., Huang, S.C., and Kuhl, D.E. ECAT: A new computerized tomographic imaging system for positron-emitting radiopharmaceuticals. *J. Nucl. Med.* **19**: 635, 1978.
23. Schelbert, H.R., Phelps, M.E., Hoffman, E.J., Huang, S.C., Selin, C.E., and Kuhl D.E. Regional myocardial perfusion assessed with N-13 labeled ammonia and positron emission computerized axial tomography. *Am. J. Cardiol.* **43**: 209, 1979.
24. Schelbert, H.R., Phelps, M.E., Huang, S.C., MacDonald, N.S., Hansen, H., Selin, C., and Kuhl, D.E. N-13 ammonia as an indicator of myocardial blood flow. *Circulation* **63**: 1259, 1981.
25. Grover-McKay, M., Huang, S.C., Hoffman, E.J., Phelps, M.E., and Schelbert, H.R. Noninvasive quantification of myocardial blood flow in dogs with rubidium-82 and PET. *J. Nucl. Med.* **27**: 976, 1986 (abst).
26. Gould, K.L., Goldstein, R.A., Mullani, N.A., Kirkeeide, R.L., Wong, W., Tewson, T.J., Berridge, M.S., Bolomey, L.A., Hartz, R.K., Smalling, R.W., Ruentes, F., and Nishikawa, A. Noninvasive assessment of coronary stenoses by myocardial perfusion imaging during pharmacologic coronary vasodilation. VIII. Clinical feasibility of positron cardiac imaging without a cyclotron using generator-produced rubidium-82. *J. Am. Coll. Cardiol.* **7**: 775–789, 1986.
27. Schon, H.R., Schelbert, H.R., Najafi, A., Robinson, G., Huang, S.C., Barrio, J., and Phelps, M.E. C-11 labeled palmitic acid for the nonivasive evaluation of regional myocardial fatty acid metabolism with positron computed tomography. I. Kinetics of C-11 palmitic acid in normal myocardium. *Am. Heart J.* **103**: 532, 1982.
28. Schon, H.R., Schelbert, H.R., Najafi, A., Hansen, H., Robinson, G.R., Huang, S.C., Barrio, J., and Phelps, M.E. C-11 labeled palmitic acid for the noninvasive evaluation of regional myocardial fatty acid metabolism with positron computed tomography. II. Kinetics of C-11 palmitic acid in acutely ischemic myocardium. *Am. Heart J.* **103**: 548, 1982.
29. Schelbert, H.R., Henze, E., Schon, H.R., Keen, R., Hansen, H.W., Selin, C., Huang, S.C., Barrio, J.R., and Phelps, M.E. C-11 palmitate for the noninvasive evaluation of regional

myocardial fatty acid metabolism with positron computed tomography. III. *In vivo* demonstration of the effects of substrate availability on myocardial metabolism. *Am. Heart J.* **105**: 492, 1983.

30. Schelbert, H.R., Henze, E., Schon, H.R., Najafi, A., Hansen, H., Huang, S.C., Barrio, J.R., and Phelps, M.E. C-11 palmitate for the noninvasive evaluation of regional myocardial fatty acid metabolism with positron computed tomography. IV. *In vivo* demonstration of impaired fatty acid oxidation in acute myocardial ischemia. *Am. Heart J.* **106**: 736, 1983.
31. Grover-McKay, M., Schelbert, H.R., Schwaiger, M., Sochor, H., Guzy, P.M., Krivokapich, J., Child, J.S., and Phelps, M.E. Identification of impaired metabolic reserve in patients with significant coronary artery stenosis by atrial pacing. *Circulation* **74**: 281–292, 1986.
32. Ratib, O., Phelps, M.E., Huang, S.C., Henze, E., Selin, C.E., and Schelbert, H.R. Positron tomography with deoxyglucose for estimating local myocardial glucose metabolism. *J. Nucl. Med.* **23**: 577, 1982.
33. Schwaiger, M., Huang, S.C., Krivokapich, J., Phelps, M.E., and Schelbert, H.R. Myocardial glucose utilization measured noninvasively in man by positron tomography. *J. Am. Coll. Cardiol.* **6**: 336, 1983 (abst).
34. Kattus, A.A., Jorgensen, C.R., Worden, R.E., and Alvaro, A.B. S-T segment depression with near-maximal exercise in detection of preclinical coronary heart disease. *Circulation* **41**: 585–595, 1971.
35. Vaalburg, W., Kamphius, J.A., Beerlingvan der Molus, H.B., Reiffers, S., Rijskamp, A., and Woldring, M.G. An improved method for the cyclotron production of N-13 labeled ammonia. *Int. J. Appl. Radiat. Isot.* **26**: 316–318, 1975.
36. Padgett, H.C., Robinson, G.D., and Barrio, J.R. [1–11C]palmitic acid: Improved radiopharmaceutical preparation. *Int. J. Appl. Radiat. Isot.* **33**: 1471–1472, 1982.
37. Bida, G.T., Satyamurthy, N., and Barrio, J.R. The synthesis of 2-[F-18]fluoro-2-deoxy-d-glucose using glycals: A reexamination. *J. Nucl. Med.* **25**: 1327–1334, 1984.
38. Marshall, R.C., Tillisch, J.H., Phelps, M.E., Huang, S.C., Carson, R., Henze, E., and Schelbert, H.R. Identification and differentiation of resting myocardial ischemia and infarction in man with positron computed tomography, F-18 labeled fluorodeoxyglucose and N-13 ammonia. *Circulation* **67**: 766–778, 1983.
39. Schwaiger, M., Schelbert, H.R., Ellison, D., Hansen, H., Yeatman, L., Vinten-Johansen, J., Selin, C., Barrio, J., and Phelps, M.E. Sustained regional abnormalities in cardiac metabolism after transient ischemia in the chronic dog model. *J. Am. Coll. Cardiol.* **6**: 336–347, 1985.
40. Tillisch, J., Brunken, R., Marshall, R., Schwaiger, M., Mandelkern, M., Phelps, M., and Schelbert, H. Prediction of the reversibility of cardiac wall motion abnormalities using positron tomography, F-18 fluorodeoxyglucose and N-13 ammonia. *N. Engl. J. Med.* **314**: 884–888, 1986.
41. Weiss, M.B., Ellis, K., Sciacca, R.R., Johnson, L.L., Schmidt, D.H., and Cannon, P.J. Myocardial blood flow in congestive and hypertrophic cardiomyopathy. *Circulation* **54**: 484–494, 1976.
42. Nagata, S., Park, Y., Minamikawa, T., Yutani, C., Kamiya, T., Nishimura, T., Kozuka, T., Sakakibara, H., and Nimura, Y. Thallium perfusion and cardiac enzyme abnormalities in patients with familial hypertrophic cardiomyopathy. *Am. Heart J.* **109**: 1317–1322, 1985.
43. Hoffman, E.J., Huang, S.C., and Phelps, M.E. Quantitation in positron computed tomography. 1. Effect of object size. *J. Comput. Assist. Tomogr.* **3**: 299–308, 1979.
44. James, T.N. and Marshall, T.K. De subitaneis mortibus XII. Asymmetrical hypertrophy of the heart. *Circulation* **51**: 1149–1166, 1975.
45. Maron, B.J., Wolfson, J.K., Epstein, S.E., and Roberts, W.C. Intramural ("small vessel") coronary artery disease in hypertrophic cardiomyopathy. *J. Am. Coll. Cardiol.* **8**: 545–547, 1986.
46. Bulkley, B.H., Rouleau, J., Strauss, H.W., and Pitt, B. Idiopathic hypertrophic subaortic

stenosis: Detection by thallium-201 myocardial perfusion imaging. *N. Engl. J. Med.* **293**: 1113–1116, 1975.

47. Camici, P., Araujo, L.I., Spinks, T., Lammertsma, A.A., Kaski, J.C., Shea, M.J., Selwyn, A.P., Jones, T., and Maseri, A. Increased uptake of F-18 fluorodeoxyglucose in postischemic myocardium of patients with exercise-induced angina. *Circulation* **74**: 81–88, 1986.
48. Morgan, H.E., Neely, J.R., and Kira, Y. Factors determining the utilization of glucose in isolated rat hearts. *Basic Res. Cardiol.* **79**: 292–299, 1984.
49. Haworth, R.A. and Berkoff, H.A. The control of sugar uptake by metabolic demand in isolated adult rat heart calls. *Circ. Res.* **58**: 157–165, 1986.
50. Suzuki, K. and Kono, T. Evidence that insulin causes translocation of glucose transport activity to the plasma membrane from an intracellular storage site. *Proc. Natl. Acad. Sci. USA* **77**: 2542–2545, 1980.
51. Cushman, S.W. and Wardzala, L.J. Potential mechanism of insulin action on glucose transport in the isolated rat adipose cell. *J. Biol. Chem.* **255**: 4758–4762, 1980.
52. Siegel, J. and Olefsky, J.M. Role of intracellular energy in insulin's ability to activate 3–0-methylglucose transport by rat adipocytes. *Biochemistry* **19**: 2183–2190, 1980.

Exercise Performance in Hypertrophic Cardiomyopathy

Benno Lösse and Franz Loogen

Department of Cardiology, University of Düsseldorf, Federal Republic of Germany

SUMMARY

This overview is based on more than 500 symptom-limited exercise tests in patients with hypertrophic obstructive and nonobstructive cardiomyopathy. The data demonstrate: (1) Exercise tests can be safely performed. (2) Exercise tests with simultaneous hemodynamic measurements help to assess the degree of functional limitation more accurately than clinical judgement alone. (3) Exercise tests including measurements of hemodynamic parameters (stroke volume, cardiac output and pulmonary artery pressure) and minimal transit times of a radioactive tracer through the heart support the concept of impaired left ventricular diastolic function as the predominant pathophysiological alteration in hypertrophic cardiomyopathies, and expand it to the right ventricle. (4) Serial exercise tests with simultaneous hemodynamic measurements are valuable to assess the efficacy of therapy more precisely. Although the symptomatic and hemodynamic response to medical therapy with propranolol or verapamil may individually vary, verapamil appears on average to be superior to propranolol with respect to changes in clinical symptoms and exercise capacity as well as in stroke volume, cardiac output, mean pulmonary artery pressure and arterio-venous oxygen difference during exercise. The most impressive improvements with respect to symptoms and hemodynamics, however, are achieved with surgery. As far as long-term results are concerned, surgically treated patients experience more frequent, more substantial and, of utmost importance, more long-lasting benefits from therapy than do medically treated patients.

Exercise tests are extensively used for diagnosis, prognostication and evaluation of therapy in patients with suspected or proven coronary artery disease. Their use in hypertrophic cardiomyopathies is uncommon, possibly due to an anticipated increased risk of serious ventricular arrhythmias and sudden cardiac death induced by strenuous exercise.[1–3] We have performed more than 500 exercise tests in patients with hypertrophic cardiomyopathies to assess the degree of hemodynamic impairment and observed no serious complications. In the following overview we want to focus on four issues: (1) safety of exercise tests; (2) use of exercise tests for the validation of symptoms; (3) changes of hemodynamic and cardiac volume parameters during exercise; (4) use of exercise tests for the evaluation of therapy.

Methods: All exercise tests were performed in an uniform manner with the patients in the supine position on a bicycle ergometer. Work load was increased in steps of 25 W to a maximum terminated by angina, dyspnea or exhaustion. Continuous measurements of heart rate (from electrocardiogram), pulmonary artery pressure (Swan Ganz catheter), systemic artery pressure (cannulated radial or brachial artery) and total body oxygen consumption (paramagnetic method, Oxycon, Mijnhardt) were performed as well as discontinuous measurements of pulmonary artery wedge pressure and oxygen content in pulmonary and systemic arteries (Lex-O_2-Con, Lexington Instruments), allowing calculations of cardiac output (Fick principle) and of stroke volume. In a few cases, the thermodilution method was used for measurement of cardiac output. Each exercise level was maintained for 5 to 10 minutes to reach steady-states of constant heart rate and oxygen consumption. Depending on the number of exercise steps, the total duration of exercise varied between 6 and more than 40 minutes.

I. Safety of Exercise Tests

Sudden death accounts for the majority of deaths in patients with hypertrophic cardiomyopathy.[3-9] Although its mechanisms are complex and probably not uniform in all patients, there is strong evidence that serious ventricular arrhythmias are the most common precipitating events of sudden death.[1,2,4,8-12] Furthermore, a considerable number of sudden deaths has been observed during or immediately after strenuous exercise.[1-3] Symptom-limited exercise tests should, therefore, be carefully performed, especially in patients with antecedent syncopes.

In a study of 245 exercise tests in 136 patients with hypertrophic cardiomyopathy (106 obstructive, 30 nonobstructive) of New York Heart Association (NYHA) class I to IV we observed ventricular arrhythmias in a considerable number of tests.[13] Figure 1 illustrates that the incidence and severity of ventricular arrhythmias (modified Lown-

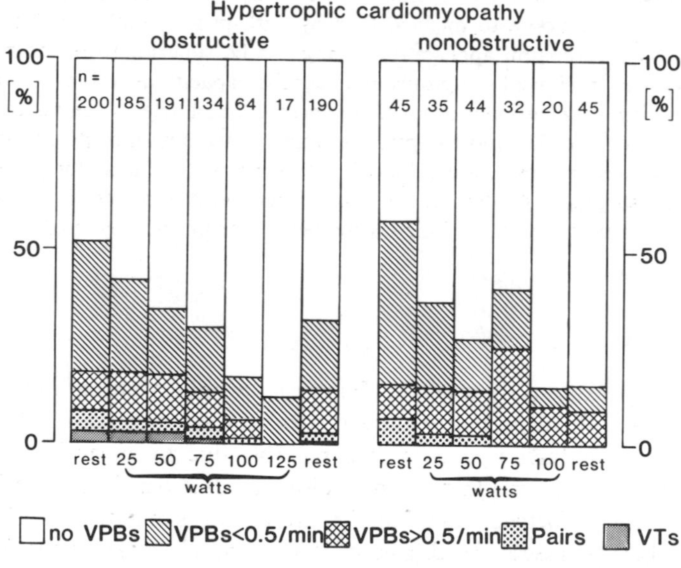

Fig. 1. Incidence of ventricular arrhythmias of different severity at rest and during exercise in 245 exercise tests, performed in 136 patients with hypertrophic obstructive cardiomyopathy (200 tests) and 30 patients with hypertrophic nonobstructive cardiomyopathy (45 tests). For each test, only the highest degree of ventricular arrhythmias (modified Lown classification) was taken into account. The resting phases under electrocardiographic observation lasted a mean of 18 $\pm$ 7.8 minutes before exercise, and a mean of 5.0 $\pm$ 3.0 minutes after exercise. Each exercise level was maintained for 5 to 10 minutes. Abbreviations: VPB: ventricular premature beat, VT: self terminating ventricular tachycardia.

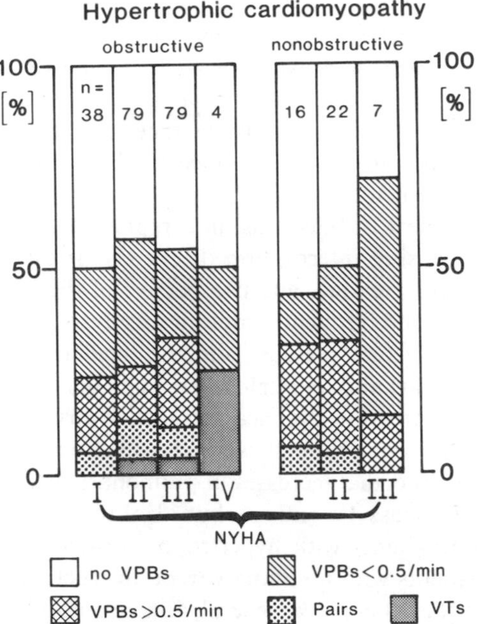

Fig. 2. Correlation of the incidence of ventricular arrhythmias of different severity, documented during exercise, with the degree of functional impairment (NYHA classification). Same patient population as in Fig. 1. Numbers of patients belonging to each NYHA group are indicated in the head of the figure. Abbreviations: see Fig. 1.

classification) decreased with increasing work load. No significant intensification of ventricular tachycardias was documented during the ensuing resting period. Self-terminating ventricular tachycardias (3 or more premature beats) of maximally 17 QRS complexes were observed only in 7 of 200 tests in hypertrophic obstructive, and not at all in 45 tests in hypertrophic nonobstructive cardiomyopathy. This finding appears remarkable since 31 (=23%) patients with hypertrophic obstructive cardiomyopathy had one or more antecedent syncopes. Furthermore, only in 3 of 54 tests (=6%) performed in this subgroup of patients with syncopes, ventricular pairs or tachycardias were observed. One may suppose that the observation of decreasing incidence and severity of ventricular arrhythmias with increasing work load is biased by the fact that the higher exercise levels were reached only by the less compromised patients. A correlation between the degree of ventricular hypertrophy and the incidence of asymptomatic ventricular tachycardias has been described.[12] On the other hand, as demonstrated in Fig. 2, we found no significant differences between the different functional classes. The apparent accumulation of ventricular tachycardias in class IV patients is based on one single observation in a small number of patients.

In conclusion it can be said that symptom-limited (angina pectoris, dyspnea or exhaustion) exercise tests can be safely performed in patients with hypertrophic cardiomyopathies without fear of serious complications. In at present more than 500 exercise tests we were forced to interrupt the test only in one case because of atrial fibrillation with rapid conduction to the ventricles, but never because of ventricular tachycardias or hemodynamic collapse.

II. Evaluation of Symptoms

The chief symptoms of hypertrophic cardiomyopathy are exertional dyspnea, angina, fatigue and transient impairment of consciousness. The intensity of symptoms is usually estimated from the patients' reports and may be aggravated or alleviated. Exercise tests may therefore help to assess more accurately the true severity of symptoms and, when hemodynamic parameters are simultaneously measured, to correlate them with the degree of hemodynamic impairment.

As can be seen from Table 1, fatigue was, in a representative group of patients, the most frequent symptom causing interruption of exercise irrespective of the degree of increase in pulmonary artery pressure, and irrespective of the behaviour of cardiac output during exercise. The second frequent symptom was dyspnea. Its frequency increased with the rise in pulmonary artery pressure and the incidence of subnormal increases in cardiac output, but, remarkably enough, even in patients with excessive increases in mean pulmonary artery pressure dyspnea was not invariably present at the end of the test. On the other side, when patients were classified according to reported symptoms (Table 2), we found abnormal increases in pulmonary artery pressure during exercise not only in all NYHA class IV patients but also, to values as high as 63 mmHg, in 40% of asymptomatic patients with hypertrophic obstructive cardiomyopathy and 23% of asymptomatic patients with no outflow tract obstruction.

It has been described that there is a general, but not absolute correlation between symptoms and the magnitude of left ventricular hypertrophy.[12,14] Our data extend this concept in so far as there is no absolute coincidence of symptoms and the severity of hemodynamic impairment. With regard to therapeutic implications it seems, therefore, reasonable to include data from exercise tests in the assessment of functional impairment, although it is not proven as yet whether an asymptomatic patient with markedly elevated pulmonary artery pressure has a worse prognosis than a patient classified as

TABLE 1. Symptoms Causing Interruption of Exercise Test in 144 Patients with Hypertrophic Obstructive Cardiomyopathy, Correlated with the Increase in Pulmonary Artery Pressure

P_{PA} (mmHg)	*n*	Dyspnea	Angina	Fatigue	CO below normal
20–29	35	20%	6%	100%	3%
30–39	59	31%	17%	95%	8%
40–49	24	33%	29%	96%	17%
50–59	16	75%	31%	94%	25%
60–71	10	80%	20%	90%	50%

Abbreviations: P_{PA}: mean pulmonary artery pressure, CO: cardiac output.

TABLE 2. Proportion of Increase in Mean Pulmonary Artery Pressure during Exercise in 63 Patients with Hypertrophic Obstructive Cardiomyopathy (HOCM) and 29 Patients with Hypertrophic Nonobstructive Cardiomyopathy, Classified according to the New York Heart Association (NYHA)

NYHA class	HOCM		HNCM	
	n	%	*n*	%
I	10	40	13	23
II	14	64	12	58
III	36	86	4	75
IV	3	100	–	–

NYHA class III according to reported symptoms who presents with normal pulmonary artery pressures during exercise. However, according to other investigators who recommend therapy for asymptomatic patients with marked hypertrophy, marked obstruction or a family history of premature sudden death,[6,12] we believe that this recommendation can be based on a yet firmer foundation when hemodynamic data from exercise tests are considered, too.

III. Hemodynamic and Cardiac Volume Parameters

Hypertrophic cardiomyopathies occur with and without outflow tract pressure gradients. The clinical and pathophysiological significance of the outflow tract gradient is debated,[5,12,14–19] whereas the impairment of diastolic ventricular relaxation and distensibility[5,12,20–28] is more uniformly considered as a major determinant of pathophysiologic alterations in hypertrophic cardiomyopathies. All these factors are suitable to affect ventricular performance especially during exercise.

In a study on 50 patients with hypertrophic obstructive cardiomyopathy (NYHA classes I to IV) and 19 patients with hypertrophic nonobstructive cardiomyopathy (NYHA classes I to III) we found no fundamental differences between both forms of the disease as far as the behaviour of hemodynamic parameters (heart rate, stroke volume, cardiac output, pulmonary artery pressure) and cardiac volume parameters is concerned.[29] The common pattern, observed in both forms of hypertrophic cardiomyopathy, included: (1) With increasing degree of clinical symptoms, the mean values of stroke volume and cardiac output became lower, and the mean values of pulmonary artery pressure became higher on the different exercise levels (Fig. 3). (2) Stroke volume failed to increase on exercise in a substantial proportion of patients (48% of patients with obstruction, 26% of patients without obstruction). This is in contrast to the normal behaviour of stroke volume which increases on supine exercise by 10 to 30% in so far as resting stroke volume index is not in excess of 50 to 60 ml/m^2.[30–35] (3) The reduction

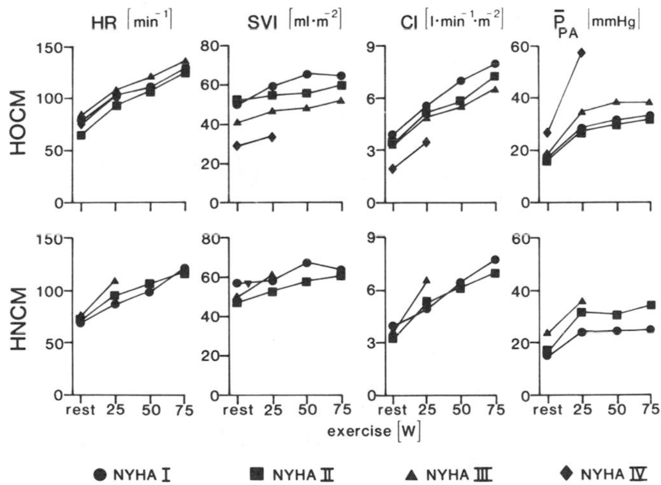

Fig. 3. Mean changes in heart rate (HR), stroke volume index (SVI), cardiac index (CI), and mean pulmonary artery pressure ($\bar{P}_{PA}$) during exercise in 50 patients with hypertrophic obstructive cardiomyopathy (HOCM) and 19 patients with hypertrophic nonobstructive cardiomyopathy classified according to New York Heart Association criteria for clinical severity.

of stroke volumes with increasing degree of functional impairment and the failure to increase stroke volume was in part compensated for by an increase in heart rate. Thus, even patients of NYHA class III were on average capable of increasing cardiac output during exercise within the lower normal range. (4) Pulmonary artery pressure rose into the pathological range in a very large proportion of patients. The greatest part of pulmonary pressure increase occured already at the lowest exercise level, with only minor changes at increasing workload. The proportions of pathologically increased pulmonary artery pressure in the different NYHA classes were similar to those reported in Table 2 for a larger group of patients. (5) Minimal cardiac transit times of a radioactive tracer, as an indicator inversely related to the ejection fraction of a volume compartment of interest,[36–39] demonstrated an identical pattern both in patients with the obstructive and the nonobstructive form of hypertrophic cardiomyopathy (Fig. 4): normal left and right ventricular minimal transit times at rest and during exercise, but prolonged left and right atrial minimal transit times at rest with further prolongation during exercise.

Minimal cardiac transit times of an intravenously injected radioactive tracer (we used ^{113m}Indium-EDTA and measured externally with a multicrystal gammacamera) are defined as differences between the appearance times of the indicator in consecutive segments of the cardiopulmonary circulation.[36–39] They are directly proportional to the ratio of the volume of interest (e.g. right atrium, right ventricle, lungs, left atrium, left ventricle, or total heart) to cardiac output. Since cardiac output equals the product of heart rate and stroke volume, cardiac minimal transit times are, after correction for heart rate, inversely proportional to the ejection fraction of the volume compartment of interest; this means that, for a given atrial or ventricular enddiastolic volume, an increase in ejection fraction is reflected by a shortening of the corresponding minimal transit time, and vice versa. A formula[37] allows the calculation of ejection fractions directly from the corresponding (atrial, ventricular, or pulmonary) minimal transit times

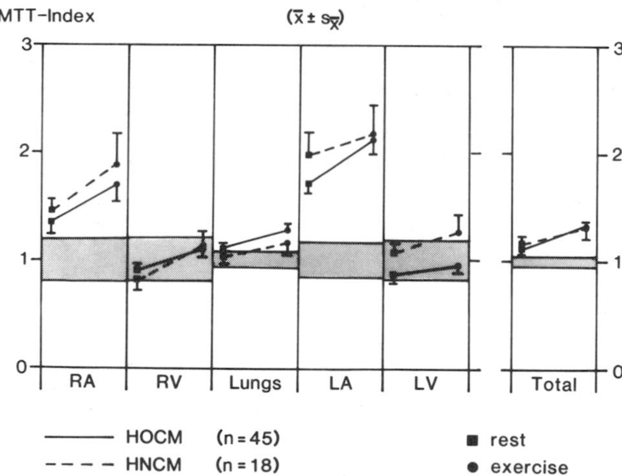

Fig. 4. Minimal transit times (MTT) of a radioactive bolus tracer through the entire heart including the lungs (=Total) as well as through the individual cardiac compartments and the lungs in patients with hypertrophic obstructive (HOCM) and nonobstructive (HNCM) cardiomyopathy. The MTT-index designates the percentage deviation of the mean value for healthy control subjects which is regarded as unity. Measurements at rest and during exercise of 25 to 50 W. RA: right atrium, RV: right ventricle, LA: left atrium, LV: left ventricle.

and has been experimentally validated by comparison with simultaneous biplane cine-angiographic determinations of left ventricular ejection fractions ranging from 17 to 80%; evaluation by independent investigators yielded a correlation coefficient of 0.92.[40)]

According to the just mentioned theoretical considerations, normal left ventricular and markedly prolonged left atrial minimal transit times are indicative of normal left ventricular and reduced left atrial ejection fractions. Since stroke volumes, except in patients of NYHA class IV, were usually normal (Fig. 3), these findings can on lybe explained by increased left atrial volumes. Together with the increase in pulmonary artery pressure, the left atrial enlargement may be explained either by mitral regurgitation or by impaired blood inflow into the left ventricle. Since moderate or severe mitral regurgitation was present, however, only in 7 of 45 patients with outflow tract obstruction and in one of 19 patients without outflow obstruction, impaired inflow into the left ventricle appears of predominant importance.

Our data of slightly prolonged right atrial minimal transit times in connection with normal right ventricular minimal transit times suggest that the pathophysiological concept of impaired ventricular inflow may be also applied, to a lesser degree, to the right ventricle. The marked increase in both left and right atrial minimal transit times during exercise suggests that inflow obstruction to both ventricles is aggravated during exercise. Furthermore, our data of a slight prolongation of right and left ventricular minimal transit times on exertion towards the upper border of the normal range indicate a decrease in right and left ventricular ejection fractions during exercise. Other investigators,[41)] using radionuclide ventriculography, described in patients with hypertrophic obstructive cardiomyopathy a corresponding pattern for the left ventricle, with a slight decrease in the supernormal resting ejection fraction during exercise. Since stroke volume remained constant or rose in the majority of our patients (Fig. 3), the transit time data suggest that both ventricles are, in spite of the impaired distensibility caused by hypertrophy and fibrosis, capable of a certain enlargement of their enddiastolic volumes during exercise.

In conclusion, our findings correlate well with the generally accepted understanding of impaired left ventricular relaxation and filling as a major determinant of pathophysiologic alterations in hypertrophic cardiomyopathies[5,12,14,20–28)] and expand it in so far as the right ventricle appears to be involved in a similar manner. Increased left ventricular filling pressures (as derived from pulmonary artery pressures) and impaired right and left atrial emptying into the ventricles, which showed no quantitative differences between patients with and without obstruction of the left ventricular outflow tract in our study, can be explained sufficiently by an impaired ventricular diastolic function alone. The similarity of exercise hemodynamics both in patients with and without outflow tract gradient further supports the concept of impaired diastolic function as the predominant pathophysiologic alteration in hypertrophic cardiomyopathies. An additional influence of ventricular outflow obstruction, the importance of which as a further pathophysiologic determinant of hypertrophic obstructive cardiomyopathy is debated,[5,12,14–19)] on exercise hemodynamics is, however, not completely ruled out by our data.

IV. Evaluation of Therapy

The primary effort of therapy is directed at ameliorating the patients' disabling symptoms, increasing the reduced exercise capacity, and prolonging life. Since functional limitation is primarily caused by hemodynamic impairment and rhythm disturbances, hemodynamic measurements, especially when performed during exercise, are valuable for quantifying and comparing the efficacy of different forms of therapy.

Experience with surgical therapy dates back to the late 1950s. Medical therapy with beta-adrenergic blocking drugs has been employed since the mid 1960s, with calcium-antagonistic drugs since the mid 1970s, whereas the potential use of disopyramide has only recently been reported.[12,42]

There are numerous reports on the long-term effects of betablocking and calcium-antagonistic drugs and of surgery on clinical symptoms and resting hemodynamics.[8,12,29,43–68] However, only few published data are available concerning the long-term hemodynamic effects during exercise;[29,41,46,51,59–61,63,66] moreover, these studies are usually limited to follow-up periods of only several weeks or months.

In recent studies we have published our experience with short- and long-term medical therapy and with surgical therapy with regard to clinical symptoms, exercise capacity, exercise hemodynamics and the incidence of ventricular arrhythmias during exercise.[13,39,69]

Follow-up below one year

In this study[69] we compared the clinical and hemodynamic effects of three therapeutic regimens in patients with hypertrophic obstructive cardiomyopathy confirmed by heart catheterization, all of whom had basal and/or provocable pressure gradients of 30 mm Hg or more within the left ventricle, either typically in the subvalvular region, or atypically in the midventricular region: propranolol (198 ± 20 mg for 3.0 ± 0.6 months, 13 patients), verapamil (432 ± 11 mg for 5.5 ± 0.3 months, 68 patients), and surgical therapy (9.1 ± 1.3 months after transaortic subvalvular septal myectomy with additional myotomy,[70,71] 31 patients). Inclusion into the study was not through a special selection. Surgery was advised when medical treatment failed to improve symptoms. In view of their clinical symptoms and initial heart catheterization data (Table 3), patients admitted to surgery were on an average in a more advanced stage of the disease than the medically treated patients. Four patients of the propranolol group and nine patients of the verapamil group later had to be admitted to surgery and are included in the myectomy group.

Figure 5 illustrates the hemodynamic changes which were observed in each individual patient at the highest common exercise level in the pre- and post-treatment exercise test. The differences in the initial control values reflect the different mean workloads caused by the different degree of severity of disease in the three patient groups. Although individual responses to therapy were quite heterogeneous (especially in the medically treated patients), propranolol induced on average a much more pronounced fall in heart

TABLE 3. Hemodynamic Characteristics at Heart Catheterization and Maximal Exercise Capacity of Patients with Hypertrophic Obstructive Cardiomyopathy before Therapeutic Intervention

	Propranolol	Verapamil	Myectomy
No. of patients	13	68	31
Sex (male: female)	7:6	46:22	25:6
Age (years)	41.1 ± 2.4	43.1 ± 1.6	43.9 ± 2.2
EDP_{LV} (mm Hg)	16.3 ± 2.0	14.3 ± 0.8	19.1 ± 1.2
P_{LV}, basal (mm Hg)	40.8 ± 11.6	28.7 ± 4.5	60.3 ± 6.8
P_{LV}, provoked (mm Hg)	129.2 ± 12.9	115.1 ± 7.0	139.1 ± 7.6
P_{RV}, basal (mm Hg)	17.5 ± 5.2	18.7 ± 3.4	20.6 ± 4.2
	(n = 4)	(n = 22)	(n = 13)
Exercise capacity (W)	75.0 ± 7.4	83.5 ± 3.5	66.9 ± 3.7

Abbreviations: EDP_{LV} = left ventricular end diastolic pressure: P_{LV} = left ventricular outflow tract gradient; P_{RV} = right ventricular outflow tract gradient.

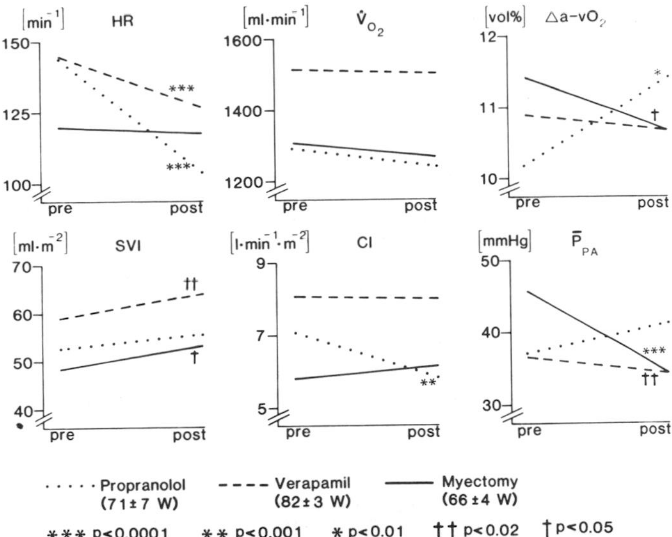

Fig. 5. Comparison of hemodynamic changes (mean $\pm$ standard error of the mean) induced by propranolol (3.0 $\pm$ 0.6 months, 13 patients), verapamil (5.5 $\pm$ 0.3 months, 68 patients) and surgical therapy (9.1 $\pm$ 1.3 months after operation, 31 patients) in patients with hypertrophic obstructive cardiomyopathy. Comparisons were made individually for each patient at the highest common exercise level reached before and after therapeutic intervention. Mean maximal work loads were different in the three patient groups and are indicated at the bottom. Upper row (from the left): heart rate, total body oxygen consumption, arterio-venous oxygen difference. Lower row: stroke volume index, cardiac index, mean pulmonary artery pressure. For statistical comparison Student's two-tailed *t*-test for paired data was used.

rate than verapamil, whereas surgery did not affect heart rate. The fall in heart rate was compensated for by a significant increase in stroke volume in the verapamil group, but not by the slight increase in stroke volume in the propranolol group. As a consequence, cardiac output fell significantly with a concomitant increase in arterio-venous oxygen difference in propranolol-treated patients, whereas both parameters remained fairly constant during verapamil treatment. Surgery caused also a significant increase in stroke volume resulting in a slight (just below level of significance) increase in cardiac output accompanied by a significant fall in arteriovenous oxygen difference. Of utmost importance for the patients' symptoms, verapamil and, much more pronounced, surgical therapy induced a significant fall in the originally pathologically elevated mean pulmonary artery pressures, whereas a tendency towards a further increase was observed after propranolol. The hemodynamic responses to verapamil treatment were independent of the site (subvalvular or midventricular) of intraventricular obstruction.

These different hemodynamic responses to therapy were reflected by different responses of clinical symptoms and exercise capacity. Figure 6 and Table 4 illustrate that verapamil induced more often symptomatic improvement than propranolol, but was not as effective as surgical therapy. Two patients deteriorated on treatment with propranolol, one patient on treatment with verapamil. After surgery all except two unchanged patients improved. Of even greater importance is the fact that, in contrast to the medically treated patients, a considerable number of patients (about one third) im-

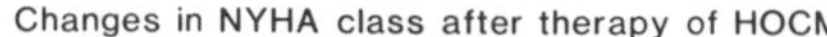

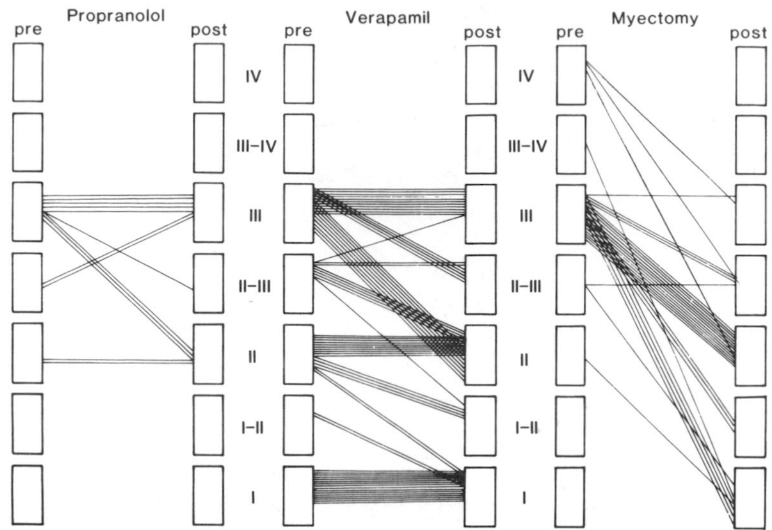

Fig. 6. Changes in functional class (NYHA classification) after propranolol, verapamil and surgical therapy. Same patients as in Fig. 5. (Reprinted with permission[69]).

TABLE 4. Changes in Clinical Symptoms after Different Forms of Therapy for Hypertrophic Obstructive Cardiomyopathy. Figures in parentheses represent patient proportions of the verapamil-treated group considering only initially symptomatic patients (i.e. NYHA class I patients excluded)

	Dose (mg)	Follow-up (months)	No. of pts.	Improved	Symptoms unchanged	Worsened
Propranolol	198 ± 20	3.0 ± 0.6	13	31%	54%	15%
Verapamil	432 ± 11	5.5 ± 0.3	68	41%	58%	1%
			(52)	(54%)	(44%)	(2%)
Myectomy		9.1 ± 1.3	31	94%	6%	0%

proved by more than one NYHA class after surgery. This improvement correlated well with a significant increase in exercise capacity, which was much more pronounced after surgery than after verapamil treatment, whereas propranolol on average induced no change in exercise capacity (Fig. 7).

Follow-up of more than 3 years

Another study served to answer the clinically important question of how long the early therapeutic benefits persist.[69] Included were patients of the foregoing short-term study who agreed to undergo repeat exercise tests several years after begin of verapamil treatment or after surgical therapy. Thus, the short- and long-term effects of both forms of therapy could be compared. In the case of verapamil, the exercise tests to be compared were performed in 29 patients a mean of 5.4 ± 0.5 months and a mean of 46.5 ± 3.3 months after begin of therapy. The drug dosage of 450.4 ± 11.3 mg at the first year study was not significantly changed until the late study. In the case of surgical treatment, the exercise tests to be compared were performed in 10 patients a mean of 12.2 ± 3.1 months and a mean of 52.4 ± 6.3 months after surgery. Postoperative medication, in-

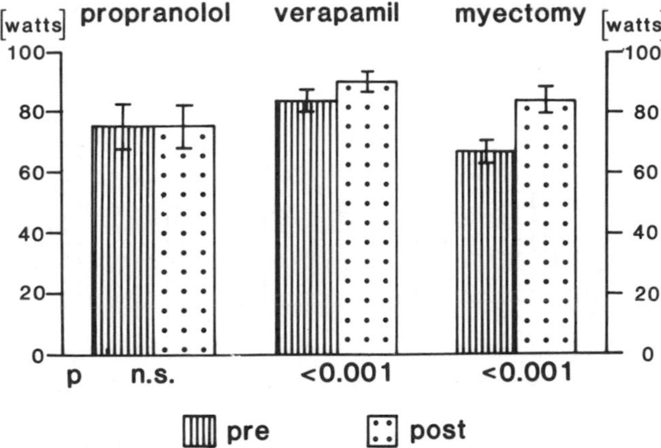

Fig. 7. Changes in exercise tolerance (mean ± standard error of the mean) after therapy with propranolol, verapamil or myectomy. Same patients as in Fig. 5. For statistical comparison Student's two-tailed t-test for paired data was used. (Reprinted with permission[69]).

troduced in some patients in the early postoperative period to control tachyarrhythmias, was changed during the follow-up period in three patients.

Figure 8 illustrates the changes in functional limitation. The improvement observed during the first year of verapamil treatment in 16 of the 29 patients continued only in 9 cases, whereas a re-deterioration to the pre-treatment level was observed in the other 7 patients. Furthermore, there were two initially unchanged patients who became even more symptomatic until the late exercise test. In the surgically treated patients, in contrast, re-deteriorations in functional limitation were counterbalanced by further improvements and never reached the preoperative level.

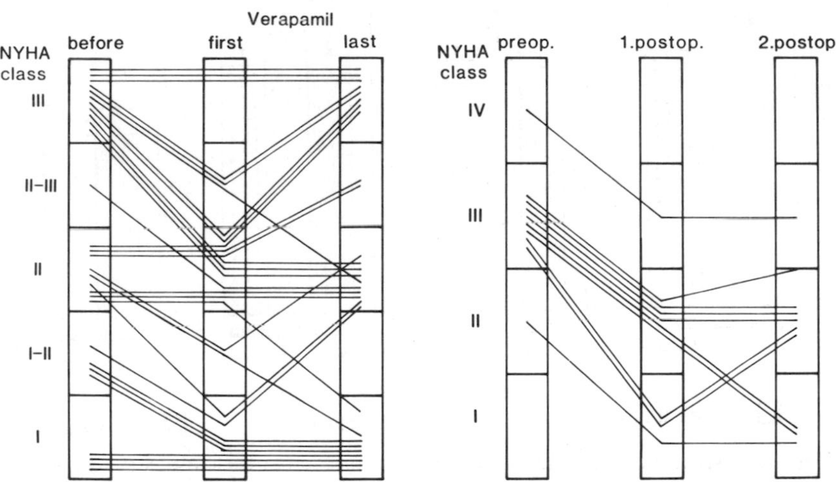

Fig. 8. Serial changes in functional limitation (NYHA classification) in 29 patients with hypertrophic obstructive cardiomyopathy during therapy with verapamil (5.4 ± 0.5 months and 46.5 ± 3.3 months after beginning of therapy) and in 10 patients after surgical therapy (12.2 ± 3.1 months and 52.4 ± 6.3 months after operation).

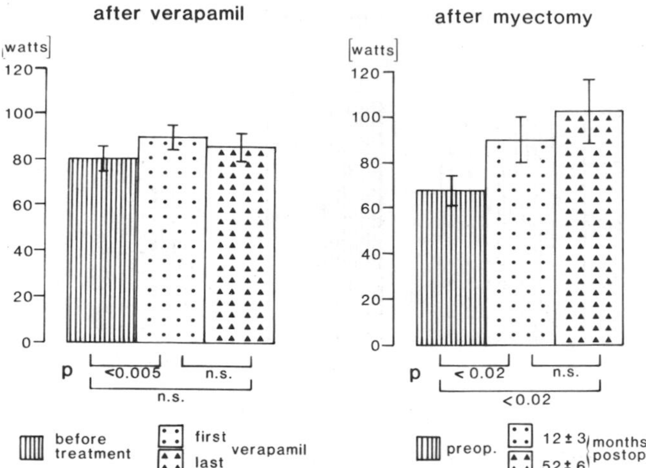

Fig. 9. Serial changes in exercise tolerance (mean ± standard error of the mean) after treatment of hypertrophic obstructive cardiomyopathy with verapamil or surgery. Same patients as in Fig. 8. For statistical comparison Student's two-tailed *t*-test for paired data was used.

The changes in exercise capacity (Fig. 9) corresponded to the changes in functional limitation. The small increase in exercise tolerance observed during the first year of verapamil treatment was not maintained during later follow-up. Again in strong contrast, surgically treated patients experienced a substantial increase in exercise capacity during the first postoperative year and a further increase up to the late study. As a con-

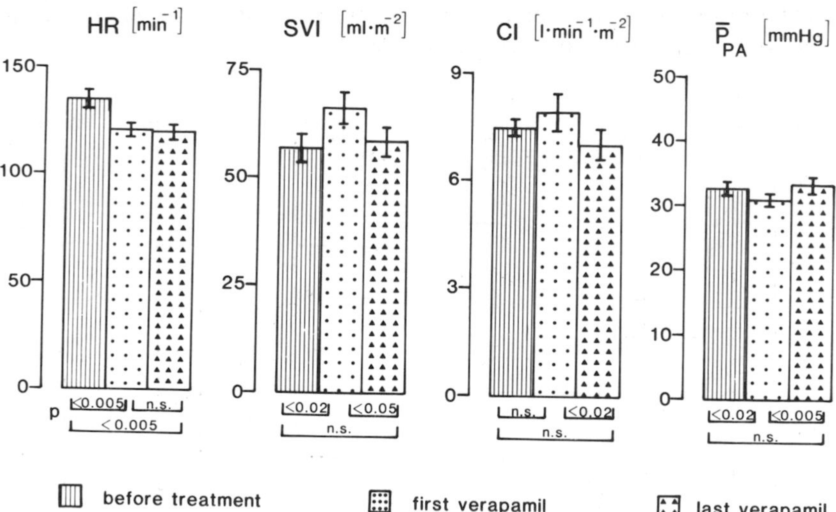

Fig. 10. Serial hemodynamic changes (from the left: heart rate, stroke volume index, cardiac index, mean pulmonary artery pressure) during therapy with verapamil in 29 patients with hypertrophic obstructive cardiomyopathy (same patients as in Fig. 8). Measurements were made in each individual at the highest common exercise level reached in all three exercise tests (average for all studies: 75 ± 6 W). Mean values ± standard error of the mean. For statistical comparison Student's two-tailed *t*-test for paired data was used.

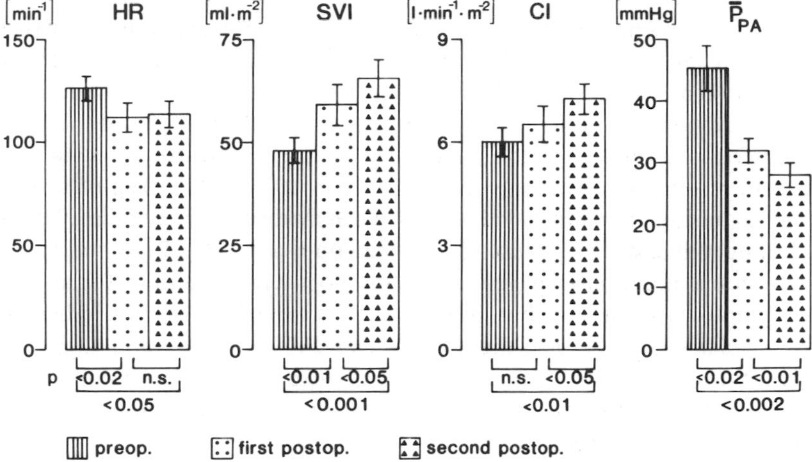

Fig. 11. Serial hemodynamic changes (same parameters as in Fig. 10, mean $\pm$ standard error of the mean) after surgical therapy (12.2 $\pm$ 3.1 months and 52.4 $\pm$ 6.3 months after operation) in 10 patients with hypertrophic obstructive cardiomyopathy (same patients as in Fig. 8). Measurements were made in each individual at the highest common exercise level reached in all three exercise tests (average for all studies: 68 $\pm$ 7 W). For statistical comparison Student's two-tailed t-test for paired data was used. (Reprinted with permission[69]).

sequence, operated patients ultimately reached higher exercise levels than the verapamil-treated patients, although they had been more restricted before therapy.

As explanation for these findings, a different behavior of hemodynamic parameters was observed. Although individual hemodynamic changes were quite heterogeneous, on average the initial beneficial effects observed during the first year of verapamil treatment—i.e. significant fall in heart rate and pulmonary artery pressure, increase in stroke volume and cardiac output during exercise—were diminished or even abolished at the late study, except the persisting fall in heart rate (Fig. 10). In contrast to these disappointing results, the beneficial hemodynamic changes observed during the first year after surgery—i.e. significant fall in heart rate and pulmonary artery pressure, increase in stroke volume and cardiac output during exercise—not only persisted but were even more pronounced in the late postoperative study (Fig. 11).

Clinical and pathophysiological considerations

As a consequence of these studies, the symptomatic and hemodynamic response to verapamil appears on average to be superior to propranolol. The most impressive improvements, however, are achieved with surgery. As far as long-term results are concerned, surgically treated patients experience more frequent, more substantial and, of utmost importance, more long-lasting benefits from therapy than medically treated patients. In addition, surgery appears of prognostic benefit, too.[72–74]

Exercise tests of the described manner facilitate the quantification and comparison of therapeutic efficacy of different approaches. They do, however, not clarify the mechanism by which the different therapeutic procedures influence the basic underlying disease process. Probably several different pathophysiologic alterations (systolic obstruction, diastolic dysfunction, ischemia, arrhythmias) play a quantitatively different role in the individual patient.[6,12] This may explain the individually different response to therapy and makes it difficult to compare exactly the efficacy of different therapy. To our knowledge, only one randomized study is available comparing different therapeutic procedures.[55] These authors found verapamil to be superior to propranolol with regard to clinical and echocardiographic findings and side effects, but they were not able to anticipate the response to either form of therapy. As in other published therapy studies, we did not perform a randomization but defined therapy empirically. Due to disappointing long-term results, we abandoned propranolol in 1978 as the drug of first choice in favor of verapamil and recommended surgery when medical therapy failed. Nevertheless, patients feeling well under propranolol, remained on that treatment. A strict randomization should in our mind only be considered for short-term studies or for asymptomatic or mildly symptomatic patients but, in view of the marked differences in hemodynamic response to medical and surgical therapy presented in this study and also reported by other institutions,[12,44,57,62,64] should not cause exclusion of symptomatic patients, unresponsive to a trial of medical therapy, from the more substantial benefits of surgery, merely from experimental reasons.

Neither the mode of action of the employed pharmacological agents propranolol and verapamil nor that of surgery is as yet fully understood. The administration of propranolol is based on its negative inotropic effects and on the demonstration of reduced left ventricular outflow tract gradients at rest and during mild exercise,[47,66,75] whereas there are controversial opinions as to whether left ventricular diastolic dysfunction is also favorably affected.[26,76,77] Verapamil has also been shown to reduce left ventricular outflow tract gradients,[52,53,78] and its beneficial effects on left ventricular diastolic dysfunction are well established.[24–26,76,79–81] Surgical therapy in the form of septal myectomy is usually thought to exert its beneficial effects by reducing or abolishing the dynamic obstruction to left ventricular outflow and by relieving mitral regurgitation.[6,12,28,45,62–64,67] Whether and to what extent an improvement in diastolic ventricular function contributes to symptomatic benefits, is still debated.[6,12,63,64]

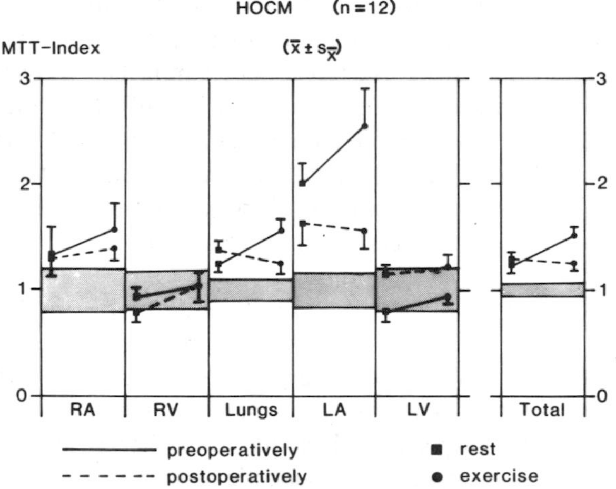

Fig. 12. Minimal transit times (MTT) of a radioactive bolus tracer through the entire heart and the lungs (= Total) as well as through the individual cardiac compartments in 12 patients with hypertrophic obstructive cardiomyopathy. The MTT-index designates the percentage deviation from the mean value for healthy control subjects which is regarded as unity. Measurements at rest and during exercise of 25 to 50 W. RA: right atrium, RV: right ventricle, LA: left atrium, LV: left ventricle.

In a recent study continuing our measurements of cardiac minimal transit times (see chapter 3) we found after surgical therapy significant changes in the cardiac volume ratios, with a prolongation of left ventricular minimal transit times and a reduction in left atrial and pulmonary and, to a lesser degree, right atrial minimal transit times (Fig. 12). The prolongation of left ventricular minimal transit times indicates a decrease in the preoperatively supernormal left ventricular ejection fractions towards the lower normal range, which is in agreement with recent radionuclide studies.[41] Together with the postoperative increase in stroke volume (Fig. 11), these findings suggest an increase in left ventricular enddiastolic volume. Since usually an impressive reduction in left ventricular enddiastolic pressures[62,82,83] and mean pulmonary artery pressures (Figs. 5, 11) is observed, an improvement in left atrial ejection can be assumed, which explains the substantial shortening of left atrial and pulmonary minimal transit times. Thus, exercise tests add information to the pathophysiological understanding of the mode of action of therapy.

REFERENCES

1. Krelhaus, W., Kuhn, H., and Loogen, F. Analysis of deaths in the course of hypertrophic obstructive cardiomyopathy. In: Cardiomyopathy and Myocardial Biopsy, Kaltenbach, M., Loogen, F. and Olsen, E.G.J. (eds.), Springer-Verlag, Berlin-Heidelberg-New York, 1978, pp. 300–307.
2. Maron, B.J., Roberts, W.C., Edwards, J.E., McAllister, H.A., Foley, D.D., and Epstein, S.E. Sudden death in patients with hypertrophic cardiomyopathy: Characterization of 26 patients without functional limitation. *Am. J. Cardiol.* **41**: 803–810, 1978.
3. Maron, B.J., Roberts, W.C., and Epstein, S.E. Sudden death in hypertrophic cardiomyopathy: A profile of 78 patients. *Circulation* **65**: 1388–1394, 1982.
4. Frank, S. and Braunwald, E. Idiopathic hypertrophic subaortic stenosis: Clinical analysis of 126 patients with emphasis on natural history. *Circulation* **37**: 759–788, 1968.
5. Goodwin, J.F. The frontiers of cardiomyopathy. *Br. Heart J.* **48**: 1–18, 1982.
6. Maron, B.J., Bonow, R.O., Cannon, R.O., Leon, M.B., and Epstein, S.E. Hypertrophic cardiomyopathy. Interrelations of clinical manifestations, pathophysiology, and therapy (second of two parts). *New Engl. J. Med.* **316** : 844–852, 1987.
7. Koga, Y., Itaya, K., and Toshima, H., Prognosis in hypertrophic cardiomyopathy. *Am. Heart J.* **108**: 351–359, 1984.
8. Shah, P.M., Adelman, A.G., Wigle, E.D., Gobel, F.L., Burchell, H.B., Hardarson, T., Curiel, R., De la Calzada, C., Oakley, C.M., and Goodwin, J.F. The natural (and unnatural) history of hypertrophic obstructive cardiomyopathy. *Circ. Res.* 34/35, Suppl. II: 179–195, 1974.
9. McKenna, W.J., Deanfield, J., Faruqui, A., England, D., Oakley, C., and Goodwin, J.F. Prognosis in hypertrophic cardiomyopathy: Role of age and clinical, electrocardiographic and hemodynamic features. *Am. J. Cardiol.* **47**: 532–538, 1981.
10. Maron, B.J., Savage, D.D., Wolfson, J.K., and Epstein, S.E. Prognostic significance of 24 hour ambulatory electrocardiographic monitoring in patients with hypertrophic cardiomyopathy: A prospective study. *Am. J. Cardiol.* **48**: 252–257, 1981.
11. Loogen, F., Krelhaus, W., and Kuhn, H. Natural history of hypertrophic obstructive cardiomyopathy. In: Cardiomyopathy and Myocardial Biopsy, Kaltenbach, M., Loogen F. and Olsen, E.G.J. (eds.), Springer-Verlag, Berlin—Heidelberg—New York 1978, pp. 286–299.
12. Wigle, E.D., Sasson, Z., Handerson, M.A., Ruddy, T.D., Fulop, J., Rakowski, H., and Williams, W.G., Hypertrophic cardiomyopathy. The importance of the site and the extent of hypertrophy. *A review. Progr. Cardiovasc. Dis.* **28**: 1–83, 1985.
13. Lösse, B., Christoph, I., Borggrefe, M., and Königer, H.-H. Das Risiko belastungsindu-

zierter ventrikulärer Arrhythmien bei hypertrophischen kardiomyopathien. *Z. Kardiol.* **73**: 304–312, 1984.
14. Murgo J.P., Alter, B.R., Dorethy, J.F., Altobelli, S.A., and McGranahan Jr., G.M. Dynamics of left ventricular ejection in obstructive and nonobstructive hypertrophic cardiomyopathy. *J. Clin. Invest.* **66**: 1369–1382, 1980.
15. Maron, B.J., Gottdiener, J.S., and Epstein, S.E. Patterns and significance of left ventricular hypertrophy in hypertrophic cardiomyopathy: A wide angle, two dimensional echocardiographic study of 125 patients. *Am. J. Cardiol.* **48**: 418–428, 1981.
16. Jenni, R., Ruffmann, K., Vieli, A., Anliker, M., and Krayenbuehl, H.P. Dynamics of aortic flow in hypertrophic cardiomyopathy. *Eur. Heart J.* **6**: 391–398, 1985.
17. Criley, M.J. and Siegel, R.J. Has 'obstruction' hindered our understanding of hypertrophic cardiomyopathy? *Circulation* **72**: 1148–1154, 1985.
18. Maron, B.J. and Epstein, S.E. Clinical significance and therapeutic implications of the left ventricular outflow tract pressure gradient in hypertrophic cardiomyopathy. *Am. J. Cardiol.* **58**: 1093–1096, 1986.
19. Wigle, E.D. and Rakowski, H. Evidence for true obstruction to left ventricular outflow in obstructive hypertrophic cardiomyopathy (muscular or hypertrophic subaortic stenosis). *Z. Kardiol.* **76**, Suppl. 3: 61–68, 1987.
20. Spiller, P., Brenner, C., Neuhaus, K.L., and Sauer, G. Disorders of left ventricular performance in congestive and hypertrophic obstructive cardiomyopathy. In: Cardiomyopathy and Myocardial Biopsy, Kaltenbach, M., Loogen, F. and Olsen, E.G.J. (eds.), Springer-Verlag, Berlin—Heidelberg—New York 1980, pp. 186–195.
21. St. John Sutton, M.G., Tajik, A.J., Gibson, D.G., Brown, D.J., Seward, J.B., and Giuliani, E.R. Echocardiographic assessment of left ventricular filling and septal and posterior wall dynamics in idiopathic hypertrophic subaortic stenosis. *Circulation* **57**: 512–520, 1978.
22. Sanderson, J.E., Traill, T.A., St. John Sutton, M.G., Brown, D.J., Gibson, D.G., and Goodwin, J.F. Left ventricular relaxation and filling in hypertrophic cardiomyopathy: an echocardiographic study. *Br. Heart J.* **40**: 596–601, 1978.
23. Hanrath, P., Mathey, D.G., Siegert, R., and Bleifeld, W. Left ventricular relaxation and filling in different forms of left ventricular hypertrophy: an echocardiographic study. *Am. J. Cardiol.* **45**: 15–23, 1980.
24. Betocchi, S., Bonow, R.O., Bacharach, S.L., Rosing, D.R., Maron, B.J., and Green, M.V. Isovolumic relaxation period in hypertrophic cardiomyopathy: Assessment by radionuclide angiography. *J. Am. Coll. Cardiol.* **7**: 74–81, 1986.
25. Bonow, R.O., Frederick, T.M., Bacharach, S.L., Green, M.V., Goose, P.W., Maron, B.J., and Rosing, D.R. Atrial systole and left ventricular filling in patients with hypertrophic cardiomyopathy: Effect of verapamil. *Am. J. Cardiol.* **51**: 1386–1391, 1987.
26. Bonow, R.O., Rosing, D.R., Bacharach, S.L., Green, M.V., Kent, K.M., Lipson, L.C., Maron, B.J., Leon, M.B., and Epstein, S.E. Effects of verapamil on left ventricular systolic function and diastolic filling in patients with hypertrophic cardiomyopathy. *Circulation* **64**: 787–796, 1981.
27. Spirito, P., Maron, B.J., Chiarella, F., Bellotti, P., Tramarin, R., Pozzoli, M., and Vecchio, C. Diastolic abnormalities in patients with hypertrophic cardiomyopathy: relation to magnitude of left ventricular hypertrophy. *Circulation* **72**: 310–316, 1985.
28. Maron, B.J., Bonow, R.O., Cannon, R.O., Leon, M.B., and Epstein, S.E. Hypertrophic cardiomyopathy. Interrelations of clinical manifestations, pathophysiology, and therapy (first of two parts). *New Engl. J. Med.* **316**: 780–789, 1987.
29. Lösse, B., Kuhn, H., Loogen, F., and Schulte, H.D. Exercise performance in hypertrophic cardiomyopathies. *Eur. Heart J.* **4**, Suppl. 4: 197–208, 1983.
30. Bevegard, S., Holmgren, A., and Jonsson, B. The effect of body position on the circulation at rest and during exercise, with special reference to the influence on the stroke volume. *Acta Physiol. Scand.* **49**: 279–298, 1960.
31. Holmgren, A., Jonsson, B., and Sjöstrand, T. Circulatory data in normal subjects at rest

and during exercise in recumbent position, with special reference to the stroke volume at different work intensities. *Acta Physiol. Scand.* **49**: 343–363, 1960.

32. Hartley, L.H., Alexander, J.K., Modelski, M., and Grover, R.F. Subnormal cardiac output at rest and during exercise in residents at 3100 m altitude. *J. Appl. Physiol.* **23**: 839–848, 1967.
33. Blümchen, G., Hoffmann, G., and Battke, K. Simultaner Vergleich von radiokardiographischer Funktionsanalyse und Farbstoff-Verdünnungsmethode/Cardiogreen). Verhalten des Schlagvolumens in Ruhe und während Arbeit bei Normalpersonen. *Z. Kardiol.* **62**: 638–653, 1973.
34. Thadani, U. and Parker J.O. Hemodynamics at rest and during supine and sitting bicycle exercise in normal subjects. *Am. J. Cardiol.* **41**: 52–59, 1978.
35. Poliner, L.R., Dehmer, G.J., Lewis, S.E., Parkey, R.W., Blomqvist, C.G., and Willerson J.T. Left ventricular performance in normal subjects: a comparison of the responses to exercise in the upright and supine positions. *Circulation* **62**: 528–534, 1980.
36. Schicha, H., Vyska, K., Becker, V., Seipel, L., and Feinenedegen, L.E. Minimale kardiale Transitzeiten bei gesunden und herzkranken Personen: Untersuchungen mit Indium-113m und der Gamma-Retina. *Atomkernenergie* **15**: 150–156, 1970.
37. Vyska, K., Profant, M., Schicha, H., Becker, V., Freundlieb, C., and Feinendegen, L.E. Theoretische Grundlagen der Anwendung der minimalen kardialen Transitzeiten für die Bestimmung der Ejektionsfraktion in der Herzkammer. In: Nuklearmedizin—Fortschritte der Nuklearmedizin in klinischer und technologischer Sicht, Pabst, H.W., Hör, G., Schmidt, H.A.E. (ed.), Schattauer-Verlag, Stuttgart—New York, 1975, pp. 68–72.
38. Feinendegen, L.E., Becker, V., Vyska, K., Schicha, H., Freundlieb, C., Bosiljanoff, P., Lösse, B., and Gleichmann, U. Bestimmung globaler und regionaler Herzfunktion mit den minimalen Transitzeiten. *Verh. Dtsch. Ges. Herz- und Kreislaufforsch.* **46**: 118–129, 1980.
39. Lösse, B. and Feinendegen, L.E. Effects of therapeutic interventions on minimal cardiac transit times and volume parameters in hypertrophic cardiomyopathy. *Z. Kardiol.* **76**, Suppl. 3: 46–52, 1987.
40. Sigwart, U., Schicha, H., Schmidt, H., Becker, V., Mertens, H.M., Gleichmann, U., and Feinendegen, L.E. Vergleich minimaler kardialer Transitzeiten mit invasiv erhaltenen hämodynamischen Parametern. Ergebnisse aus simultaner Isotopen-Herzfunktionsanalyse und Herzkatheteruntersuchung. *Herz/Kreisl.* **10**: 15–20, 1978.
41. Borer, J.S., Bacharach, S.L., Green, M.V., Kent, K.M., Rosing, D.R., Seides, S.F., Morrow, A.G., and Epstein, S.E. Effect of septal myotomy and myectomy on left ventricular systolic function at rest and during exercise in patients with IHSS. *Circulation* **60**, Suppl. I: 82–87, 1979.
42. Pollick, C. Muscular subaortic stenosis. Hemodynamic and clinical improvement after disopyramide. *New Engl. J. Med.* **307**: 997–999, 1982.
43. Adelman, A.G., Wigle, E.D., Ranganathan, N., Webb, G.D., Kidd, B.S.L., Bigelow, W.G., and Silver, M.D. The clinical course in muscular subaortic stenosis: A retrospective and prospective study of 60 hemodynamically proved cases. *Ann. Intern. Med.* **77**: 515–524, 1972.
44. Beahrs, M.M., Tajik, A.J., Seward, J.B., Giuliani, E.R., and McGoon, D.C. Hypertrophic obstructive cardiomyopathy: Ten- to 21-year follow-up after partial septal myectomy. *Am. J. Cardiol.* **51**: 1160–1166, 1983.
45. Bigelow, W., Trimble, A.S., Wigle, E.D., Adelman, A.G., and Felderhof, C. The treatment of muscular subaortic stenosis. *J. Thorac. Cardiovasc. Surg.* **68**: 384–391, 1974.
46. Edwards, R.H.T., Kristinsson, A., Warrell, D.A., and Goodwin, J.F. Effects of propranolol on response to exercise in hypertrophic obstructive cardiomyopathy. *Br. Heart J.* **32**: 219–225, 1970.
47. Flamm, M.D., Harrison, D.C., and Hancock, E.W. Muscular subaortic stenosis. Prevention of outflow obstruction with propranolol. *Circulation* **38**: 846–858, 1968.
48. Frank, M.J., Abdulla, A.M., Canedo, M.I., and Saylors, R.E. Long-term medical manage-

ment of hypertrophic obstructive cardiomyopathy. *Am. J. Cardiol.* **42**: 993–1001, 1978.
49. Frank, M.J., Abdulla, A.M., Watkins, L.O., Prisant, L., and Stefadouros, M.A. Long-term medical management of hypertrophic cardiomyopathy: Usefulness of propranolol. *Eur. Heart J.* **4**, Suppl F: 155–164, 1983.
50. Haberer, T., Hess, O.M., Jenni, R., and Krayenbühl, H.P. Hypertrophe obstruktive Kardiomyopathie: Spontanverlauf im Vergleich zur Langzeittherapie mit Propranolol und Verapamil. *Z. Kardiol.* **72**: 487–493, 1983.
51. Hanrath, P., Schlüter, M., Sonntag, F., Diemert, J., and Bleifeld, W. Influence of verapamil therapy on left ventricular performance at rest and during exericse in hypertrophic cardiomyopathy. *Am. J. Cardiol.* **52**: 544–548, 1983.
52. Kaltenbach, M. and Hopf, R. Treatment of hypertrophic cardiomyopathy: Relation to pathological mechanisms. *J. Mol. Cell Cardiol.* **17**: 59–68, 1985.
53. Kaltenbach, M., Hopf, R., Kober, G., Bussmann, W.D., Keller, M., and Petersen, Y. Treatment of hypertrophic obstructive cardiomyopathy with verapamil. *Br. Heart J.* **42**: 35–42, 1979.
54. Hopf, R. and Kaltenbach, M. 10-year results and survival of patients with hypertrophic cardiomyopathy treated with calcium antagonists. *Z. Kardiol.* **76**, Suppl. 3: 137–144, 1987.
55. Kober, G. Hopf, R., Biamino, G., Bubenheimer, P., Förster, K., Kuck, K.H., Hanrath, P., von Olshausen, K.-E., Schlepper, M., and Kaltenbach, M. Long-term treatment of hypertrophic cardiomyopathy with verapamil or propranolol in matched pairs of patients: Results of a multicenter study. *Z. Kardiol.* **76**, Suppl. 3: 113–118, 1987.
56. Kuhn, H., Thelen, U., Leuner, C., Köhler, E., and Bluschke, V. Langzeitbehandlung der hypertrophischen nicht obstruktiven Kardiomyopathie (HNCM) mit Verapamil. *Z. Kardiol.* **69**: 669–675, 1980.
57. von der Lohe, E., Müller-Haake, C., Minale, C., von Essen, R., Effert S., and Messmer, B.J. Septumresektion bei hypertropher obstruktiver Kardiomyopathie: Langzeitergebnisse bei 33 Patienten. *Dtsch. Med. Wschr.* **109**: 1749–1753, 1984.
58. Loogen, F., Kuhn, H., Gietzen, F., Lösse, B., Schulte, H.D., and Bircks, W. Clinical course and prognosis of patients with typical and atypical hypertrophic obstructive and with hypertrophic non-obstructive cardiomyopathy. *Eur. Heart J.* **4**, Suppl F: 145–153, 1983.
59. Lösse, B., Kuhn, H., Krönert H. Rafflenbeul, D., Kirschner, P., Schulte, H.D., and Loogen, F. Hämodynamische Auswirkungen konservativer und operativer Therapie bei hypertrophischer obstruktiver Kardiomyopathie. *Z. Kardiol.* **69**: 470–477, 1980.
60. Lösse, B., Kuhn, H., and Loogen, F. Klinische und hämodynamische Effekte von Verapamil bei hypertrophischer obstruktiver Kardiomyopathie. *Z. Kardiol.* **71**: 813–189, 1982.
61. Lösse, B., Loogen, F., and Schulte, H.D. Frühe und späte hämodynamische Veränderungen nach operativer Therapie der hypertrophischen obstruktiven Kardiomyopathie. *Z. Kardiol.* **73**: 654–662, 1984.
62. Maron, B.J., Merrill, W.H., Freier, P.A., Kent, K.M., Epstein, S.E., and Morrow, A.G. Long-term clinical course and symptomatic status of patients after operation for hypertrophic subaortic stenosis. *Circulation* **57**: 1205–1213, 1978.
63. Redwood, D.R., Goldstein, R.E., Hirshfeld, J., Borer, J.S., Morganroth, J., Morrow, A.G., and Epstein, S.E. Exercise performance after septal myotomy and myectomy in patients with obstructive hypertrophic cardiomyopathy. *Am. J. Cardiol.* **44**: 215–220, 1979.
64. Rothlin, M.E., Gobet, D., Haberer, T., and Krayenbuehl, H.P. Surgical treatment versus medical treatment in hypertrophic obstructive cardiomyopathy. *Eur. Heart J.* **4**, Suppl. F: 215–223, 1983.
65. Spicer, R.L., Rocchini, A.P., Crowley, D.C., and Rosenthal, A. Chronic verapamil therapy in pediatric and young adult patients with hypertrophic cardimyopathy. *Am. J. Cardiol.* **53**: 1614–1619, 1984.
66. Stenson, R.E., Flamm, M.D. Jr., Harrison, D.C., and Hancock, E.W. Hypertrophic subaortic stenosis: Clinical and hemodynamic effects of long-term propranolol therapy. *Am. J. Cardiol.* **31**: 763–773, 1973.

67. Tajik, A.J., Giuliani, G.R., Weidman, W.H., Brandenburg, R.D., and McGoon, D.C. Idiopathic hypertrophic subaortic stenosis. Long-term surgical follow-up *Am. J. Cardiol.* **34**: 815–822, 1974.
68. Turina, J., Jenni, R., Krayenbuehl, H.P., Turina, M., and Rothlin, M. Echocardiographic findings late after myectomy in hypertrophic obstructive cardiomyopathy. *Eur. Heart J.* **7**: 685–692, 1986.
69. Lösse, B., Loogen, F., and Schulte H.D. Hemodynamic long-term results after medical and surgical therapy of hypertrophic cardiomyopathies. *Z. Kardiol.*, Suppl. **3**: 119–130, 1987.
70. Schulte, H.D., Bircks, W., Körfer, R., and Kuhn, H. Surgical aspects of typical subaortic and atypical midventricular hypertrophic obstructive cardiomyopathy (HOCM). *Thorac. Cardiovasc. Surg.* **29**: 375–380, 1981.
71. Schulte, H.D., Bircks, W., and Lösse, B. Techniques and complications of transaortic subvalvular myectomy in patients with hypertrophic obstructive cardiomyopathy (HOCM). *Z. Kardiol.* **76**, Suppl. 3: 145–151, 1987.
72. Cooper, M., W., McIntosh, Ch. L., Tucher, E., and Clark, R.E. Operation for hypertrophic subaortic stenosis in the aged. *Ann. Thorac. Surg.* **44**: 370–378, 1987.
73. Williams, W.G., Wigle, E.D., Rakowski, H., Smallhorn, J., Leblanc, J., and Trusler, G.A. Results of surgery for hypertrophic obstructive cardiomyopathy. *Circulation* **76**, Suppl. V: 104–108, 1987.
74. Lösse, B., Schulte, H.D., Loogen, F., and Bircks, W. Long-term survival after transaortic subvalvular septal myectomy in patients with hypertrophic obstructive cardiomyopathy. In preparation.
75. Harrison, D.C., Braunwald, E., Glick, G., Mason, D.T., Chidsey, C.A., and Ross, J. Jr. Effects of beta adrenergic blockade on the circulation, with particular reference to observations in patients with hypertrophic subaortic stenosis. *Circulation* **29**: 84–98, 1964.
76. Hess, O.M., Grimm, J., and Krayenbuehl, H.P. Diastolic function in hypertrophic cardiomyopathy: Effects of propranolol and verapamil on diastolic stiffness. *Eur. Heart J.* **4**, Suppl F: 47–56, 1983.
77. Swanton, R.H., Brooksby, I.A.B., Jenkins, B.S., and Webb-Peploe, M.M. Hemodynamic studies of β blockade in hypertrophic obstructive cardiomyopathy. *Eur. J. Cardiol.* 5/4: 327–341, 1977.
78. Rosing, D.R., Kent, K.M., Borer, J.S., Seides, S.F., Maron, B.J., and Epstein, S.E. Verapamil therapy: A new approach to the pharmacologic treatment of hypertrophic cardiomyopathy. I. Hemodynamic effects. *Circulation* **60**: 1201-1207, 1979.
79. Anderson, D.M., Raff, G.L., Ports, T.A., Brundage, B.H., Parmley, W.W., and Chatterjee, K. Hypertrophic obstructive cardiomyopathy. Effects of acute and chronic verapamil treatment on left ventricular systolic and diastolic function. *Br. Heart J.* **51**: 523–529, 1984.
80. Bonow, R.O., Rosing, D.R., and Epstein, S.E. The acute and chronic effects of verapamil on left ventricular function in patients with hypertrophic cardiomyopathy. *Eur. Heart J.* **4**, Suppl F: 57–65, 1983.
81. Hanrath, P., Mathey, D.G., Kremer, P., Sonntag, F., and Bleifeld, W. Effect of verapamil on left ventricular isovolumic relaxation time and regional left ventricular filling in hypertrophic cardiomyopathy. *Am. J. Cardiol.* **45**: 1258–1264, 1980.
82. Kuhn, H., Krelhaus, W., Bircks, W., Schulte, H.D., and Loogen, F. Indication for surgical treatment in patients with hypertrophic obstructive cardiomyopathy. In: Cardiomyopathy and Myocardial Biopsy, Kaltenbach, M., Loogen, F. and Olsen, E.G.J. (eds.), Springer-Verlag, Berlin—Heidelberg—New York 1978, pp. 308–315.
83. Morrow, A.G., Reitz, B.A., Epstein, S.E., Henry, W.L., Conkle, D.M., Itscoitz, S.B., and Redwood, D.R. Operative treatment in hypertrophic subaortic stenosis: Techniques and the results of pre- and postoperative assessments in 83 patients. *Circulation* **52**: 88–102, 1975.

Color Flow Mapping in Hypertrophic Cardiomyopathy

Seiki Nagata, Kunio Miyatake, and Yasuharu Nimura

National Cardiovascular Center, Suita, Osaka, Japan

Hypertrophic cardiomyopathy is characteristically accompanied by inappropriate hypertrophy of the interventricular septum and ventricular free walls, narrowness of the ventricular cavity, impaired distensibility of the ventricular wall in diastole, systolic anterior motion of the mitral valve and some other anatomical and functional features of the ventricle.[1–3] These abnormalities in morphology and dynamics of the heart may be reflected in intracardiac flow patterns. Some special features of intracardiac flow pattern have been demonstrated by conventional Doppler echocardiography in hypertrophic cardiomyopathy.[4–6]

Color flow mapping—that is, Doppler flow imaging—enables us to visualize the intracardiac flow distribution on an anatomical basis, so it can provide significant information on intracardiac flow which has not been obtained by other techniques up to now. Therefore, color flow imaging may be very significant for understanding the pathophysiology of the heart in hypertrophic cardiomyopathy.

Intracardiac hemodynamics, especially intraventricular pressure gradient, can now be noninvasively measured by the pulsed and continuous wave Doppler techniques in hypertrophic cardiomyopathy.[7,8] In order to enhance the accuracy of measurement, it is essential to know the orientation of the target flow. Color flow imaging is advantageous for this purpose.

1. Ejection Flow in Hypertrophic Nonobstructive Cardiomyopathy

In hypertrophic nonobstructive cardiomyopathy, the left ventricular outflow tract tends generally to be narrow because of hypertrophy of the interventricular septum and free wall. The flow image is monochromatic, without showing the reddish-bluish mosaic pattern that indicates a high velocity corresponding to a localized stenosis (Fig. 1).

Doppler flow pattern on the velocity spectrogram obtained by the Fast Fourier Transformation, FFT, sampled at the central part of the outflow tract, exhibits peak velocity in the early part of the ejection time, which is similar to that in healthy subjects (Fig. 2).

2. Left Ventricular Outflow Obstruction and Flow (I)

In hypertrophic obstructive cardiomyopathy, left ventricular obstruction usually occurs between the mitral valve and the interventricular septum. The distal parts of the anterior mitral leaflet and the posterior one are lifted anterosuperiorly toward the interventricular septum.[9,10] They appear to be oriented in such a manner as to intersect the left ventricular outflow tract (Fig. 3a). A pressure gradient is noted at the level of the tips of the mitral leaflets.

Corresponding to such anatomical and functional conditions, in the two-dimensional Doppler image from the apical approach, the distal part of the outflow tract from the

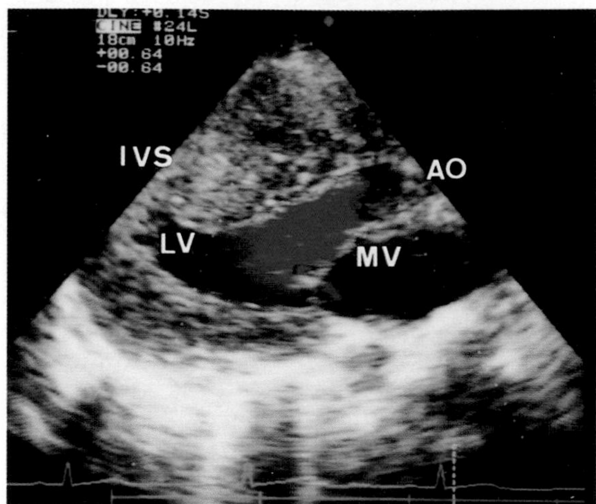

Fig. 1. Left ventricular ejection flow in hypertrophic nonobstructive cardiomyopathy

Long-axis view of the left ventricle. While the interventricular septum is diffusely hypertrophied into the left ventricular outflow tract, the anterior mitral leaflet exhibits the usual orientation. The image of ejection flow is monocolored, showing no localized stenosis in the outflow tract. LV: left ventricle, IVS: interventricular septum, MV: anterior mitral leaflet, AO: aorta

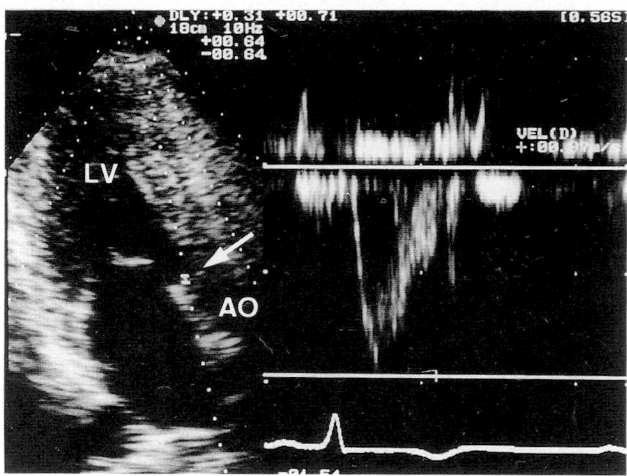

Fig. 2. Flow pattern of the left ventricular ejection in hypertrophic nonobstructive cardiomyopathy

Left panel: Apical long-axis view of the left ventricle. The sample volume for the Doppler is set in the left ventricular outflow tract (arrow). Right panel: Flow pattern of ejection. The peak of the flow velocity is noted in the early stage of the ejection time. LV: left ventricle, AO: aorta.

intersecting mitral valve is coded by a reddish-bluish mosaic pattern, while the proximal part is coded by blue[11,12] (Fig. 3b). Such a phenomenon is not observed in hypertrophic nonobstructive cardiomyopathy, but appears in the Doppler flow image to be one of the characteristic features of obstructive cardiomyopathy. The mosaic area is interpreted as showing a jet spurting from the stenotic site toward the aorta.

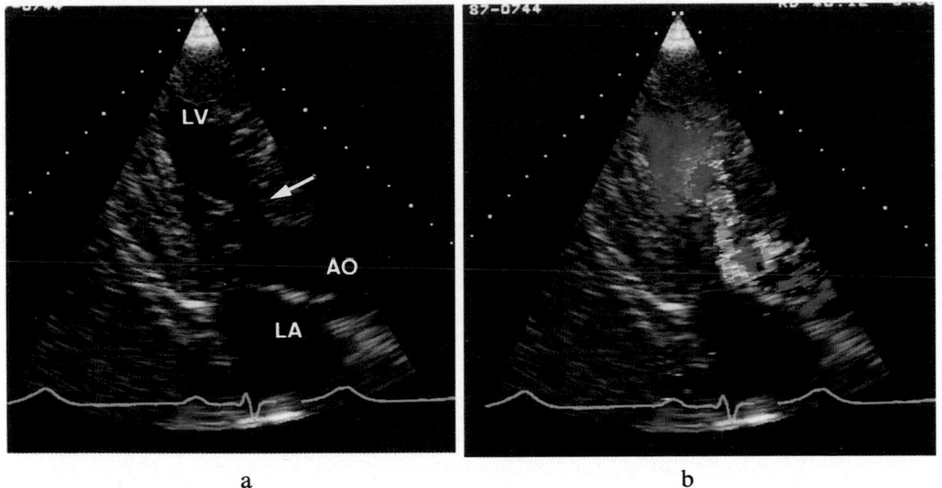

Fig. 3. Left ventricular ejection flow in hypertrophic obstructive cardiomyopathy
a: Apical long-axis view of the left ventricle. The distal part of the mitral valve is bent toward the interventricular septum, resulting in a localized stenosis in the outflow tract (arrow). It is manifested as SAM in the M-mode echocardiogram. LA: left atrium, LV: left ventricle, IVS: interventricular septum, AO: aorta
b: Ejection flow is markedly accelerated at the site of stenosis, exhibiting a reddish-bluish mosaic pattern in the distal outflow tract. The ejection flow is already accelerated before the stenosis, exhibiting color reversal due to aliasing.

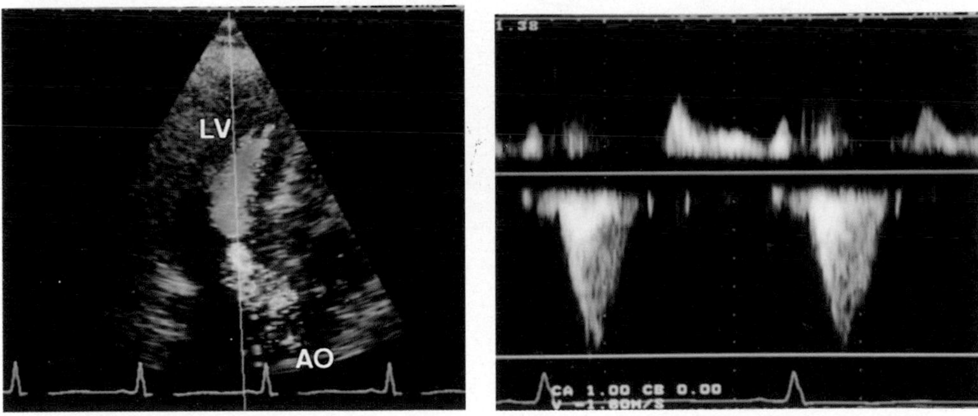

Fig. 4. Flow pattern of the left ventricular ejection in hypertrophic obstructive cardiomyopathy
Left panel: Flow image in the apical long-axis view. The yellow line indicates the beam direction of the continuous wave Doppler. LV: left ventricle, AO: aorta
Right panel: Flow pattern in the FFT spectrogram. The peak of the flow velocity is noted in the middle of the ejection time. The peak pressure gradient calculated from the flow velocity is about 15 mmHg.

The distinct appearance of the mosaic pattern from the level of the intersecting mitral valve toward the aorta shows that a sharp pressure gradient occurs at this level, supporting the assumption from the echo image. The pressure gradient can be calculated from the flow velocity measured by the pulsed or continuous wave Doppler technique at the site just distal to the intersecting mitral valve (Fig. 4), referring to the modified Bernoulli equation.[7]

The FFT spectrogram is advantageous to demonstrate temporal relationships on the accelerated jet. The peak of flow velocity during one cardiac period is noted in mid-systole on the accelerated jet, while it is noted at early systole in the left ventricular outflow tract of nonobstructive cases, as mentioned above (Fig. 4). The reasons for this delay in the peak of flow velocity are considered to be as follows: (1) it may take longer to accelerate the flow against the resistance through the stenotic site than against that in the outflow tract of the nonobstructive form, and (2) the outflow obstruction is maximum in mid-systole, as understood from the configuration of the systolic anterior motion of the mitral valve in the M-mode echocardiogram.

3. Left Ventricular Outflow Obstruction and Flow (II)

In hypertrophic cardiomyopathy, the left ventricular outflow obstruction is also caused at the level of the papillary muscle.[9] The hypertrophied papillary muscles occupy a large

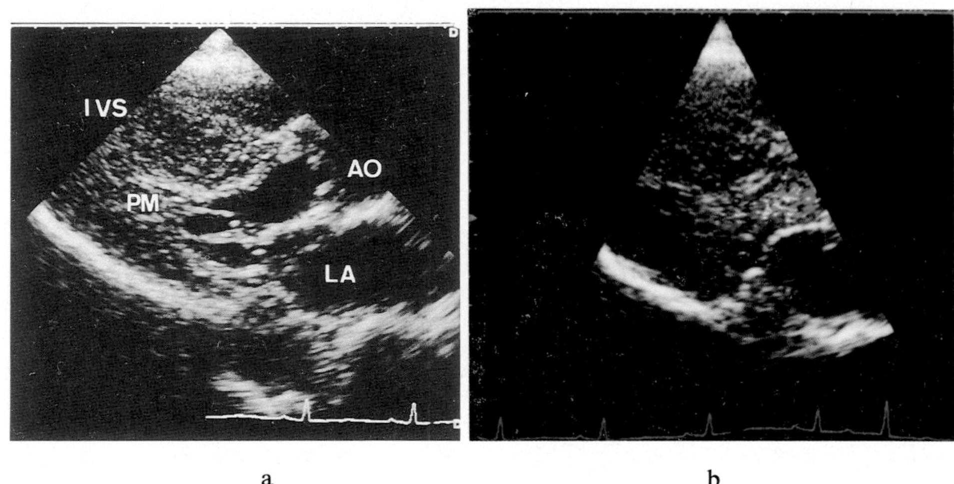

a b

Fig. 5. Left ventricular ejection flow in hypertrophic obstructive cardiomyopathy
a: Parasternal long-axis view of the left ventricle. The hypertrophied papillary muscle obliterates the left ventricular cavity, showing a pressure gradient at this level. The mitral chordae tendineae is shifted anteriorly, following the anteriorly shifted papillary muscle. It is manifested as SAM in the M-mode echocardiogram, while the anterior mitral leaflet is oriented in almost the usual position. LA: left atrium, PM: papillary muscle, IVS: interventricular septum, AO: aorta
b: Flow image. The ejection flow exhibits a reddish-bluish mosaic pattern already from the papillary muscle level, indicating the existence of pressure gradient at this level. The orientation of the anterior mitral leaflet does not look much different from the normal one.

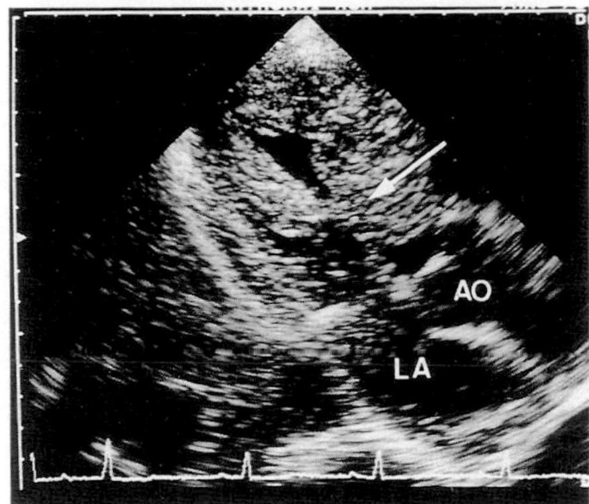

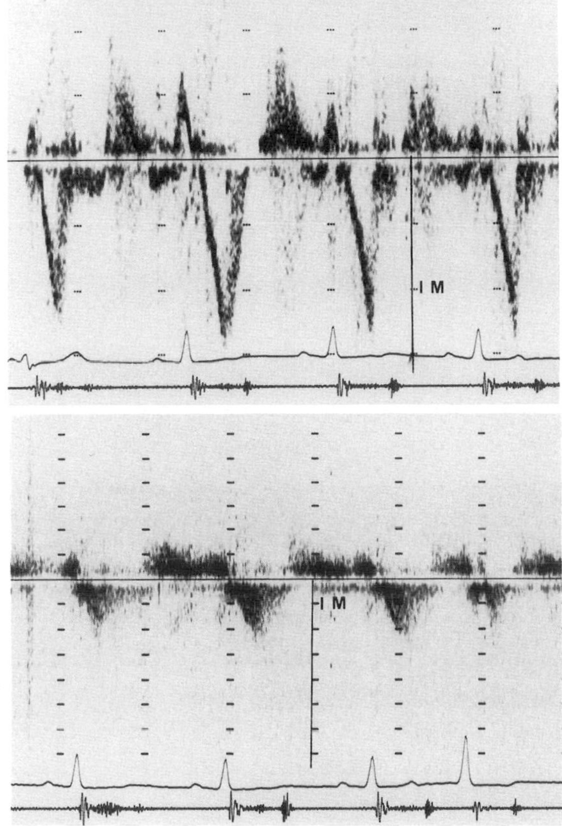

Fig. 6. Flow velocity at the papillary muscle level
Top: Apical long-axis view of the left ventricle. The papillary muscle is so hypertrophied that it occupies a large percentage in the left ventricular cavity, especially at the level of its tip (arrow). LA: left atrium, AO: aorta. Middle: Flow velocity measurement by the pulsed Doppler at the level of the tip of the papillary muscle (arrow on the top). The velocity peak is near 1.5 m/sec.
Bottom: Flow velocity measured by the CW Doppler. The peak velocity is about 3 times of normal, being 2.5 m/sec. The difference between the result by the CW Doppler and that by the pulsed Doppler may be because the sample volume of the latter is positioned further to the proximal side than the most narrow level of the cavity.

part during systole in the cross-section of the left ventricular cavity, already narrowed because of hypertrophy of the interventricular septum and other ventricular walls, making the remaining part of the cavity cross-section even narrower, resulting in the occurrence of pressure gradient at the level of the papillary muscles. In this case, the mitral valve is almost normally oriented and the echo source of the SAM is mainly the chordae (Fig. 5).[9] Of course, in some cases, pressure gradient is noted both at the level of the tip of the mitral valve and at the level of the papillary muscles.

In the Doppler image, a reddish-bluish mosaic pattern appears clearly at the level of the papillary muscles and extends toward the aorta, indicating a pressure gradient at this level (Figs. 5 and 6).

4. *Left Ventricular Inflow Pattern*

There have been many papers which report that the diastolic distensibility of the left ventricular wall is impaired in hypertrophic cardiomyopathy.[4–7] Although the left ventricular inflow pattern shows a variety of configurations, it tends to show reduced velocity, slow acceleration, and slow deceleration in the mitral rapid filling wave and increased height of the presystolic filling wave. The flow signal area covered by the presystolic filling flow tends to be wider than usual (Fig. 7). In hypertrophic cardiomyopathy, mitral regurgitation is often demonstrated, which may heighten the rapid filling wave of the mitral ostium. The impaired distensibility of the left ventricular wall and mitral regurgitation may influence the mitral rapid filling wave in opposite directions, so that the rapid filling wave may exhibit a variety of configurations depending upon the contributions of these two factors.

5. *Mitral Regurgitation*

Mitral regurgitation is often noted in patients of hypertrophic cardiomyopathy, especially in cases of the obstructive form, in which the distal parts of the mitral leaflets

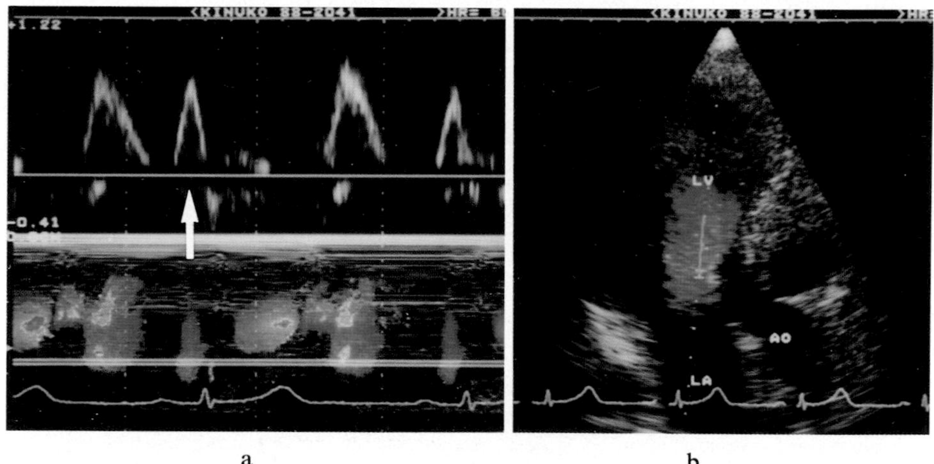

Fig. 7. Left ventricular inflow
a: The presystolic filling wave generally tends to be enlarged in hypertrophic cardiomyopathy (arrow).
b: In correspondence to the enlargement of the presystolic wave, the signal area of the presystolic filling is also wide in the flow image. LA: left atrium, LV: left ventricle, AO: aorta.

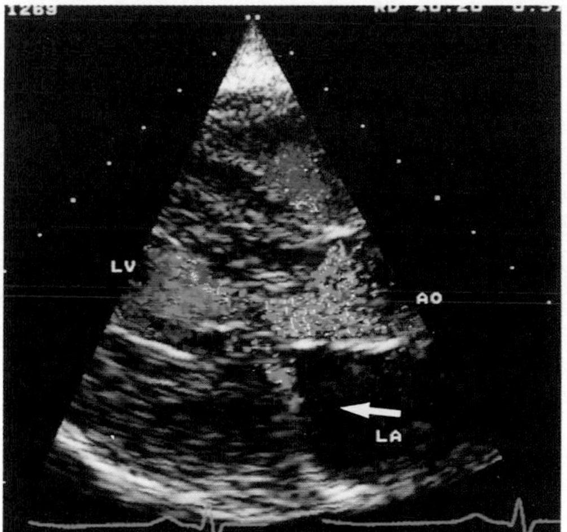

Fig. 8. Mitral regurgitation in hypertrophic obstructive cardiomyopathy
Parasternal long-axis view. Slight regurgitant jet is noted along the posterior mitral leaflet toward the posterior atrial wall (arrow). Ejection flow exhibits a reddish-bluish mosaic pattern from the level of the mitral valve toward the aorta. LV: left ventricle, LA: left atrium, AO: aorta

cause obstruction of the left ventricular outflow tract.[13,14] It is slight in early systole and then exhibits its maximum, decreasing to middle grade in mid-systole, when the unusual orientation of the mitral leaflets also reaches the maximum. Therefore, these two phenomena are considered to be closely related. The mitral regurgitant jet mostly runs along the atrial side of the posterior mitral leaflet toward the posterior wall of the atrium (Fig. 8).

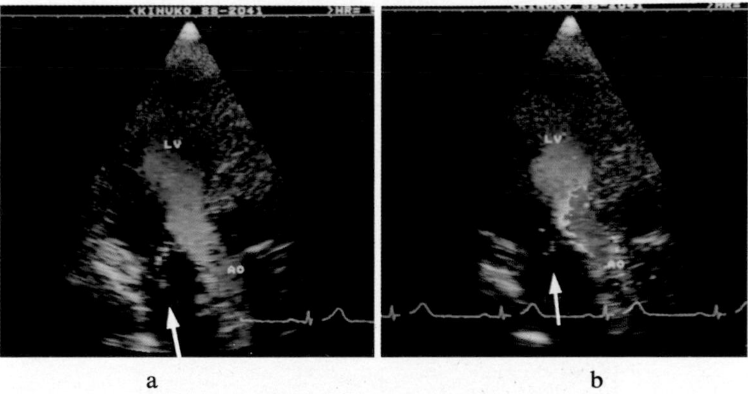

a b

Fig. 9. Mitral regurgitation in hypertrophic nonobstructive cardiomyopathy
a: Apical long-axis view. In early systole, a trivial regurgitant jet is noted along the posterior mitral leaflet (arrow). Ejection flow in the outflow tract is coded in blue. LV: left ventricle, AO: aorta
b: Mid-systole. While the ejection flow is accelerated, exhibiting color aliasing, the mitral regurgitant jet is reduced.

The factors causing mitral regurgitation are not yet determined in hypertrophic obstructive cardiomyopathy. There may be many factors involved in causing systolic anterior motion of the mitral valve.[9,10] However, it appears to be ultimately determined by the malorientation of the inappropriately hypertrophied papillary muscles.[9] Such unusual circumstances may lead to some distortion of mitral coaptation, resulting in mitral regurgitation.

Mitral regurgitation is observed also in about half of all cases of hypertrophic nonobstructive cardiomyopathy[13] (Fig. 9). In slight cases, it is limited to within early systole. The factors promoting mitral regurgitation are also not yet unknown in the nonobstructive form. The left ventricular cavity is likely to be narrowed and deformed by inappropriate hypertrophy of the interventricular septum and free walls, so that this condition may influence mitral coaptation to some extent, leading to slight regurgitation. In hypertrophic cardiomyopathy, the anterior mitral leaflet contacts with the interventricular septum in diastole, resulting in fibrotic changes on the leaflet.[15] Such a fibrous lesion on the mitral leaflet is another possible factor causing mitral regurgitation.

6. Aortic Regurgitation

Aortic regurgitation is observed in some cases of hypertrophic cardiomyopathy, especially of the obstructive form, although no organic lesion is clearly noted in the echogram.[16,17] It is usually slight in severity (Fig. 10). In the obstructive form, the aortic valve is exposed to a high-velocity jet coming through the stenotic site of the outflow tract, as understood from the Doppler flow image, so that it is likely to be more or less damaged, leading to slight regurgitation. Unusual anatomical conditions, such as hypertrophy of the interventricular septum, may result in some deformation of the aortic ring.

There are some papers reporting that aortic regurgitation appears after transaortic

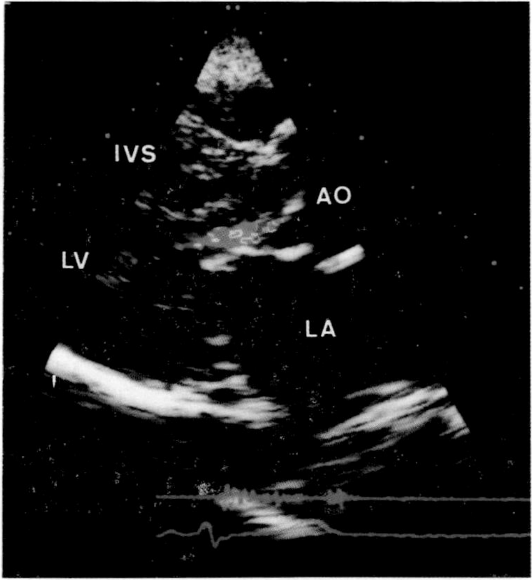

Fig. 10. Aortic regurgitation in hypertrophic cardiomyopathy
Parasternal long-axis view. While the anterior mitral leaflet is almost normally oriented, the hypertrophied interventricular septum diffusely protrudes into the left ventricular tract, resulting in narrowing of the latter. Slight aortic regurgitation is noted. LA: left atrium, LV: left ventricle, IVS: interventricular septum, AO: aorta

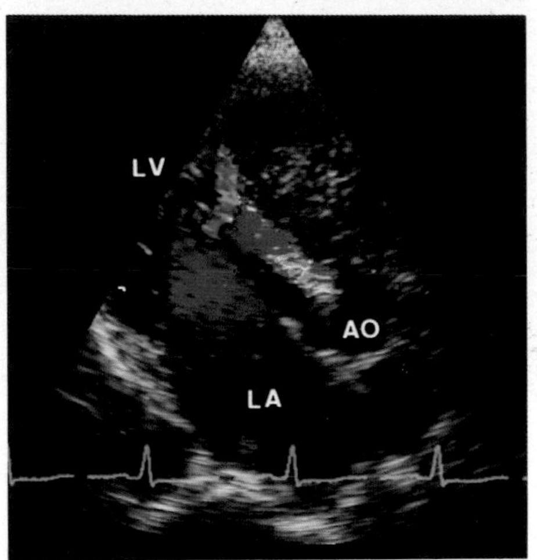

Fig. 11. Aortic regurgitation after transaortic septal myotomy in hypertrophic obstructive cardiomyopathy
Apical long-axis view. Moderate aortic regurgitation is noted. The mitral inflow is also noted in red with its rebound from the apical region in blue. AO: aorta, LV: left ventricle, LA: left atrium

septal myectomy and myotomy against hypertrophic obstructive cardiomyopathy (Fig. 11). The aortic valve may be unexpectedly damaged to some extent by surgical procedures, leading to regurgitation.[18] Abrupt changes in mechanical circumstances surrounding the aortic ring may have some influence on aortic coaptation. These are possible factors causing postsurgical aortic regurgitation. However, they should be further studied in future.

7. Other Unusual Intracardiac Flows in Hypertrophic Cardiomyopathy

a. Unusual flow in mid-ventricular obstruction: Mid-ventricular obstruction is considered to result from marked hypertrophy of the left ventricular wall at the level of the attachment of the papillary muscles.[20] The left ventricular cavity is apparently separated into two chambers, apical and basal. In some cases, scar formation is noted in the wall of the apical chamber.

In one of the authors' patients with mid-ventricular obstruction, a thin reddish-bluish mosaic pattern was noted during systole in the left ventricle, which had never been noted in healthy subjects (Fig. 12). It was interpreted as showing that blood was ejected with high velocity from the apical chamber through the mid-ventricular stenotic site. It was further worthy of note that this thin flow remained until late diastole. This was also observed on the FFT spectrogram. Although the basal chamber was already in a state of relaxation, the apical chamber continued ejection, so that diastolic filling of the apical chamber barely began in the following period of atrial systole. The Doppler flow image led one to consider that both chambers presented primary or secondary asynchrony.

b. Accompanying abnormalities in right ventricular flow: A Doppler flow image with a reddish-bluish mosaic pattern is observed at the right ventricular outflow tract in some cases of hypertrophic cardiomyopathy (Fig. 13). This is interpreted as indicating that

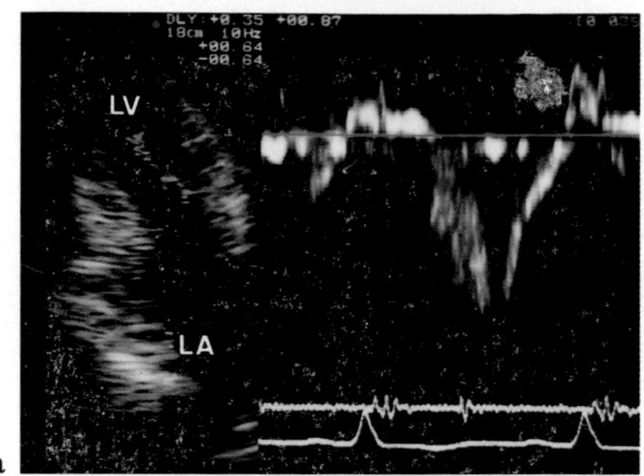

a

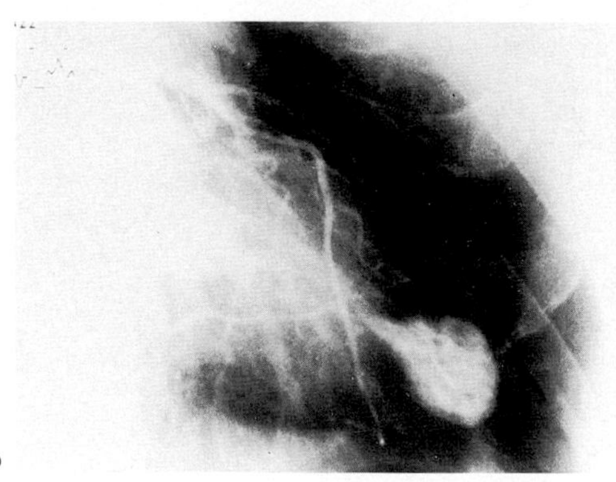

b

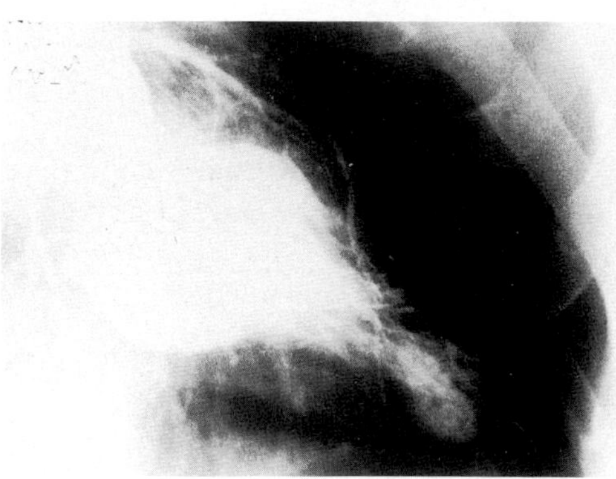

c

Fig. 12. Unusual flow in the left ventricular chamber in a case of mid-ventricular obstruction
a: Left panel: Apical long-axis view. A thin flow of reddish-bluish mosaic pattern is observed in the left ventricular cavity. It is interpreted to be the flow running through the mid-ventricular stenotic site. Right panel: FFT spectrogram of the above-mentioned flow. It is worthy to note that this flow continues from mid-systole up to late diastole, running in the direction from the apex toward the aorta.

there is such an intraventricular obstruction as to accelerate blood flow there. In practice, an intraventricular pressure gradient is usually demonstrated in such cases by catherization.

REFERENCES

1. Maron, B.J., Gottdiener, J.S., and Epstein, S.E. Patterns and significance of distribution of left ventricular hypertrophy in hypertrophic cardiomyopathy. *Am. J. Cardiol.* **48**: 418–428, 1981.
2. Shapiro, L.M. and Mckenna, W.J. Distribution of left ventricular hypertrophy in hypertrophic cardiomyopathy: A two-dimensional echocardiographic study. *J. Am. Coll. Cardiol.* **2**: 437–444, 1983.
3. Nimura, Y., Nagata, S., and Sakakibara, H. Newer aspect in hypertrophic cardiomyopathy studied with cross sectional echocardiography. In: Cardiomyopathy; clinical pathological and theoretical aspect. Sekiguchi, M., Olsen, E.G.L. (eds) p. 13, University of Tokyo Press, Tokyo, University Park Press, Baltimore, 1980.
4. Bryg, R.J., Pearson, A.C., Williams, G.A., and Labovitz, A.J. Left ventricular systolic and diastolic flow abnormalities determined by Doppler echocardiography in obstructive hypertrophic cardiomyopathy. *Am. J. Cardiol.* **59**: 925–931, 1987.
5. Takenaka, K., Dabestani, A., Gardin, J.M., Russell, D., Clark, S., Allfie, A., and Henry,

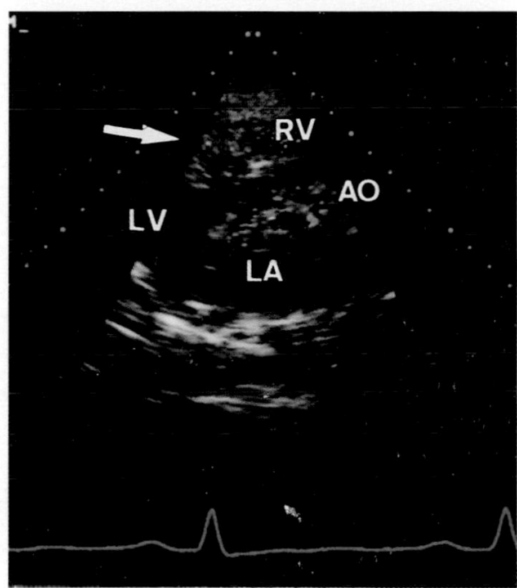

Fig. 13. Unusual rapid flow in a case of hypertrophic obstructive cardiomyopathy
An unusual rapid flow is noted in the right ventricular outflow tract, exhibiting a reddish-bluish mosaic pattern (arrow). It is considered to be due to stenosis of the right ventricular outflow tract. RV: right ventricular outflow tract, LV: left ventricle, AO: aorta, LA: left atrium

---

b: Left ventriculogram in systole. Mid-ventricular stenosis is clearly noted with the apical part which looks like a diverticulum.
c: Left ventriculogram in diastole. While the basal part of the left ventricular chamber is spread in comparison with that in systole, the apical part appears to be still in contraction. This condition corresponds well to the above-mentioned unusual flow, showing asynchrony between the basal part and apical parts of the left ventricle.

W.L. Left ventricular filling in hypertrophic cardiomyopathy: A pulsed Doppler echocardiographic study. *J. Am. Coll. Cardiol.* **7**: 1263–1271, 1986.

6. Spirito, P., Maron. B.J., and Bonow, R.O. Noninvasive assessment of left ventricular diastolic function: Comparative analysis of Doppler echocardiographic and radionuclide angiographic techniques. *J. Am. Coll. Cardiol.* **7**: 518–526, 1986.
7. Hatle, J., Brubakk, A., Tromsdol, A., and Angelsen, B. Noninvasive assessment of pressure drop in mitral stenosis by Doppler ultrasound. *Br. Heart J.* **40**: 131–140, 1987.
8. Sasson, Z., Yock, P.G., Hatle, L.K., Alderman, E.L., and Popp, R.L. Doppler echocardiographic determination of the pressure gradient in hypertrophic cardiomyopathy. *J. Am. Coll. Cardiol.* **11**: 752–756, 1988.
9. Nagata, S., Nimura, Y., Beppu, S., Park, Y.D., and Sakakibara, H. Mechanism of systolic anterior motion of mitral valve and site of intraventricular pressure gradient in hypertrophic obstructive cardiomyopathy. *Br. Heart J.* **49**: 234–243, 1983.
10. Maron, B.J., Harding, A.M., Spirito, P., Roberts, W.C., and Waller, B.F. Systolic anterior motion of the posterior mitral leaflet: a previously unrecognized cause of dynamic subaortic obstruction in patients with hypertrophic cardiomyopathy. *Circulation* **68**: 282–293, 1983.
11. Kudo, T., Mikami, T., Sakurai, N., Akutsu, M., Sakamoto, S., Tanabe, Y., and Yasuda, H. Study on left ventricular ejection flow patterns in hypertrophic cardiomyopathy by real-time two-dimensional blood flow imaging system (2-D Doppler). Proceedings of the 44th Scientific Meeting of the Japanese Society of Ultrasonics in Medicine, p. 297–298, 1984. (in Japanese)
12. Stewart, W.J., Schiavone, W.A., Salcedo, E.E., Lever, H.M., Cosgrove, D.M., and Gill, C.C. Intraoperative Doppler echocardiography in hypertrophic cardiomyopathy: Correlations with the obstructive gradient. *J. Am. Coll. Cardiol.* **10**: 327–335, 1987.
13. Kinoshita, N., Nimura, Y., Okamoto, M., Miyatake, K., Nagata, S., and Sakakibara, H. Mitral regurgitation in hypertrophic cardiomyopathy. Noninvasive study by two-dimensional Doppler echocardiography. *Br. Heart J.* **49**: 574–583, 1983.
14. Prieur, T., Fulop, J.C., Sasson, Z., Wigle, E.D., and Rakowski, H. The relationship between mitral regurgitation and LV outflow obstruction in hypertrophic cardiomyopathy. (Abstract) *Circulation* **72**: III-156, 1985.
15. Moreyra, E., Klein, J.J., Schimada, H., and Segal, B.L. Idiopathic hypertrophic subaortic stenosis diagnosis by reflected ultrasound. *Am. J. Cardiol.* **23**: 32–37, 1969.
16. Theard, M.A., Bhatia, S., Plappert, T., and Sutton, M.G. Doppler echocardiographic study of the frequency and severity of aortic regurgitation in hypertrophic cardiomyopathy. *Am. J. Cardiol.* **60**: 1143–1147, 1987.
17. Shiota, T., Sakamoto, T., Amano, K., Hada, Y., Takenaka, K., Hasegawa, I., Takahashi, T., Suzuki, J., Takahashi, H., and Sugimoto, T. Aortic regurgitation in hypertrophic cardiomyopathy as detected by color Doppler echocardiography. *J. Cardiogr.* **17**: 759–768, 1987. (in Japanese)
18. Sasson, Z., Prieur, T., and Skrobik, Y. Aortic regurgitation following surgery for muscular subaortic stenosis. A newly recognized phenomenon. (Abstract) *Circulation* **72**: III-395, 1985.
19. Rakowski, H., Sasson, Z., and Wigle, E.D. Echocardiographic and Doppler assessment of hypertrophic cardiomyopathy. *J. Am. Soc. Echo.* **1**: 31–47, 1988.
20. Falicov, R.E., Resnekov, L., Bharati, S., and Lev, M. Mid-ventricular obstruction: A variant of obstructive cardiomyopathy. *Am. J. Cardiol.* **37**: 432–437, 1976.

Various Patterns of Left Ventricular Hypertrophy in Hypertrophic Cardiomyopathy

Harry Rakowski, Zion Sasson, Peter Liu, and E. Douglas Wigle

Division of Cardiology, Department of Medicine, Toronto General Hospital and University of Toronto, Canana

ABSTRACT

Variations in the degree of asymmetric hypertrophy have been recognised since Teare's original pathologic description of the disease. Echocardiography and more recently Magnetic Resonance Imaging have allowed us to define the great variability that may exist between patients and in the different hemodynamic subgroups of hypertrophic cardiomyopathy. The site and extent of hypertrophy is important to document in each patient since there is a significant correlation between the degree of hypertrophy and the severity of symptoms and prognosis.

Variations in the degree of asymmetric hypertrophy have been recognised since Teare's[1] original pathologic studies which showed asymmetric hypertrophy of the heart involving the ventricular septum and sometimes extending to the anterolateral free wall. The development of echocardiography led to easier antemortem diagnosis of the condition, the recognition of non obstructive forms of the disease and unusual sites of hypertrophy localized to the apex or causing mid ventricular obstruction. As well it led to the ability to establish the diagnosis in relatively asymptomatic patients who often had more localized forms of disease. Since initial M-mode studies[2] were limited to assessing only the basal septum and posterior wall, the variations in the patterns of asymmetric hypertrophy were not well recognised until studied by 2-dimensional echocardiography[3–7] and more recently Magnetic Resonance Imaging.[8,9]

Two-dimensional echocardiographic studies from our laboratory[6,7] as well as by Maron *et al.*,[4] and Shapiro and McKenna[5] have demonstrated significant anatomic variations in the degree of hypertrophy. In addition the hypertrophied muscle may have a ground glass appearance involving 20–100% of the length of the septum and 16–40% of its circumference,[3] likely representing areas of myocardium with the greatest amount of myocardial fibre disarray and/or fibrosis. The hypertrophy is usually maximal in the proximal septum and may be localized to the subaortic region or extend to the apex. In adult patients with hypertrophic cardiomyopathy, proximal septal thickness is generally greater than 15mm and occasionally exceeds 40mm. Circumferential extent of the hypertrophy medially and laterally from the septum is also variable. Occasionally apical[10–13] or mid ventricular hypertrophy[7,14] predominates. In patients with resting obstruction the hypertrophied septum causes greater narrowing of the LV outflow tract and often there is posterior wall hypertrophy.

Echocardiographic Assessment of Asymmetric Hypertrophy

The distribution of hypertrophy can vary greatly from patient to patient and in dif-

TABLE 1. Extent of Hypertrophy in Hypertrophic Cardiomyopathy According to an Echocardiographic Point Score System

Extent of hypertrophy		Points
Septal thickness (mm)	15–19	1
(Basal 1/3 of septum)	20–24	2
	25–29	3
	>30	4
Extension to papillary muscles		
(Basal 2/3 of septum)		2
Extension to apex		
(Total spetal involvement)		2
Anterolateral wall extension		2
Total		10

ferent centres depending on the population studied. In studies by Maron *et al.*,[4] four types of asymmetric hypertrophy were described. In 10% of cases, the anterior half of the septum alone was involved (type 1). In 20% of cases, both the anterior and posterior septum was thickened (type 2). Septal plus anterolateral wall involvement (type 3) was seen in 52% of cases, whereas only 18% had postero-septal, apical-septal, or anterolateral wall involvement (type 4), which could be missed by M-mode studies alone. Type 4 involvement is much less common in our experience and may reflect differences in patient selection with fewer patients included in our work[6,7] who were studied for screening purposes.

Concentric LV hypertrophy was relatively rare in Maron's study[4] as it is in our experience, but was more common in the study of Shapiro and McKenna[5] of 89 patients with hypertrophic cardiomyopathy where 31% had concentric hypertrophy. In their series, 49 patients had asymmetric septal hypertrophy, with the hypertrophy confined to the anterior septum in 14%, the anterior and posterior septum in 35% and involving both the septum and free wall in 51% of patients. Notably, 55% of these patients had a region of the left ventricle that was thicker than the upper anterior septum.

To better define the degree of asymmetric hypertrophy and its relationship to hemodynamic subgroups and symptoms, we studied 100 patients with good quality 2-dimensional echocardiograms who had undergone hemodynamic classification.[6] The degree of asymmetric hypertrophy was semiquantitated with a 2D echo point score with a maximum of 10 points given as shown in Table 1. One to 4 points is given to septal thickness measured at the leaflet tips in the parasternal long axis view, up to 4 points for the length of ASH from parasternal and apical views (Fig. 1), and 2 points for anterolateral extension of hypertrophy seen on the short axis view (Fig. 2). This echocardiographic point score has correlated well with Magnetic Resonance quantitation of LV mass.[8]

As shown in Table 2, the asymmetric hypertrophy was confined to the basal one third of the septum (subaortic area) in 25%, extended to the papillary muscle level in 27% and involved the whole septum from base to apex in 48% (Fig. 1). Extension to the anterolateral wall was not observed in cases of localized hypertrophy, but was seen in 35% of cases where the hypertrophy extended to the papillary muscles, and in 91% of patients where the full length of the septum was involved. Overall, 54% of patients had anterolateral extension of the hypertrophy, a percentage similar to that originally described by Teare[1] and as seen in other echocardiographic studies.[4–6] Thus, tremen-

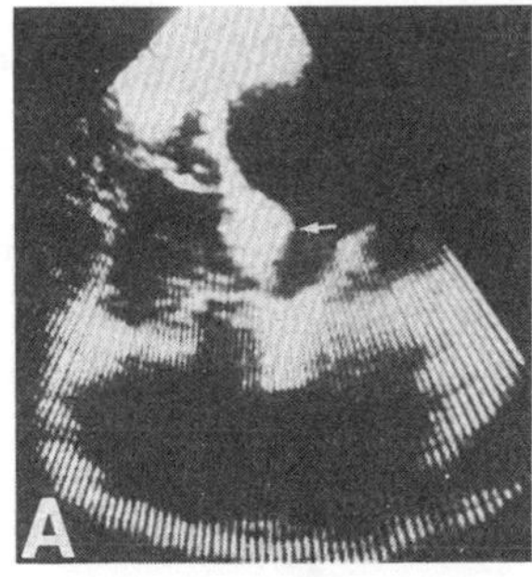

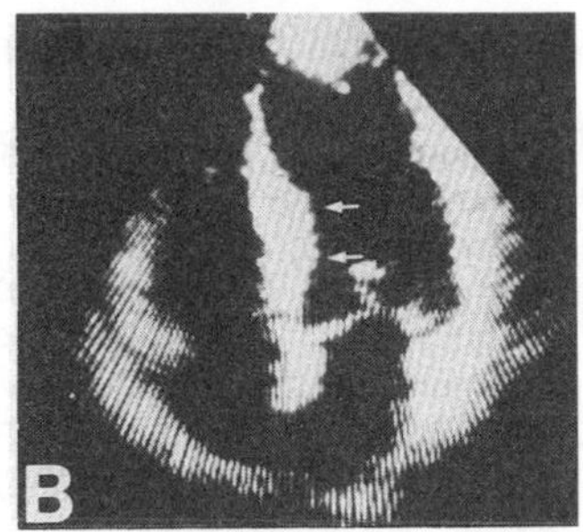

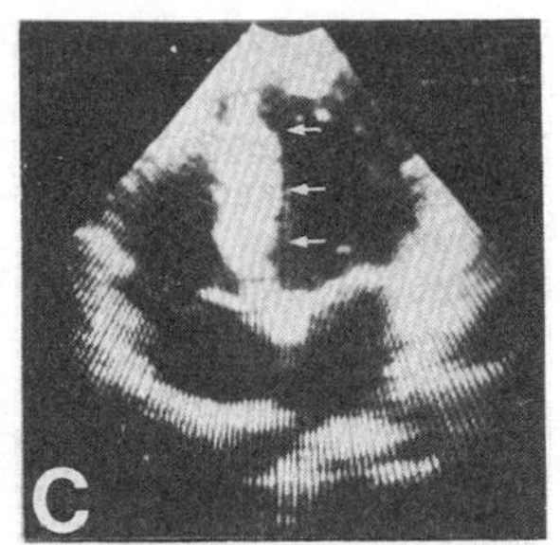

Fig. 1. The length of septal hypertrophy can be assessed from apical 4 chamber views. The horizontal arrows point to the extent of hypertrophy in each instance. Septal hypertrophy may involve (A) the basal one-third of the septum in 25% of cases or (B) the basal two-thirds of the septum (extending down to the papillary muscles) in 25% of cases, or the septal hypertrophy may involve (C) the whole septum from base to apex in approximately 50% of cases. (Reprinted with permission from Wigle *et al.* Hypertrophic cardiomyopathy: the importance of the site and extent of hypertrophy. A review. *Prog. Cardiovasc. Dis.* **28**: 1–83, 1985.)

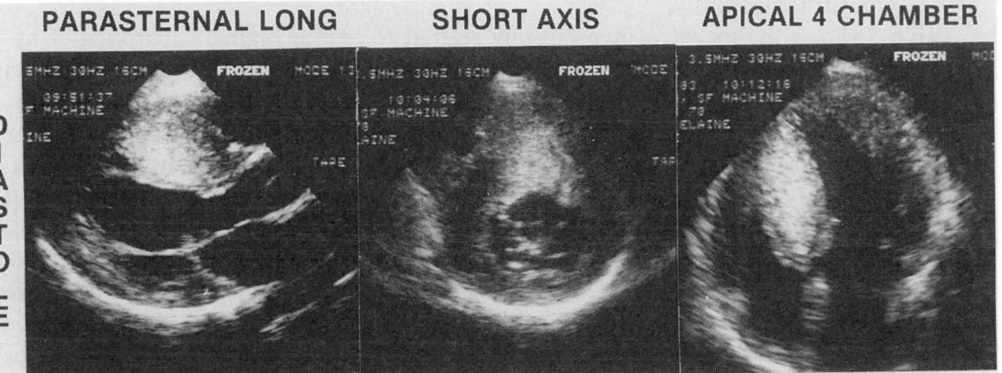

Fig. 2. Diastolic parasternal and apical 4 chamber frames from a patient with hypertrophic cardiomyopathy and severe hypertrophy are shown. The septum is thickened along its full length with a portion of it demonstrating a brighter ground glass appearance. In the short axis view extension of hypertrophy to the anterolateral wall can be seen. In the 4 chamber view the full length of septal hypertrophy can be best appreciated as well as hypertrophy of the apex.

TABLE 2. Extent of Hypertrophy in 100 Cases of Ventricular Septal Hypertrophy[a] Determined by Two-dimensional Echocardiography

Extent of hypertrophy	Number of cases	Anterolateral wall extension[b]
Basal 1/3 of septum (subaortic area)	25	0/23– 0%
Basal 2/3 of septum (down to papillary muscles)	27	8/23–35%
Whole septum (from base to apex)	48	42/46–91%
Total	100	50/92–54%

[a] The presence of septal hypertrophy was determined by one-dimensional echocardiographic criteria in all cases. (Ventricular septum ≥ 15 mm and septal-posterior wall ratio ≥ 1.5:1)[53]
[b] In eight case it was not possible to comment on anterolateral wall extension, thus only 92 of these cases were analyzed in this respect.

TABLE 3. Extent of Asymmetric Hypertrophy Related to Hemodynamic Subgroups in Hypertrophic Cardiomyopathy

Hemodynamic subgroup	No. of cases	Extent of septal hypertrophy				Anterolateral extension	Mean echo point score
		IVS (mm)	Basal 1/3	Basal 2/3	Whole septum		
Obstruction at rest	39	2.45 ± 0.55	8%	20%	72%	83%	8.57
Latent obstruction	34	1.89 ± 0.35	53%[a]	35%	12%[a]	13%[a]	2.88[a]
No obstruction	27	2.09 ± 0.57	14%[b]	26%	59%[b]	63%[b]	6.04[b]

IVS, Interventricular septum.
[a] $p < 0.001$, Latent vs both obstruction at rest and no obstruction.
[b] $p < 0.05$, No obstruction vs obstruction at rest.

dous variability in the extent of hypertrophy can be seen in different patients with hypertrophic cardiomyopathy.

Table 3 shows the extent of hypertrophy related to hemodynamic subgroups of hypertrophic cardiomyopathy with marked differences noted. Patients with obstruction at rest had the greatest degree of septal thickness and the most extensive hypertrophy. At least two-thirds of the length of the septum was involved in 92% of these patients with anterolateral extension in 83%, and a mean hypertrophy point score of 8.57. Patients with latent obstruction had a less severe form of hypertrophy with the smallest septal thickness and hypertrophy localised to the basal third of the septum in 53%. Anterolateral extension was seen in only 13% with a mean point score of only 2.88. Patients without obstruction had an intermediate degree of hypertrophy with some patients having mild hypertrophy and others more severe hypertrophy. These dramatic differences in the extent of hypertrophy in the three major hemodynamic subgroups of hypertrophic cardiomyopathy help explain the differences in symptoms and natural history between the groups.

Importance of the Extent of Hypertrophy

Patients with resting obstruction and those without obstruction with extensive hypertrophy are likely to be more symptomatic, with impaired relaxation and delayed diastolic filling,[15] a higher incidence of atrial and ventricular arrhythmias and a poorer prognosis. While latent obstruction has often been thought to be of intermediate severity, between those with resting and those without obstruction, most cases are at the mild end of the hypertrophic spectrum. This is in keeping with our previous observations that these patients have less severe symptoms and rarely die of ventricular arrhythmias.

The site and extent of hypertrophy is important to document in each patient since there is a significant association with symptoms and prognosis.[6] Patients with outflow tract obstruction and the greatest degree of hypertrophy have a higher LVEDP when compared to patients with latent obstruction with the least hypertrophy (18.4 vs 12.4 mm Hg; $P<0.001$) and those without obstruction and intermediate degrees of hypertrophy (18.4 < 16.6 mm Hg; $P<0.05$). Severe symptoms (NYHC 3–4) are more common in patients with resting obstruction compared to those without obstruction (46 vs 12%; $P<0.001$) with the degree of hypertrophy likely playing an important role.[6] The degree of hypertrophy also affects prognosis. In our study of 36 patients with hypertrophyic cardiomyopathy undergoing 72 hour ambulatory holter monitoring, the incidence of ventricular tachycardia (3 beats or more) was compared to the echocardiographically determined extent of hypertrophy. The occurrence of ventricular tachycardia correlated with septal width ($P<0.002$) and an echocardiographic point score of >5.

Post-Operative Assessment

Surgical myectomy is often required to decrease or abolish the outflow tract obstruction and to improve symptoms. The site and extent of the septal myectomy can be visualized as shown in Fig. 3.

Right Ventricular Involvement

Right ventricular involvement in hypertrophic cardiomyopathy is common, but the manifestations of this involvement are usually much less evident than those in the left side of the heart. Occasional cases have been described however, in which right sided involvement occurred in apparent isolation or was the dominant presenting feature. Obstruction to right ventricular outflow may occur as a result of hypertrophy of the

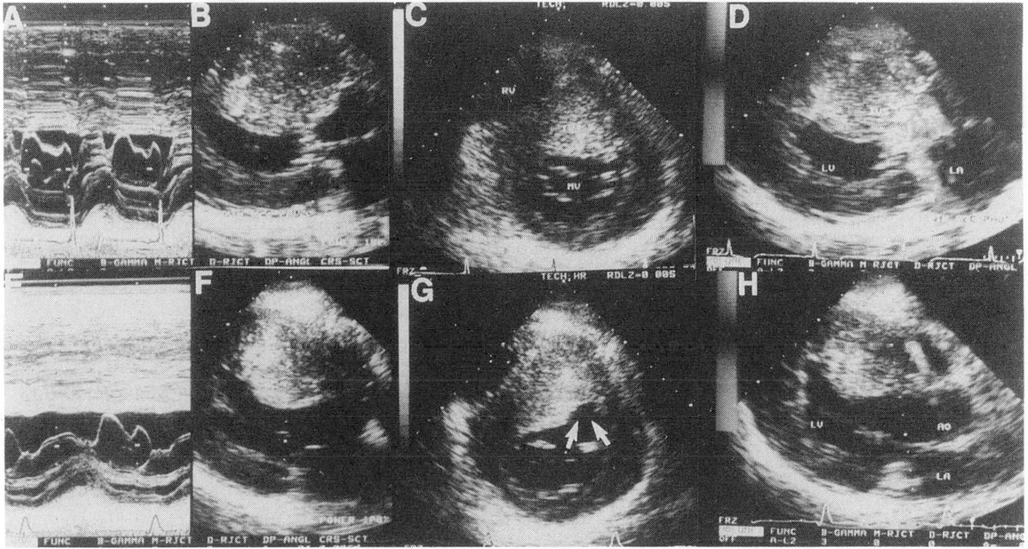

Fig. 3. This study is from a patient with obstructive hypertrophic cardiomyopathy (A-D) who underwent successful septal myectomy (E-H). Pre-operatively there was evidence of marked hypertrophy and severe systolic anterior motion of the mitral apparatus with septal contact, as can be seen from the M-mode (A) and parasternal long axis (B) images. Circumferential extent of septal hypertrophy can be seen in the parasternal short axis view at the level of the mitral leaflets (C). Colour flow imaging (D) revealed a high velocity outflow tract jet and an eccentric posteriorly directed jet of mitral regurgitation. Post operatively, the myectomy site can be seen (G, arrows), resulting in widening of the outflow tract (F&G) with regression of SAM (E) and disappearance of the turbulent outflow tract and mitral regurgitation jets (H). (Reprinted with permission from Rakowski *et al.* Echocardiographic & Doppler assessment of hypertrophic cardiomyopathy. *J. Am. Soc. Echocardiography*, Vol. 1, No. **1**, pp. 31–47, Jan-Feb 1988.

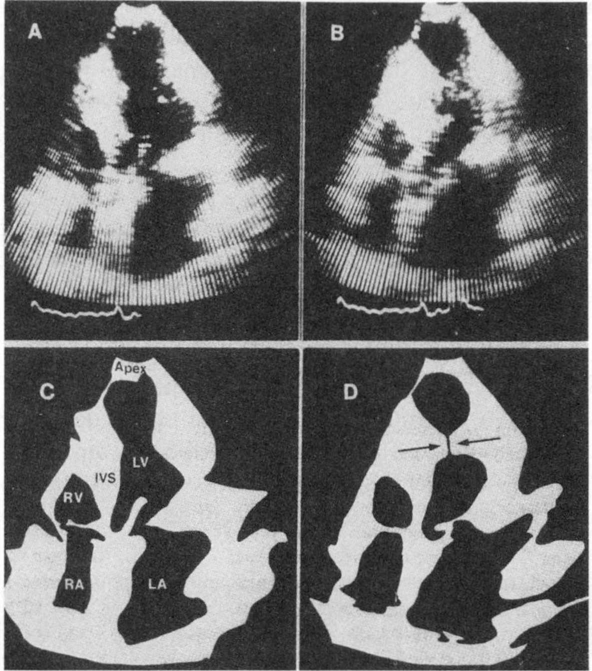

Fig. 4. Apical 4 chamber 2-Dimensional echocardiographic views (A&B) and corresponding line diagram (C&D) from a patient with mid ventricular obstruction with apical infarction and aneurysm formation is shown. Note mid ventricular obstruction at end systole (arrows, panel D) and poorly contractile, partially diskinetic apical motion. Cine angiographic ejection fraction of the basal chamber was 91% but only 16% in the apical chamber (from Wigle, E.D., *et al. Prog. Cardiovasc. Dis.* **28**: 13, 1985. Reprinted with permission).

crista supraventricularis and it's septal and parietal bands or at the mid right ventricular level, where at times, the hypertrophied septum bulges into the right ventricular cavity to such an extent that the cavity is virtually occluded.

Mid Ventricular Obstruction

Mid ventricular obstruction[14] is a rare manifestation of hypertrophic cardiomyopathy. Mid cavity obliteration is due to the systolic apposition of hypertrophied walls and papillary muscles at the mid ventricular level, producing two distinct left ventricular chambers, a hypokinetic basal chamber and a normal or poorly contracting, partially dyskinetic apical chamber (Fig. 4). We have seen only 5 such patients and in 3 patients apical infarction with aneurysm formation without obstructive coronary artery disease was present.

Asymmetric Apical Hypertrophy

Sakamoto *et al.*[10] and Yamaguchi *et al.*[11] first described an unusual variant of nonobstructive HCM that was characterized by giant T wave negativity (>10 mm) on the electrocardiogram and echocardiographic evidence of asymmetric apical hypertrophy, with a spadelike appearance of the LV at end diastole. This condition is present in about 2% of patients with HCM, predominantly in men, and is usually associated with a good prognosis. Reports that deal with populations other than the Japanese have defined a wider spectrum of disease and expanded the definition to include all patients with echocardiographic evidence of asymmetric apical hypertrophy, regardless of whether giant T negativity is present. We use a ratio of apex to posterior wall thickness of 1.5:1 as our criterion for apical hypertrophy. In our own series of 22 patients it appears that giant negativity may define patients with more severe apical hypertrophy, since marked negativity is present only in patients with an apical wall thickness of > 20 mm. Careful echocardiographic examination of the apex should be done in patients suspected of having the disorder, since the apical hypertrophy may be confined to a localized portion of the apex.

Magnetic Resonance Imaging

Magnetic resonance imaging has provided an alternative method of obtaining high resolution tomographic images of the heart in hypertrophic cardiomyopathy. The images are obtained by placing the patient inside a high field magnet and stimulating the protons within the body with specially encoded radio frequency pulses. Information can be collected regarding the proton containing chemical characteristics and location. The contrast from the MR images is the result of interactions amongst proton density relaxation parameters (T_1 and T_2) and blood flow.

The patient is usually placed supine in the imaging magnet, with the right shoulder rotated away from the horizontal at 30 degrees. In this position the long axis of the heart will be close to horizontal. To precisely localise the true cardiac long and short axes, initial standard multislice coronal and/or sagital views are obtained without initial viewing angle rotation. From these localizing images, true orthogonal cardiac long and short axes can be located. The angles can be precisely entered into the computer and subsequent true cardiac short and long axial plane images can be precisely acquired at desired thickness and separation. At our centre, multislice imaging is usually carried out along the true cardiac short and long axis with a thickness of 5mm and the slice located at 1 cm apart from centre to centre. The slices are acquired in an interleaved manner to avoid interslice interference. For large hearts or images in systole, multiple acquisitions may be necessary in order to cover the entire myocardium from apex to base.

The images are then reconstructed using standard 2-D Fourier transform and specific wall thickness measurements and chamber dimensions can be obtained right from the image display, since these slices represent true axial views. Furthermore, since these views are identical to those acquired in 2-D echocardiography, direct image comparison and hypertrophy localization can be carried out with ease. The tomographic outlines of the endocardium and epicardium can be stacked and fitted with a smooth surface to calculate the precise endocardial and epicardial volume. Validation with cast filled canine hearts have confirmed that this technique is extremely reproducible, and accurate to within 10 mls in calculating the precise myocardial volume. After correction with a density factor, precise myocardial mass can be derived for each patient.

Comparison of NMR with 2-D Echocardiography

Quantitative visual comparisons to localize myocardial hypertrophy in patients with hypertrophic cardiomyopathy have been carried out previously. We have performed this comparison by having two unbiased observers classifying the location of hypertrophy into upper and lower septum, anterior, posterolateral, inferior or apical locations. From a series of 19 patients, standard echocardiographic views were able to iden-

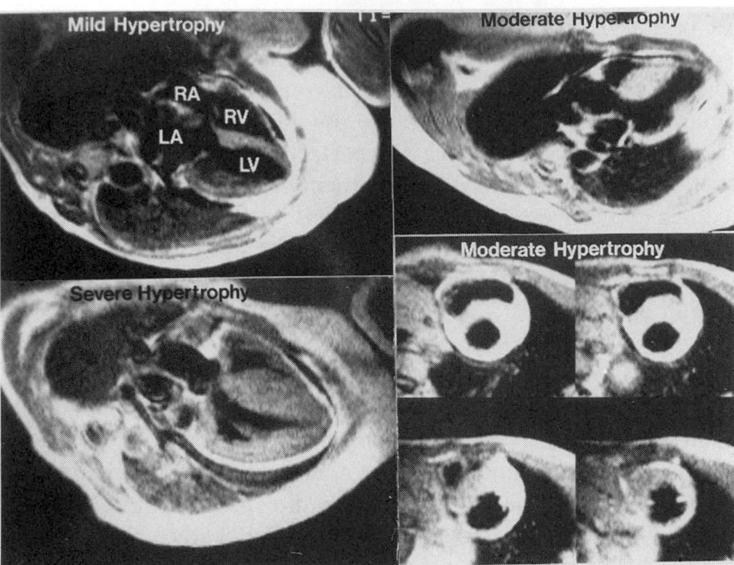

Fig. 5. Magnetic resonance imaging in 3 patients with hypertrophic cardiomyopathy with variable degrees of asymmetric hypertrophy is shown. The upper left panel is taken analogous to an apical 4 chamber view showing the septal hypertrophy combined to the basal one-third (subaortic region) of the septum. The upper right panel shows more extensive hypertrophy involving the upper two-thirds of the septum to the level of the papillary muscles. Serial short axis views from the same patient are shown in the bottom right panel, demonstrating involvement of both the anterior and posterior septum, anterolateral extension and sparing of the posterior and inferior walls. The bottom left panel is from a patient with severe hypertrophy with involvement of the full length of the septum, apex and distal posterolateral wall and is analogous to the apical 4 chamber view in Fig. 2.

tify the location of hypertrophy (Figs. 5 and 6) in all but one patient in this group. On the other hand, combined multiplane MR imaging was able to identify the site of hypertrophy in all patients, including the echo indeterminant case, which turned out to be a case of very localized hypertrophy near the base of the papillary muscle. Comparing the various MR views that can be used to localize hypertrophy, the coronal view was most inefficient, in that it can only detect 50% of hypertrophy, while the long axis and short axis can detect 75% and 85% respectively alone. The combination of various views thus allowed the precise localization in all cases.

Semiquantitative comparison was then carried out by correlating the echocardiographic hypertrophy score with MR derived myocardial mass measurements. This correlation was good with an R value of 0.89.

Comparing the various axial views, the short axis views are most accurate to detect hypertrophy at multiple levels circumferentially, as it is least prone to tangential sectioning and partial volume effects. It is also extremely useful to detect the extent of septal, posterolateral and anterior wall hypertrophy, and can precisely localize bands of hypertrophy that run from the upper septum to the posterolateral wall. The long axis views on the other hand are excellent for localizing mid ventricular and apical hyper-

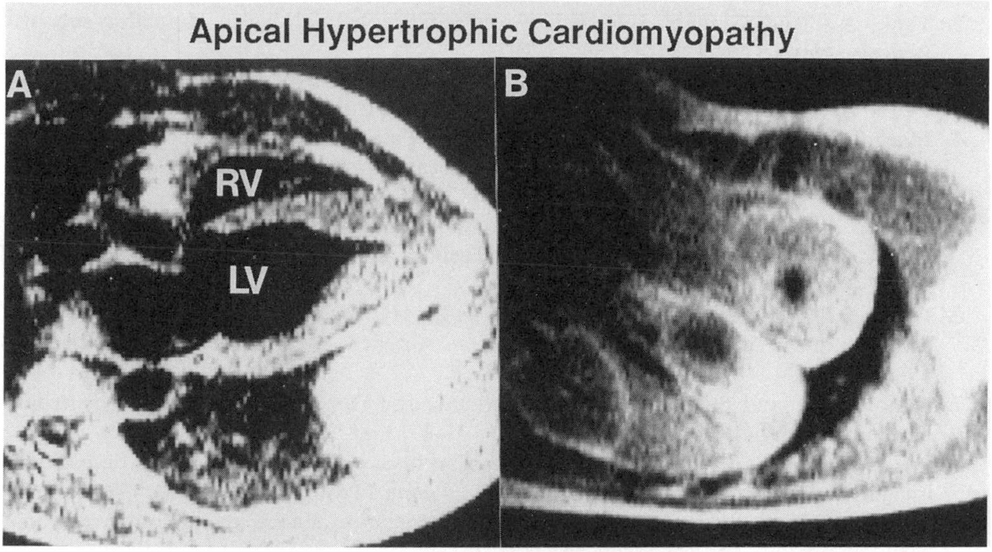

Fig. 6. Magnetic Resonance Imaging in a patient with apical hypertrophic cardiomyopathy is shown. In the long axis view (panel A) the upper half of the septum is spared and the hypertrophy is localized to the distal one half of the left ventricle involving the apex. A diastolic short axis view taken at the distal third of the LV shows the concentric apical hypertrophy and small LV cavity.

trophy. It is therefore extremely important to precisely and accurately place the cardiac axes, to properly assess the location and extent of hypertrophy in hypertrophic cardiomyopathy.

SUMMARY

Patients with hypertrophic cardiomyopathy can have great variability in the site and extent of asymmetric hypertrophy. While the upper septum is most commonly involved, the hypertrophy may involve the full length of the septum as well as the anterolateral free wall. Occasionally the hypertrophy may be maximal at the mid ventricular level or at the apex. Patients with resting obstruction have the most severe hypertrophy, those with latent obstruction a much lesser degree of hypertrophy and those without obstruction an intermediate degree of hypertrophy. Magnetic resonance imaging studies can provide high resolution tomographic images of the heart with good correlation between MRI determination of myocardial mass and echo hypertrophy point score. The site and extent of hypertrophy is important to document echocardiographically in each patient since it has important implications for symptoms and prognosis.

Acknowledgment

This was supported in part by the Heart & Stroke Foundation of Ontario.

REFERENCES

1. Teare, R.D. Asymmetrical hypertrophy of the heart in young adults. *Br. Heart J.* **20**: 1–8, 1958.

2. Tajik, A.J. and Giuliani, E.R. Echocardiographic observations in idiopathic subaortic stenosis. *Mayo. Clin. Proc.* **49**: 89–97, 1974.
3. Martin, R.P., Rakowski, H., French, J., *et al.* Idiopathic hypertrophic subaortic stenosis viewed by wide angle phased-array echocardiography. *Circulation* **59**: 1206–17, 1979.
4. Maron, B.J., Gottdiener, J.S., and Epstein, S.E. Patterns and significance of distribution of left ventricular hypertrophy in hypertrophic cardiomyopathy. *Am. J. Cardiol.* **48**: 418–28, 1981.
5. Shapiro, L.M. and McKenna, W.J., Distribution of left ventricular hypertrophy in hypertrophic cardiomyopathy: A two-dimensional echocardiographic study. *J. Am. Coll. Cardiol.* **2**: 437–44, 1983.
6. Wigle, E.D., Sasson, Z., Henderson, M.A., *et al.* Hypertrophic cardiomyopathy: The importance of the site and extent of hypertrophy. A review. *Prog. Cardiovasc. Dis.* **28**: 1–83, 1985.
7. Rakowski, H. and Sasson, Z. Echocardiographic and Doppler assessment of hypertrophic cardiomyopathy. *J. Am. Soc. Echocardio.* **1**: 31–47, 1988.
8. Liu P., Willansky S., Poon P., *et al.* Myocardial mass quantitation by magnetic resonance imaging in hypertrophic cardiomyopathy. *Circulation* **74** (Suppl): 226 (abst), 1986.
9. Higgins, C.B., Byrd, B.F., Stark, D., *et al.* Magnetic resonance imaging in hypertrophic cardiomyopathy. *Am. J. Cardiol.* **55**: 1121–26, 1985.
10. Sakamoto, T., Tei, C., Muramaya, M., *et al.* Giant negative T-wave inversion as a manifestation of asymmetric apical hypertrophy (AAH) of the left ventricle. Echocardiographic and ultrasonocardiotomographic study. *Jpn. Heart J.* **17**: 611–29, 1976.
11. Yamaguchi, H., Ishimura, T., Nishiyama, S., *et al.* Hypertrophic non-obstructive cardiomyopathy with giant negative T-waves (apical hypertrophy): Ventriculographic and echocardiographic features in 30 patients. *Am. J. Cardiol.* **44**: 401–11, 1979.
12. Keren, G., Belhassen, B., Sherez, J., *et al.* Apical hypertrophic cardiomyopathy: Evaluation by non-invasive and invasive technique in 23 patients. *Circulation* **71**: 45–56, 1985.
13. Louie, E.K. and Maron, B.J. Apical hypertrophic cardiomyopathy: Clinical and two-dimensional echocardiographic assessment. *Ann. Intern. Med.* **106**: 663–70, 1987.
14. Falicov, R.E. and Resnekov, L. Midventricular obstruction in hypertrophic obstructive cardiomyopathy. New diagnostic and therapeutic challenge. *Br. Heart J.* **39**: 701–05, 1977.
15. Sasson, Z. and Lefkowitz, C.A. Langer, G., *et al.* Diastolic dysfunction in hypertrophic cardiomyopathy. Importance of the extent of hypertrophy. *Clin. Invest. Med.* **8**: 60 (abst), 1985.

Two Forms of Apical Hypertrophic Cardiomyopathy: Japanese and Western Forms

Yoshinori Koga, Masatoshi Nohara,** Yoshitaka Miyazaki,* and Hironori Toshima**

* The Third Department of Internal Medicine, Kurume University School of Medicine, Kurume, Japan
** Institute of Cardiovascular Diseases, Kurume University School of Medicine, Kurume, Japan

ABSTRACT

Studies from Japan have identified a morphologic variant of hypertrophic cardiomyopathy in which wall thickening is confined to the most apical portion of the left ventricle, and several reports have since described apical hypertrophy or apical hypertrophic cardiomyopathy. Whereas the form of apical hypertrophy identified in Japan is characterized by a striking electrocardiographic pattern of giant negative T-waves and a spade deformity of the left ventricle, nonoriental patients often fail to manifest such features. Both the diagnostic criteria and disease entity of apical hypertrophic cardiomyopathy, therefore, remain a subject of controversy. This paper describes the two forms of apical hypertrophic cardiomyopathy, as the Japanese and the Western forms, that present characteristically different clinical manifestations, prognosis and genetic background. The Western form of apical hypertrophic cardiomyopathy appears to lie within disease spectrum of classical hypertrophic cardiomyopathy, while the Japanese form may represent a separate disease entity. A left ventriculographic demonstration of a spade-shaped deformity appcarcs to be essential to identify Japanese form of apical hypertrophy, and to distinguish such from the Western form of apical hypertrophic cardiomyopathy.

1. INTRODUCTION

Hypertrophic cardiomyopathy (HCM) is most frequently characterized by an asymmetric increase in the thickness of the interventricular septum with or without outflow obstruction. Asymmetric septal hypertrophy was therefore initially considered to be a pathognomonic echocardiographic sign of HCM.[1,2] Subsequent studies,[3–9] however, have revealed that the morphological spectrum of HCM can vary considerably from localized hypertrophy of almost any region of the left ventricle to diffuse left ventricular hypertrophy. Japanese investigators, Sakamoto *et al.*[10] in 1976 and Yamaguchi *et al.*[11] in 1979, first described a specific morphologic variant of the disease in which wall thickening is confined to the most apical portion of the left ventricle and called it as asymmetric apical hypertrophy or apical hypertrophy. They also have noted that this variant is characterized by a striking electrocardiographic pattern of "giant" negative T-waves and a "spade" deformity of the left ventricle, as detected by left ventricular angiography. From the United States, Maron *et al.*[12] reported in 1982 five patients with apical hypertrophic cardiomyopathy in whom ventricular hypertrophy was virtually confined to the distal portion of the left ventricle. It is, however, of note that none of their patients presented giant negative T-waves or a spade-shaped configuration. These initial studies have interested several investigators from centers outside Japan and a total of almost 100 non-Japanese patients with apical hypertrophy or apical hypertrophic cardiomyopathy[13–29] have been described as having those clinical features similar to those reported as the Japanese form of apical hypertrophy. However, Louie and Maron[30] recently noted by reviewing these patients reported in the literature, that the majority (82 patients) did not convincingly show both giant negative T-waves and a spade deformity of the left ventricle, although two-dimensional echocardiography demonstrated ventricular hypertrophy confined to the apical portion of the left ventricle. These patients rather appeared more similar morphologically and clinically to those patients with apical hypertrophic cardiomyopathy described by Maron *et al.*[12] We have also reported in 1984[31] using two-dimensional echocardiography and left ventriculography that there exist two forms of apical hypertrophic cardiomyopathy; being conveniently termed as a Japanese form and the Western form. We have since proposed to call the Western form, as "apical asymmetric septal hypertrophy" (apical ASH), since the majority of these patients presented asymmetric hypertrophy in the apical region, mainly involving the apical ventricular septum, and they appeared to be included in the disease spectrum of classical HCM.

The different methods and criteria for identifying apical HCM or apical hypertrophy among investigators seem to be the main reason for variance and controversy. The majority of Western investigators identified apical HCM through a two-dimensional echocardiographic demonstration of ventricular hypertrophy being confined to the apical portion of the left ventricle. On the other hand, Japanese investigators have described apical hypertrophy as requiring a spade-shaped deformity of the left ventricle or giant negative T-waves, or both. Nevertheless, controversies with regard to diagnostic criteria for apical hypertrophy still remain even in Japan. Yamaguchi *et al.*[11,32] have relied on an electrocardiographic sign of giant negative T-waves, while Sakamoto *et al.*[10,33] have described that a two-dimensional echocardiographic demonstration of asymmetric hypertrophy in the apical portion with obliterated apical cavity is essential to identify apical hypertrophy. Therefore, both investigators included in their patients with apical hypertrophy those with ASH at the basal portion of the left ventricle, if these patients met their diagnostic criteria. On the other hand, we[34,35] defined apical hypertrophy based on the angiographic demonstration of the spade-shaped deformity of the left ventricle, and excluded those with ASH observed by echocardiogram at the mitral chordal level. These discrepancies in the hallmark of apical hypertrophy have possibly led to controversy regarding whether the condition represented part of the HCM spectrum or was indeed a separate disease entity.

This paper describes clinical profiles of our patients with apical HCM, separating apical hypertrophy of the Japanese form from the Western form. We then propose that the apical hypertrophy of Japanese form is different from Western apical HCM and represents an etiologically distinct disease entity different from the classical form of HCM.

2. MORPHOLOGICAL APPEARANCE

Figure 1 presents M-mode and two-dimensional echocardiograms as well as a left ventriculogram for a representative patient with Japanese form of apical hypertrophy. On the two-dimensional echocardiogram, no clear hypertrophy is found in the left ventricular septum nor in the left ventricular posterior wall. The septal thickness is 11 mm on the M-mode echocardiogram, while the ratio of apical thickness to middle anterior free wall thickness is 1.4 on the left ventriculogram, presenting a typical spade-shaped configuration. Figure 2 depicts a patient with the other form of apical HCM. While

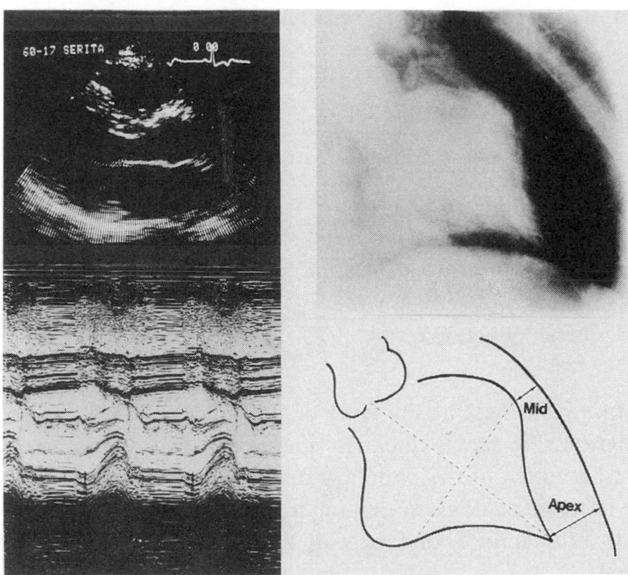

Fig. 1. A representative patient with Japanese form of apical hypertrophy presenting a spade-shaped deformity of the left ventricle on the left-anterior oblique projection of cineangiogram (right). Note that no asymmetric septal hypertrophy is observed both on two-dimensional and M-mode echocardiograms (left).

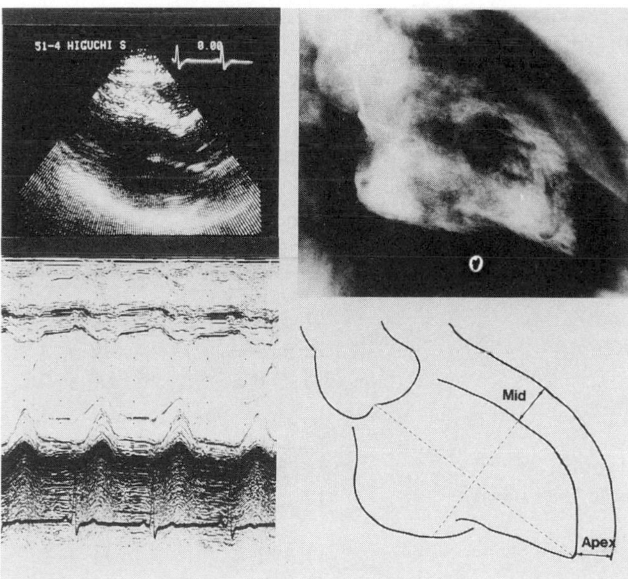

Fig. 2. A representative patient with Western form of apical hypertrophic cardiomyopathy (apical ASH). The septal thickness increases towards the apex and is 22 mm at papillary muscle level on the two-dimensional echocardiogram, while no asymmetric septal hypertrophy is seen on the M-mode echocardiogram. The left ventriculogram presents a "kidney-shaped" appearance, rather than a spade-shaped deformity.

TABLE 1. Patterns of Left Ventricular Hypertrophy in 152 Patients with Hypertrophic Cardiomyopathy

	ASH by 2-D Echo	Left ventricular Configuration	No. of patients
Typical ASH	Basal & Apical	Banana, Kidney or Oval	72
Apical ASH	Apical	Banana, Kidney or Oval	26
Spade-like ASH	Basal & Apical	Spade-like	20
Apical Hypertrophy	No	Spade	29
Others	Posterobasal septum, Lateral free wall	Various	5

ASH = asymmetric septal hypertrophy

the ventricular septal thickness at the level of the mitral chordae is 11 mm on the M-mode echocardiogram, the septal thickness increases towards the apex, and septal hypertrophy (22 mm) is noted at the papillary muscle level on the two-dimensional echocardiogram. The left ventriculogram demonstrates no spade-shaped deformity with an apical thickness to middle anterior free wall thickness ratio of 1.1. Rather an inward indentation of the left ventricular inferior wall is observed into the left ventricular cavity (giving a "kidney-shaped" appearance) which is possibly manifested by distal septal hypertrophy. We therefore postulate that this patient has asymmetric hypertrophy in the apical portion of the left ventricle, mainly involving the apical septum, and propose to call this form of HCM as apical asymmetric septal hypertrophy (apical ASH).

Table 1 presents our current experience of patterns of left ventricular hypertrophy. In 152 patients with HCM who had both two-dimensional echocardiographic and left ventriculographic examinations sufficient for analysis, we found 26 patients with apical ASH and 29 with apical hypertrophy. All patients with apical hypertrophy (Japanese form) demonstrated a spade-shaped deformity of the left ventricle, the ratio of apical

TABLE 2. Patterns of Left Ventricular Hypertrophy among Apical Hypertrophy vs. Apical ASH

	Apical hypertrophy (n = 29)	Apical ASH (n = 26)	p
1) Cineangiogram			
Mid free wall (mm)	14 ± 3	12 ± 5	NS
Apical free wall (mm)	22 ± 4	12 ± 3	<0.001
Apex/Mid	1.6 ± 0.3	1.0 ± 0.2	<0.001
2) Echocardiogram			
IVST			
Chordal level (mm)	11 ± 2	12 ± 3	NS
Papillary muscle level (mm)	17 ± 3	19 ± 3	<0.05
PWT			
Chordal level (mm)	11 ± 1	11 ± 2	NS
Papillary muscle level (mm)	16 ± 2	13 ± 2	<0.001
IVST/PWT			
Chordal level	1.1 ± 0.1	1.1 ± 0.1	NS
Papillary muscle level	1.1 ± 0.6	1.5 ± 0.2	<0.01

Values are as mean ± SD.
ASH = asymmetric septal hypetrophy, IVST = interventricular septal thickness, PWT = posterior wall thickness.

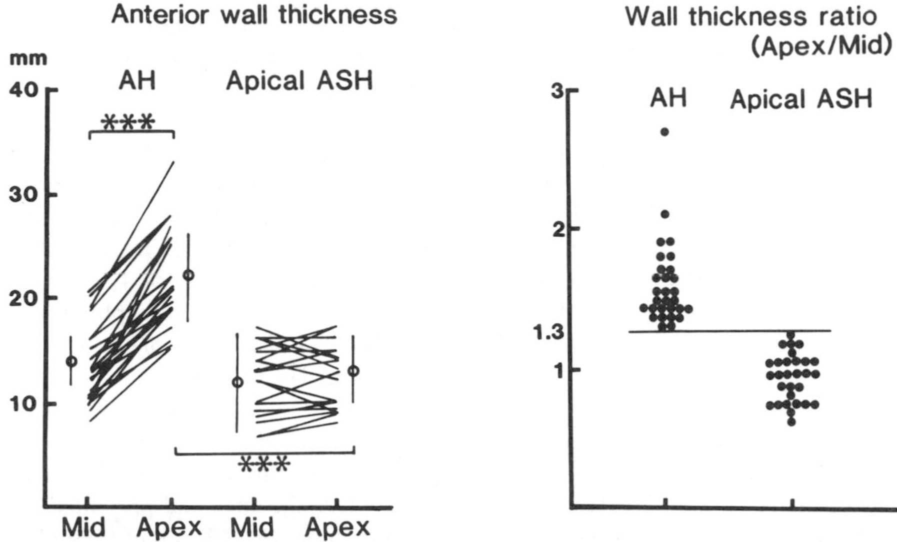

Fig. 3. In left ventricular cineangiography, the anterior free wall thickness increases towards the apex and the ratio of apical to mid-free wall thickness exceeds 1.3 in patients with the Japanese form of apical hypertrophy (AH). Mid: mid-free wall, ***p < 0.001

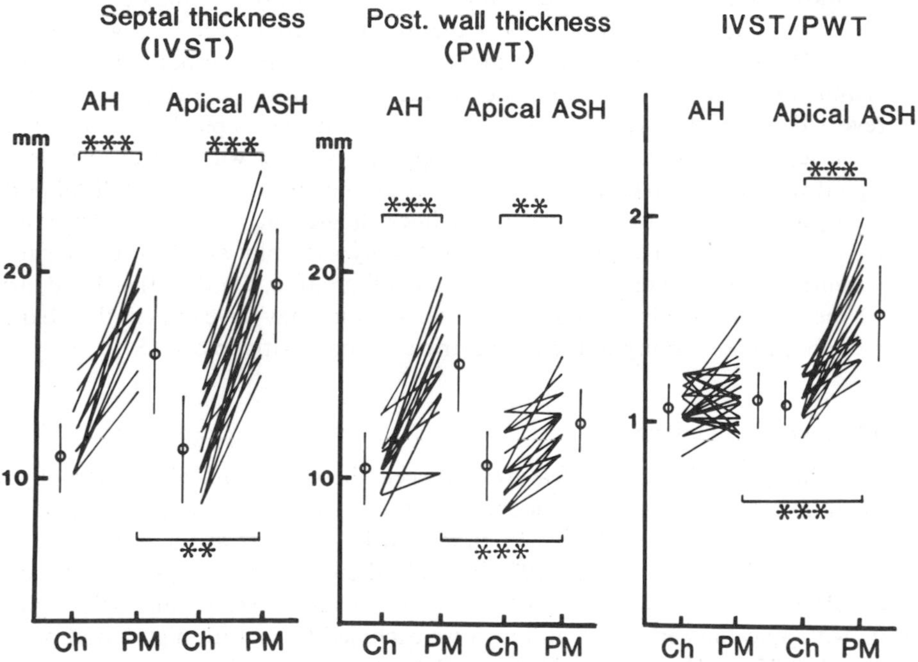

Fig. 4. In two-dimensional echocardiography, the septal thickness increases at the papillary muscle level in both those with apical hypertrophy (AH) and those with apical ASH, while the posterior wall thickness increases to the greater extent in those with apical hypertrophy. Therefore a patient with apical ASH presents asymmetric septal hypertrophy at the papillary muscle level, while those with apical hypertrophy show symmetric hypertrophy. Ch: chordal level, PM: papillary muscle level, **p < 0.01, ***p < 0.001

wall thickness to anterior free wall thickness being 1.3 or greater as described by Yamaguchi *et al.*[11] The apical ASH group presented asymmetric thickening of the ventricular septum of 15 mm or more at the papillary muscle level on two-dimensional echocardiogram. None of the patients of the two groups presented a typical form of ASH at the mitral chordal level. Of the 92 patients with the typical form of ASH presenting a ventricular septal thickness of 15 mm or more and a ratio of septal to posterior wall thickness of more than 1.3 at the mitral chordal level, 20 patients showed a spade-like configuration on the left ventriculogram (spade-like ASH). However in these patients, only 6 demonstrated the apical to anterior free wall thickness ratio of 1.3 or greater. The remaining 5 patients presented other forms of left ventricule hypertrophy, involving the posterobasal septum, lateral free wall or the most basal portion of the ventricular septum. These 97 patients other than those with apical HCM were excluded from the further analyses.

Table 2 presents the morphological characteristics of patients with apical hypertrophy and of those with apical ASH. In left ventriculograhy, patients with apical hypertrophy showed an increased anterior free wall thickness towards the apex and presented a ratio of apical free wall to mid-free wall thickness of 1.3 or more (Fig. 3), all of these demonstrating spade-shaped deformity of the left ventricle by definition. On the other hand, no patients with apical ASH gave the appearance of a spade-shaped deformity with the ratio averaging 1.0 ± 0.2. Of these patients with apical ASH, 3 demonstrated "banana-shaped" deformity and 17 showed "kidney-shaped" deformity. In the echocardiographic study, patients of both groups showed no, or mild, thickening of both the ventricular septum and the posterior wall at the mitral chordal level (Fig. 4). Therefore, classical ASH was not identified by M-mode echocardiography in both groups. On the other hand, two-dimensional echocardiographic examination at the papillary muscle level revealed asymmetric septal hypertrophy in patients with apical ASH, contrasting symmetric septal and posterior wall hypertrophy in patients with apical hypertrophy. Although it was difficult to determine the exact wall thickness at the more distal portion of the left ventricle, these two-dimensional echocardiographic observations suggest that patients with apical hypertrophy have symmetric hypertrophy at the distal portion of the left ventricle, thus giving the spade-shaped configuration. On the other hand, asymmetric hypertrophy, mainly involving the distal septum, may have caused the "banana- or kidney-shaped" deformity of the left ventricle in those with apical ASH.

3. CLINICAL FEATURES

Table 3 compares the clinical features between those with apical hypertrophy and those with apical ASH. On the demographic profile, patients with apical hypertrophy were significantly older than those with apical ASH and were at the same time characterized by a male predominance (90%), while there was no sex predilection in the apical ASH group. Systolic and diastolic blood pressures were significantly higher in patients with apical hypertrophy, although we excluded those with high-blood pressure exceeding 160/95 mmHg during admission. Patients with apical hypertrophy were not, or were only minimally, symptomatic, while 31% of those with apical ASH were classified in NYHA functional class III or IV. In electrocardiogram, striking "giant" negative T-waves exceeding -10 mm were noted in 93% of those with apical hypertrophy, while in only 4% for apical ASH. The R-wave amplitude was increased at V_5 for those with apical hypertrophy, while was so at V_1 for those with apical ASH. The negative P-wave at V_1 was significantly deeper in apical ASH, 8 (31%) of them being associated

TABLE 3. Clinical Features for Apical Hypertrophy vs. Apical ASH

	Apical hypertrophy (n = 29)	Apical ASH (n = 26)	p
Age	53 ± 7	32 ± 13	<0.001
Sex (Male:Female)	26 : 3	16 : 10	<0.05
Blood pressure (mmHg)			
Systolic	131 ± 20	116 ± 11	<0.01
Diastolic	81 ± 14	67 ± 12	<0.001
NYHA class III or IV (%)	0	31	<0.01
Electrocardiogram			
Negative P in V_1 (mm)	−0.5 ± 0.4	−1.0 ± 0.8	<0.01
Atrial fibrillation			
Persistent (%)	6.9	7.7	NS
Transient (%)	0	23.1	<0.01
R in V_1 (mm)	3 ± 2	11 ± 11	<0.001
R in V_5 (mm)	41 ± 10	29 ± 13	<0.001
T in V_5 (mm)	−16 ± 6	−3 ± 5	<0.001
Echocardiogram			
LVIDs (mm)	26 ± 4	30 ± 6	<0.01
LVIDd (mm)	45 ± 5	46 ± 5	NS
FS (%)	44 ± 6	34 ± 9	<0.001
LVEDP (mmHg)	14 ± 5	23 ± 8	<0.001
Exercise stress test			
FAI	27 ± 18	45 ± 18	<0.001
ST depression (%)	0	36	<0.001

Values are as mean ± SD or percent.
ASH = asymmetric septal hypertrophy, NYHA = New York Heart Association, LVIDs = left ventricular internal dimension at end-systole, LVIDd = left ventricular internal dimension at end-diastole, FS = fractional shortening, FAI = functional aerobic impairment, LVEDP = left ventricular end-diastolic pressure.

with persistent or transient atrial fibrillation. Figure 5 depicts representative electrocardiograms from patients with apical hypertrophy and apical ASH. The left ventricular systolic function as determined by M-mode echocardiography was mildly impaired and the left ventricular end-diastolic pressure was markedly elevated in patients with apical ASH. The exercise tolerance was also severely impaired in those with apical ASH, 36% developing ST-depression on exercise stress testing.

These observations clearly indicate that patients with apical ASH manifest clinical features completely distinct from those of apical hypertrophy. Although our findings further confirmed that giant negative T-waves associated with a high QRS amplitude are the characteristic electrocardiographic sign for apical hypertrophy, exceptions did also occur in our experience. The giant negative T-waves can be observed in patients with classical ASH with or without outflow obstruction, while patients with apical hypertrophy do not always present giant negative T-waves.[10,34–41] It is therefore apparent that giant negative T-waves are neither pathognomonic nor highly specific to apical hypertrophy of Japanese type. The electrocardiographic changes are in striking contrast with the rather milder functional limitation and hemodynamic impairment in patients with apical hypertrophy. There have been no reports describing the occurrence of sudden death until recently in the Japanese form of apical hypertrophy as far as we know.[33,42] Therefore,

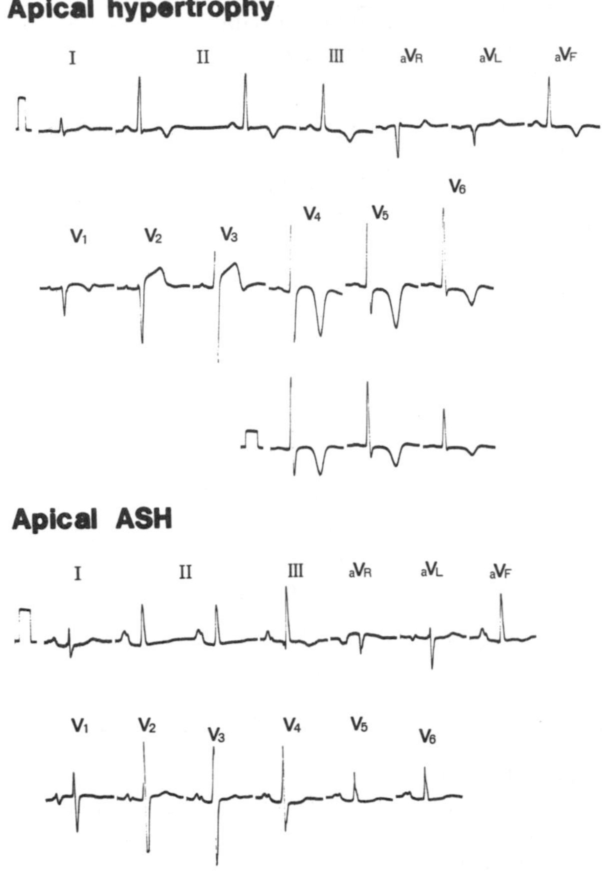

Fig. 5. An electrocardiogram from a patient with apical hypertrophy (upper) demonstrates a characteristic pattern of giant negative T-waves, associated with high QRS amplitudes. A patient with apical ASH (lower) shows left atrial overload and increased R-waves in V_1 and V_2 but no giant negative T-waves

there appears to be general agreement among Japanese investigators[11,32–35,38,40,45] that the Japanese form of apical hypertrophy appears to be a benign condition.

On the other hand, patients with apical ASH presented marked elevation in left ventricular end-diastolic pressure and a reduction in fractional shortening. One third of them were severely symptomatic (NYHA functional class III or IV), being frequently associated with atrial fibrillation which leads to embolic events, often fatal, or intractable heart failure. These impairment in the left ventricular compliance associated with systolic dysfunction in patients with apical ASH were more pronounced than in those with apical hypertrophy or even in those with typical ASH.[31,35] These observations appear to be consistent with reports by Spirito *et al.*[9,47] that HCM patients with mild left ventricular hypertrophy, rather than those with marked hypertrophy, present more severe functional limitation and left ventricular dysfunction. Hence the distinction is necessary with the two forms of apical HCM separately having clinical importance as well.

4. GENETIC AND ENVIRONMENTAL BACKGROUNDS

To further investigate a relationship between these two forms of apical HCM and also with the classical form of HCM, we conducted a family survey (Table 4). Electrocardiographic examination was initially performed in 74 first degree relatives in 22 families for apical hypertrophy and in 54 first degree relatives in 19 families for apical ASH. For those who showed abnormal electrocardiograms such as abnormal Q or negative T-waves, we further undertook two-dimensional echocardiographic examinations.

In the relatives of those with apical hypertrophy, three (4%) presented an abnormal electrocardiogram: an abnormal Q-wave in one, and negative T-waves in two (including giant negative T-waves in one). None of these three relatives demonstrated ASH on two-dimensional echocardiography although we could not perform left ventriculogram and were thereby unable to find a spade-shaped deformity in those relatives. These results clearly indicate that familial occurrence is rare, if at all, in apical hypertrophy, which is consistent with previous reports from Japan.[33–35,38,40,41] Although we could not eliminate the possibility of a sex-linked recessive inheritance, as suggested by Yamaguchi *et al.*,[11] by tracing the family tree recorded in the population register, none of the patients reported consanguinity in their parents. From these observations, we would suggest that apical hypertrophy of Japanese form can occur sporadically.

In contrast, patients with apical ASH presented a high frequency of familial occurrence (74%), with 35% of examined relatives showing abnormal findings in both electrocardiographic and two-dimensional echocardiographic examinations. Such observations appear consistent to an autosomal dominant inheritance. Furthermore, two-dimensional echocardiography revealed a typical classical ASH in 7 relatives, in addition to apical ASH in 8. Three of these suggested a left ventricular outflow obstruction, presenting systolic anterior motion of the mitral valve approaching the ventricular septum and a loud systolic murmur. Sudden death was reported in 3 additional relatives. It was of note that no relatives demonstrated any giant negative T-wave. Maron *et al.*[12] also examined 20 relatives in 4 families of patients with apical HCM, and found hypertrophic cardiomyopathy in 11. Four of these presented hypertrophy of the anterior basal septum, producing typical ASH in M-mode echocardiography. In a recent report by Louie and Maron,[30] 9 out of 23 patients with apical HCM demonstrated a familial occurrence of HCM or sudden death, although in the remaining 14 patients a family survey

TABLE 4. Familial Occurrence for Apical Hypertrophy vs. Apical ASH

	Apical hypertrophy	Apical ASH
No. of index cases	22	19
No. of relatives examined	74	54
Abnormal ECG		
No. of family	3 (14%)	14 (74%)
No. of relatives	3 (4%)	19 (35%)
Abnormal 2-D echocardiogram		
Typical ASH	0	7
Apical ASH	0	8
Non-obstructive	0	12
Obstructive	0	3
Sudden death	0	3

ASH = asymmetric septal hypertrophy.

was not available. They then proposed that apical HCM is transmitted by autosomal dominant inheritance and represent part of spectrum of classic HCM, rather than as a separate and etiologically distinct disease entity. The consistent pattern of inheritance in our patients with apical ASH indicates that apical ASH is the same condition with apical HCM by Maron *et al.*[12,30] On the other hand, sporadic occurrence without any evidence of ASH in relatives may indicate that apical hypertrophy of the Japanese form is distinct from our apical ASH or apical HCM by Maron *et al.*[12,30]

Another feature of apical hypertrophy that is distinct from apical ASH as well as from the classic form of HCM is the peculiar demographic profile of these patients. All Japanese investigators[10,11,31-46] have agreed that apical hypertrophy occurs exclusively in the middle-aged or elderly males. The development of giant negative T-waves from almost normal electrocardiograms over several years has been well described by us[31] and other investigators in Japan.[10,11,33,38] The evidence has raised the possibility that patients with apical hypertrophy have developed abnormal hypertrophy during middle-aged or elderly life in association with some environmental factors. The postulation has been supported by many studies from Japan[10,32-34,36-40,42,44,45] that have reported a high prevalence of mild hypertension in those with apical hypertrophy (33 ~ 54%). It is of note that the original study by Yamaguchi *et al.*[11] excluded such patients associated with systemic hypertension to avoid the confusion with hypertensive heart disease, but 34% of those with giant negative T waves were hypertensive in their following report.[32]

In our patients with apical hypertrophy, 50% reported a history of hypertension, even after excluding those demonstrating high blood pressure exceeding 160/95 mmHg during admission. In contrast, only 8% of those with apical ASH reported a history of hypertension. The case-control studies have clearly shown that hypertension and apical

TABLE 5. Response of Systolic Blood Pressure during Exercise in Apical Hypertrophy

	Apical hypertrophy (n = 25)	Control* (n = 25)	p
At rest			
SBP (mmHg)	128 ± 16	128 ± 15	NS
HR (beats/min)	68 ± 13	71 ± 11	NS
$\dot{V}O_2$ (ml/min/kg)	4.6 ± 0.7	4.6 ± 0.8	NS
At maximal exercise			
SBP (mmHg)	212 ± 31	203 ± 21	NS
HR (beats/min)	141 ± 18	155 ± 21	<0.05
$\dot{V}O_2$ (ml/min/kg)	25.7 ± 7.7	31.4 ± 5.7	<0.01
Slope⁺: SBP vs HR	1.2 ± 0.4	0.9 ± 0.3	<0.01
SBP vs $\dot{V}O_2$	4.3 ± 1.7	2.8 ± 0.8	<0.001
With Hx of hypertension			
Slope⁺: SBP vs HR	1.4 ± 0.4	1.0 ± 0.3	<0.01
SBP vs $\dot{V}O_2$	4.9 ± 1.6	2.9 ± 0.7	<0.001
Without Hx of hypertension			
Slope⁺: SBP vs HR	1.0 ± 0.4	0.8 ± 0.3	NS
SBP vs $\dot{V}O_2$	3.8 ± 1.6	2.9 ± 0.8	<0.10

Values are means ± SD.

* age (within ± 5 years) and sex-matched healthy volunteers

⁺ slope of the linear regression between systolic blood pressure and heart rate or oxygen uptake.

SBP = systolic blood presure, HR = heart rate, $\dot{V}O_2$ = oxygen uptake.

hypertrophy are significantly associated, as described in detail elsewhere in this monograph. We further studied the response of systolic blood pressure during bicycle ergometer stress testing (Table 5). As the maximal exercise capacity differed among individual patients, a response of systolic pressure during exercise was evaluated by deriving slopes of systolic pressure elevation against increase in heart rate or oxygen uptake by linear regression analysis. While at rest, the systolic blood pressure, heart rate and oxygen uptake did not differ between the patients with apical hypertrophy and their age- and sex-matched healthy volunteers. At peak exercise, the systolic blood pressure was not different between the two groups, whereas maximal heart rate and oxygen uptake were significantly lower in the patients with apical hypertrophy indicating impaired exercise tolerance. The slope of the systolic pressure elevation during exercise against either heart rate or oxygen uptake was significantly greater in those with apical hypertrophy. These trends were observed in both those with and those without a history of hypertension. The above collective evidence would strongly suggest that hypertension is related in the development of apical hypertrophy. However, since it is apparent that hypertension alone cannot be a sole causative factor for the remarkable hypertrophy observed in this condition, we must consider additional factors, possibly genetic while distinct from autosomal dominant inheritance.

5. APICAL HCM IN THE DISEASE SPECTRUM OF HCM

From these observations, our patients with apical ASH appeared to be similar both morphologically and clinically to those with apical HCM described by Maron *et al.*[12,30] The pattern of familial occurrence of patients with apical ASH was consistent with that observed in apical HCM by Maron *et al.*[12,30,48] with typical ASH being identified in their relatives. These observations suggest that both conditions have a disease entity that is part of the spectrum of classical HCM. The data also indicate that the Western form of apical HCM occurs in Japan, in addition to the apical hypertrophy of Japanese form.

The majority of our patients with apical ASH manifested more severe cardiac symptoms and functional limitation than those with apical hypertrophy and more so than those with classical HCM with typical ASH.[31,35] These patients often presented an impaired left ventricular systolic function in addition to a marked elevation in the left ventricular end-diastolic pressure. These findings suggest that primary cardiomyopathic process is more advanced in patients with apical ASH and has led to myocardial degeneration rather than hypertrophy, resulting in the atypical morphologic expression of the disease. Alternatively, myocardial ischemia may be an independent important determinant of these morphological and functional alteratious, as discussed in detail elsewhere in this monograph. Furthermore, the patients with apical ASH may include, particularly in younger patients, those who are in the process of developing abnormal hypertrophy and have not yet fully expressed typical ASH.

In contrast, our patients with apical hypertrophy with a spade-shaped deformity in the left ventricle demonstrated clinical features distinct from those with apical ASH. The condition appeared to be benign with minimal symptoms, less functional limitation and no reported sudden death. The majority of these patients were non-familial and ASH was detected in none of their relatives, while an association with systemic hypertension was suggested. We would therefore propose that apical hypertrophy of Japanese type is a distinct form of disease from the classical HCM, and from apical HCM by Maron *et al.*[12,30]

There are several explanations leading us to conclude there must be two distinct form of apical HCM. First, we used both two-dimensional echocardiography and left ventriculography to identify apical hypertrophy. On the other hand, the majority of Western investigators have primarily based the morphologic diagnosis of apical HCM on the echocardiographic demonstration of left ventricular hypertrophy that is situated almost entirely distal to the chordal level. In our exprience, however, it is sometimes difficult with two-dimensional echocardiography to assess a precise morphology of the distal portion of the left ventricle and to distinguish apical hypertrophy from apical ASH or apical HCM. To avoid this uncertainty, we defined apical hypertrophy only for those who demonstrated spade-shaped deformity on left ventriculography. Second, giant negative T-waves associated with high QRS amplitudes have been used as an electrocardiographic hallmark for apical hypertrophy. This electrocardiographic pattern, however, can occur in patients with various cardiac conditions, including HCM patients with typical ASH but no spade-shaped deformity. We did not therefore use this criteria to define apical hypertrophy. Third, we excluded from apical hypertrophy those patients who presented ASH on M-mode echocardiogram at the chordal level even if they showed a spade-shaped deformity on left ventriculography. In our experience however, patients who manifested the both signs were rare (approximately 4%). The selection of only those patients having a spade-shaped deformity and exclusion of those with typical ASH to identify apical hypertrophy therefore help to explain why we were able to distinguish clinical features of the two forms of apical HCM. We therefore believe that apical hypertrophy of Japanese type could be better diagnosed by requiring both the angiographic demonstration of a spade-shaped configuration of the left ventricle and the echocardiographic exclusion of asymmetric septal hypertrophy at the basal portion of the left ventricle. The giant negative T-waves may be neither characteristic nor highly specific to apical hypertrophy.

As indicated by Louie and Maron,[30] the majority of the previously described non-Japanese patients with apical HCM appear more similar morphologically and clinically to those reported by Maron *et al.*[12] However, some patients in the literature from Western countries closely resemble those having the Japanese form of apical hypertrophy. It is therefore likely that apical hypertrophy of Japanese type does additionally exist in any population and in any race throughout the world, although the prevalence rates differ considerably between Japan and the Western countries. In consecutive patients who underwent cineangiography, Yamaguchi *et al.*[32] found apical hypertrophy in 74 out of 2,100 (3.5%), while Bertrand in France[22] noted it in only 7 out of 6,264 (0.1%). In 965 patients with hypertrophic cardiomyopathy, Louie and Maron[30] found only one patient who showed spade-like configuration, while the prevalence rate of apical hypertrophy among HCM in Japan has been reported as 15 to 51%.[32,33,49] In a large-scale population survey using electrocardiography, Morimoto *et al.*[37] described that a prevalence of giant negative T-waves in the adult population was 0.085% (11 out of 12,898) for men and 0.028% (6 out of 21,232) for women. Eleven subjects underwent cardiac catheterization and cineangiography, and 3 disclosed spade-shaped deformity, consistent with apical hypertrophy. These results indicate an estimate for the prevalence rate of apical hypertrophy in the Japanese general adult population to be approximately 0.014%.

The reason for having such a high prevalence rate of apical hypertrophy in Japan is not known. Genetic, racial or environmental factors may account for such variance. The more popular application of electrocardiography in screening a large proportion of the adult working population for heart diseases could be another explanation. We might further consider that a much higher incidence of coronary artery disease in the

Western population has possibly preempted or hindered the development of apical hypertrophy. Giant negative T-waves may also be often taken as a sign of myocardial ischemia in the presence of coronary artery disease.

The present analyses have excluded patients with other various patterns of left ventricular hypertrophy that have been described in HCM by Western investigators,[6,50] while we have observed these patients, including localized hypertrophy to the posterobasal septum, lateral free wall, or to the most basal portion of the ventricluar septum. It should be recognized in this regard that apical hypertrophy occurs as a distinct form from any of these morphologic varieties of HCM previously described.

In conclusion, apical hypertrophy of Japanese form appears to be both morphologically and clinically distinct from the majority of patients with apical HCM described in the Western literature. The left ventriculographic demonstration of a spade-shaped deformity seems to be necessary to distinguish these two forms of apical hypertrophy. Apical hypertrophy of Japanese type may represent a different disease entity, rather than part of spectrum of classical HCM along with ASH.

This study was supported in part by the Research Grant for the Intractable Diseases from the Ministry of Health and Welfare of Japan.

REFERENCES

1. Henry, W.L., Clark, C.E., and Epstein, S.E. Asymmetric septal hypertrophy. Echocardiographic identification of the pathognomonic anatomic abnormality of IHSS. *Circulation* **47**: 225–33, 1973.
2. Epstein, S.E., Henry, W.L., Clark, C.E., Roberts, W.C., Maron, B.J., Ferrans, V.J., Redwood, D.R., and Morrow, A.G. Asymmetric septal hypertrophy. *Ann. Intern. Med.* **81**: 650–80, 1974.
3. Maron, B.J., Gottdiener, J.S., and Epstein, S.E. Patterns and significance of distribution of left ventricular hypertrophy in hypertrophic cardiomyopathy: a wide angle, two dimensional echocardiographic study of 125 patients. *Am. J. Cardiol.* **48**: 418–28, 1981.
4. Maron, B.J., Gottdiener, J.S., Bonow, R.O., and Epstein, S.E. Hypertrophic cardiomyopathy with unusual locations of left ventricular hypertrophy undetectable by M-mode echocardiography: identification by wide-angle two-dimensional echocardiography. *Circulation* **63**: 409–18, 1981.
5. Shapiro, L.M. and McKenna, W.J. Distribution of left ventricular hypertrophy in hypertrophic cardiomyopathy: a two-dimensional echocardiographic study. *J. Am. Coll. Cardiol.* **2**: 437–44, 1983.
6. Wigie, E.D., Sasson, Z., Henderson, M.A., Ruddy, T.D., Fulop, J., Rakowski, H., and Williams, W.G. Hypertrophic cardiomyopathy. The importance of the site and the extent of hypertrophy: a review. *Prog. Cardiovasc. Dis.* **28**: 1–83, 1985.
7. Loule, E.K. and Maron, B.J. Hypertrophic cardiomyopathy with extreme increase in left ventricular wall thickness: functional and morphologic features and clinical significance. *J. Am. Coll. Cardiol.* **8**: 57–65, 1986.
8. Maron, B.J., Spirito. P., Chiarella, F., and Vecchio, C. Unusual distribution of left ventricular hypertrophy in obstructive hypertrophic cardiomyopathy: Localized posterobasal free wall thickening in two patients. *J. Am. Coll. Cardiol.* **5**: 1474–7, 1985.
9. Spirito, P., Maron, B.J., Bonow, R.O., and Epstein, S.E., Severe functional limitation in patients with hypertrophic cardiomyopathy and only mild localized left ventricular hypertrophy. *J. Am. Coll. Cardiol.* **8**: 537–44, 1986.
10. Sakamoto, T., Tei, C., Murayama, M., Ichiyasu, H., Hada, Y. Hayashi, T., and Amano, K. Giant T wave inversion as a manifestation of asymmetrical apical hypertrophy (AAH) of the left ventricle: echocardiographic and ultrasono-cardiotomographic study. *Jpn. Heart J.* **17**: 611–29, 1976.

11. Yamaguchi, H., Ishimura, T., Nishiyama, S., Nagasaki, F., Nakanishi, S., Takatsu, F., Nishijo, T., Umeda, T., and Machii, K. Hypertrophic non-obstructive cardiomyopathy with giant negative T waves (apical hypertrophy): ventriculographic and echocardiographic features in 30 patients. *Am. J. Cardiol.* **44**: 401–12, 1979.
12. Maron, B.J., Bonow, R.O., Seshagiri, T.N.R., Roberts, W.C., and Epstein, S.E. Hypertrophic cardiomyopathy with ventricular septal hypertrophy localized to the apical region of the left ventricle (apical hypertrophic cardiomyopathy). *Am. J. Cardiol.* **49**: 1838–48, 1982.
13. Tilmant, P.Y., Lablanche, J.M., Laurent, J.M., Hethuin, J.P., Folliot, J.P., and Bertrand, M.E. Myocardiopathie hypertrophique apicale nonobstructive. A propos de 5 observations. *Arch. Mal. Coeur.* **73**: 1269-78, 1980.
14. Chia, B.L., Ng, R., Oh, V., Ee, B., and Tan, L. Apical hypertrophic cardiomyopathy in an Indian male. *Singapore Med. J.* **22**: 298–301, 1981.
15. Sheikhzadeh, A., Ghabusi, P., and Afraz, M.R. Apikale linksventrikulaere Hypertrophie, eine Form der hypertrophen nicht-obstruktiven Kardiomyopathie mit extrem grossen negativen T-Wellen. *Herz.* **6**: 369–76, 1981.
16. Steingo, L., Dansky, R., Pocock, W.A., and Barlow, J.B. Apical hypertrophic non-obstructive cardiomyopathy. *Am. Heart J.* **104**: 635–7, 1982.
17. Sheikhzadeh, A. and Ghabussi, P. A case of asymmetrical apical hypertrophy which is a form of hypertrophic non-obstructive cardiomyopathy with giant negative T-waves. *Jpn. Heart J.* **23**: 843–9, 1982.
18. Krishnaraj, N., Rajan, S., Jayakrishnan, T.K., Raghuram, A.R., Moorthy, J.S., Abraham, K.A., and Subramanyam, R. Apical hypertrophic cardiomyopathy. *Indian Heart J.* **34**: 133–7, 1982.
19. Abinader E.G., Rauchfleisch, S., and Naschitz, J. Hypertrophic apical cardiomyopathy: a subtype of hypertrophic cardiomyopathy. *Isr. J. Med. Sci.* **18**: 1005–9, 1982.
20. Kereiakes, D.J., Anderson, D.J., Crouse, L., and Chatterjee, K. Apical hypertrophic cardiomyopathy. *Am. Heart J.* **105**: 855–6, 1983.
21. McDonnell, M.A. and Tsagaris, T.J. Recognition and diagnosis of apical hypertrophic cardiomyopathy. *Chest* **84**: 644–7, 1983.
22. Bertrand, M.E., Tilmant, P.Y., Lablanche, J.M., and Thieuleux, F.A. Apical hypertrophic cardiomyopathy: clinical and metabolic studies. *Eur. Heart J.* **4** (suppl. F): 127–33, 1983.
23. Bloomberg, G.B., Henderson, M.A., Rakowski, H., and Wigle, E.D. Apical hypertrophic cardiomyopathy (Abstract). *Circulation.* **70** (suppl. II): II–335, 1984.
24. Vacek, J.L., Davis, W.R., Bellinger, R.L., and McKiernan, T.L. Apical hypertrophic cardiomyopathy in American patients. *Am. Heart J.* **108**: 1501–6, 1984.
25. Przybojewski, J.Z. and Blake, R.S. Hypertrophic non-obstructive apical cardiomyopathy: a case presentation and review of the literature. *S. Afr. Med. J.* **66**: 492–8, 1984.
26. Keren, G., Belhassen, B., Sherez, J., Miller, H.I., Megidish, R., Berenfeld, D., and Laniado, S. Apical hypertrophic cardiomyopathy: evaluation by noninvasive and invasive techniques in 23 patients. *Circulation.* **71**: 45–56, 1985.
27. Keren, A., Takamoto, T., Harrison, D.C., and Popp, R.L. Left ventricular apical masses: noninvasive differentiation of rare from common ones. *Am. J. Cardiol.* **56**: 697–9, 1985.
28. Panidis I.P., Nestico, P., Hakki, A.H., Mintz, G.S., Segal, B.L., and Iskandrian, A.S. Systolic and diastolic left ventricular performance at rest and during exercise in apical hypertrophic cardiomyopathy. *Am. J. Cardiol.* **57**: 356–8, 1986.
29. Rovelli, E.G., Parenti, F., and Devizzi, S. Apical hypertrophic cardiomyopathy of "Japanese type" in a Western European person. *Am. J. Cardiol.* **57**: 358–9, 1986.
30. Louie, E.K. and Maron, B.J. Apical hypertrophic cardiomyopathy: clinical and two-dimensional echocardiographic assessment. *Ann. Intern. Med.* **106**: 663–70, 1987.
31. Koga, Y., Takahashi, H., Ifuku, M., Itaya, M., Adachi, K., and Toshima, H. Hypertrophic cardiomyopathy with ventricular septal hypertrophy localized to the apical region of the left ventricle (apical ASH). *J. Cardiogr.* **14**: 301–10, 1984.

32. Yamaguchi, H., Nishiyama, S., Nakanishi, S., and Nishimura, S. Electrocardiographic, echocardiographic and ventriculographic characterization of hypertrophic non-obstructive cardiomyopathy. *Eur. Heart J.* **4**: (suppl. F): 105–19, 1983.
33. Sakamoto, T., Amano, K., Hada, Y., Tei, C., Takenaka, K., Hasegawa, I., and Takahashi, T. Asymmetric apical hypertrophy: ten years experience. *Postgrad. Med. J.* **62**: 567–70, 1986.
34. Koga, Y., Itaya, M., Takahashi, H., Koga, M., Ikeda, H., Itaya, K., and Toshima, H. Apical hypertrophy and its genetic and acquired factors. *J. Cardiogr.* **15** (suppl. VI): 65–74, 1985.
35. Miyazaki, Y., Shida, M., Matsuyama, K., Chiba, M., Nakata, M., Sakai, S., Inuzuka, S., Nohara, M., Toshima, H., and Koga, Y. Japanese apical hypertrophy is distinct from apical hypertrophic cardiomyopathy (by Maron). *Shinzoh* **19**: 559–68, 1987 (in Japanese).
36. Ueno Y., Suruda, H. Ohta, A., Fujimoto, A., Arita, M., Mohara, O., Miyamoto, Y., Nishio, I., and Masuyama, Y. Left ventricular function and characteristics of hypertension in juvenile hypertension with marked ST.T changes: With respect to idiopathic cardiomyopathy. *Shinzoh* **11**: 1082–89, 1979 (in Japanese).
37. Morimoto, S., Osamura, Y., Matsumura, K., Harada, M., Komatsu, Y., Hiroe, M., and Sekiguchi, M. On the incidence of giant negative T waves of the electrocardiograms among 34,000 population and a cardiac study including ventriculography and endomyocardial biopsy. *Kokyu To Junkan* **29**: 1337–46, 1981.
38. Morimoto, S. Incidence and clinical significance of giant negative T waves: A multidimensional study including endomyocardial biopsy. *J. Tokyo Wom. Med. Coll.* **51**: 1967–88, 1981.
39. Kudo, K. Histopathological study of the so-called apical hypertrophy type myocardial disease. *Nippon Naika Gakkai Zasshi* **71**: 1410–19, 1982 (in Japanese).
40. Morimoto, S., Sekiguchi, M., Hasumi, M., Inagaki, Y., Takimoto, H., Ohtsubo, K., Hiroe, M., Hirosawa, K., Matsuda, M., and Komatsu, Y. Do giant negative T waves represent apical hypertrophic cardiomyopathy? Left ventriculographic and cardiac biopsy studies. *J. Cardiogr.* **15** (suppl. VI): 35–51, 1985.
41. Fujii, J., Saihara, S., Sawada, H., Aizawa, T., and Kato, K. Distribution of left ventricular hypertrophy and electrocardiographic findings in patient with so-called apical hypertrophic cardiomyopathy. *J. Cardiogr.* **15** (suppl. VI): 23–33, 1985.
42. Koga, Y., Itaya, K., and Toshima, H. Prognosis in hypertrophic cardiomyopathy. *Am. Heart J.* **108**: 351–59, 1984.
43. Ryono, M. Left ventricular function and cardiac hypertrophy in the case of mild hypertension with marked ST-T changes in electrocardiogram. *J. Wakayama Med. Soc.* **32**: 151–64, 1981.
44. Suzuki, Y., Kadota, K., Nohara, R., Tamaki, S., Kambara, H., Yoshida, A., Murakami, T., Osakada, G., Kawai, C., Tamaki, N., Mukai, T., and Torizuka, K. Recognition of regional hypertrophy in hypertrophic cardiomyopathy using thallium-201 emission-computed tomography: Comoparison with two-dimensional echocardiography. *Am. J. Cardiol.* **53**: 1095–1102, 1984.
45. Fujiwara, S., Umemoto, M., Miyamoto, Y., Ota, A., Arita, M., Yokote, Y., Nakamura, Y., Ueno, Y., Nishio, I., and Masuyama, Y. The role of hypertension in apical hypertrophy. *J. Cardiogr.* **15** (suppl. VI): 53–64, 1985.
46. Kishimoto, C., Kadota, K., Nonogi, H., Sasayama, S., Matsumori, A., Sakurai, T., Wakabayashi, A., Kawai, C., Murakami, T., and Fujita, M. Interventricular septal configurations and motions in patients with hypertrophic cardiomyopathy by angled biventriculography. *J. Cardiogr.* **15** (suppl. VI): 13–21, 1985.
47. Spirito, P. Maron, B.J., Bonow, R.O., and Epstein, S.E. Occurrence and significance of progressive left ventricular wall thinning and relative cavity dilatation in hypertrophic cardiomyopathy. *Am. J. Cardiol.* **59**: 123–29, 1987.
48. Maron, B.J., Nichols, P.F., Pickle, L.W., Wesley, Y.E., and Mulvihill, J.J. Patterns of in-

heritance in hypertrophic cardiomyopathy: Assessment by M-mode and two-dimensional echocardiography. *Am. J. Cardiol.* **53**: 1087–94, 1984.

49. Kawai, C., Sakurai, T., Kishimoto, C., and Tomioka, S. Prognosis of idiopathic cardiomyopathy. Annual report of the idiopathic cardiomyopathy research committee, the Ministry of Health and Welfare of Japan. 63–66, 1983 (in Japanese).
50. Maron, B.J., Bonow, R.O., Cannon, R.O., Leon, M.B., and Epstein, S.E. Hypertrophic cardiomyopathy. Interrelations of clinical manifestations, pathophysiology, and therapy. *N. Engl. J. Med.* **316**: 780–89, 844–52, 1987.

INTRAVENTRICULAR PRESSURE GRADIENT

The Evidence for True Obstruction to Left Ventricular Outflow in Obstructive Hypertrophic Cardiomyopathy (Muscular or Hypertrophic Subaortic Stenosis)

E.D. Wigle, B.P. Kimball, Z. Sasson, and H. Rakowski

Division of Cardiology, Department of Medicine, Toronto General Hospital, University of Toronto, Toronto, Ontario, Canada

SUMMARY

In obstructive hypertrophic cardiomyopathy (muscular or hypertrophic subaortic stenosis), there is rapid early systolic ejection through an outflow tract that is narrowed by ventricular septal hypertrophy. This results in Venturi forces acting on the mitral leaflets, which cause mitral leaflet systolic anterior motion. Subsequent mitral leaflet-septal contact results in subaortic obstruction to left ventricular outflow and concomitant mitral regurgitation. Evidence is provided that the subaortic pressure gradient in obstructive hypertrophic cardiomyopathy reflects true obstruction to left ventricular outflow. Recent pulsed, continuous-wave, and color Doppler studies confirm this conclusion, which was previously based on clinical, echocardiographic, hemodynamic, and cineangiographic evidence. It is important to distinguish the truly obstructive subaortic pressure gradient due to mitral leaflet-septal contact from an early systolic impulse gradient as well as from the intraventricular pressure difference that may be encountered in midventricular obstruction or cavity obliteration.

INTRODUCTION

Hypertrophic cardiomyopathy (HCM) is characterized by symmetrical or asymmetrical hypertrophy of the left and/or right ventricles. It is a primary disorder of heart muscle, in which the site and extent of the hypertrophic process are believed to be of importance in determining the disease manifestations.[1] In this discussion, we will limit our remarks to the commonest form of HCM, which is associated with ventricular (asymmetrical) septal hypertrophy. It has been traditional to classify this form of HCM hemodynamically into obstructive and nonobstructive types, depending on whether or not there is a systolic pressure gradient across the left ventricular outflow tract, due to mitral leaflet-septal contact. In obstructive HCM, this pressure gradient may be persistent (gradient at rest), labile (spontaneously variable), or latent (provocable).[1,2] In discussing whether there is true obstruction to left ventricular outflow in obstructive HCM, we will focus our attention on the situation in which there is a persistent subaortic pressure gradient at rest.

TYPES OF SYSTOLIC PRESSURE DIFFERENCE IN HCM

Prior to reviewing the evidence for true obstruction to left ventricular outflow caused by mitral leaflet-septal contact in obstructive HCM, it is necessary to define the four different types of systolic pressure difference that may be encountered in HCM (Table 1, Fig. 1).[1,2] An early systolic impulse gradient across the aortic valve results from flow

TABLE 1. Differentiation of Intraventricular Pressure Differences That May be Encountered in Hypertrophic Cardiomyopathy

	Obstructive HCM	Cavity obliteration	Impulse gradient	Midventricular obstruction
Hemodynamics				
Elevated LV inflow pressure	+	–	+	–
Entrapment criteria*	–	+	–	–
Time of peak systolic gradient	Late	Late	Early	Late
Spike- and-dome aortic pressure	+	–	–	–
Spike- and-dome aortic flow	+	–	–	–
LV ejection time	Increased	Normal (or short)	Normal (or short)	Increased
Cineangiography				
Mitral leaflet-septal contact (ML-SC) (radiolucent line)	+	–	–	–
LV end-systolic volume	Variable	Small	Normal	Base small Apex Large
Mitral regurgitation (MR)	++	±	–	–
LV cavity obliteration	± Late if +	+ Early	–	–
Echocardiography				
1D				
Severe SAM	+	–	–	–
Left atrial enlargement	+	–	–	±
Aortic valve notch	+	–	–	–
2D				
Mitral leaflet-septal contact	+	–	–	–
Doppler				
LV peak velocity at	ML-SC ($\propto$pressure gradient)	Papillary muscle level (Late peak)	–	Midventricular ($\propto$pressure gradient)
Left atrium	Posteriorly directed MR	MR ±	–	MR ±
Clinical				
Apical murmur	3–4/6	0–2/6	±	2–4/6
Reversed split S_2	+	–	–	+

* See text. LV = left ventricle; SAM = systolic anterior motion of mitral leaflet; 1D and 2D = one- and two-dimensional echocardiography.

acceleration in early systole.[3] This gradient may be greater than normal in HCM, due to very rapid early systolic ejection, but it ends by mid-systole, when flow acceleration decreases.[3] A second type of systolic pressure difference within the left ventricle in HCM is that produced by midventricular obstruction at the level of the papillary muscles (Fig. 1, right).[1,2,4] This hemodynamic variant of HCM may occur with or without apical myocardial infarction and aneurysm formation.[1,4] In midventricular obstruction, the apical systolic pressure is elevated, but both the left ventricular inflow and outflow tract pressure are low and equal to aortic systolic pressure (Table 1, Fig. 1, right).[1,2,4] Left ventricular cineangiography reveals mid-cavity obliteration (occlusion)

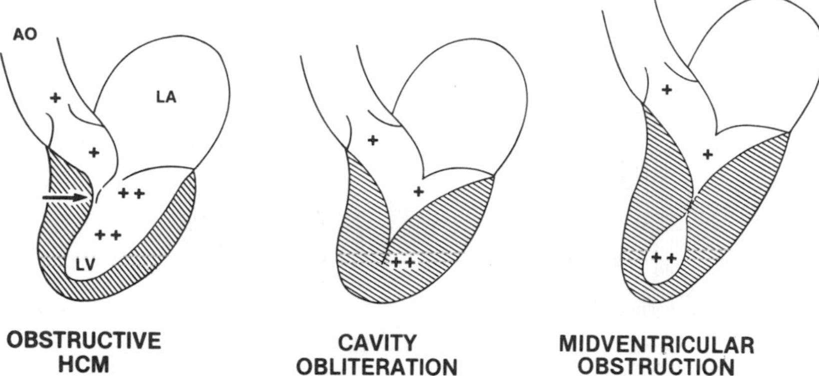

Fig. 1. The left ventricular (LV) inflow tract pressure concept.[7] In obstructive HCM, all LV pressures proximal to the outflow tract obstruction, caused by mitral leaflet-septal contact (arrow), are elevated, including the inflow tract pressure, just inside the mitral valve. In cavity obliteration and midventricular obstruction,[4] the pressure at the apex of the LV is elevated, but the inflow tract pressure is not (see text). AO = aorta; LA = left atrium.
Reproduced with permission from Wigle, E.D. and Rakowski, H. Z. *Kardiol.* **76**: suppl. 3, 61–68, 1987.

at the level of the papillary muscles. This cineangiographic appearance in midventricular obstruction must be distinguished from end-systolic papillary muscle approximation (without obstruction) that occurs in HCM when there is extensive left ventricular and papillary muscle hypertrophy. An impulse gradient and the gradient that occurs in midventriuclar obstruction should be readily recognized (Table 1).[1,4]

The third type of pressure difference that may be encountered in HCM is the intraventricular pressure difference that may be associated with cavity obliteration (Table 1, Fig. 1, center). In this situation the apical cavity obliteration occurs early in systole,[5] and the catheter recording the elevated apical systolic pressure is usually observed to be outside the end-systolic cineangiographic silhouette of the left ventricle.[5–7] The apical left ventricular pressure is elevated (Fig. 1, center), whereas all other pressures in the left ventricle, including the left ventricular inflow tract pressure, are low and equal to the outflow tract and aortic systolic pressures.[7] The intraventricular pressure difference of cavity obliteration is not associated with echocardiographic or cineangiographic evidence of mitral leaflet-septal contact (Table 1).[1,2]

The elevated apical systolic pressure in cavity obliteration was originally attributed to the apical catheter being enfolded,[6] engulfed,[6] or entrapped[7] by isometrically contracting myocardium in the obliterated apex of the ventricle. More recently, it has been suggested that the intraventricular pressure difference in cavity obliteration is the result of a high pressure being generated by the rapidly contracting apex, and that this pressure is somehow not transmitted to the hypocontractile base of the left ventricle.[8] However, Doppler velocity signals recorded at the junction between the rapidly contracting apex and the poorly contracting base (D in Fig. 2, right) do not correlate in time or magnitude with the measured intraventricular pressure difference.[2] Thus, it would seem most likely that the elevated left ventricular systolic pressure in cavity obliteration is due to the apical catheter being enfolded,[6] engulfed,[6] or entrapped[7] by isometrically

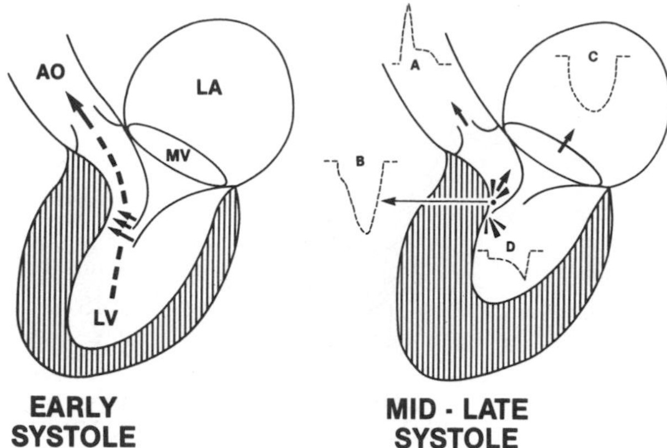

Fig. 2. Left: In obstructive HCM there is rapid, early systolic ejection (dashed line) through the outflow tract that is narrowed by septal hypertrophy. This results in Venturi forces (three short oblique arrows in the outflow tract) drawing the anterior (upper two arrows) and/or posterior (lower arrow) mitral leaflet(s) toward the septum (systolic anterior motion).[9] Subsequent mitral leaflet-septal contact results in obstruction to left ventricular (LV) outflow and concomitant mitral regurgitation, as seen on the right.
Right: By mid-systole, anterior mitral leaflet-septal contact causes obstruction to LV outflow resulting in a decreased forward aortic flow (smaller arrow) and mitral regurgitation (oblique arrow arising from the mitral orifice). Converging and diverging lines represent color flow imaging abnormalities at the site of obstruction[21,22] (see text and Fig. 5).

A, B, C, and D indicate Doppler velocity recordings throughout systole in the ascending aorta[15,26,29] (A) (flow toward the transducer); at the level of mitral leaflet-septal contact[1,11,19,20] (B); in the left atrium[1,11,22] (C); and near LV apex[11] (D). In B, C, and D, flow is away from the transducer. Peak velocities recorded at B correlate accurately with simultaneously measured obstructive subaortic pressure gradients,[1,11,19,20] whereas late peaking velocities at D do not. AO = aorta; LA = left atrium; MV = mitral valve; LV = left ventricle (see text).
Reproduced with permission of the American Heart Association, from Wigle, E.D., *Circulation* (Editorial) **75**:311–322, 1987.

contracting myocardium, as was originally suggested. In these circumstances, the high pressure recorded may be a reflection of intramyocardial tissue pressure.[7]

The fourth type of intraventricular pressure difference that may be encountered in HCM is the subaortic pressure gradient, due to mitral leaflet-septal contact in obstructive HCM (Fig. 1, left; Fig. 2; Table 1). In this situation (Fig. 1, left), the left ventricular outflow tract pressure, distal to mitral leaflet-septal contact (and proximal to the aortic valve) is low and equal to aortic systolic pressure, whereas all ventricular pressures proximal to the obstruction, including the left ventricular inflow tract pressure, just inside the mitral valve, are elevated.[7] This type of subaortic pressure gradient is associated with echocardiographic and cineangiographic evidence of mitral leaflet-septal contact (Fig. 1, left; Fig. 2, right; Fig. 3), and an elevated left ventricular inflow tract pressure (Fig. 1, left), whereas in cavity obliteration, or in midventricular obstruction, the left ventricular inflow tract pressure is not elevated (Fig. 1, center and right) and there is no evidence of mitral leaflet-septal contact(Table 1).[1,2,4,5,7] It is essential in the manage-

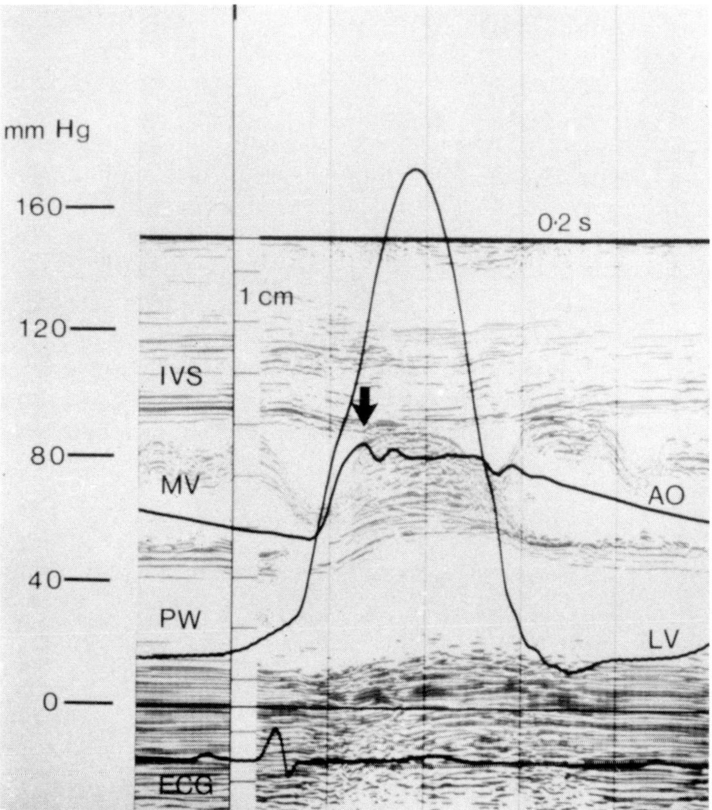

Fig. 3. Simultaneous hemodynamic and one-dimensional echocardiographic recordings in a patient with severe obstructive HCM (gradient = 86 mmHg). The arrow indicates the onset of mitral leaflet-septal contact and the onset of the pressure gradient (defined as the peak of the aortic percussion wave), which are virtually simultaneous. Note how early in systole the onset of mitral leaflet-septal contact and the pressure gradient occur in patients with severe outflow tract obstruction. IVS = interventricular septum; MV = mitral valve; PW = posterior wall; AO = central aortic pressure; LV = left ventricular pressure.
Reprinted with permission of the American Heart Association Inc., from Pollick *et al.*, *Circulation* **66**: 1087–1093, 1982.

ment of patients with HCM to distinguish an obstructive subaortic pressure gradient due to mitral leaflet-septal contact from the intraventricular pressure difference that may be associated with cavity obliteration or midventricular obstruction.[1,2,4,7)]

The remainder of this discussion will be directed at deciding whether the subaortic pressure gradient due to mitral leaflet-septal contact in obstructive HCM represents true obstruction to left ventricular outflow.

MECHANISM OF MITRAL LEAFLET SYSTOLIC ANTERIOR MOTION AND MITRAL LEAFLET-SEPTAL CONTACT IN OBSTRUCTIVE HCM

In 1971, we first suggested that mitral leaflet systolic anterior motion could result from Venturi forces acting on the mitral leaflets, due to the rapid nonobstructed early systolic ejection jet passing closer to the mitral leaflets than is normal, as a result of the outflow tract being narrowed by ventricular septal hypertrophy[9] (Fig. 2, left). Evidence in support of this concept is as follows[1,2,4]:

HCM patients with obstructive pressure gradients generally have a greater degree of subaortic septal hypertrophy and a narrower left ventricular outflow tract at the onset of systole than do patients without obstructive pressure gradients, setting the stage for the Venturi mechanism to be operative.[10]

Early systolic ejection in obstructive HCM is rapid and unobstructed before the onset of the pressure gradient (Fig. 2, left) and the velocity of ejection accelerates just before the onset of mitral leaflet systolic anterior motion.[11]

To test the hypothesis that mitral leaflet systolic anterior motion was caused by Venturi forces, Bellhouse and Bellhouse built a model of the left ventricle to resemble dynamic subaortic stenosis and were able to demonstrate mitral leaflet systolic anterior motion when the ejection velocities were rapid enough, as well as close enough to the mitral leaflets.[12]

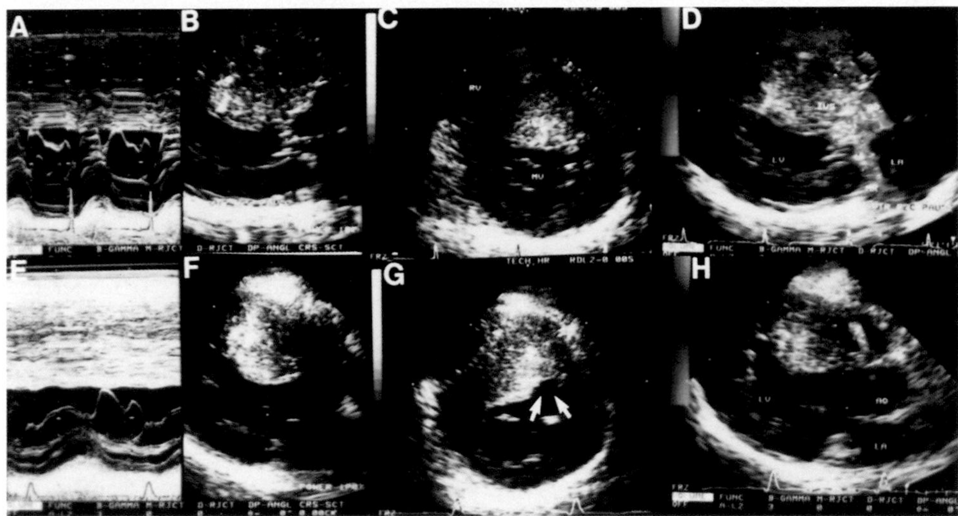

Fig. 4. Combined one- and two-dimensional echocardiographic and color Doppler study in a patient with obstructive HCM(A-D) who underwent successful ventriculomyectomy (E-H). Preoperatively, there was early and prolonged mitral leaflet-septal contact, as can be seen from the M-mode (A) and parasternal long axis (B) images. Circumferential extent of septal hypertrophy can be seen in parasternal short axis view, at the level of the mitral leaflects (C). Color flow imaging (D) revealed a high velocity outflow tract jet arising from the site of mitral leaflet-septal contact and an eccentric posteriorly directed jet of mitral regurgitation (MR) into the left atrium (LA). Postoperatively, the myectomy site can be seen (G, arrows), resulting in widening of the left ventricular (LV) outflow tract (F and G) with abolition of mitral leaflet-septal contact (E and F) and disappearance of the turbulent outflow tract and mitral regurgitation jets (H). Note the absence of cavity obliteration at the time of mitral leaflet-septal contact in B and D.
Reproduced with permission from Rakowski, H., *et al*., *J. Am. Soc. Echo*. **1**: 31–47, 1988.

Widening of the outflow tract by surgery (ventriculomyectomy) (Fig. 4) or increased preload (transfusion) reduces or abolishes mitral leaflet systolic anterior motion because the rapid early systolic ejection path is no longer in close proximity to the mitral leaflets.[1,2] Surgical widening of the lateral half of the left ventricular outflow tract will abolish systolic anterior motion of the lateral half of the anterior mitral leaflet, whereas systolic anterior motion remains in the medial half of the leaflet, where the outflow tract remains narrow.[1,2]

Any maneuver that changes the velocity of early systolic ejection will alter the degree of systolic anterior motion and hence the severity of the pressure gradient and mitral regurgitation. Thus, increased contractility (positive inotropes) or decreased afterload (vasodilators) increases this velocity and hence the severity of mitral leaflet systolic anterior motion, the pressure gradient, and mitral regurgitation. Decreased contractility (negative inotropes) and increased afterload (vasopressors) have the opposite effect by decreasing early systolic ejection velocity.[1,2]

The Venturi mechanism can also explain the occurrence of dynamic subaortic stenosis caused by mitral leaflet systolic anterior motion in hypovolemia, hyperkinetic states, tissue mitral valve prostheses, mitral anular calcification, and Carpentier ring valvuloplasty.[1,2] In each of these instances, the left ventricular outflow tract is narrowed, setting the stage for the Venturi mechanism to be operative. Elongated mitral leaflets and/or mitral leaflets displaced anteriorly by abnormally placed papillary muscles would be more subject to Venturi effects during early systolic ejection. The Venturi mechanism can also explain systolic anterior motion of the posterior mitral leaflet (Fig. 2, left).

Mitral leaflet systolic anterior motion has been attributed to contraction of malaligned papillary muscles and/or to posterior wall hyperkinesis or cavity obliteration.[8] If any of these contraction mechanisms were responsible for systolic anterior motion and mitral leaflet-septal contact, then maximal systolic anterior motion (mitral leaflet-septal contact) should remain until the end of contraction, i.e., until end-systole. Mitral leaflet-septal contact, however, ends about three-quarters of the way through systole, making these contraction mechanisms unlikely, if not untenable.[13] In addition, the rate of development of mitral leaflet systolic anterior motion is three times the rate of inward movement of the posterior wall of the left ventricle, and mitral leaflet-septal contact occurs over 200 milliseconds before maximal inward movement of the posterior wall.[13] These considerations would render it impossible for a hyperkinetic posterior wall, whether associated with cavity obliteration or not, to play any part in the genesis of mitral leaflet systolic anterior motion.[13]

Although there is considerable evidence to support the Venturi mechanism initiating mitral leaflet systolic anterior motion, it is presently unclear whether mitral leaflet-septal contact is maintained by continuing Venturi forces and/or by the left ventricular systolic pressure, proximal to the site of obstruction.[1,2]

EVIDENCE THAT MITRAL LEAFLET-SEPTAL CONTACT IS THE CAUSE OF THE OBSTRUCTIVE SUBAORTIC PRESSURE GRADIENT AND MITRAL REGURGITATION IN OBSTRUCTIVE HCM

HCM patients with severe systolic anterior motion with early and prolonged leaflet-septal contact have obstructive subaortic pressure gradients, whereas patients with moderate, mild, or no systolic anterior motion do not.[10,13]

Combined hemodynamic-echocardiographic[13,14] and hemodynamic-cineangiographic studies[5] reveal that the onset of the obstructive subaortic pressure gradient (defined as the peak of the aortic percussion wave) begins just before or simultaneously with the onset of echocardiographic or cineangiographic mitral leaflet-septal contact (Fig. 3). The mitral leaflet strikes the septum with considerable force, as is evidenced by the septal fibrotic plaque, the fibrous thickening on the ventricular surface of the mitral leaflet that strikes the septum, and the occasional occurrence of an audible sound at the onset of mitral leaflet-septal contact.[1,2]

A number of characteristic features of obstructive HCM occur in close time proximity to the onset of mitral leaflet-septal contact: the peak of the aortic percussion wave,[5,13,14] the onset of flow deceleration in the ascending aorta,[15] the point of inflexion on the rising left ventricular pressure tracing[16] and on the continuous wave Doppler recording from the level of mitral leaflet-septal contact, the onset of partial aortic valve closure, as well as an abrupt mid-systolic slowing of left ventricular emptying[17] and velocity of inward left ventricular wall movement.[18] This combination of near simultaneous events strongly suggests a sudden alteration of systolic hemodynamics, i.e., the onset of outflow tract obstruction.[1,2]

The time of onset in systole of mitral leaflet-septal contact determines the magnitude of the obstructive pressure gradient, the degree of prolongation of left ventricular ejection time, the degree of mitral regurgitation, and the percentage of left ventricular stroke volume that is ejected in the presence of the obstruction.[1,14] Thus, early and prolonged mitral leaflet-septal contact is associated with a high pressure gradient, marked prolongation of the left ventricular ejection time, a significant amount of mitral regurgitation, and a large percentage of left ventricular stroke volume ejected against the obstruction. In contrast, mitral leaflet-septal contact of late onset and short duration is associated with a small pressure gradient, mild prolongation of left ventricular ejection time, a lesser degree of mitral regurgitation, and only a small percentage of left ventricular stroke volume ejected against the obstruction. If mitral leaflet-septal contact occurs after 55% of the systolic ejection period,[1] or if the duration of mitral leaflet-septal contact is less than 30% of echocardiographic systole,[10] no pressure gradient develops.

Recently, pulsed,[1,11] continuous-wave,[11,19,20] and color[19,21,22] Doppler studies have provided important new confirmatory evidence that the site of the obstruction, and hence the origin of the pressure gradient in obstructive HCM, is at the level of mitral leaflet-septal contact (Fig. 2, right; Figs. 4–6). Pulsed and continuous-wave Doppler techniques permit accurate measurement of the peak flow velocity across a stenotic orifice, allowing calculation of the pressure gradient by the modified Bernoulli equation ($PG = 4 \times \text{peak velocity}^2$).[11] Both pulsed Doppler and sequential continuous-wave and color Doppler studies in obstructive HCM localize the origin of the high outflow tract velocities to the site of mitral leaflet-septal contact[1,11,19–22] (B in Fig. 2, right; Figs. 4–6). When pressure gradients are derived from these peak flow velocities across the outflow tract in obstructive HCM, there is a highly significant correlation with the simultaneously measured hemodynamic pressure gradients, whether recorded in the heart catheterization laboratory[1,20] or intraoperatively.[19] This close correlation between flow velocity measured by pulsed or continuous-wave Doppler and the simultaneously measured pressure gradient represent strong confirmatory evidence of the obstructive nature of the left ventricular outflow tract pressure gradient in HCM. These same strong correlations between flow velocity and pressure are present in valvular aortic stenosis.

Color Doppler studies demonstrate two other important features in obstructive HCM: (A) acceleration of the jet just proximal to the obstruction, i.e., mitral leaflet-septal contact (in valvular aortic stenosis the jet accelerates just proximal to the valve), and

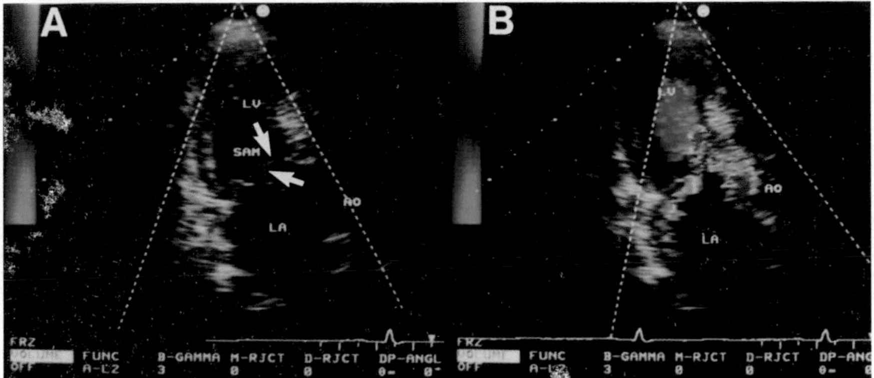

Fig. 5. Panels A and B are apical long axis views with and without color flow imaging in a patient with obstructive HCM. In panel A, two arrows indicate the site of mitral leaflet-septal contact with marked narrowing of the left ventricular (LV) outflow tract. In panel B, ejection dynamics can be better understood with color flow imaging. Flow toward the transducer is shown in red, and flow away from the transducer is in blue, with brighter hues indicating higher velocity of flow. There is acceleration of flow just proximal to the site of mitral leaflet-septal contact, with blue outflow becoming brighter and finally aliasing. At the site of mitral leaflet-septal contact, the outflow jet is narrowed and then diverges into two turbulent high-velocity jets, one directed toward the posterior outflow tract and the other an eccentric posteriorly directed jet of mitral regurgitation that is layered along the posterior left atrial wall and might easily be underestimated by pulsed Doppler studies alone. Note large LV systolic size at the time of mitral leaflet-septal contact, i.e., there is no cavity obliteration at the time of the development of obstruction to LV outflow.
Reproduced with permission from Rakowski H., *et al.*, *J. Am. Soc. Echo* **1**: 31–47, 1988.

(B) significant systolic narrowing of the jet at the level of mitral leaflet-septal contact, presumably caused by mitral leaflet systolic anterior motion[21,22] (Fig. 2, right; Fig. 5).

Mitral regurgitation invariably accompanies the obstructive subaortic pressure gradient in obstructive HCM, and in the absence of an independent mitral valve abnormality, the severity of the obstruction and the mitral leak are directly related to the degree of mitral leaflet systolic anterior motion[1,2,23] (Figs. 2, 4, 5). Both cineangiography[1] and color Doppler[22] studies reveal an eject/obstruct/leak sequence in systole, i.e., there is rapid unobstructed early systolic ejection into the aorta (Fig. 2, left), the onset of mitral leaflet septal contact, and the obstruction (Figs. 2, 4, 5), followed by posteriorly directed, predominantly mid-to late systolic mitral regurgitation (Figs. 4, 5), which is a principle determinant of the end-systolic size of the left ventricle.[1] A decrease or abolition of mitral leaflet systolic anterior motion by pharmacological or surgical means results in a decrease or abolition of both the outflow obstruction and mitral regurgitation[1,2,23] (Fig. 4).

The presence of an independent mitral valve abnormality in obstructive HCM often results in the mitral regurgitation becoming pansystolic and more severe[1,2,23] (Fig. 6).

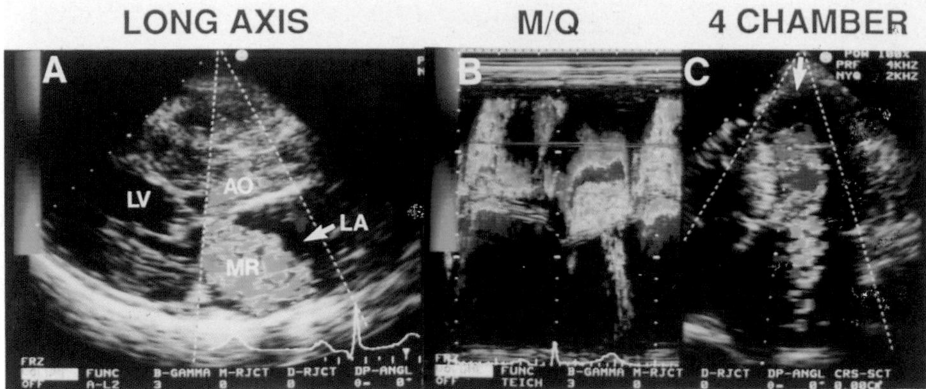

Fig. 6. Study from a patient with severe obstructive HCM and severe mitral regurgitation, some of which was independent of the outflow tract obstruction. Panel A is a parasternal long axis view, showing severe mitral leaflet-septal contact (to left of color sector) with turbulent left ventricular (LV) outflow tract and aortic (AO) jet, and severe mitral regurgitation (MR) directed toward posterior left atrial (LA) wall. Panel B is a color M-mode study taken from an apical four-chamber view with the color M-mode line highlighted by the white arrow in panel C. Flow toward transducer is shown in red and flow away in blue. Depth at which flow velocity is shown on the M-mode corresponds to its position on simultaneous four-chamber view in panel C. Systolic flow at midventricular level is homogenously blue and thus laminar. As flow approaches area of outflow obstruction at the site of mitral leaflet-septal contact, alaising to red occurs over a depth of 1 cm. Obstructed area of outflow tract then has mosaic pattern indicative of turbulent flow within it. Systolic timing of events can be made with reference to electrocardiogram in panel B. In very early systole, there is a narrow band of blue flow, with a brief duration of alaising to red, followed by turbulent flow, indicating early development of turbulent flow, which was timed with the onset of mitral leaflet-septal contact. Note the absence of cavity obliteration in panels A and C in the presence of outflow tract obstruction as indicated by mitral leaflet-septal contact.

Reproduced with permission from Rakowski, H., *et al.*, *J. Am. Soc. Echo.* **1**: 31–47, 1988.

EVIDENCE OF TRUE OBSTRUCTION TO LEFT VENTRICULAR OUTFLOW DUE TO MITRAL LEAFLET-SEPTAL CONTACT IN OBSTRUCTIVE HCM

1. Elevation of All Ventricular Systolic Pressures Proximal to Mitral Leaflet-Septal Contact

As in the case with valvular aortic stenosis, in obstructive HCM, all ventricular systolic pressures proximal to the subaortic obstruction caused by mitral leaflet-septal contact are elevated, including the left ventricular inflow tract pressure (Fig. 1, left).[1,2,4,7,24] Catheters recording these high pressures can be freely moved about within the left ventricular cavity without altering the high systolic pressures, and indeed multiple catheters may be placed in the left ventricle proximal to the obstruction, and equally elevated pressures are recorded.[7,24] When the proximal end of these catheters is open, blood "shoots out" in systole, indicating that the distal tip of the catheter is in a high pressure, blood-filled area of the left ventricle.[7)]

2. Prolongation of Left Ventricular Ejection Time

One of the most characteristic features of any form of obstruction to left ventricular outflow is a prolongation of left ventricular ejection time. We have previously demonstrated that the degree of prolongation of left ventricular ejection time in obstructive HCM is directly related to the magnitude of the pressure gradient[25)] and that both are related to the time of onset of mitral leaflet-septal contact in systole.[1,14)] This direct relationship between the magnitude of the pressure gradient and the degree of prolongation of left ventricular ejection time is maintained whether the gradient is increased or decreased by pharmacological or surgical means.[1)] Some authors, who have adopted a nonobstructive viewpoint of obstructive HCM, have suggested that the prolonged ejection time is related to impairment of left ventricular relaxation.[3,8)] However, prolongation of left ventricular ejection time does not occur in nonobstructive HCM with impairment of left ventricular relaxation. A prolonged ejection time only occurs in obstructive HCM and the degree of prolongation is related to the severity of the obstruction, as is the case with valvular aortic stenosis.[1,25)]

3. Percentage of Left Ventricular Stroke Volume Ejected in the Presence of the Obstructive Subaortic Pressure Gradient

It is recognized that there is rapid, nonobstructed early systolic ejection in obstructive HCM (Fig. 2, left). If this were not the case, there would be no Venturi effect to cause mitral leaflet systolic anterior motion.[9)] The question to be answered here is: What percentage of left ventricular stroke volume leaves the left ventricle after the onset of mitral leaflet-septal contact and the pressure gradient? No fewer than five different techniques have been used to study this question, and the results are very similar. Thus, cineangiographic,[1)] echocardiographic,[15)] combined micromanometric and nuclear angiographic,[16)] as well as Doppler[26)] and electromagnetic[24,27)] flow studies have indicated that between 40% and 70% of left ventricular stroke volume leaves the left ventricle after the onset of the mitral leaflet-septal contact and/or the subaortic pressure gradient. With the onset of the obstruction to outflow, the calculated resistance across the outflow tract increases dramatically[28)] and this is accompanied by a sudden deceleration in ascending aortic flow,[15,29)] a decrease in the rate of left ventricular emptying,[17)] and a sudden decrease in inward left ventricular wall motion.[18)] Ascending aortic and left ventricular outflow tract velocity flow studies indicate continued but reduced ejection into the left ventricular outflow tract and aorta (A and B in Fig. 2, right; Figs. 4–6) during the presence of the subaortic pressure gradient.[26,30)] Cineangiographic[1,31)] as well as color[21,22)] and continuous wave[11)] Doppler studies (C in Fig. 2, right) indicate that the major portion of mitral regurgitation occurs in the last half of systole, after the onset of mitral leaflet-septal contact and the subaortic obstruction. Thus, there is overwhelming evidence to indicate that a very significant percentage of left ventricular stroke volume leaves the left ventricle as forward or regurgitant flow during the presence of the obstructive subaortic pressure gradient. The actual percentage of left ventricular stroke volume that is ejected in the presence of the subaortic obstruction is determined by the time of onset of mitral leaflet-septal contact in systole, which also determines the magnitude of the pressure gradient, the amount of mitral regurgitation, and the degree of prolongation of left ventricular ejection time?[1,14)]

This systolic overload is not only of hemodynamic importance in obstructive HCM, but is also of metabolic and clinical significance (see below).

4. Myocardial Ischemia Associated with Obstructive Subaortic Pressure Gradients in Obstructive HCM

In patients with obstructive HCM, large pressure gradients are associated with increased myocardial oxygen consumption and metabolic evidence of myocardial ischemia during pacing. Surgical abolition of the pressure gradient results in a marked reduction in myocardial oxygen consumption and alleviation of myocardial ischemia. These observations are consistent with the elevated left ventricular systolic pressure causing increased myocardial oxygen consumption and resulting in myocardial ischemia.[32]

5. Symptoms Related to the Presence of the Obstructive Subaortic Pressure Gradient

Although it is recognized that HCM patients with and without obstructive pressure gradients may have similar symptoms, we have recently reported that patients with obstructive HCM have a significantly higher incidence of class III-IV New York Heart Association symptomatology, as well as a significantly higher overall incidence of angina and dyspnea.[1] Patients with obstructive pressure gradients also have a significantly higher incidence of grade III-IV/VI apical systolic murmurs and reversed splitting of the second heart sound. These observations provide evidence that the obstructive pressure gradients in HCM are not only of hemodynamic and metabolic significance, but also of profound clinical significance and are in keeping with the dramatic clinical benefits derived from a successful ventriculomyectomy operation (Fig. 4).

6. A Brief Comment on the Nonobstructive Viewpoint in HCM

The nonobstructive viewpoint suggests that left ventricular emptying in HCM occurs faster and more completely than normal, that an intraventricular pressure difference develops between the rapidly contracting apex and poorly contracting base of the left ventricle, and that forward aortic flow and left ventricular emptying virtually cease well before end-systole, i.e., the left ventricle is essentially isovolumetric during the last half of systole.[8] Mitral leaflet-septal contact is attributed to left ventricular cavity obliteration, right up to the submitral area.[8]

Although superficially plausible, this nonobstructive viewpoint does not stand up to careful scrutiny[1,2,4]: (1) The authors make no attempt to distinguish the subaortic pressure gradient due to mitral leaflet-septal contact in obstructive HCM from the intraventricular pressure difference that may be encountered in cavity obliteration (Fig. 1). (2) Doppler flow velocity studies (D in Fig. 2, right) do not support the concept that an early pressure gradient develops between the rapidly contracting apex and poorly contracting base of the left ventricle, but Doppler studies do provide conclusive evidence that the subaortic pressure gradient in obstructive HCM arises at the site of mitral leaflet-septal contact (B in Fig. 2, right; Figs. 4–6). (3) Although catheter-mounted velocity flow probe studies suggest that in late systole there is no significant forward aortic flow in obstructive or nonobstructive HCM,[3] four other methods of investigating forward aortic flow in obstructive HCM have failed to confirm this finding.[15,24,26–30] These other methods indicate that there is a rapid deceleration of ascending aortic flow in early systole that occurs virtually simultaneously with the onset of mitral leaflet-septal contact.[15] Subsequently, there is reduced but definite forward aortic flow throughout the rest of systole[29] (A in Fig. 2, right). Both continuous wave[33] and multigated[29] Doppler studies in obstructive HCM reveal that ascending aortic flow is very nonuniform after the onset of the obstruction. Multigated studies reveal cessation of forward aortic flow prior to the end of systole near the posterior aortic wall, whereas forward flow continues near the anterior aortic wall.[29] These observations dictate extreme caution in the interpretation of aortic velocity-flow measurements when they are recorded from a single aortic site by a technique such as a catheter-mounted velocity flow probe.[3] (4) The nonobstructive viewpoint suggests that mitral leaflet systolic anterior motion and subsequent mitral leaflet-septal contact is due to cavity obliteration of the submitral area of the left ventricle, i.e., very little left ventricular emptying occurs after the onset of mitral leaflet septal contact. However, we have shown that mitral leaflet systolic anterior motion bears no relation to the inward motion of the left ventricular posterior wall or to cavity obliteration,[1,13] and that mitral leaflet-septal contact occurs about 200 milliseconds prior to minimal left ventricular diameter.[13] In addition, large obstructive pressure gradients due to mitral leaflet-septal contact have been observed to occur in the absence of any cavity obliteration[1] (Figs. 4–6). Finally a number of studies have documented that a significant percentage of left ventricular emptying into the aorta and left atrium occurs after the onset of mitral leaflet-septal contact and the obstructive pressure gradient, i.e., the left ventricle is not isovolumetric during the last half of systole,[1,15,16,26–29] as suggested by those holding the nonobstructive viewpoint.[8]

CONCLUSIONS

As a result of the foregoing analysis, one can only conclude that true obstruction to left ventricular outflow does exist in obstructive HCM and is caused by prolonged mitral leaflet-septal contact. Recent pulsed, continuous-wave, multigated, and color Doppler studies only reinforce this conclusion, which was previously based on clinical, phonocardiographic, echocardiographic, hemodynamic, and cineangiographic evidence. Appropriate care must continue to be exercised in distinguishing the subaortic pressure gradient in obstructive HCM from the intraventricular pressure difference encountered in cavity obliteration or in midventricular obstruction. Fortunately, there are now clinical and echo-Doppler criteria that permit clear distinction between these different types of intraventricular pressure difference in HCM without resorting to invasive studies. The latter should be reserved for diagnostic problems and/or when surgery is being considered.

To deny the presence of true obstruction to left ventricular outflow in obstructive HCM is to deny these patients appropriate medical and/or surgical therapy.

Acknowledgments

This work was supported in part by the Heart & Stroke Foundation of Ontario and the Canadian Heart Foundation.

REFERENCES

1. Wigle, E.D., Sasson, Z., Henderson, M.A., Ruddy, T.D., Fulop, J., Rakowski, H., and Williams, W.G. Hypertrophic cardiomyopathy. The importance of the site and the extent of hypertrophy. A review. *Prog. Cardiovasc. Dis.* **28**: 1–83, 1985.
2. Wigle, E.D. Hypertrophic cardiomyopathy. A 1987 viewpoint. (editorial) *Circulation* **75**: 311–322, 1987.
3. Murgo, J.P., Alter, B.R., Dorethy, J. F., Altobelli, S.A., and McGranahan, G.M., Jr. Dynamics of left ventricular ejection in obstructive and nonobstructive hypertrophic cardiomyopathy. *J. Clin. Invest.* **66**: 1369–1382, 1980.

4. Wigle, E.D. and Rakowski, H. Evidence for true obstruction to left ventricular outflow in obstructive hypertrophic cardiomyopathy (muscular or hypertrophic subaortic stenosis). *Z. Kardiol.* **76**: 61–68, 1987.
5. Grose, R.M., Strain, J.E., and Spindola-Franco, H. Angiographic and hemodynamic correlations in hypertrophic cardiomyopathy. *Am. J. Cardiol.* **58**: 1085–1092, 1986.
6. Criley, M.J., Lewis, K.S., White, R.I., and Ross, R.S. Pressure gradients without obstruction: a new concept of "hypertrophic subaortic stenosis." *Circulation* **22**: 881–887, 1965.
7. Wigle, E.D., Marquis, Y., and Auger, P. Muscular subaortic stenosis: Initial left ventricular inflow tract pressure in the assessment of intraventriuclar pressure differences in man. *Circulation* **35**: 1100–1117, 1967.
8. Criley, M.J. and Seigel, R.J. Has 'obstruction' hindered our understanding of hypertrophic cardiomyopathy? *Circulation* **72**: 1148–1154, 1985.
9. Wigle, E.D., Adelman, A.G., and Silver, M.D. Pathophysiological considerations in muscular subaortic stenosis. In: Wolstenholme GEW, O'Connor, M. (eds.), Hypertrophic Obstructive Cardiomyopathy. Ciba Foundation Study Group 47. London, pp. 63–76, 1971.
10. Gilbert, B.W., Pollick, C., Adelman, A.G., and Wigle, E.D. Hypertrophic cardiomyopathy: Subclassification by M-Mode echocardiography. *Am. J. Cardiol.* **45**: 861, 1980.
11. Hatle, L. and Angelsen, B. (eds.) Doppler ultrasound in cardiology. Philadelphia, Lea & Febiger, pp. 205–217, 1985.
12. Bellhouse, B.J. and Bellhouse, F.H. The fluid mechanics of subaortic stenosis in a model left ventricle. University of Oxford, Department of Engineering Science, Report No. 1032/72, 1982.
13. Pollick, C., Gilbert, B.W., Rakowski, H., Morgan, C.D., and Wigle, E.D. Muscular subaortic stenosis: The temporal relationship between systolic anterior motion of the anterior mitral leaflet and the pressure gradient. *Circulation* **66**: 1087, 1982.
14. Pollick, C., Rakowski, H., and Wigle, E.D. Muscular subaortic stenosis: The quantitative relationship between systolic anterior motion and the pressure gradient. *Circulation* **69**: I-43, 1984.
15. Glasgow, G.A., Gardin, J.M., Burns, C.S., Childs, W.J., and Henry, W.L. Echocardiographic and Doppler flow observations in idiopathic hypertrophic subaortic stenosis (IHSS). *Circulation* **62**: III–99, 1980 (abstr.).
16. Bonow, R.O., Ostrow, H.G., Rosing, D.R., Cannon, R.O., Leon, M.B., Watson, R.M., Bacharach, S.L., Green, M.V., and Epstein, S.E. Dynamic pressure-volume alterations during left ventricular ejection in hypertrophic cardiomyopathy: Evidence for true obstruction to left ventricular outflow. *Circulation* **70**: II–17, 1984 (abstr.).
17. Bonow, R.O., Crawford-Green, C., Betocci, S., Rosing, D.R., and Maron, B.J. Left ventricular ejection dynamics in hypertrophic cardiomyopathy: Comparison with valvular aortic stenosis. *J. Am. Coll. Cardiol.* **5**: 394, 1985 (abstr.).
18. Pouleur, H., Van Eyll, C., Gurne, O., Hanet, C., and Rousseau, M.F. Regional velocity of shortening in hypertrophic cardiomyopathy: Evidence for true impedance to shortening in the presence of outflow gradients. *Circulation* **72**: III–448, 1985 (abstr.).
19. Stewart, W.J., Schiavone, W.A., Salcedo, E.E., Lever, H.M., Cosgrove, D.M., and Grill, C.C. Intraoperative Doppler velocity correlates with outflow gradient in HOCM pre- and postmyectomy. *Circulation* **72**: III–447, 1985 (abstr.).
20. Sasson, Z., Yock, P.G., Hatle, L.K., Alderman, E.L., and Popp, R. Non-invasive determination of the pressure gradient in hypertrophic cardiomyopathy. *Circulation* **74**: II–215, 1986 (abstr.).
21. Holt, B., Sahn, D.J., Dalton, N., Smith, S.C., Yun, Y., and Dittrich, H. Color Doppler flow mapping studies of jet formation in hypertrophic cardiomyopathy (HCM). *Circulation* **72**: III–447, 1985 (abstr.).
22. Rakowski, H., Sasson, Z., and Wigle, E.D. Echocardiographic and Doppler Assessment of hypertrophic cardiomyopathy. *J. Am. Soc. Echo.* **1**: 31–47, 1988.

23. Wigle, E.D., Adelman, A.G., Auger, P., and Marquis, Y. Mitral regurgitation in muscular subaortic stenosis. *Am. J. Cardiol.* **24**: 698–706, 1969.
24. Ross, J. Jr., Braunwald, E., Gault, J.H., Mason, D.T., and Morrow, A.G. The mechanism of the intraventricular pressure gradient in idiopathic hypertrophic subaortic stenosis. *Circulation* **43**: 558–578, 1966.
25. Wigle, E.D., Auger, P., and Marquis, Y. Muscular subaortic stenosis: The direct relation between the intraventricular pressure gradient and left ventricular ejection time. *Circulation* **36**: 36–44, 1967.
26. Maron, B.J., Gottdiener, J.S., Arce, J., Rosing, D.R., Wesley, Y.E., and Epstein, S.E. Dynamic subaortic obstruction in hypertrophic cardiomyopathy: analysis by pulsed Doppler echocardiography. *J. Am. Coll. Cardiol.* **6**: 1–15, 1985.
27. Pierce, G.E., Morrow, A.G., and Braunwald, E. Idiopathic hypertrophic subaortic stenosis III. Intraoperative studies of the mechanism of obstruction and its hemodynamic consequences. *Circulation* **30**: IV, 152–207, 1964.
28. Bircks, W., Bostroem, B., Gleichmann, U., Kreuzer, H., and Loogen, F. Electromagnetic flow measurement in the ascending aorta before and after repair of valvular and subvalvular lesions including IHSS. Proceedings of the Vth European Congress of Cardiology (Athens), pp. 13–22, 1968.
29. Jenni, R., Ruffmann, K., Vieli, A., Anlinker, M., and Krayenbuehl, H.P. Dynamics of aortic flow in hypertrophic cardiomyopathy. *Eur. Heart J.* **6**: 391–398, 1985.
30. Hernandez, R.R., Greenfield, J.C. Jr., and McCall, B.W. Pressure-flow studies in hypertrophic subaortic stenosis. *J. Clin. Invest.* **43**: 401–407, 1964.
31. Adelman, A.G., McLoughlin, M.J., Marquis, Y., Auger, P., and Wigle, E.D. Left ventricular cineangiographic observations in muscular subaortic stenosis. *Am. J. Cardiol.* **24**: 689, 1969.
32. Cannon, R.O., Rosing, D.R., McIntosh, C.L., and Epstein, S.E. Hypertrophic cardiomyopathy (HCM): Improved hemodynamics, metabolism, and anginal threshold following surgical relief of obstruction. *Circulation* **72**: III–447 (abstr.).
33. Yock, P.G., Hatle, L., and Popp, R.L. Dispersion of high-velocity left ventricular outflow jets in hypertrophic obstructive cardiomyopathy. *J. Am. Coll. Cardiol.* **5**: II–394 (abstr.), 1985.

The Influence of the Brock Bias on Our Current Understanding of Hypertrophic Cardiomyopathy

John Michael Criley, Robert J. Siegel,* and Peter C.D. Pelikan***

* Divisions of Cardiology at Harbor-UCLA Medical Center and Cedars-Sinai Medical Center, and the Saint John's Heart Institute, U.S.A.

** Clinician-Scientist of the American Heart Association, Greater Los Angeles Affiliate, U.S.A.

The Brock Bias

When the entity now commonly called hypertrophic cardiomyopathy was first brought to the attention of the readership of cardiology literature in the late 1950s it stimulated a rapid multinational quest for knowledge about this previously unappreciated cardiac disorder. Its discovery and characterization were byproducts of three newly emerging technologies: left heart catheterization, selective angiography, and cardiac surgery. Although the condition was initially described by a cardiac surgeon, Russell Brock, it was his hemodynamic findings and not his surgical explorations that were responsible for the indelible characterization of the disease as a form of functional or dynamic left ventricular outflow tract obstruction.[1,2]

Brock did not question or temper his conviction that an outflow tract obstruction was present despite some disturbing and compelling evidence to the contrary which he summarized in this enigmatic statement: "The functional nature of the obstruction is concealed in death. Indeed it is concealed in life unless we are able to document its presence with a pressure withdrawal record." The concealment of the "nature of the obstruction" occurred when he tried to localize the "obstruction" in the beating heart with bougies and expanding dilators which "encountered no obstruction."[1,2]

Investigators who followed Brock's seminal investigations did not question the wisdom of Brock's conclusion that the pressure gradient in the left ventricle was sole and sufficient proof to confirm the presence of an obstruction to outflow. The large body of literature on the disease that followed Brock's confirmed this indelible conviction. Over 40 names for the condition were coined, the vast majority promulgating the unquestioned presence and importance of "obstruction" in the pathophysiology of the disease.

It is the purpose of this chapter to suggest that the readers consider what our understanding of this disease entity might now be if the same body of investigations that occurred in the last three decades were not biased by Brock's predominant conviction that gradient = obstruction. It is our belief that investigations that preceded Brock's, had they been more widely publicized, might have led to an entirely different perception of hypertrophic cardiomyopathy.

The Gauer-Henry Phenomenon

During and after World War II, Otto Gauer, a German investigator was concerned with the causes and prevention of blackouts in aviators resulting from centrifugal force encountered during high speed aircraft maneuvers. Following expatriation to the United States he continued his work at the aerospace facility at Wright-Patterson Field in Dayton, Ohio with Dr. James P. Henry. In the course of their investigations on experimental animals subjected to negative gravitational forces along the long axis of the body (-Gz) they found that the body of the left ventricle generated high pressures while the aortic pressure was markedly reduced. Cineangiocardiograms obtained during generation of these pressure differences revealed that the ventricle emptied rapidly and completely, so that "... the ventricle continues to contract after having expelled its pathologically small blood content." Left ventricular pressure gradients were also noted to occur during hemorrhagic shock. The pulse contours from these experiments resemble those of hypertrophic cardiomyopathy: the aortic pressures have a rapid upstroke followed by a rapid decline while the left ventricular pressure rises generating the largest gradient in mid and late systole.[3,4]

These investigators therefore described and characterized a nonobstructive mechanism responsible for intraventricular pressure differences resulting from the antithesis of obstruction, namely a gradient that is generated by the excessively rapid and complete emptying of the left ventricle (cavity obliteration). Because many of these experiments were withheld from publication because of their classified (military secret) nature, they were published in abstract form in 1950, and more fully in 1964.[3,4]

Brock's Observations Revisited

Let us now return to Brock's observations in 1957 and 1959. Had he realized that a hypercontractile left ventricle with a pathologically small cavity size could generate an intracavitary gradient would he have concluded, despite his inability to find an obstruction in the beating heart, that a pressure gradient was tantamount to obstruction? Contemporaneously, in 1958 Teare described the autopsy findings in 9 young patients, 8 of whom had died suddenly and were found to have asymmetrical hypertrophy of the heart with pathologically small ventricular cavitary volumes. He was not prejudiced by hemodynamic data and therefore did not invoke "outflow tract obstruction" as the cause for the inordinate hypertrophy and sudden death in these patients.[5]

The Angiographic "Cone" and the "Contraction Ring"

Studies that followed Brock's were clearly influenced by his conviction that pressure gradients within the left ventricle were sufficient proof that the ventricle was obstructed. This conviction was so prevalent that ventricular angiocardiograms demonstrating an hourglass, conical narrowing of the mid ventricle were portrayed as "systolic" frames.[6,7] The closed aortic valve and open mitral valve (responsible for the conical narrowing) in these published figures unequivocally confirm that these were in fact diastolic frames.[8] Would these misinterpretations have occurred if there was not a need to confirm by angiocardiography that the gradient was associated with an "obstruction?"

The Brock bias was also manifest in later characterizations by surgeons who attributed the "obstruction" to a muscular sphincter or "contraction ring" that firmly gripped their exploring fingers. Some of these descriptions leave no doubt of the nature of this "obstruction" when encountered by passing a finger through the aortic valve. Morrow stated: "Forceful contraction of the outflow tract on the exploring finger is evident during systole."[6] Dobell was even more dramatic: "That this obstruction is dynamic is immediately appreciated by the surgeon who passes his finger through the obstruction in a beating heart. The compression around the finger is nothing short of painful."[9] Julian, who entered the ventricle from the apex made the following observations: "Upon making a small apical ventriculotomy, palpation with the finger of the ventricular chamber showed a small apical chamber. During systole, the musculature of the outflow tract contracted over a long segment, squeezing the operator's finger to a degree which could only be duplicated with some effort within the fist of the other hand."[10] Had these surgeons been aware of Gauer and Henry's experiments they might have entertained the possibility that the pressure gradients were generated by "... the ventricle (which) continues to contract after having expelled its pathologically small blood content."[3,4] However, the angiographic "cone" and Brock's bias greatly influenced their conclusion that a muscular "contraction ring" was responsible for the gradient and that an operation analogous to a pyloroplasty for hypertrophic pyloric stenosis was indicated.[6,11]

The New Mechanism of "Obstruction"

The reader of the current articles on hypertrophic cardiomyopathy may well wonder what happened to this "contraction ring" which was so indelibly described during the first decade of investigations about hypertrophic cardiomyopathy. This mythical entity was replaced in the mid 1960s by mitral-septal apposition, an event that would be unlikely to produce "... compression around the finger (that) is nothing short of painful."[9] This new site and mechanism of "obstruction" is thought to result from Venturi forces generated by high velocity outflow which cause the mitral valve to contact the interventricular septum and thus narrow or occlude the outflow tract.[12,13]

This concept is supported by several observations which have resulted from echo and Doppler ultrasonographic studies. The presence and duration of contact between the mitral valve and septum can be correlated with the presence and magnitude of the pressure gradient,[14] and the timing of the onset of the pressure gradient can be correlated with the timing of mitral-septal contact.[12,13] Doppler studies have demonstrated high velocity outflow in the left ventricle anterior to the mitral valve, and Doppler-derived pressure gradients correlate with hemodynamic measurements.[15,16] It is now conceded that not only can one equate pressure gradients with "obstruction", but the presence of mitral septal apposition can be equated with "obstruction" as well.

Evidence That the Ventricle is Not Obstructed

An obstruction is by definition an impediment or hindrance. The ventricle in hypertrophic cardiomyopathy does not exhibit any discernable impediment or hindrance to emptying when studied by radionuclide or contrast angiography and echocardiography.[17–20] The left ventricle is able to empty more rapidly and to a greater degree than a normal ventricle.[18] When the ejection characteristics of a hypertrophic cardiomyopathy ventricle are compared before and after the provocation of a gradient, it empties more rapidly and more completely when the gradient is present.[19] This response is the antithesis of what would be expected if an obstruction were responsible for the gradient.

Conversely, when the ejection pattern in aortic stenosis is compared with normal ventricles, the rate of emptying is impaired. When the magnitude of the gradient is correlated with the rate of emptying, those with higher gradients empty more slowly.[18] When aortic stenosis is relieved by valve replacement the ejection fraction rises. In contrast, pre- and postoperative comparisons in patients undergoing septal myotomy-myectomy for hypertrophic cardiomyopathy demonstrate a postoperative fall in ejection fraction.[21] Pressure gradients have been abolished as a result of myocardial infarction concomitant with a fall in ejection fraction and rate of ventricular emptying.[22]

Whether the "obstruction" is a result of a muscular sphincter or mitral-septal apposition, it would be expected to result in a decreased rate of ejection when present and enhanced ejection when absent. Alternatively, if the pressure gradient is the result of the Gauer-Henry phenomenon, the more rapidly and completely the ventricle is able to empty, the more likely would a gradient be present. In keeping with this concept, when we compared three groups of patients with hypertrophic cardiomyopathy, those with resting gradients had the highest ejection fractions (92 ± 6.4%), those with inducible gradients had intermediate ejection fractions of 85 ± 9%, and those without resting or inducible gradients had the lowest ejection fractions (75.5 ± 9%). These differences between groups were significant ($p<0.05$ to <0.01), as was the fact that all groups had higher than normal ejection fractions for our laboratory (60 ± 8%, $p<0.05$).[19]

Perhaps because of the Brock bias there has been a reluctance to accept the fact that pressure gradients can occur in the absence of obstructions. However, the Gauer-Henry phenomenon, or cavity obliteration, can be readily reproduced in hydrodynamic models of hypercontractile ventricles.[23–25] If a conical latex model ventricle is designed to have a rigid cylindrical outflow tract and to taper from base to apex, it will rapidly and progressively obliterate all but the outflow tract cavity when subjected to external compressive force. Pressure gradients of well over 100 mmHg can be generated in these model ventricles, which respond to perturbations in a manner similar to the ventricle in hypertrophic cardiomyopathy. When the impedance to ejection or the degree of ventricular filling are reduced and the contractile force is held constant, the gradient increases. Similarly if the contractile force is increased, the gradient increases. When continuous wave Doppler ultrasonography is applied to the model, the magnitude of the gradients measured with matched micromanometer catheters track closely with the Doppler-derived gradients.[24,25] These studies convincingly show the validity and reproducibility of the Gauer-Henry phenomenon, and refute the notion that the catheter is "entrapped" when high pressures are recorded in the obliterating cavity.

The high pressures are recorded from the obliterating portions of the model ventricle, which in hypertrophic cardiomyopathy represent the entire submitral region. The low pressure is recorded from the noncontractile outflow tract, which comprises the "dead space" or residual end systolic volume in the model and in the HCM ventricle. Although high velocities are recorded in mid and late systole emanating from the interstices of the obliterating ventricle, the volumetric flow through the downstream outflow tract is trivial. These findings also closely reproduce flowmeter recordings from the aortic root in hypertrophic cardiomyopathy which demonstrate little or no outflow after mid systole.[6,26,27]

Summary and Conclusions

Despite a large body of evidence that ventricular emptying is not hindered or impeded in hypertrophic cardiomyopathy, the prevalent view reflected in the medical literature and medical terminology continues to support the primacy of "obstruction." The durability of this obstructive concept is a testimonial to the preeminence of Brock's conviction. It is interesting to speculate what Brock might have written had he known of the work of Gauer and Henry when he found only a pressure gradient to suggest a "functional obstruction" and was unable to find any anatomical confirmation in the beating heart. Similarly, when surgeons encountered a "painful" squeeze of the exploring finger, cognizance of the Gauer-Henry phenomenon would have provided an alternative, nonobstructive explanation to the mythical "contraction ring" for the mechanism of the pressure gradient.

As our knowledge base of hypertrophic cardiomyopathy increases we have learned that premature mortality and disabling symptomatology are as likely to occur in the absence as in the presence of pressure gradients, and that arrhythmias and impaired filling of the left ventricle are the principal causes. Obstruction is therefore no longer necessary to invoke as an important or necessary feature in the pathophysiology of hypertrophic cardiomyopathy.[25)]

The enlightened cardiologist would do well to study and understand the Gauer-Henry phenomenon. The technology and methodology not available in Brock's time are now readily available to explore its manifestations *in vitro* and *in vivo*. A through understanding of the phenomenon will provide the investigator with a more rational explanation than "obstruction" when a ventricle is seen to empty rapidly and completely in the presence of a pressure gradient.

Acknowledgment

This work was supported by the Sarah and Matthew Rosenhaus Peace Foundation.

REFERENCES

1. Brock, R. Functional obstruction of the left ventricle (acquired aortic subvalvular stenosis). *Guy's Hospital Reports.* **106**: 221–238, 1957.
2. Brock, R. Functional obstruction of the ventricle (acquired aortic subvalvular stenosis). *Guy's Hospital Reports.* **108**: 126–142, 1959.
3. Teare, D. Asymmetrical hypertrophy of the heart in young adults. *Br. Heart J.* **21**: 1–8, 1958.
4. Gauer, O.H. Evidence in circulatory shock of an isometric phase following ejection. Federation Proceedings, (abstract) **9**: 47, 1950.
5. Gauer, O.H. and Henry, J.P. Negative (-Gz) acceleration in relation to arterial oxygen saturation, subendocardial hemorrhage and venous pressure in the forehead. *Aerospace Medicine* **35**: 533–544, 1964.
6. Braunwald, E., Lambrew, C.T., Morrow, A.G., Pierce, G.E., Rockoff, S.D., and Ross, J.Jr. Idiopathic hypertrophic subaortic stenosis. *Circulation* **30**: (Suppl IV) 1–213, 1964.
7. Bristow, J.D. Recognition of left ventricular outflow tract obstruction. *Circulation* **31**: 600–611, 1965.
8. Criley, J.M., Lewis, K.B., White, R.I., and Ross, R.S. Pressure gradients without obstruction. A new concept of "hypertrophic subaortic stenosis". *Circulation* **32**: 881–887, 1965.
9. Dobell, A.R.C. and Scott, H.J. Hypertrophic subaortic stenosis: evolution of a surgical technique. *J. Thorac. Cardiovasc. Surg.* **47**: 26–39, 1964.
10. Julian, O.C., Dye, W.S., Javid, H., Hunter, J.A., Muenster, J.J. Jr., and Najafi, H. Apical ventriculotomy in subaortic stenosis due to a fibromuscular hyperplasia. *Circulation* **31, 32**: (Suppl I) 44–56, 1965.
11. Morrow, A.G., Reitz, B.A., Epstein, S.E., Henry, W.L., Conkle, D.M., Itscoitz, S.B., and Redwood, D.R. Operative treatment in hypertrophic subaortic stenosis. Techniques and the results of pre- and postoperative assessment in 83 patients. *Circulation* **52**: 88–102, 1975.
12. Pollick, C., Morgan, C.D., Gilbert, B.W., Rakowski, H., and Wigle, E.D. Muscular subaortic stenosis: The temporal relationship between systolic anterior motion of the anterior mitral leaflet and the pressure gradient. *Circulation* **66**: 1087–1094, 1982.
13. Pollick, C., Rakowski, H., and Wigle, E.D. Muscular subaortic stenosis: The quantitative relationship between systolic anterior motion and the pressure gradient. *Circulation* **69**: 43–49, 1984.
14. Henry, W.L., Clark, C.E., Glancy, D.L., and Epstein, S.E. Echocardiographic measurement of the ventricular outflow gradient in idiopathic hypertrophic subaortic stenosis. *N. Engl. J. Med.* **288**: 989–993, 1973.

15. Yock, P.G., Hatle, L., and Popp, R.L. Pattern and timing of Doppler-detected intracavitary and aortic flow in hypertrophic cardiomyopathy. *J. Am. Coll. Cardiol.* **8**: 1047–1058, 1986.
16. Maron, B.J., Gottdeiner, J.S., Arce, J., Rosing, D.R., Wesley, Y.E., and Epstein, S.E. Dynamic subaortic obstruction in hypertrophic cardiomyopathy: analysis by pulsed Doppler echocardiography. *J. Am. Coll. Cardiol.* **6**: 1–15, 1985.
17. Sugrue, D.D., McKenna, W.J., Dickie, S., Myers, M.J., Lavender, J.P., Oakley, C.M., and Goodwin, J.F. The relation of left ventricular gradient and relative stroke volume ejected in early and late systole in hypertrophic cardiomyopathy: assessment with radionuclide cineangiography. *Br. Heart J.* **52**: 602–607, 1984.
18. Wilson, W.S., Criley, J.M., and Ross, R.S. Dynamics of left ventricular emptying in hypertrophic subaortic stenosis: a cineangiographic and hemodynamic study. *Am. Heart J.* **73**: 4–16, 1967.
19. Siegel, R.J. and Criley, J.M. Comparison of ventricular emptying with and without a pressure gradient in patients with hypertrophic cardiomyopathy. *Br. Heart J.* **53**: 283–291, 1985.
20. Ginzton, L.E. and Criley, J.M. "Obstructive" systolic anterior motion of the mitral valve in cavity obliteration. (abstract) **64**: IV–30, 1981.
21. Borer, J.S., Bacharach, S.L., Green, M.V., Kent, K.M., Rosing, D.R., Seides, S.F., Morrow, A.G., and Epstein, S.E. Effect of septal myotomy and myectomy on left ventricular systolic function at rest and during exercise in patients with IHSS. *Circulation* **60**: (Suppl I) 81–87, 1979.
22. Caplan, J., Boltwood, C.M., Tei, C., and Shah, P.M. Clinical improvement in hypertrophic cardiomyopathy after inferior myocardial infarction. *J. Am. Coll. Cardiol.* **5**: 797–802, 1985.
24. Siegel, R.J., Ellis, P.S., Pelikan, P.C.D., Maurer, G., and Criley, J.M. Pressure, flow, and velocity studies of experimentally produced intracavitary pressure gradients. *Circulation* **74**: II–298, 1986.
25. Criley, J.M. and Siegel, R.J. Obstruction is unimportant in the pathophysiology of hypertrophic cardiomyopathy. *Postgrad. Med. J.* **62**: 515–529, 1986.
26. Murgo, J.P., Alter, B.R., Dorethy, J.F., Altobelli, S.A., and McGranahan, G.M. Jr. Dynamics of left ventricular ejection in obstructive and nonobstructive hypertrophic cardiomyopathy. *J. Clin. Invest.* **66**: 1369–1382, 1980.
27. Murgo, J.P. and Miller, J.W. Hemodynamic, angiographic, and echocardiographic evidence against impeded ejection in hypertrophic cardiomyopathy. In: Heart Muscle Disease, Goodwin, J.F. (ed.) Lancaster: MTP Press Ltd., 187–212, 1985.

MANAGEMENT OF HYPERTROPHIC CARDIOMYOPATHY

The Management of Hypertrophic Cardiomyopathy Based on Symptoms, Natural History, and Prognosis

John F. Goodwin

Emeritus Professor of Cardiology, Royal Postgraduate Medical School, Hammersmith Hospital, London, U.K.

There are five basic abnormalities of structure and function in hypertrophic cardiomyopathy. Consideration of them is essential for rational and effective management. They are (1) ventricular hypertrophy, myofibrillar disarray, and fibrosis; (2) over-powerful contraction of the left ventricle with elimination of the cavity; (3) intraventricular systolic pressure gradients; (4) impaired relaxation and filling of the ventricles; and (5) marked tendency to serious arrhythmia and sudden death.

These abnormalities account for the manifestations of the disease, its hazards, and its prognosis.

MANAGEMENT BASED ON SYMPTOMS

Angina, which usually occurs on effort, may occasionally develop spontaneously and last for several hours; even myocardial infarction may occur.[1] The cause is likely to be reduced diastolic coronary blood flow as a result of the massive hypertrophy and impaired relaxation of the left ventricle. Compression of the septal perforating arteries,[2] occlusive changes in the intramuscular arterioles,[3] and failure to increase coronary flow sufficiently to meet demand may be additional factors.[4]

Relief of angina is obtained by beta-adrenergic or calcium-blocking agents, which reduce oxygen demand and improve diastolic function.[5–7] An important effect of β-blocking agents is slowing of the heart rate, which allows more time for ventricular filling. Most important of all is the catecholamine-blocking effect which reduces the excessive contractile force of the ventricle and improves compliance. A notable, but less important factor is reduction of outflow tract systolic gradients. A nonselective β-adrenergic blocking agent should be chosen because it has a greater effect than a selective agent in reducing the outflow tract gradient. This is probably because of release of peripheral vasoconstrictor impulses which increase left ventricular afterload. Propranolol is the agent of choice.

If propranolol is not tolerated, oxprenolol can be tried. This has the disadvantage of having intrinsic sympathomimetic action, which may limit the reduction of the heart rate, and also may increase the force of contraction of the left ventricle. Other alternatives are the selective β-blocking agents, atenolol and metoprolol, which are often effective and do not have intrinsic sympathomimetic action. Acebutalol, which is β-1 selective and has intrinsic sympathomimetic activity, may be useful for the rare patient who prefers tachycardia to bradycardia.

Calcium-blocking agents are useful second-line drugs for the relief of angina, but care should be taken with verapamil, because of the dangers of pulmonary edema, severe hypotension, and sudden death.[8] Care is also needed with nifedipine because of vasodilatation, which by reducing left ventricular afterload, may increase the outflow tract gradient. The vasodilatation produced by nifedipine can be blocked to some extent by the use of a nonselective β-adrenergic blocking agent.[9] For the same reasons cited for nifedipine, nitrates should be avoided if possible. Neither β-blocking nor calcium-blocking agents are always successful in relieving angina. Alternative drugs that may be tried are sotalol and amiodarone, but in general amiodarone is indicated only for symptomatic or life-threatening arrhythmia. Disopyramide may occasionally help angina because of its negative inotropic action.[10] Refractory angina is an indication to consider surgical treatment in patients who have substantial outflow gradients.

Occlusive coronary artery disease is associated with hypertrophic cardiomyopathy in a larger proportion of patients than is realized[11]: perhaps up to 15–20%. It cannot be distinguished symptomatically from hypertrophic cardiomyopathy alone, nor is effort testing (which may show dramatic ST segment depression in hypertrophic cardiomyopathy) of great value in detecting associated coronary artery disease. Coronary arteriography is needed, and should always be considered in any patient with hypertrophic cardiomyopathy who has severe angina.

Dyspnea is thought to be due to high left ventricular end-diastolic pressure consequent upon the stiffness of the poorly relaxing left ventricle, and is worse on effort, though spontaneous attacks of dyspnea may occur with or without arrhythmia.

In some patients, dyspnea on effort is associated with severe fatigue, which may be due to peripheral blood flow anomalies or biochemical defects in exercising muscle.

Dyspnea is usually reduced by β-adrenergic or calcium-blocking agents, but occasionally may be made worse. Commonly, patients with hypertrophic cardiomyopathy benefit by relative bradycardia, and become more symptomatic with tachycardia, but occasionally the reverse is true. Effort testing may be of value in identifying such patients who may benefit from β-blocking agents with intrinsic sympathomimetic activity like alprenolol or oxprenolol.

Palpitation may result merely from the powerful contraction of the hypertrophied left ventricle, but is often due to ectopic beats or runs of atrial fibrillation. Undue bradycardia, occurring naturally or due to β-blocking agents, may aggravate the sense of palpitation, as may unduly rapid heart rates.

The treatment of palpitation depends upon the cause; 48-hr electrocardiographic ambulatory monitoring is essential in all patients with hypertrophic cardiomyopathy. If ectopic rhythm coincides with a sensation of palpitation, then antiarrhythmic treatment is appropriate. Palpitations not due to arrhythmia will usually respond to explanation and β-adrenergic blockade.

Syncope or near-syncope may be due to arrhythmia,[12] or be caused by hemodynamic factors[13] as a result of acute reduction of left ventricular volume due to elimination of the cavity and decrease in compliance leading to impairment both of filling and emptying. Perhaps in some patients syncope or sudden death may be due to combined hemodynamic causes and arrhythmic causes. Acute ischemia might be an important trigger.[14]

Management of syncope requires electrocardiographic monitoring to detect arrhythmia. The investigation may have to be repeated; at least 48 hr of monitoring is essential. If serious arrhythmia consists of frequent multifocal premature ventricular contractions, runs of nonsustained ventricular tachycardia, or atrial fibrillation with very rapid ventricular rate, then amiodarone is indicated. It should be a first-line drug for the treatment of arrhythmias in hypertrophic cardiomyopathy, because other antiarrhythmic agents, notably β-blocking agents, verapamil, and class-1 agents, are usually unavailing.[12,15,16] Additional advantages of amiodarone are its lack of negative inotropic effect and noncompetitive sympathetic blocking action. Implantable defibrillators may have a place in treating tachycardia and fibrillation. Arrhythmias are likely to be due to increased automaticity and local re-entry circuits induced by myofibrillar disarray, although pre-excitation can be a mechanism when abnormal tissue sets up a re-entrant pathway between atrium and ventricle.[17,18]

Since syncope or fainting may be due to hemodynamic factors, treatment aimed at improving left ventricular compliance and reducing left ventricular systolic cavity elimination should be given. First-line drugs are β-blocking agents. Calcium-blocking agents may be used to improve both systolic and diastolic function,[7,19,20] but precautions already mentioned must be borne in mind.

Heart block may very rarely be a cause of syncope.[21,22] Patients with atrial fibrillation may be found to have a tachycardia-bradycardia syndrome and require a pacemaker in addition to antiarrhythmic drugs. If a pacemaker is needed, it is important to ensure sequential atrioventricular pacing, since the loss of atrial drive resulting from a VVI pacemaker may have significant deleterious hemodynamic effects.[14]

MANAGEMENT BASED ON SYMPTOMS

The natural history of hypertrophic cardiomyopathy is highly variable and depends on the site, extent, and distribution of the myofibrillar disarray, hypertrophy, and fibrosis. Many patients pursue an uneventful course for many years with few, if any, symptoms, and may live to old age. These patients have modest hypertrophy, few arrhythmias, and often no family history. Experience suggests that the apical type of hypertrophic cardiomyopathy[23] often carries a benign prognosis, although no detailed trials have been carried out to check this impression.

In a personal study of 254 patients, followed from 1–23 years (mean 6 years) the mortality was 28.6%.[21] The average annual mortality was 2.6%, but patients at special risk had double the death rate.[21] In most patients, the diagnosis was made between the ages of 11 and 15 years, but in 2% it was made in the first five years of life, and in 16% between the ages of 50 and 60 years. Only in 1% was the patient over 60 years when the diagnosis was first made. However, it is likely that hypertrophic cardiomyopathy is underdiagnosed and that there are patients masquerading as aortic valve stenosis or mitral regurgitation with atrial fibrillation of rheumatic origin.

Fifty percent of patients who die from the disease do so suddenly, other modes of death being congestive heart failure, systemic embolism, and infective endocarditis. Atrial fibrillation, commonly, but not always, causes severe deterioration and can be fatal.

No special clinical, electrocardiographic, or hemodynamic abnormalities aid prognosis[21] except perhaps the deep T-wave inversion seen in the apical type, which appears to carry a favorable outlook. The combination of four features—age less than 14 years at diagnosis, previous syncopal episodes, severe symptoms (dyspnea), and family history of hypertrophic cardiomyopathy and/or sudden death—provides the best predictor of sudden death in an individual.[14] Other features that affect natural history and prognosis are atrial fibrillation and systemic embolism. Mitral valve calcification or regurgitation may predispose to infective endocarditis. Extreme mitral regurgitation may result in pulmonary edema that can be fatal, especially if acute. Urgent valve replacement may be needed.

Assessment of natural history and prognosis influences treatment. Thus the asymptomatic or minimally symptomatic patient in whom the disease is diagnosed in adult life and who has evidence only of moderate hypertrophy, no arrhythmia on ECG monitoring, and no family history may not need any treatment. But such patients must be kept under regular observation by Holter monitoring and echocardiography. In a minority of children, severe hypertrophy may progress in a relatively short period.[24] Control of arrhythmia may be expected to improve prognosis and favorably influence the natural history. Unfortunately, although both β- and calcium-blocking agents can improve systolic and diastolic function, neither can be expected to improve prognosis. Furthermore, initial hopes that β-blocking agents might reduce or delay ventricular hypertrophy have not been realized: the same is true of calcium-blocking agents. Nor does surgery influence survival rate.[25,26]

Prognosis based on the extent of hypertrophy may not be entirely reliable, since it can depend more on the extent of myofibrillar disarray and cellular disorganization than upon the degree of hypertrophy,[17] and patients dying of hypertrophic cardiomyopathy do not always have marked hypertrophy.

Patients who are found to have significant arrhythmias, as defined earlier, require antiarrhythmic therapy. Amiodarone has been shown to improve prognosis in hypertrophic cardiomyopathy in a small series of patients with ventricular tachycardia.[28] This is the only evidence of any treatment increasing survival in hypertrophic cardiomyopathy. If amiodarone is not tolerated, then alternative antiarrhythmic treatment is indicated, as mentioned earlier. If patients have both serious arrhythmia and symptoms, then additional symptomatic treatment may also be necessary. The combination of propranolol and amiodarone is both logical and effective. Treatment should be tailored to the individual patient along the lines suggested.

Exercise, physical exertion, and competitive sports of a violent nature should be avoided, as should sympathomimetic drugs. Antibiotic prophylaxis against infective endocarditis before dental work and abdominal or pelvic procedures is essential for all patients.

Situations that can precipitate hypotension should be avoided, as reduction in peripheral resistance can reduce left ventricular volume and provoke hemodynamic syncope.

SPECIAL SITUATIONS

Atrial fibrillation can be a serious emergency; the loss of atrial drive lowers effective cardiac output and patients may develop severe hypotension or pulmonary edema. Treatment is therefore urgent. The patient should be anticoagulated at once with heparin, and amiodarone started, and if sinus rhythm is not achieved, cardioversion is indicated. Since oral amiodarone takes several days to exert its effect, it should be given intravenously and followed by immediate cardioversion if the situation is urgent. As an alternative, verapamil may stabilize atrial fibrillation, but has certain disadvantages, as already mentioned. If needed, cardioversion can be attempted without amiodarone, but is less likely to succeed.

Congestive cardiac failure occurs when systolic failure is added to diastolic impairment of the left ventricle. The ejection fraction and effective cardiac output fall away precipitously and the patient becomes highly incapacitated. Congestive heart failure, unless precipitated by a treatable cause such as myocardial infarction, atrial fibrillation, ventricular tachycardia, or acute mitral regurgitation, usually indicates an advanced state of the disease and a poor prognosis. Beta-adrenergic blocking agents should be avoided except in small doses to control heart rate. Diuretics will be needed. Since the powerful overaction of the left ventricle in systole has diminished, there is little fear of augmenting left ventricular cavity elimination by reducing afterload or extracellular blood volume. If rapid atrial fibrillation is present, amiodarone is indicated because, despite recent reports,[29] it probably has little, if any, negative inotropic effect at rest.[30] In intractable cases, transplantation should be considered.

Digitalis has a bad reputation in hypertrophic cardiomyopathy, and may provoke outflow "obstruction" or sudden death. The dangers have probably been exaggerated, but nevertheless, digitalis should not usually be used, mainly because it may provoke ventricular arrhythmia. It must be employed very cautiously in congestive heart failure with rapid atrial fibrillation, and amiodarone is preferable.

Pregnancy is well tolerated in hypertrophic cardiomyopathy. Beta-adrenergic blocking therapy may be used, but doses should be kept low in order to avoid fetal hypoglycemia and bradycardia. In patients on β-blocking agents, signs of mild congestive heart failure may develop toward the end of pregnancy and require diuretic therapy. Epidural anesthesia and hypovolemia must be avoided during delivery.[31]

Hypertrophic cardiomyopathy should not be a contraindication to pregnancy on genetic grounds, unless there is already a strong family history of the disease with sudden death at an early age.

Surgical treatment is indicated in a minority of patients.[32] Operations available are septal resection, mitral valve replacement using a low-profile mechanical or biological prosthesis, and cardiac transplantation.

Septal resection is indicated for severe symptoms that cannot be relieved by medical means. Although it is usually accompanied by reductions in gradients, left ventricular end-diastolic pressure, and symptoms,[33] it is not clear how the operation works, and true obstruction to outflow is probably confined to only a few patients who have a very small left ventricular cavity, with very large papillary muscles. In the great majority of patients, there is rapid, early and almost complete emptying of the left ventricle whether or not there is a gradient.[34] Occasionally patients with large gradients and early systolic anterior motion of the mitral valve may have considerable residual ventricular volume consistent with obstruction.[35]

Children pose a special problem. While β-blocking agents and even amiodarone are fully warranted when indications are clear, the use of these and similar drugs over long periods during the growth period must occasion anxiety. Asymptomatic children with no arrhythmia and no family history should not inevitably be treated initially, but should be kept under regular observation by clinical examination, echocardiography, and ECG monitoring. Exercise testing to assess the effect of exertion on blood pressure, heart rate, and arrhythmia may be of help.

CONCLUSIONS

Treatment must be directed individually to each patient, aimed at relief of symptoms, reduction in hemodynamic faults, and prevention of arrhythmia and sudden death. Unfortunately, no method is available at the present time to influence the progress of the underlying pathology or to prevent the disease.

REFERENCES

1. Maron, B.J., Epstein, S.E., and Roberts, W.C. Hypertrophic cardiomyopathy and transmural myocardial infarction without significant atherosclerosis of the extramural coronary arteries. *Am. J. Cardiol.* **43**: 1086–1091, 1979.

2. Brugada, P., Bar, F.W.H.M., de Zwaan, C., Roy, D., Green, M., and Wellens, H.J.J. "Saw-fish" systolic narrowing of the left anterior descending coronary artery: An angiographic sign of hypertrophic cardiomyopathy. *Circulation* **67**: 191–197, 1983.
3. Maron, B.J., Wolfson, J.K., Epstein, S.E., and Roberts, W.C. Intramural (small vessel) coronary artery disease in hypertrophic cardiomyopathy. *J. Am. Coll. Cardiol.* **8**: 545–557, 1986.
4. Cannon, R.O., Rosing, D.R., Maron, B.J., *et al.* Myocardial ischemia in hypertrophic cardiomyopathy: Contribution of inadequate vasodilator reserve and elevated left ventricular filling pressures. *Circulation* **71**: 234–243, 1985.
5. Frank, M.J., Abdulla, A.M., Canedo, M.I., and Saylors, R.E. Long-term medical management of hypertrophic obstructive cardiomyopathy. *Am. J. Cardiol.* **42**: 993–1001, 1978.
6. Webb-Peploe, M.M. Beta-blockade in the treatment of hypertrophic cardiomyopathy. *Postgrad. Med. J.* **61**: 1120–1122, 1985.
7. Bonow, R.O., Ostrow, H.G., Rosing D.R., *et al.* Effects of verapamil on left ventricular systolic and diastolic function in patients with hypertrophic cardiomyopathy: Pressure-volume analysis with a non-imaging scintillation probe. *Circulation* **68**: 1062–1073, 1983.
8. Epstein, S.E. and Rosing, D.R. Verapamil: Its potential for causing serious complications in patients with hypertrophic cardiomyopathy. *Circulation* **64**: 437–441, 1981.
9. Landmark, K., Sire, S., Thaulow, E., *et al.* Haemodynamic effects of nifedipine and propranolol in patients with hypertrophic obstructive cardiomyopathy. *Br. Heart J.* **48**: 19–26, 1982.
10. Pollick, C. Muscular subaortic stenosis: Hemodynamic and clinical improvement after disopyramide. *N. Engl. J. Med.* **307**: 997–999, 1982.
11. Cokkinos, D.V., Krajcer, Z., and Leachman, R.D. Coronary artery disease in hypertrophic cardiomyopathy. *Am. J. Cardiol.* **55**: 1437–1438, 1985.
12. McKenna, W.J., England, D., Doi, Y.L., Deanfield, J.E., Oakley, C.M., and Goodwin, J.F. Arrhythmia in hypertrophic cardiomyopathy: I. Influence on prognosis. *Br. Heart J.* **46**: 168–172, 1981.
13. McKenna, W.J., Harris, L., and Deanfield, J. Syncope in hypertrophic cardiomyopathy. *Br. Heart J.* **47**: 177–179, 1982.
14. Sugrue, D.D. and McKenna, W.J. Hypertrophic cardiomyopathy: treatment and prognosis. In: Goodwin, J.F. (ed.), Heart Muscle Disease. Lancaster, MTP Press, pp. 35–36, 1985.
15. McKenna, W.J., Chetty, S., Oakley, C.M., and Goodwin, J.F. Arrhythmia in hypertrophic cardiomyopathy: Exercise and 48 hour ambulatory electrocardiographic assessment with and without beta adrenergic blocking therapy. *Am. J. Cardiol.* **45**: 1–5, 1980.
16. McKenna, W.J., Harris, L., Perez, G., Krikler, D.M., Oakley, C.M., and Goodwin, J.F. Arrhythmia in hypertrophic cardiomyopathy. II. Comparison of amiodarone and verapamil in treatment. *Br. Heart J.* **46**: 173–178, 1981.
17. Goodwin, J.F. and Krikler, D.M. Arrhythmias as a cause of sudden death in hypertrophic cardiomyopathy. *Lancet* ii: 937–940, 1976.
18. Krikler, D.M., Davies, M.J., Rowland, E., Goodwin, J.F., Evans, R.C., and Shaw, D.B. Sudden death in hypertrophic cardiomyopathy: Associated accessory atrioventricular pathways. *Br. Heart J.* **43**: 245–251, 1980.
19. Suwa, M., Hirota, Y., and Kawamura, K. Impairment in left ventricular diastolic function during intravenous and oral diltiazem therapy in patients with hypertrophic cardiomyopathy: an echocardiographic study. *Am. J. Cardiol.* **54**: 1047–1052, 1984.
20. Colle, J.P., Ohayon, J., and Besse, P. Effects of intravenous calcium antagonists on systolic and diastolic function in left ventricular hypertrophy. *Arch. Mal. Coeur* **78**: 1843–1852, 1985.
21. McKenna, W.J., Deanfield, J., Faruqui, A., England, D., Oakley, C.M., and Goodwin, J.F. Prognosis in hypertrophic cardiomyopathy: Role of age and clinical, electrocardiographic and hemodynamic features. *Am. J. Cardiol.* **47**: 532–538, 1981.

22. Louie, E.K. and Maron, B.J. Familial spontaneous complete heart block in hypertrophic cardiomyopathy. *Br. Heart J.* **55**: 469–474, 1986.
23. Yamaguchi, H., Ichinura, T., Nishiyawa, S., Nagasaki, S., Takatsu, F., Nakanishi, S., Nishijo, T., Umeda, T., and Machii, K. Hypertrophic cardiomyopathy with giant negative T waves (apical hypertrophy): ventriculographic and echocardiographic features in 30 patients. *Am. J. Cardiol.* **44**: 401–411, 1979.
24. Maron, B.J., Spirito, P., Wesley, Y., and Arce, J. Development and progression of left ventricular hypertrophy in children with hypertrophic cardiomyopathy. *N. Engl. J. Med.* **315**: 610–614, 1986.
25. Kuhn, H. Myocardial hypertrophy: regression of hypertrophic cardiomyopathies. *Z. Kardiol.* **74**: 179, 1985.
26. Healy, B. Hypertrophic cardiomyopathy. *Curr. Opinion Cardiol.* **2**: 475–485, 1987.
27. McKenna, W.J. and Goodwin, J.F. The natural history of hypertrophic cardiomyopathy. *Curr. Probl. Cardiol.* **6**: 1–26, 1981.
28. McKenna, W.J., Oakley, C.M., Krikler, D.M., and Goodwin, J.F. Improved survival with amiodarone in patients with hypertrophic cardiomyopathy and ventricular tachycardia. *Br. Heart J.* **53**: 412, 1985.
29. Paulus, W.J., Wellens, P., Hyndrickx, G.R., and Andries, E. Effects with long term treatment with amiodarone on exercise, hemodynamics and left ventricular relaxation in patients with hypertrophic cardiomyopathy. *Circulation* **74**: 544–554, 1986.
30. Sugrue, D.D., Dickie, S., Myers, M.J., Lavender, J.P., and McKenna, W.J. Effect of amiodarone on left ventricular ejection and filling in hypertrophic cardiomyopathy as assessed by radionuclide angiography. *Am. J. Cardiol.* **54**: 1054–1058, 1984.
31. Oakley, G.D.C., McGarry, K., Limb, D.G., and Oakley, C.M. Management of pregnancy in patients with hypertrophic cardiomyopathy. *Br. Med. J.* **1**: 1749–1750, 1979.
32. Goodwin, J.F. Ergebnisse der Inneren Medizin und Kinderheilkunde, Bd 55. Springer-Verlag: Berlin, 1987, pp. 42–79.
33. Maron, B.J., Merrill, W.H., Freier, P.A., *et al.* Long-term clinical course and symptomatic status of patients after operation for hypertrophic subaortic stenosis. *Circulation* **57**: 1205–1213, 1978.
34. Criley, J.M. and Siegel, R.J. Obstruction is unimportant in the pathophysiology of hypertrophic cardiomyopathy. *Postgrad. Med. J.* **62**: 515–529, 1986.
35. Wigle, E.D., Sasson, Z., Henderson, M.A., Ruddy, T.D., Fulop, J., Rakowski, H., and Williams, W.G. Hypertrophic cardiomyopathy: The importance of the site and extent of hypertrophy. A review. *Prog. Cardiovasc. Dis.* **28**: 1–83, 1985.

Medical Treatment of Hypertrophic Cardiomyopathy: Influence on Outflow Obstruction and Filling Pressure

Rüdiger Hopf and Martin Kaltenbach

Zentrum der Inneren Medizin, Abteilung für Kardiologie, Klinikum der Johann Wolfgang Goethe-Universität, Frankfurt, F.R.G.

ABSTRACT

Any therapeutic intervention in hypertrophic cardiomyopathy should be aimed at a reduction of symptoms, improvement of exercise tolerance, retardation or prevention of disease progression, and improvement of the prognosis. Beta-adrenergic blocking agents, calcium antagonists, and the antiarryhthmic drug amiodarone have been recommended for medical treatment. In patients treated with β-blockers, initial reduction of outflow obstruction can be seen, but during long-term therapy subsequent deterioration has been common. Without doubt, amiodarone is effective in patients with hypertrophic cardiomyopathy and concomitant ventricular tachycardia, but no hemodynamic effects could be demonstrated. Overall, present studies related to hemodynamic and clinical results and to prognosis are demonstrating verapamil to be the most efficient drug therapy in patients with hypertrophic cardiomyopathy, due to its favorable effects on left ventricular systolic and diastolic function.

INTRODUCTION

In 1907, Schmincke was the first to describe diffuse "hyperplasia" of the heart muscle, involving predominantly the wall of the left ventricular outflow tract, in two female patients.[1] Teare presented in 1958 pathologic findings of asymmetrical hypertrophy of the heart in young adults; eight of whom died from sudden death, seven during physical activity.[2] Braunwald *et al.* in 1964 described the findings of 64 patients with hypertrophic cardiomyopathy (HCM), emphasizing angiographically determined normal or even supernormal left ventricular function and hemodynamically documented large variations of outflow tract gradient.[3] Today there seems to be no doubt that impaired diastolic function of the left ventricle is the predominant hemodynamic characteristic in HCM.[4,5]

By 1962 it was demonstrated that drugs with positive inotropic action augment the outflow tract gradient in hypertrophic obstructive cardiomyopathy (HOCM),[6] so that various degrees of obstruction were thought to be under β-adrenergic modulation, as, for example, during physical activity.[7] After it had been shown that the positive inotropic effects of isoprenaline administration could be acutely counteracted by pronethalol,[8] β-blockade seemed to be a reasonable concept in medical treatment of HCM.

The importance of the calcium ion in the pathogenesis of myocardial hypertrophy and its role in myocardial contraction and relaxation had been repeatedly emphasized, so that we, ourselves, initiated calcium antagonist therapy in patients with HCM in 1973 and first presented our results in 1976 and 1979.[9–11] The effects of combined therapy with nifedipine and propranolol we described in 1987.[12] With regard to the role of ventricular arrhythmia associated with sudden death,[13] antiarrhythmic drugs, especially amiodarone, have been given to patients with HCM since 1981.[14]

Therapy with β-Adrenergic Blocking Agents

It has been discussed that increased activity of sympathetic nerves in the heart or a disorder of inotropic catecholamine stimulation might be closely associated with the systolic features in HCM.[8,15] Hemodynamic measurements seemed to confirm this hypothesis, because exercise, tachycardia, emotion, and circulatory active drugs augmented contractility as well as outflow tract obstruction.[3,6] It therefore appeared to be a rational concept to treat patients with HCM with β-adrenergic blocking agents.

A reduction of heart rate at rest and a modulation of rate increase during exertion is expected because of the negative chronotropy which in turn may improve exercise tolerance.[8] The effects of pronethalol had not been marked at rest, but due to negative inotropic action, hemodynamic studies uncovered a slight decrease in ventricular systolic pressure and outflow obstruction.[16] In addition, persistent dynamic outflow tract obstruction was associated with deterioration of symptoms.[17] A reduction of the basal gradient in the left ventricle was observed only in a few patients,[18,19] whereas an increase in gradient with sympathetic stimulation usually could be prevented, the spontaneous variation of the obstruction decreased, and the effective outflow orifice presumably widened.[17,20–22] Left ventricular end-diastolic and end-systolic volume showed a significant increase, and ejection fraction was reduced,[16] but cardiac index usually did not change.[8,17] Depending on early hemodynamic or noninvasive studies, it was suggested that propranolol might decrease left ventricular filling pressure and improve left ventricular diastolic function by shortening the isovolumic relaxation time and increasing myocardial distensibility.[16,22,23] In contrast, other investigators could demonstrate that β-blocking agents did not importantly influence on ventricular diastolic function, but could increase filling pressure at rest and during exercise.[21,24,25]

In HOCM, as well as in the nonobstructive form (HNCM), β-blocking agents can relieve typical symptoms such as dyspnea and angina, but seldom improve lightheadness or syncope.[26,27] Exercise tolerance was improved in only some patients.[25,27] In contrast, some patients were described as feeling better under placebo.[22] Long-term observations in some cases showed symptomatic benefit,[17] but more often complaints remained unaffected or reappeared during therapy.[19,28,29] In addition, the favorable hemodynamic effects following acute intravenous administration of β-blockers could not be reproduced during long-term oral therapy, where the obstruction was seen reappear partly.[30] End-diastolic pressure and mean pulmonary artery pressure were not influenced by long-term therapy.[25,30,31] Perhaps due to relatively low doses of β-blockers, the overall clinical course was not influenced and mortality rate remained high.[32,33] More satisfying results were reported by Frank *et al.*, who administered a mean oral dose of 500 mg propranolol per day, and whose results were interpreted as "complete β-blockade."[34,35] Unfortunately, it appears that β-blockers influence neither the disease progression nor the incidence of sudden death.[36,37]

Our own experience is related to the observation of 17 (two female and 15 male) patients (age 24–59, mean 44 years). They had been treated for three to 106 (mean 31) months with β-blockers, given doses as high as subjectively tolerated, i.e., up to 480 mg propranolol per day. In only three cases could initial and temporal improvement be seen, but in all cases slow progressive or recurrent deterioration was reported, and exercise tolerance did not improve in any case. The Sokolow index remained unchanged (4.9

and 4.8 mV, respectively). Heart size, calculated by X-ray technique,[38–40] showed enlargement from 850 to 915 ml/1.73 m^2 (for reasons of better comparability the heart volume was calculated for a body surface area of 1.73 m^2; normal: men <800, women <700 ml/1.73 m^2), paralleled by an echocardiographic increase of left atrial diameter from 42 to 44 mm, whereas left ventricular wall thickness remained unchanged (interventricular septum 24 vs 25 mm and posterior left ventricular wall 15 mm at the beginning and at the end of the follow-up period).

Therapy with Calcium Antagonists

In 1976, we presented the first data describing therapeutic results achieved with verapamil in 20 patients with HCM. During the 14 months' treatment, most patients reported impressive relief of symptoms, attended by reduction in QRS-amplitude and heart volume.[9,10] In 1979, we confirmed these results through longer studies with 22 patients.[11] Also 1979, Rosing *et al.* were able to show that intravenously administered verapamil significantly decreases outflow obstruction in HCM[41] and given orally improves exercise capacity and symptomatic status compared with placebo and propranolol.[42] In 1980, Hanrath *et al.* verified that verapamil improves left ventricular relaxation and filling.[43] These results were confirmed by radionuclide angiograms[44] and hemodynamic investigations following acute and chronic verapamil administration,[45] or acute nifedipine application.[46] Furthermore, we have presented our results of long-term verapamil treatment (more than 10 years),[47] and results following nifedipine and diltiazem therapy were also published.

Studies on Verapamil

For more than 10 years now, verapamil has been shown to be an effective therapeutic agent in the medical treatment of HCM, relieving dyspnea and angina and achieving sustained improvement in exercise capacity.[47–49] Following intravenous administration of verapamil, left ventricular outflow tract gradient, filling pressure, and contractility are significantly reduced.[41,50] An oral dose of 160 mg verapamil affected a reduction of filling pressure despite angiography with controversial effects.[50] Hemodynamic effects have also been evident during exercise.[25,50–52] The good clinical results from verapamil in patients with HCM can probably be explained by the improvement in systolic and particularly in diastolic left ventricular function, whether there is an outflow tract obstruction or not.[24,43,44,54–56]

We ourselves investigated the hemodynamic effects of verapamil following intracoronary, intravenous, and oral administration.

Effects of intracoronary administration: To evaluate its exclusive myocardial effects, verapamil was administered into the left coronary artery in seven patients with HOCM (five males and two females; age 41–65, mean 49 years). The mean dose was 1.6 mg (1.5–2.0 mg). Following slow administration, no verapamil could be detected in the plasma. Hemodynamic measurements were performed after five minutes. Heart rate fell from 75.4 to 71/min (n.s.), and systolic left ventricular pressure went from 128.3 to 107.9 mmHg (n.s.). Left ventricular filling pressure was 25.7 mmHg before and 21.6 mmHg after verapamil, significantly different ($2p<0.02$) (Fig. 1). The basal left ventricular outflow tract gradient was reduced from 45.4 to 25.9 ($2p<0.02$) (Fig. 2), and the maximal gradient (following provocation: nitroglycerin, Valsalva maneuver, and postextrasystolic augmentation) fell from 107 to 63.9 mmHg ($2p<0.01$) (Fig. 3). Contractility was diminished from 2,107 to 1,650 mmHg/sec (n.s.).

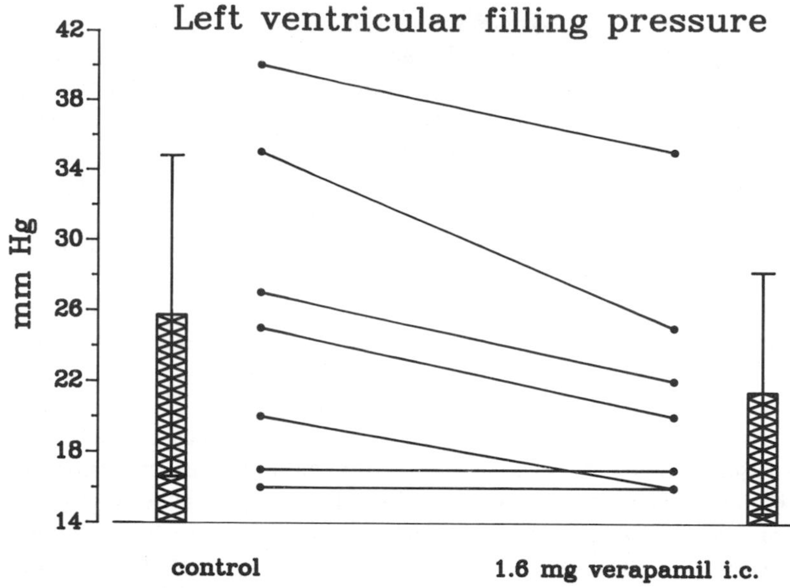

Fig. 1. Hemodynamic effects in patients with HCM following intracoronary administration of 1.6 mg verapamil. Left ventricular filling pressure was significantly reduced from 25.7 ± 9.1 to 21.1 ± 6.8 mmHg.

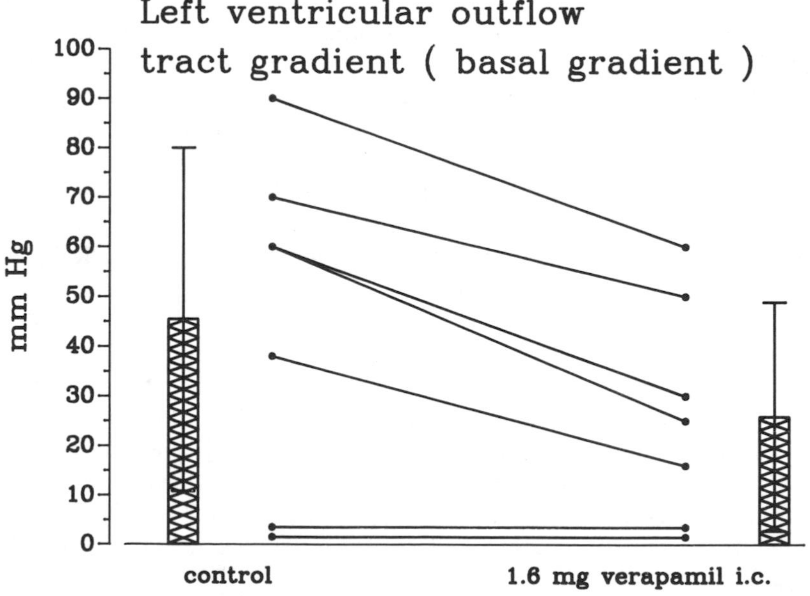

Fig. 2. Hemodynamic effects in patients with HCM following intracoronary administration of 1.6 mg verapamil. Left ventricular basal gradient was significantly reduced from 45.4 ± 34.6 to 25.9 ± 23.1 mmHg.

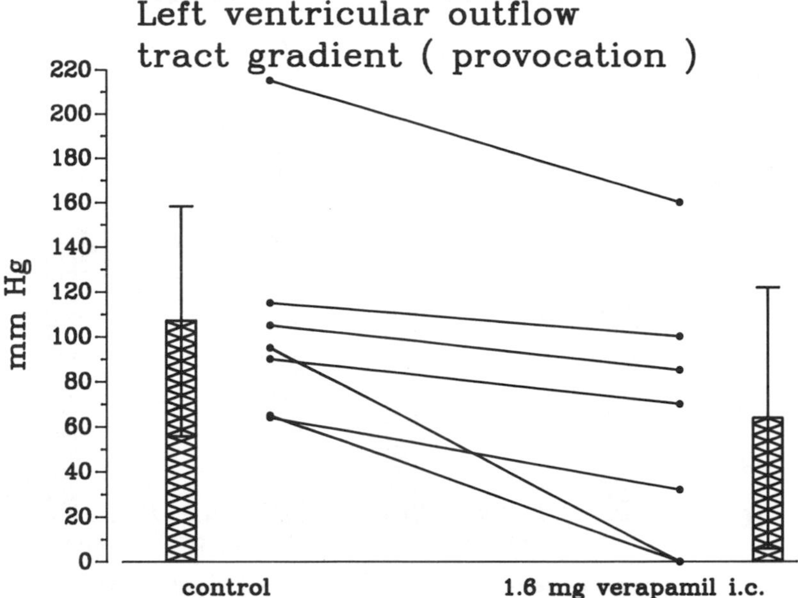

Fig. 3. Hemodynamic effects in patients with HCM following intracoronary administration of 1.6 mg verapamil. Maximal left ventricular gradient (following provocation maneuvers) was significantly reduced from 107.0 ± 51.3 to 63.9 ± 58.0 mmHg.

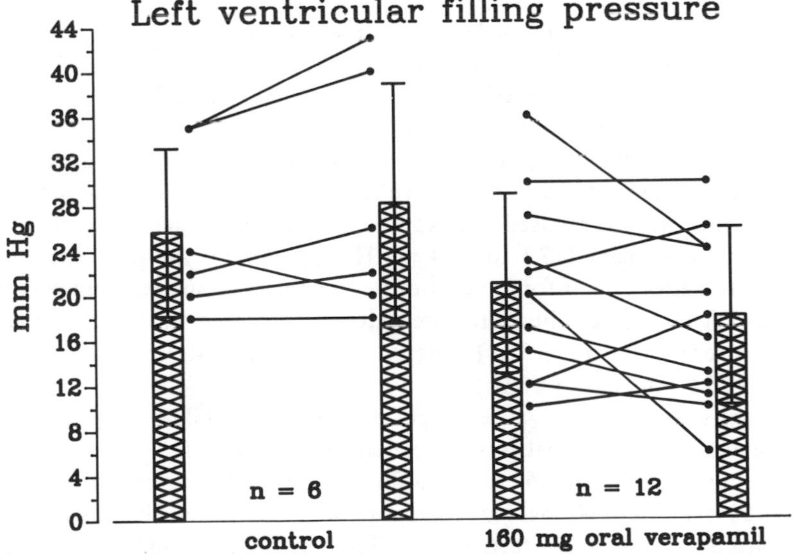

Fig. 4. Hemodynamic effects of 160 mg oral verapamil in patients with HCM. In the control group, following diagnostic angiography, there was an increase in left ventricular filling pressure from 25.7 ± 7.5 to 28.2 ± 10.7 mmHg. In contrast, patients taking verapamil showed a significant reduction from 20.3 ± 7.8 to 17.5 ± 7.4 mmHg, although they had angiography as well.

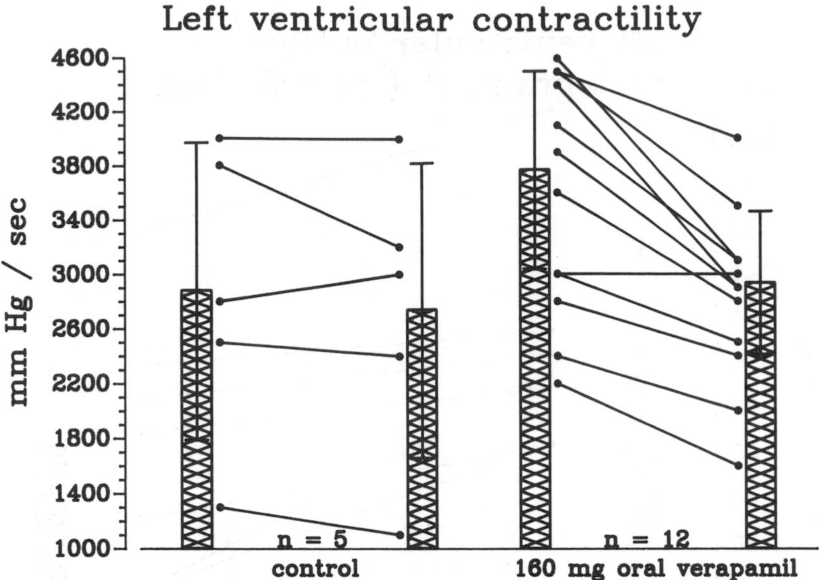

Fig. 5. Hemodynamic effects of 160 mg oral verapamil in patients with HCM. Angiography alone (control) had no clear influence on left ventricular contractility, but oral verapamil reduced dp/dt max significantly from 3770 ± 735 to 2935 ± 525 mmHg/sec.

Effects of intravenous administration: In 15 patients (14 males and one female; age 29–62, mean 45 years), we investigated the effects of slow intravenous verapamil administration (10 mg over 10 min). Hemodynamic measurements uncovered cardiac as well as reflex mechanisms due to peripheral actions. Heart rate increased from 67.7 to 75.5/min ($2p < 0.03$) while contractility remained unaffected: 2,243 and 2,231 mmHg/sec ($2p < 0.02$). Systolic left ventricular pressure fell from 118.7 to 110.6 mmHg (n.s.). Left ventricular filling pressure was 19.5 mmHg before and 16.6 mmHg after verapamil ($2p < 0.05$). In nine patients with obstructive cardiomyopathy, the basal left ventricular outflow tract gradient was reduced from 45.3 to 32.9 (n.s.) and the maximal gradient was significantly reduced from 117.1 to 80.4 mmHg ($2p < 0.01$). In 10 of the 15 patients, ergometry was performed before and after verapamil. The increases in systolic blood pressure and left ventricular filling pressure were reduced after verapamil: left ventricular systolic pressure went from 158.5 to 153.6 (n.s.), while end-diastolic pressure was reduced from 36.3 to 27.5 mmHg ($2p < 0.05$).

Effects of oral administration: The effects of oral verapamil are of greatest interest. We investigated another 12 patients (three females and nine males), six of whom had HOCM. The age range was 16–59 years (mean 39 years). Measurements were performed before and 60 min after 160 mg oral verapamil was given and diagnostic angiography and myocardial biopsy were carried out. To take into account the hemodynamic effects of the radiopaque medium, hemodynamic changes were measured before and after angiography in another six patients. This group consisted of two female and four male patients, whose age ranged from 26 to 57 years (mean 48 years); all had HOCM. In the control group, heart rate (67.3 vs 70.5/min), systolic blood pressure (141.2 vs 135.7 mmHg), dp/dt max (2,880 vs 2,740 mmHg/sec), and the degree of outflow tract obstruction (basal gradient 58.2 vs 52.0 mmHg, maximal gradient 129.2 vs 124.2

mmHg) were reduced, whereas left ventricular filling pressure increased from 25.7 to 28.2 mmHg. In the 12 patients receiving oral verapamil medication, heart rate (74.6 vs 72.8/min) and systolic blood pressure (131.0 vs 117.5 mmHg) tended to show reductions; these were not significant, however, when compared with the control group. In contrast, left ventricular filling pressure was significantly reduced from 20.3 to 17.5 mmHg ($2p < 0.05$) (Fig. 4) and contractility was reduced from 3,770 to 2,935 mmHg/sec ($2p < 0.02$) (Fig. 5). In the subgroup of six patients with HOCM, there was only a trend toward a reduction of the obstruction (basal gradient 51.0 vs 42.7 mmHg and maximal gradient 149.0 vs 111.0 mmHg) (Figs. 6 and 7), when compared with the control group (n.s.).

These results confirm other experiences: verapamil predominantly improves diastolic left ventricular function, but can also reduce high contractility and the degree of left ventricular obstruction.

Our clinical experience with verapamil covers 91 consecutive patients (20 females and 71 males; age 12 to 59, mean 43 years), 23 of whom had HNCM and 68 of whom had the obstructive form (left ventricular outflow tract pressure gradient exceeding 30 mmHg). The patients were treated as follows: a mean oral daily dose of 515 mg verapamil in 77 cases, 160 mg gallopamil in 27, and 30 mg nifedipine in one. The follow-up period was between two and 150 months (mean 70 months). Thus our experience is based on a total of 525 patient treatment years. For each patient, the mean values for all data acquired during calcium antagonist therapy were calculated and compared with individual primary values. Complete echocardiographic measurements have been included since 1976.

Results: Prior to therapy with calcium antagonists, most patients complained of typical symptoms, in particular, dyspnea and angina pectoris. Only 10 patients were symptom free. During therapy, 63 of the previously symptomatic patients (69%) re-

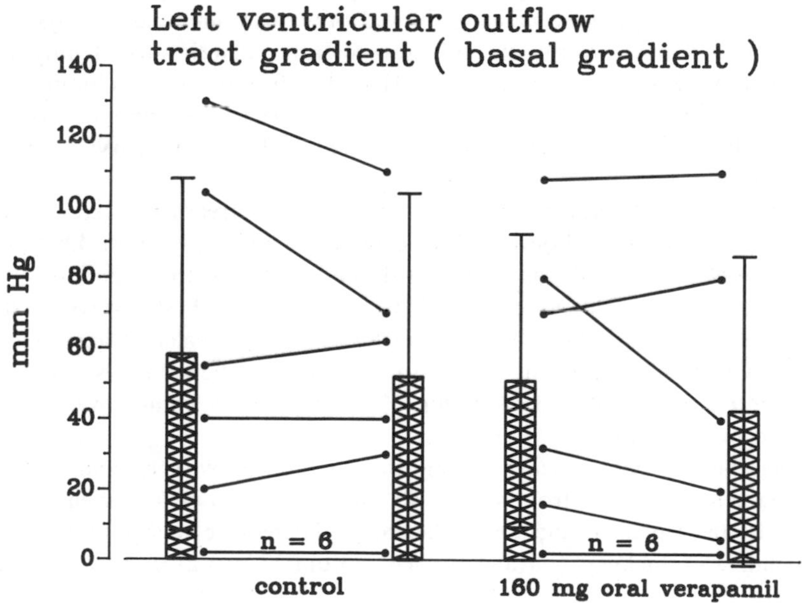

Fig. 6. Hemodynamic effects of 160 mg oral verapamil in patients with HCM. The medication with verapamil had no influence on basal left ventricular gradient in the subgroup of patients with the obstructive form (51.0 ± 41.6 vs 42.7 ± 43.9 mmHg).

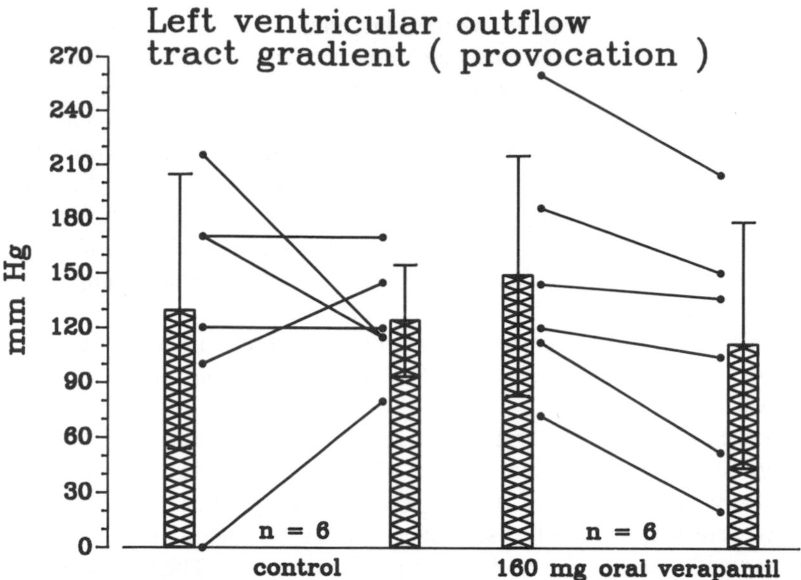

Fig. 7. Hemodynamic effects of 160 mg oral verapamil in patients with HCM. When compared with the control group (measurement before/after angiography), verapamil in all patients reduced the maximal left ventricular outflow tract gradient (following provocation maneuvers) from 149.0 ± 66.1 to 111.0 ± 67.2 mmHg. The differences were not significant with the administered dose, however.

ported improvement or even complete relief of symptoms. In 20 patients there was no change; however, nine of these patients showed previously unimpaired physical stress tolerance. In nine patients symptoms and stress tolerance deteriorated slightly. According to the New York Heart Association (NYHA) classification, a mean improvement of all patients from functional class 2.6 to 1.9 was achieved. The annual mortality rate related to cardiomyopathy was 1.5% in our patients. The 10-year survival probability (Kaplan-Meier test) was 81.4%.

Follow-up electrocardiograms during calcium antagonist treatment were documented in 89 patients. The mean Sokolow index decreased significantly from 4.8 to 4.4 mV within the first 24 months and was 4.4 mV at the end of the treatment period.

The cardiac configuration, as evaluated by conventional chest X-rays in standing position as well as cardiac size, remained unchanged during calcium antagonist treatment. Heart volume measurements were available in 85 patients and showed it to be reduced from 932 to 897 ml/1.73 m^2 within 24 months. Heart volume was 902 ml/1.73 m^2 at the end of observation.

Paralleling the changes in heart volume during therapy with calcium antagonists, left atrial diameter decreased from 42.5 to 40.7 mm in a total of 63 patients within the first 24 months and remained unchanged thereafter. There were no significant changes in left ventricular wall thickness (intraventricular septum 22.8 vs 21.0; posterior wall 14.4 vs 13.4 mm).

Studies on Diltiazem

In 1983, Nagao *et al.* demonstrated with echocardiography in 11 patients that intravenously administered diltiazem decreases isovolumic left ventricular relaxation time and thus may improve impaired diastolic filling patterns in HCM.[57] Suwa *et al.* compared diltiazem and propranolol, and found left ventricular diastolic function improved following acute intravenous or chronic oral diltiazem administration.[58] Although no controlled clinical trials have been reported as yet, it could be expected that diltiazem might have effects on HCM similar to those of verapamil, because of its similar hemodynamic actions.

Studies on Nifedipine

Nifedipine has also been reported to improve diastolic ventricular function in patients with HCM. Lorell *et al.* first demonstrated modification of left ventricular filling pattern in a patient with HNCM.[46] This was confirmed by systematic studies.[59,60] In contrast, Betocchi *et al.* were unable to see these effects on systolic and diastolic function in 36 patients with HCM, including 17 with HOCM.[61] Nifedipine diminishes peripheral vascular resistance and can thereby produce hemodynamic instability with provocation or augmentation of outflow tract obstruction.[61,62] Following acute administration or short-term therapy with sublingual nifedipine, cardiac index usually increases in association with a fall in blood pressure and filling pressure,[55,61,63,64] whereas the behavior of the left ventricular outflow tract gradient is nonuniform.[55,64]

Combination of Calcium Antagonists and β-Blockers

It could be supposed that the hemodynamic effects of propranolol on supernormal left ventricular systolic function and those of nifedipine on impaired diastolic function together might improve cardiac function and consequently symptoms as well. Although clinical investigations only showed minor effects on ventricular systolic function at rest, augmentation of obstruction, following provocation, could be prevented. Calcium antagonists predominantly improve diastolic left ventricular function. Therefore it has been suggested that the combination of β-blockers and calcium antagonists might constitute a beneficial therapeutic approach.[65–67] Combined therapy should be especially effective with a β-blocker like propranolol, because there is no intrinsic sympathomimetic activity which could produce attenuation of the desired effects. It seems to be rational then to use nifedipine as a calcium antagonist, thereby improving especially diastolic features without additional negative chronotropic or dromotropic effects. In addition, data have shown that nifedipine has beneficial acute effects on ventricular dynamics; these are further improved by propranolol and vice versa.[68]

Our study comparised 15 patients with HCM (14 males and one female; age 22–67, mean 45.5 years). HNCM was present in five and HOCM in 10 patients. Left ventricular filling pressures ranged from 5 to 32 mmHg (mean 16 mmHg). Twelve patients had undergone pretreatment with verapamil, one with propranolol; two had no previous therapy. Combined medication was initiated with a daily oral dose of 30 mg nifedipine and 240 mg propranolol. The duration of combined therapy was six to 24 months (mean 18 months). Due to side effects, premature termination became necessary in three patients after six months, and in two patients after 12 months. The other 10 patients tolerated the combined treatment well. The study was stopped when eight patients had been treated for 24 months and two for 18 months.

Results: During treatment with nifedipine and propranolol, improvement occurred in two patients, there was no change in five and there was deterioration in eight. Two patients exhibited syncope for the first time while under this therapy. The symptomatic status, according to the NYHA classification, was 1.9 before and 2.1 at the end of therapy.

The Sokolow index of all patients showed no significant change during nifedipine-propranolol therapy, but the heart volume increased significantly from 887 to 947 ml/1.73 m^2 body surface area. On echocardiogram, a significant increase in left atrial diameter from 40 to 42 mm was evident, whereas left ventricular wall thickness did not change (intraventricular septum: 20.5 vs. 21.5 mm; posterior wall: 13.1 vs. 13.6 mm).

Our results indicate that the combination of nifedipine and propranolol has no favorable clinical effects in patients with HCM.[12]

Therapy with Antiarrhythmic Agents

Arrhythmias, including supraventricular tachyarrhythmias, bradyarrhythmias, and heart block, are frequent in patients with HCM.[69] Nonsustained ventricular tachycardia can be present even in patients with normal exercise tolerance and without symptomatic episodes, and may be associated with cardiac arrest.[70–73] The aim of anti-arrhythmic therapy is prevention of sudden cardiac death. But the combination of conventional agents, such as quinidine or mexiletine, when used alone or in combination with moderate doses of β-blockers was unsuccessful and not well tolerated.[74]

Studies on Disopyramide

Disopyramide has also been proven in patients with HCM to be potentially effective in the treatment of supraventricular and ventricular arrhythmias. The observation that negative inotropic action is able to reduce the degree of outflow tract obstruction seemed to be an additional argument for introduction into the therapeutic regimen.[75] Following acute administration, improvement in symptoms and exercise capacity can be seen, but long-term results are not yet available. In addition, the effectiveness of disopyramide on rhythm disturbances has been reported to be poor in patients with HCM.[74]

Studies on Amiodarone

Because amiodarone is effective in prevention and conversion of supraventricular as well as serious ventricular arrhythmias, it can assumed an important role in the therapy of HCM.[76] Supraventricular arrhythmias have been suppressed or even abolished. Ventricular tachycardia was almost completely preventable.[77] In comparison to conventional antiarrhythmic treatment, amiodarone reduced mortality rate.[78] However, inefficacy and a potential increase in the rate of sudden death have also been described.[79] Independent of antiarrhythmic effects, systolic anterior motion of the mitral valve was seen to disappear after treatment,[80] and improvement of symptoms and prolongation of exercise tolerance has been described in some patients;[81] this was, however, not seen during long-term treatment.[82] In addition, hemodynamic measurements and radionuclide angiography did not show any beneficial effects.[82,83] Side effects are well documented, so that individual dose titration is advised.[84] Amiodarone might thus be useful in patients with refractory arrhythmias[49]: the combination with calcium antagonists seems, in our experience, to be useful and without major complications.

Other Medications

Formerly diuretics were assumed to be dangerous in HOCM because of a possible reduction in preload and subsequent augmentation of outflow tract obstruction. In our experience, however, this agents have proved to be useful, especially in patients with pulmonary congestion and peripheral edema. Today diuretics are usually included in the therapeutic regimen and are thought to have mainly beneficial effects due to a reduction of left ventricular filling pressure.[49]

However, drugs which cause rapid reduction in preload, such as nitroglycerin, or with positive inotropy are potentially dangerous in HOCM, but in some special cases with tachyarrhythmia, digitalis might become necessary to delay av-conduction.

There are HCM patients with normal systolic ventricular function who develop pulmonary congestion due to "diastolic heart failure." In these cases, it can be helpful to administer sublingual verapamil or nifedipine in addition to saluretic basic medication. In later stages of the disease, some patients with HCM may also have severely impaired systolic left ventricular function and therefore congestive heart failure. Our experience indicates that, even for such patients, the combination of verapamil with diuretics is able to improve symptoms and exercise tolerance.

Comparison of Different Treatment Regimens and Conclusions

There are the following goals of therapeutic intervention which are the basis for comparison of treatment regimens and their value: (1) a reduction of symptoms and thereby an improvement of exercise tolerance, (2) a retardation or even prevention of disease progression, and (3) improvement of the patient's prognosis.

High-risk patients with the obstructive form of HCM are characterized by familial history or episodes of syncope and/or rapid subjective and objective progression, manifestation in childhood. In these cases surgery with myotomy/myectomy must be discussed, although in many of them impressive improvement can be seen following verapamil treatment.

Kober *et al.* compared a two-year treatment with verapamil or propranolol in patients with HCM. On the basis of symptoms and electrocardiogram, verapamil showed better results than patients treated with high doses of propranolol. Side effects and deterioration were also seen more often in the propranolol group.[86] However, in some patients verapamil was seen to have serious side effects.[87] We ourselves cannot confirm this. Usually verapamil was well tolerated. Only one of our patients developed first degree atrioventricular block, and we did not observe pulmonary edema due to verapamil in any patient, including those with high outflow tract gradients or markedly increased left ventricular filling pressure.[88] Verapamil improved maximal exercise tolerance and also hemodynamics; no comparable effects were brought about by propranolol.[25] This is in agreement with the results of Suwa *et al.*, who found diastolic left ventricular function only improved following long-term diltiazem therapy, but not with long-term propranolol therapy.[58] Similar results have been reported when verapamil has been compared to pindolol, with the calcium antagonist found superior to the β-blocker.[89] In contrast, nifedipine alone was not seen to be more effective than propranolol,[65] but the combined acute administration of both drugs had favorable hemodynamic effects.[66]

The symptomatic status and clinical results of amiodarone therapy are contradictory; thus it is considered as a therapeutic option only in those patients in whom conventional treatment has failed.[49]

It is not yet clear whether any therapeutic intervention is potent enough to stop the process of hypertrophy or hyperplasia in HCM, but results indicate at least a probable retardation of the disease progression with surgery or verapamil therapy.[10,54] Perhaps this is only the consequence of hemodynamic effects, which can be shown in children and adolescents[90] to lead to relief of the left ventricle, or the result of cellular calcium antagonistic mechanisms that directly half the increase in cardiac mass.

The natural history of HCM is characterized by slow progression, and sudden death may occur independent of objective findings and symptomatic status. It has been shown that annual mortality is about 3.5% in untreated patients.[91–93] Medical or surgical treatment may improve prognosis.[94] Only Frank *et al.* has reported a better prognosis in patients treated with propranolol,[35,67] which has shown no improvement,[32,33,93] or only minor effects.[94] Prognosis was significantly better in patients who successfully underwent surgery or were treated with verapamil.[30,32,33,92,93] It has been shown that verapamil has antiarrhythmic effects.[95] In addition to improved left ventricular funcncy, there might be better tolerance, in the case of arrhythmia, as the reason for a better prognosis. When compared with verapamil, amiodarone was shown to have more pronounced antiarrhythmic effects,[76] but it has not been clearly demonstrated to improve life expectancy in HCM.[49,79]

It therefore seems rational to treat patients with HCM medically with calcium antagonists, especially with verapamil. With regard to a probable improvement in life expectancy, we consider that it is reasonable to also treat patients without symptoms. Rhythm disturbances should be treated with additional antiarrhythmics, for example, amiodarone. We saw no problems with this combination, but repeat studies of its effectiveness are necessary. If patients do not respond to medical treatment, surgery must always be considered an alternative.

REFERENCES

1. Schmincke, A. Über linksseitige muskuläre Conusstenosen. *Dtsch. Med. Wschr.* **33**: 2082–2083, 1907.
2. Teare, D. Asymmetrical hypertrophy of the heart in young adults. *Br. Heart J.* **20**: 1–8, 1958.
3. Braunwald, E., Lambrew, C.T., Rockoff, S.D., Ross, J. Jr., and Morrow, A.G. Idiopathic hypertrophic subaortic stenosis: A description of the disease based upon an analysis of 64 patients. *Circulation* **30**, (Suppl. 4) IV3–IV119, 1964.
4. Wigle, E.D., Heimbecker, R.O., and Gunton, R.W. Idiopathic ventricular septal hypertrophy causing muscular subaortic stenosis. *Circulation* **26**: 325–340, 1962.
5. Wigle, E.D. and Wilansky, S. Diastolic dysfunction in hypertrophic cardiomyopathy. *Heart Failure* **2**: 82–93, 1987.
6. Braunwald, E. and Ebert, P.A. Hemodynamic alterations in idiopathic hypertrophic subaortic stenosis induced by sympathomimetic drugs. *Am. J. Cardiol.* **10**: 489–500, 1962.
7. Gorlin, R., Cohen, L.S., Elliott, W.C., Klein, M.D., and Lane, F.J. Haemodynamics of muscular subaortic stenosis (Obstructive Cardiomyopathy). In: Cardiomyopathies, Wolstenholme, G.E.W. and O'Connor, M. (eds.), J. & A. Churchill, Ltd., London, 1964, pp. 76–99.
8. Goodwin, J.F., Shah, M., Oakly, C.M., Cohen, J., Yipintsoi, T., and Pocock, W. The clinical pharmacology of hypertrophic obstructive cardiomyopathy. In: Cardiomyopathies, Wolstenholme, G.E.W. and O'Connor, M. (eds.), J. & A. Churchill, Ltd., London, 1964, pp. 189–213.
9. Hopf, R., Keller, M., and Kaltenbach, M. Die Behandlung der hypertrophen obstruktiven Kardiomyopathie mit Verapamil. *Verh. Dtsch. Ges. Inn. Med.* 82, Bd. II, 1054–1057, 1976.
10. Kaltenbach, M., Hopf, R., and Keller, M. Calciumantagonistische Therapie bei hypertroph obstructiver Kardiomyopathie. *Dtsch. Med. Wschr.* **101**: 1907–1911, 1976.
11. Kaltenbach, M., Hopf, R., Kober, G., Bussmann, W.-D., Keller, M., and Petersen, Y. Traetment of hypertrophic obstrucive cardiomyopathy with verapamil. *Br. Heart J.* **42**: 35–42, 1979.

12. Hopf, R., Thomas, J., Klepzig, H., and Kaltenbach, M. Behandlung der hypertrophischen Kardiomyopathie mit Nifedipin und Propranolol in Kombination. *Z. Kardiol.* **76**: 469–478, 1987.
13. McKenna, W.J., England, D., Oakley, C., and Goodwin, J. Detection of arrhythmia in hypertrophic cardiomyopathy: prospective study (abstr.). *Circulation* **62** (suppl. III): 187, 1980.
14. McKenna, W.J., Harris, L., Perez, G., Krikler, D.M., Oakley, C., and Goodwin, J.F. Arrhythmia in hypertrophic cardiomyopathy. II: Comparison of amiodarone and verapamil in treatment. *Br. Heart J.* **46**: 173–178, 1981.
15. Linden, R.J. Related physiology of cardiac contraction. In: Cardiomyopathies, Wolstenholme, G.E.W. and O'Connor, M. (eds.), J. & A. Churchill, Ltd., London, 1964, pp. 100–131.
16. Swanton, R.H., Brooksby, I.A.B., Jenkins, B.S., and Webb-Peploe, M.M. Hemodynamic studies of beta-blockade in hypertrophic obstructive cardiomyopathy. *Eur. J. Cardiol.* **5/4**: 327–341, 1977.
17. Flamm, M.D., Harrison, D.C., and Hancock, E.W. Muscular subaortic stenosis: Prevention of outflow obstruction with propranolol. *Circulation* **38**: 846–858, 1968.
18. El Gamal, M., Schasfort, G.B.A., and Schrijvers, L.C.M. Relief of severe left ventricular outflow obstruction in a case of hypertrophic obstructive cardiomyopathy treated with practolol. *Br. Heart J.* **37**: 225–228, 1975.
19. Goodwin, J.F. Treatment of cardiomyopathies. *Am. J. Cardiol.* **32**: 341–351, 1973.
20. Harrison, D.C., Braunwald, E., Glick, G., Mason, D.T., Chidsey, C.A., and Ross, J. Jr. Effects of beta adrenergic blockade on the circulation, with particular reference to observations in patients with hypertrophic subaortic stenosis. *Circulation* **29**: 84–98, 1964.
21. Oakley, C.M. Beta-adrenergic blocking agents in hypertrophic cardiomyopathy (HOCM), *Singapore Med. J.* **14**: 408–409, 1973.
22. Sowton, E. Betarezeptorenblocker bei hypertropher Kardiomyopathie. In: Die Betablocker—Gegenwart und Zukunft, Schweizer, W. (ed.), Verlag Hans Huber, Bern-Stuttgart-Wien, 1976, pp. 239–258.
23. De la Calzada, C.S., Ziady, G.M., Hardarson, T., Curiel, R., and Goodwin, J.F. Effect of acute administration of propranolol on ventricular function in hypertrophic obstructive cardiomyopathy measured by non-invasive techniques. *Br. Heart J.* **38**: 798–803, 1976.
24. Hess, O.M., Grimm, J., and Krayenbuehl, H.P. Diastolic function in hypertrophic cardiomyopathy: effects of propranolol and verapamil on diastolic stiffness. *Eur. Heart J.* **4**, Suppl. F: 47–56, 1983.
25. Losse, B., Kuhn, H., Loogen, F., and Schulte, H.D. Exercise performance in hypertrophic cardiomyopathies. *Eur. Heart J.* **4**, Suppl. F: 197–208, 1983.
26. Cherian, G., Brockington, I.F., Shah, P.M., Oakley, C.M., and Goodwin, J.F. Beta-adrenergic blockade in hypertrophic obstructive cardiomyopathy. *Br. Med. J.* **1**: 895–898, 1966.
27. Cohen, L.S. and Braunwald, Amelioration of angina pectoris in idiopathic hypertrophic subaortic stenosis with beta adrenergic blockade. *Circulation* **35**: 847–851, 1967.
28. Adelman, A.G., Shah, P.M., Gramiak, R., and Wigle, E.D. Longterm propranolol therapy in muscular subaortic stenosis. *Br. Heart J.* **32**: 804–811, 1970.
29. Goodwin, J.F. Congestive and hypertrophic cardiomyopathies. A decade of study. *Lancet* **i**: 731–739, 1970.
30. Stenson, R.E., Flamm, M.D. Jr., Harrison, D.C., and Hancock, E.W. Hypertrophic subaortic stenosis: clinical and hemodynamic effects of long-term propranolol therapy. *Am. J. Cardiol.* **31**: 763–773, 1973.
31. Assmann, H., Assmann, I., Fiehring, H., Dittrich, P., and Eger, H. Verlaufsbeobachtungen bei der idiopathischen hypertrophischen subaortalen Stenose unter Propranololbehandlung. *Dt. Gesundh.-Wesen* **30**: 918–920, 1975.
32. Kuhn, H. and Loogen, F. Die anwendung von beta-rezeptorenblockern bei hypertrophis-

cher obstruktiver Kardiomyopathie (HOCM). *Internist* **19**: 527–531, 1978.

33. Loogen, F., Kuhn, H., Gietzen, F., Lösse, B., Schulte, H.D., and Bircks, W. Clinical course and prognosis of patients with typical and atypical hypertrophic obstructive and with hypertrophic non-obstructive cardiomyopathy. *Eur. Heart J.* **4** (suppl. F): 145–153, 1983.
34. Frank, M.J., Abdulla, A.M., Canedo, M.I., and Saylors, R.E. Long-term medical management of hypertrophic obstructive cardiomyopathy. *Am. J. Cardiol.* **42**: 993–1001, 1978.
35. Frank, M.J., Abdulla, A.M., Watkins, L.O., Prisant, L., and Stefadouros, M.A. Long-term medical management of hypertrophic cardiomyopathy: usefulness of propranolol. *Eur. Heart J.* **4** (suppl. F): 155–164, 1983.
36. Adelman, A.G., Wigle, E.D., Ranganathan, R., Webb, G.D., Kidd, B.S.C., Bigelow, W.G., and Silver, M.D. The clinical course of muscular subaortic stenosis. *Ann. Int. Med.* **77**: 515–525, 1972.
37. Epstein, S.E. and Maron, B.J. Hypertrophic cardiomyopathy: an overview. *Clin. Invest. Med.* **3**: 185–193, 1980.
38. Mushoff, K. and Reindell, H. Zur Rontgenuntersuchung des Herzens in horizontaler und vertikaler Korperstellung: I. Mitteilung: Der Einflu der Korperstellung auf das Herzvolumen. *Dtsch. Med. Wschr.* **81**: 1001–1008, 1956.
39. Mushoff, K. and Reindell, H. Zur Rontgenuntersuchung des Herzens in horizontaler und vertikaler Korperstellung: II. Mitteilung: Der Einflu der Korperstellung auf die Herzform. *Dtsch. Med. Wschr.* **82**: 1075–1080, 1957.
40. Hopf, R. and Kaltenbach, M. Röntgenologische Herzvolumenbestimmung: Beschreibung einer neuen Methode mit Durchfuhrung im Sitzen. *Fortschr. Rontgenstr.* **127**: 167–169, 1977.
41. Rosing, D.R., Kent, K.M., Borer, D.J., Seides, S.F., Maron, B.J., and Epstein, S.E. Verapamil therapy: A new approach to the pharmacologic treatment of hypertrophic cardiomyopathy. I. Hemodynamic effects. *Circulation* **60**: 1201–1207, 1979.
42. Rosing D.R., Kent, K.M., Maron, B.J., and Epstein, S.E. Verapamil therapy: A new approach to the pharmacologic treatment of hypertrophic cardiomyopathy. II. Effects on exercise capacity and symptomatic status. *Circulation* **60**: 1208–1213, 1979.
43. Hanrath, P., Mathey, D.G., Kremer, P., Sonntag, F., and Bleifeld, W. Effect of verapamil on left ventricular isovolumic relaxation time and regional left ventricular filling in hypertrophic cardiomyopathy. *Am. J. Cardiol.* **45**: 1258–1264, 1980.
44. Bonow, R.O., Rosing, D.R., Bacharach, S.L., Green, M.V., Kent, K.M., Lipson, L.C., Maron, B.J., and Epstein, S.E. Effects of verapamil on left ventricular systolic function and diastolic filling in patients with hypertrophic cardiomyopathy. *Circulation* **64**: 787–796, 1981.
45. Anderson, D.M., Raff, G.L., Ports, T.A., Brundage, B.H., Parmley, W.W., and Chatterjee, K. Hypertrophic obstructive cardiomyopathy: Effects of acute and chronic verapamil treatment on left ventricular systolic and diastolic function. *Br. Heart J.* **51**: 523–529, 1984.
46. Lorell, B.H., Paulus, W.J., Grossman, W., Wynne, J., Cohn, P.F., and Braunwald, E. Improved diastolic function and systolic performance in hypertrophic cardiomyopathy after nifedipine. *N. Engl. J. Med.* **303**: 801–803, 1980.
47. Hopf, R., Rodrian, S., and Kaltenbach, M. Behandlung der hypertrophen Kardiomyopathie mit Kalziumantagonisten: Eine Zehnjahresbilanz. *Therapiewoche* **36**: 1433–1454, 1986.
48. Rosing, D.R., Condit, J.R., Maron, B.J., Kent, K.M., Leon, M.B., Bonow, R.O., Lipson, L.C., and Epstein, S.E. Verapamil therapy: a new approach to the pharmacologic treatment of hypertrophic cardiomyopathy: III. Effects of long-term administration. *Am. J. Cardiol.* **48**: 545–553, 1981.
49. Maron, B.J., Bonow, R.O., Cannon, R.O., Leon, M.B., and Epstein, S.E. Hypertrophic cardiomyopathy: interrelations of clinical manifestations, pathophysiology, and therapy. *N. Engl. J. Med.* **316**: 780–789, 844–852, 1987.
50. Hopf, R. and Kaltenbach, M. Einfluß hoher Dosen von Verapamil auf die linksventrikuläre

Hämodynamik. In: Die Bedeutung der Kalzium-Antagonisten für die Hochdrucktherapie, Gross, F. (ed.), MMW Medizin Verlag, München, 1984, pp. 41–57.
51. Hopf, R. and Kaltenbach, M. Die hypertrophische Kardiomyopathie: Möglichkeiten der kalziumantagonistischen Behandlung. Georg Thieme Verlag, Stuttgart, New York, 1982, pp. 129–137.
52. Hanrath, P., Schlüter, M., Sonntag, F., Diemert, J., and Bleifeld, W. Influence of verapamil therapy on left ventricular performance at rest and during exercise in hypertrophic cardiomyopathy. *Am. J. Cardiol.* **52**: 544–548, 1983.
53. Bonow, R.O., Dilsizian, V., Rosing, D.R., Maron, B.J., Bacharach, S.L., and Green, M.V. Verapamil-induced improvement in left ventricular diastolic filling and increased exercise tolerance in patients with hypertrophic cardiomyopathy: short- and long-term effects. *Circulation* **72**: 853–864, 1985.
54. Kuhn, H., Thelen, U., Leuner, C., Köhler, E., and Bluschke, V. Lang-zeitbehandlung der hypertrophischen nicht obstruktiven Kardiomyopathie (HNCM) mit Verapamil. *Z. Kardiol.* **69**: 669–675, 1980.
55. Rosing, D.R., Idänpään-Heikkilä, U., Maron, B.J., Bonow, R.O., and Epstein, S.E. Use of calcium-channel blocking drugs in hypertrophic cardiomyopathy. *Am. J. Cardiol.* **55**: Suppl. 185B–195B, 1985.
56. Bryhn, M. and Eskilsson, J. Effects of verapamil on left ventricular diastolic function at rest and during isometric exercise in patients with hypertrophic cardiomyopathy. *Clin. Cardiol.* **10**: 31–36, 1987.
57. Nagao, M., Omote, S., Takizawa, A., and Yasue, H. Effect of diltiazem on left ventricular isovolumic relaxation time in patients with hypertrophic cardiomyopathy. *Jpn. Circ. J.* **47**: 54–58, 1983.
58. Suwa, M., Hirota, Y., and Kawamura, K. Improvement in left ventricular diastolic function during intravenous and oral diltiazem therapy in patients with hypertrophic cardiomyopathy: an echocardiographic study. *Am. J. Cardiol.* **54**: 1047–1053, 1984.
59. Lorell, B.H., Paulus, W.J., Grossman, W., Wynne, J., and Cohn, P.F. Modification of abnormal left ventricular diastolic properties by nifedipine in patients with hypertrophic cardiomyopathy. *Circulation* **65**: 499–507, 1982.
60. Senn, M., Hess, O.M., and Krayenbuhl, H.P. Nifedipin in der Behandlung der hypertrophen, nicht obstruktiven Kardiomyopathie. *Schweiz. Med. Wschr.* **112**: 1312–1317, 1982.
61. Betocchi, S., Cannon, R.O., Watson, R.M., Bonow, R.O., Ostrow, H.G., Epstein, S.E., and Rosing, D.R. Effects of sublingual nifedipine on hemodynamics and systolic and diastolic function in patients with hypertrophic cardiomyopathy. *Circulation* **72**: 1001–1007, 1985.
62. Krayenbühl, H.P., Hirzel, H.O., Hess, O.M., and Senn, M. Behandlung der hypertrophen kardiomyopathie mit Kalzium-Antagonisten. In: New Calcium Antagonists: Recent Developments and Prospects. Fleckenstein, A., Hashimoto, K., Herrmann, M., Schwartz, A., and Seipel L. (eds.), Gustav Fischer Verlag, Stuttgart, New York, 1983, pp. 199–210.
63. Paulus, W.J., Lorell, B.H., Craig, W.E., Wynne, J., Murgo, J.P., and Grossman, W. Comparison of the effects of nitroprusside and nifedipine on diastolic properties in patients with hypertrophic cardiomyopathy: altered left ventricular loading or improved muscle inactivation? *J. Am. Coll. Cardiol.* **2**: 879–886, 1983.
64. Schanzenbacher, P., Schick, K.D., and Kochsiek, K. Nifedipin bei hypertrophisch obstruktiver Kardiomyopathie. *Dtsch. Med. Wschr.* **107**: 1842–1846, 1982.
65. Cserhalmi, L., Abmann, I., Glavanow, M., Rev, J., and Kelecseneyi, Z. Langzeittherapie der hypertrophischen obstruktiven und nichtobstruktiven Kardiomyopathie mit Nifedipin im Vergleich zu Propranolol. *Zschr. Ges. Inn. Med.* **39**: 330–335, 1984.
66. Landmark, K., Sire, S., Thanlow, E., Amlie, J.P., and Nitter-Hange, S. Haemodynamic effects of nifedipine and propranolol in patients with hypertrophic obstructive cardiomyopathy. *Br. Heart J.* **48**: 19–26, 1982.
67. Frank, M.J., Watkins, L.O., and Abdulla, A.M. Management with beta-adrenergic blocking

drugs. In: Hypertrophic Cardiomyopathy: Clinical recognition and management, Ten Cate, F.J. (ed.), M. Dekker, New York, Basel, 1985, pp. 155–172.

68. Gotsman, M.S. and Lewis, B.S. Left ventricular volumes and compliance in hypertrophic cardiomyopathy. *Chest* **66**: 498–505, 1974.
69. Sonntag, F., Hanrath, P., Saal, M., Diemert, J., Mathey, D., Kupper, W., and Bleifeld, W. Untersuchungen zur Frage der Häufigkeit und Vorhersehbarkeit von ventrikulären Herzrhythmusstorungen bei Patienten mit hypertropher Kardiomyopathie. *Herz/Kreislauf* **12**: 481–489, 1980.
70. Maron, B.J., Savage, D.D., Wolfson, J.K., and Epstein, S.E. The prognostic significance of 24 hour ambulatory electrocardiographic monitoring in patients with hypertrophic cardiomyopathy. *Am. J. Cardiol.* **48**: 252–257, 1981.
71. McKenna, W.J., Chetty, S., Oakley, C.M., and Goodwin, J.F. Arrhythmia in hypertrophic cardiomyopathy: exercise and 48 hour ambulatory electrocardiographic assessment with and without beta adrenergic blocking therapy. *Am. J. Cardiol.* **45**: 1–5, 1980.
72. McKenna, W.J., England, D., Oakley, C., and Goodwin, J.F. Detection of arrhythmia in hypertrophic cardiomyopathy. I. Influence on prognosis. *Br. Heart J.* **46**: 168–172, 1981.
73. McKenna, W.J. and Kleinebenne, A. Arrhythmien bei hypertrophischer Kardiomyopathie: Bedeutung und therapeutische Konsequenzen. *Herz* **10**: 91–101, 1985.
74. McKenna, W.J. Arrhythmia and prognosis in hypertrophic cardiomyopathy. *Eur. Heart J.* **4** (suppl. F): 225–234, 1983.
75. Pollick, C. Muscular aortic stenosis: Hemodynamic and clinical improvement after disopyramide. *N. Engl. J. Med.* **307**: 997–999, 1982.
76. McKenna, W.J. Arrhythmia and prognosis in hypertrophic cardiomyopathy. *Eur. Heart J.* **4** (suppl. F): 225–234, 1983.
77. McKenna, W.J., Harris, L., Rowland, E., Kleinebenne, A., Krikler, D.M., Oakley, C.M., and Goodwin, J.F. Amiodarone for long-term management of patients with hypertrophic cardiomyopathy. *Am. J. Cardiol.* **54**: 802–810, 1984.
78. McKenna, W.J., Oakly, C.M., Krikler, D.M., and Goodwin, J.F. Improved survival with amiodarone in patients with hypertrophic cardiomyopathy and ventricular tachycardia. *Br. Heart J.* **53**: 412–416, 1985.
79. Leon, M-B., Tracy, C.M., Winkler, J., Bergamo, C., Bonow, R.O., and Epstein, S.E. Amiodarone does not prevent, and may increase, sudden death in patients with hypertrophic cardiomyopathy. *Circulation* **76**, Suppl. IV: 248 (abstr.), 1987.
80. Enia, F., Comparato, C., DiFranca, F., Ledda, A., and Mizio, G. Systolic anterior motion of the mitral valve in patients with hypertrophic cardiomyopathy: Disappearance after treatment with amiodarone. *Chest* **91**: 277–278, 1987.
81. Leon, M.B., Rosing, D.R., Maron, B.J., Bonow, R.O., Lesko, L.L., and Epstein, S.E. Amiodarone in patients with hypertrophic cardiomyopathy and refractory cardiac symptoms: an alternative to current medical therapy. *Circulation* **70**, Suppl. 2: II–18, 1984.
82. Paulus, W.J., Nellens, P., Heyndrickx, G.R., and Andries, E. Effects of long-term treatment with amiodarone on exercise hemodynamics and left ventricular relaxation in patients with hypertrophic cardiomyopathy. *Circulation* **74**: 544–554, 1986.
83. Sugrue, D.D., Dickie, S., Myers, M.J., Lavender, J.P., and McKenna, W.J. Effect of amiodarone on left ventricular ejection and filling in hypertrophic cardiomyopathy as assessed by radionuclide angiography. *Am. J. Cardiol.* **54**: 1054–1058, 1984.
84. McKenna, W.J., Harris, L., Mulrow, J.P., Rowland, E., and Holt, D.W. Amiodarone dose titration: a method to minimise side effects during long term therapy. *Br. J. Clin. Proct.* 40, Suppl. **44**: 121–127, 1986.
85. McKenna, W.J., Harris, L., Perez, G., Krikler, D.M., Oakley, C., and Goodwin, J.F. Arrhythmia in hypertrophic cardiomyopathy. II: comparison of amiodarone and verapamil in treatment. *Br. Heart J.* **46**: 173–178, 1981.
86. Kober, G., Hopf, R., Biamino, G., Bubenheimer, P., Förster, K., Kuck, K.H., Hanrath, P., Olshausen, K.-E. V., Schlepper, M., and Kaltenbach, M. Long-term treatment of hy-

pertrophic cardiomyopathy with verapamil or propranolol in matched pairs of patients. Results of a multicenter study. *Z. Kardiol.* **76** (suppl. 3): 113–118, 1987.

87. Epstein, S.E. and Rosing, D.R. Verapamil: Its potential for causing serious complications in patients with hypertrophic cardiomyopathy. *Circulation* **64**: 437–441, 1981.
88. Hopf, R. and Kaltenbach, M. 10-year results and survival of patients with hypertrophic cardiomyopathy treated with calcium antagonists. *Z. Kardiol.* **76** (suppl. 3): 137–144, 1987.
89. Masini, V., Ceci, V. Malinconico, U., and Milazzotto, F .Therapeutic evaluation of pindolol and verapamil in hypertrophic obstructive cardiomyopathy. *G. Ital. Cardiol.* **11**: 1729–1737, 1981.
90. Spicer, R.L., Rocchini, A.P., Crowley, D.C., Vasiliades, J., and Rosenthal, A. Hemodynamic effects of verapamil in children and adolescents with hypertrophic cardiomyopathy. *Circulation* **67**: 413–420, 1983.
91. Shah, P.M., Adelman, A.G., Wigle, E.D., Gobel, F.L., Burchell, H.B., Hardarson, T., Curiel, R., Calzada, C.S., and Oakley, C.M. Trophic obstructive cardiomyopathy. A multicenter study. *Circ. Res.* **34** (suppl II): 179–195, 1973.
92. Haberer, T., Hess, O.M., Jenni, R., and Krayenbühl, H.P. Hypertrophe obstruktive Kardiomyopathie: Spontanverlauf im Vergleich zur Langzeittherapie mit Propranolol und Verapamil. *Z. Kardiol.* **72**: 487–493, 1983.
93. Loogen, F., Kuhn, H., and Krelhaus, W. Natural history of hypertrophic cardiomyopathy and the effect of therapy. In: Cardiomyopathy and Myocardial Biopsy. Kaltenbach, M., Loogen, F., Olssen, E.G. (eds.), Springer-Verlag, Berlin Heidelberg New York 1978, pp. 286–299.
94. Rothlin, M.E., Gobet, D., Haberer, T., Krayenbuehl, H.P., Turina, M., and Senning, A. Surgical treatment versus medical treatment in hypertrophic obstructive cardiomyopathy. *Eur. Heart J.* **4** (suppl. F): 215–223.
95. Cranefield, P.F., Aronson, R.S., and Wit, A.L. Effect of verapamil on the normal action potential and on a calcium dependent slow response of canine Purkinje fibers. *Circ. Res.* **34**: 204–213, 1971.

Diastolic Properties in Hypertrophic Cardiomyopathy and Its Modulation with Pharmacotherapy

Yuzo Hirota

The Third Division, Department of Internal Medicine, Osaka Medical College, Takatsuki, Japan

ABSTRACT

Hypertrophic cardiomyopathy is a disease of diastolic dysfunction characterized by impaired relaxation and reduced compliance of the left ventricle. Impaired relaxation and reduced compliance are considered to be due to (1) hypertrophy of the myocardium, (2) subendocardial or global ischemia, and (3) interstitial or replacement fibrosis. Beta-blocking agents, especially propranolol. have been used for treatment, and some believe that propranolol improves abnormal diastolic properties. Others, however, believe that β-blockers do not improve diastolic dysfunction. Currently, calcium antagonists are widely employed because of their positive lusitropic effect. There are, however, certain limitations to symptomatic improvement with these agents. Congestive heart failure induced by calcium antagonists has been reported in patients with hypertrophic cardiomyopathy. Caution must be exercised when calcium antagonists are prescribed, to avoid deleterious effects such as congestive heart failure and sino-atrial or atrioventricular block. These untoward effects are usually seen in patients with severely elevated left ventricular end-diastolic pressure or bradyarrhythmias.

INTRODUCTION

It has been frequently stated that hypertrophic cardiomyopathy (HCM) is a diastolic disease. Normal or supernormal left ventricular (LV) systolic function manifested by normal or supernormal LV ejection fraction (EF), and stiff or less compliant LV evidenced by normal LV end-diastolic volume and elevated LV end-diastolic pressure have been known for more than two decades.[1] As early as 1968, Stewart and his associates[2] demonstrated impairment of the LV filling rate by analyzing diastolic left atrial pressure decay in HCM. With increased understanding of the mechanical properties of the myocardium, diastolic failure is now considered as important as systolic failure in the recognition of congestive heart failure, especially for the understanding of this disease.[3] The abnormal diastolic properties in HCM will be clarified and possible modulations with pharmacotherapy will be discussed in this paper.

EVIDENCE FOR IMPAIRED RELAXATION AND EARLY DIASTOLIC FILLING

High resistance to LV filling following hypertrophy and ventricular rigidity of unknown etiology was proposed as the most important feature of this disease by Goodwin in 1970.[4] This has been confirmed by reduced peak negative dP/dt,[5] prolonged isovolumic relaxation period as measured by echocardiography[6] and cineangiography,[7] and prolonged time constant of LV pressure fall.[8] Impaired early diastolic filling has been commonly known since the early observation of Stewart *et al.*[2] This phenomenon has been confirmed by many other investigators using different methodologies: cineangiography,[7] M-mode and Doppler echocardiography,[6,9–12] and radionuclide angiography.[13–15] As prolonged relaxation causes slow LV pressure fall, isovolumic relaxation should be prolonged. In some extreme cases, abnormally prolonged relaxation is evident by the fact that LV pressure continues to decline long after mitral valve opening, as pointed out by Lorell and her associates[16] (Fig. 1).

With the recent advance of Doppler echocardiography, numerous reports have been published dealing with the diastolic properties of HCM. It must be worthwhile to mention the results of these papers with the cautions to interplet these data. Pulsed Doppler transmitral flow velocity tracing is shown in Fig. 2. Gidding *et al.* found reduced peak early diastolic filling velocity (E) in pediatric patients with HCM compared to their normal control without any differences in peak late diastolic filling velocity (A) or these 2 ratio (E/A).[10] On the other hand, Gryg *et al.* reported marked reduction of E/A ratio when patients with mirtal regurgitation were excluded.[11] Rapid filling index which is the product of E and the cross-sectional area of the mitral anulus has been reported to be significantly reduced in patients with LV hypertrophy according to Peason *et al.*[12] They also found the ratio of the integral of early to late filling velocity (Ei/Ai) was re-

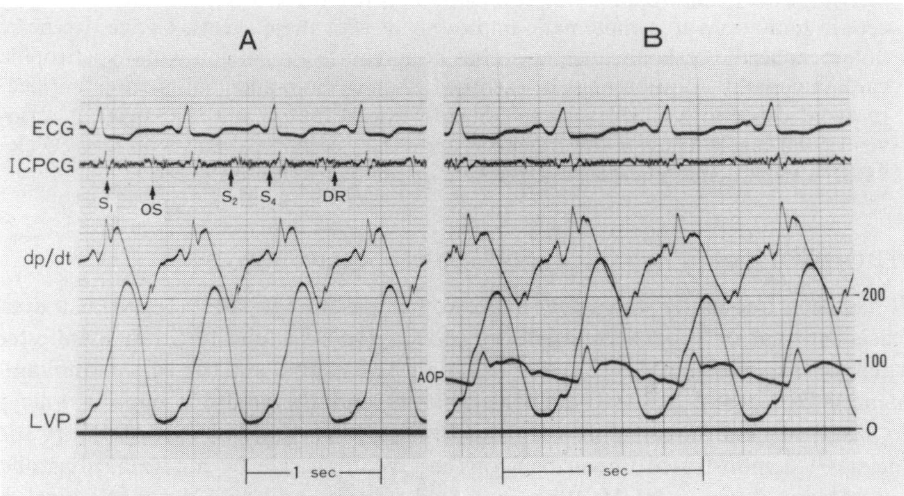

Fig. 1. A: Left ventricular pressure (LVP), its first derivative (dP/dt), and intracardiac phonocardiogram (ICPC) in a 48-year-old patient with hypertrophic obstructive cardiomyopathy, recorded in the high-pressure chamber with a catheter-tipped manometer system. LV pressure continued to decline long after the opening of the mitral valve indicated by the opening snap (OS) in ICPC. OS is not the actual opening snap, but the sound induced by the tip of the catheter being hit by the mitral valve. The form of dP/dt was markedly distorted. ECG = electrocardiogram, S1 = first heart sound, S2 = second heart sound, S4 = fourth heart sound, DR = diastolic rumble.

B: The simultaneous pressure recording of LVP and aortic pressure (AOP) in the same patient after sublingual nifedipine (10 mg) administration. AOP was recorded with a fluid-filled system. Elevation of LV end-diastolic pressure with the appearance of pulsus alternans of the LV pressure suggests deterioration of LV systolic and diastolic function with nifedipine.

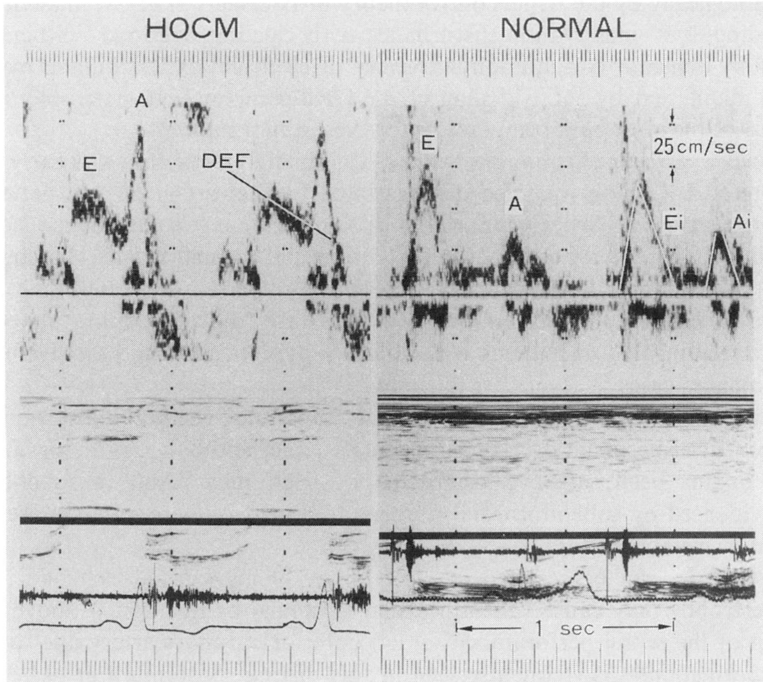

Fig. 2. Pulsed Doppler transmitral flow velocity tracing obtained from the apical position in a patient with hypertrophic obstructive cardiomyopathy (left panel: HOCM) and a normal subject (right panel: NORMAL). Peak early filling velocity (E), peak late filling velocity (A), their ratio (E/A), deceleration of early diastolic flow (DEF), integral of early (Ei) and late diastolic filling (Ai) and their ratio (Ei/Ai) are used as indexes of LV diastolic properties.

duced in hypertrophied heart. In their normal control, they found this Ei/Ai ratio had inverse correlation with age, and postulated that left ventricle become stiff by aging.[12] Marked differences of these Doppler derived diastolic indexes between patients with and without systolic anterior motion (SAM) of the mitral valve were reported by Takenaka and his associates.[17] With a large study population (111 patients with HCM), Maron and coworkers[18] have reported that in about 80% of their patients all Doppler derived indexes of diastolic properties were abnormal regardless of the presence or absence of outflow tract obstruction or cardiac symptoms. It is well known that these indexes are dependent on numerous factors such as preload, afterload and heart rate. Among these factors, preload or level of left atrial pressure seems to be the most important one.[19,20] Although precise analysis of these load depencence of diastolic properties in HCM are not yet done, we must pay cautions to interpret data of Doppler derived diastolic properties with regard to the patients' age, level of left atrial pressure, mitral regurgitation and intraventricular pressure gradient.

It has been concluded that relaxation disturbance does exist in HCM, and this prolongation of relaxation and ventricular rigidity, as discussed later, are the most important factors in impaired early diastolic filling.

The genesis and clinical significance of isovolumic relaxation and early diastolic filling disturbances are not well understood. They can be explained mechanically and electrophysiologically by the triple control theory of Brutsaert *et al.*[21]: inadequate end-systolic loading,[22-24] inactivation disturbance with calcium overload—either intrinsic or mediated by ischemia[25]—and nonuniformity of electrical excitation and mechanical contraction manifested by the widening of the QRS complex.[1] Hypertrophy and ischemia seem to be the most important factors for these abnormalities.

Hypertrophy: LV hypertrophy per se leads to impaired relaxation and early diastolic filling. Impaired LV filling was also demonstrated by Stewart *et al.*[2] in patients with valvular aortic stenosis. Hirota[8] reported a prolonged time constant of the isovolumic pressure fall in patients with essential hypertension and normal systolic function. Hanrath *et al.*[9] and Shimizu and coworkers[26] reported impaired diastolic filling in aortic stenosis and essential hypertension, respectively. Early diastolic filling abnormalities in HCM are seen in 70% of patients with mild LV hypertrophy, and the dysfunction is more prominent in cases of severe hypertrophy.[27]

Subendocardial ischemia: It is known that transient ischemia induces relaxation prolongation in experimental animal models[28] and spontaneous[29] or pacing-induced[30,31] angina pectoris. Severe hypertrophy itself may result in subendocardial ischemia, evidenced by subendocardial fibrosis,[32,33] inadequate coronary reserve,[34,35] and changes in metabolic state.[36]

Four possibilities can be counted in the etiology of myocardial ischemia in HCM. Excess hypertrophy may cause subendocardial ischemia, as mentioned above. Systolic compression of the septal perforators[37] or left anterior coronary artery due to myocardial bridge formation[38] is frequently seen in this disease. Nishimura *et al.*[39] have reported vasospasm of the large epicardial artery as a possible cause of anginal pain in patients with HCM. The presence of "small vessel disease" in HCM is one of the current interests of investigators.[40-42] Subendocardial or intramural fibrosis may be the result of a chronic ischemic process. Thus, recurrent subendocardial or global ischemia might be the major component of impaired relaxation and early diastolic filling.

EVIDENCE FOR REDUCED COMPLIANCE

Since the first description of the hemodynamic characteristics of this disease by Braunwald *et al.*[1] the importance of reduced compliance or ventricular stiffness has been repeatedly emphasized. Initially, it was demonstrated by the evidence that the majority of patients have elevated LV end-distolic pressure with normal or small end-diastolic cavity. There are two possible reasons for the reduction in ventricular compliance: one is low chamber compliance due to hypertrophy itself, with normal compliance of a unit muscle; the another is reduced compliance of a unit muscle or the reduction of muscle compliance. It must be clarified whether the ventricle is stiff due to hypertrophy itself or whether the myocardium is stiff in HCM.

Mirsky *et al.*[43] proposed the possibility of reduced muscle compliance in this disease based on their evaluation of the elastic stiffness constant (ks) derived from the theory of stress-strain relation analysis at the end-diastole. This finding was confirmed by Hirota *et al.*[24] Whereas the index of chamber stiffness derived from the analysis of pressure-volume relation (kp) is about three times higher than the normal value in HCM, the index of muscle stiffness (ks) is about 1.5 times higher than that of the normal ventricle.[3,43] Therefore, it can be concluded that the stiff left ventricle in HCM is due in part to hypertrophy itself and in part to increased myocardial stiffness. There are two possible reasons for the mechanism of reduced muscle compliance in this disease.

First, myocardial ischemia would cause reduced muscle compliance.[44,45] The direct mechanism involved in myocardial stiffness due to ischemia is not well understood, but disturbance of the calcium transport system and intracellular calcium overload have been postulated as the major cause of reduced compliance during the early phase of myocardial ischemia.[46] Cell injury and edema might also play important roles, in addition to calcium overload, in the early stage of ischemia. Development of myocardial fibrosis in the advanced stage of ischemia is also responsible for reduced muscle compliance in HCM.

Second, myocardial fibrosis is a common finding in HCM,[32,33,47] and it is generally believed that fibrosis is the major mechanism of reduced muscle compliance. There is one important question concerning the pathogenesis of myocardial fibrosis in HCM. If fibrosis is the sequela of ischemia, it must be associated with cell death, and therefore, either global or focal replacement fibrosis would be expected. The most common type is, however, interstitial or plexiform fibrosis, according to Anderson *et al.*[33] Since replacement fibrosis is usual with ischemia, the etiology of the fibrosis seen in HCM may not be ischemia.

CLINICAL SIGNIFICANCE OF DIASTOLIC DISORDER IN HCM

Although sporadic cases of progression to dilated and poorly contracting ventricle like dilated cardiomyopathy have recently been reported as the terminal stage of HCM,[40,48–50] the majority of patients with congestive heart failure have normal systolic function with elevated LV end-diastolic and left atrial pressures.[24,51,52] This can be interpreted as diastolic failure if patients do not have massive mitral regurgitation.[3] Deterioration of the patient's condition with the development of atrial fibrillation is another common finding.[4,51,55] The direct cause of atrial fibrillation could be diastolic failure, as elevated left atrial pressure is probably responsible for atrial fibrillation. Not only the absence of atrial contraction but also the presence of impaired early diastolic filling might play the critical role in the development of congestive heart failure with atrial fibrillation, since tachycardia or rapid ventricular response is a common sequela of atrial fibrillation. It is concluded that the major mechanism of congestive heart failure in HCM is diastolic failure associated with prolonged relaxation, impaired early diastolic filling, and reduced compliance.

MODULATION OF IMPAIRED DIASTOLIC PROPERTIES WITH PHARMACOTHERAPY

Before considering pharmacotherapy, the basic mechanism involved in the diastolic disturbance in HCM must be reconsidered, and possible reversible factors must be sought. As discussed above, hypertrophy, ischemia, and fibrosis seem to be the three major factors.

Hypertrophy: Hypertrophy of the myocardium is the primary disturbance in HCM. Although sympatholytic agents, angiotensin-converting enzyme inhibitors, and various other agents produce regression of hypertrophy in essential hypertension,[53] no agents which can prevent or reduce myocardial hypertrophy in HCM have been reported. Efforts to prevent myocardial hypertrophy, however, must be carried out as urgent investigations.

Fibrosis: No technique exists to remove established fibrosis from the myocardium.

The major current concern is focused on preventing the development of fibrosis, and therefore therapy should be aimed at the treatment of ischemia, as will be discussed in the next paragraph.

Ischemia: The treatment of myocardial ischemia is directed at the reduction of myocardial oxygen consumption, augmentation of blood supply by dilating arterioles, or preventing coronary artery spasms. Beta-blocking agents and calcium entry blockers have been most frequently employed in the past 10 years.

IS THERE ANY EFFECTIVE THERAPY?

As is discussed by Hopf and Kaltenbach in this volume, medical therapy for HCM was limited to β-blocking agents, mainly propranolol, in the initial decade. The rationale for treatment with β-blocking agents was based on the concept that this disease is characterized by supernormal systolic function. Catecholamine overload theory or "noradrenosis" was another important justification for the use of β-blockers.

Abolishment or reduction of the intraventricular gradient was an important landmark in determining the efficacy of treatment and in analyzing the clinical features. Several authors have postulated that propranolol might improve diastolic abnormalities in HCM.[54-57] Although myocardial relaxation and compliance can be modulated with β-adrenergic stimulants in what has been called the positive lusitropic effect, β-adrenergic blockers do not possess this effect at all.[58,59] Beta-blocker-mediated improvement of diastolic properties can be interpreted as the result of improvement in subendocardial ischemia caused by reduced myocardial oxygen consumption. Hess and his coworkers[60] and Suwa *et al.*[61] have reported that they did not observe any improvement in diastolic properties in HCM with propranolol therapy (Fig. 3).

Numerous papers have been published recently on the effects of calcium entry blockades, since Kaltenbach[62] reported the therapeutic efficacy of verapamil. This agent was initially expected to reduce the intraventricular pressure gradient.[62,63] There are three possible ways in which a calcium antagonist might improve diastolic properties: (1) improvement of ischemia by dilating arterioles, (2) improvement of ischemia by preventing spasm of the epicardial arteries, and (3) modulation of the intracellular calcium overload by blocking the entry of calcium ions.

As recently reviewed by Bonow,[64] there are numerous reports that verapamil,[13,60,65,66] nifedipine,[16,67] and diltiazem[61] favorably modulate the abnormal diastolic properties of HCM. The data, however, must be interpreted cautiously, since the indexes of LV relaxation and early diastolic filling, such as the time constant of LV pressure fall, isovolumic relaxation time, early diastolic peak filling rate, and time to peak filling, are highly sensitive to factors like loading conditions, heart rate, extent of previous systolic shortening, and level of left atrial pressure.[19,40,59] Furthermore, even a downward shift of the diastolic pressure-volume curve cannot be interpreted as a direct increase in diastolic compliance, since four chamber interactions and LV constraint must be taken into account in interpreting shifts in the diastolic pressure-volume relationship.[68]

Therefore, the evaluation of the efficacy of the treatment should be addressed to the relief of symptoms, prevention or regression of hypertrophy, and prolongation of the life, instead of evaluating these indexes of diastolic properties. In the study of double-blind crossover trial of diltiazem and verapamil, Toshima *et al.*[69] reported that both of these calcium channel blockades were equally effective in symptomatic relief and improvement of exercise capacity. Treatment of calcium entry blockades is recommended at this moment not only symptomatic but also asymptomatic patients with HCM, ex-

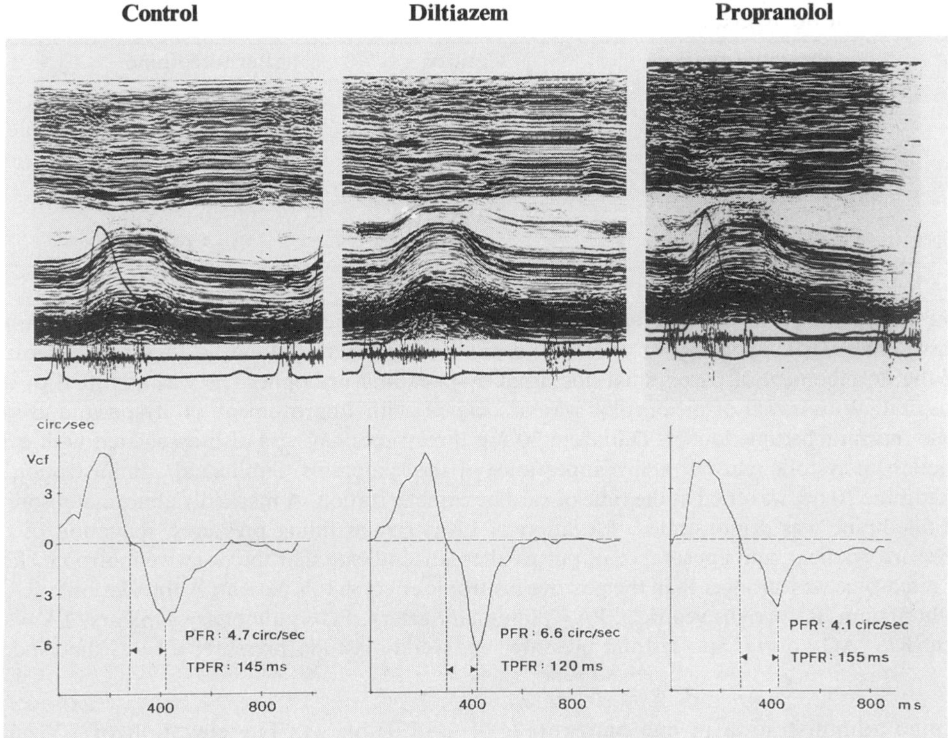

Fig. 3. M-mode echocardiograms and digitized instantaneous velocity of circumferential fiber changes (Vcf) before (left panel), 2 weeks after continuous oral diltiazem (middle panel), and 2 weeks after continuous oral propranolol treatment (right panel) in a patient with hypertrophic obstructive cardiomyopathy. Peak filling rate in diastole (PFR) was increased and the time to PFR (TPFR) was shortened with diltiazem therapy, and these diastolic indexes returned to pretreatment levels with propranolol therapy. Figure is reproduced from Reference No. 61 with the permissions of The Yorke Medical Journal and the authers.

pecting that they may prevent myocardial ischemia with dilating small and large coronary arteries, and hence, may prevent fibrosis and intracellular calcium overload.

Three areas of caution must be mentioned regarding calcium blockade therapy. First, all three major calcium antagonists, verapamil, diltiazem, and nifedipine, have a negative inotropic effect through the reduction of intracellular calcium. The manifestation of this negative inotropic action *in vivo* is stronger in verapamil and diltiazem than nifedipine. This difference is considered to be due to the difference in vasodilating action, which is strongest in nifedipine.[70] Recent report of Betocch and his associates[71] is worthwhile to be commented. They found peripheral vasodilating effect is prominent with low to medium serum nifedipine concentration, while negative inotropic effect overcome this vasodilating effect with high concentration in HCM. Verapamil-induced pulmonary edema was reported by Epstein *et al.*[72] in patients with severely elevated LV end-diastolic pressure. We have experienced six cases of pulmonary edema with diltiazem.[73] All six patients had severely elevated LV end-diastolic pressure with supernormal EF. We also experienced elevation of LV end-diastolic pressure with sublingual nife-

TABLE 1. Unusual Response of Sublingual Nifedipine in a Patient with Hypertrophic Obstructive Cardiomyopathy

Pressure (mmHg)	Control	After nifedipine
RA mean	5	7
RV sp/edp	32/9	42/13
PA sp/dp (mean)	32/14 (19)	42/20 (28)
PC mean	15	19
LV sp/edp	220/33	200/40
AO sp/dp (mean)	105/65 (90)	120/65 (92)
CI (l/min/m^2)	2.4	2.3

The patient was a 48-year-old male, shown in Fig. 1, who was diagnosed to have hypertrophic obstructive cardiomyopathy in another hospital, where metoprolol was prescribed. Because of the development of paroxysmal nocturnal dyspnea and orthopnea, he was admitted to our hospital. Withdrawal of metoprolol was associated with improvement of dyspnea, and systolic murmur became louder. Diltiazem 30 mg three times/day was also associated with a reduction in systolic murmur and reappearance of the symptoms. Sublingual administration of nifedipine 10 mg was tried at the time of cardiac catheterization. A markedly abnormal response to nifedipine was demonstrated. Elevation of biventricular filling pressures, reduction of the pressure gradient, and appearance of pulsus alternans indicate that the negative inotropic effect of nifedipine was stronger than the positive lusitropic effect in this patient. Abbreviations: RA = right atrium, RV = right ventricle, PA = pulmonary artery, PC = pulmonary capillary, LV = left ventricle, AO = aorta, sp = systolic pressure, edp = end-diastolic pressure, CI = cardiac index.

dipine administration in one patient (Fig. 1 and Table 1). The elevation of LV end-diastolic pressure due to the negative inotropic effect in these patients is considered to be stronger than afterload reduction due to peripheral vasodilation and/or the positive lusitropic effect of calcium blocking agents. Therefore, as recommended by Epstein *et al.*[71] verapamil, diltiazem, and even nifedipine must be used very cautiously in patients with elevated LV end-diastolic pressure.

Second, both diltiazem and verapamil have a strong negative chronotropic effect and cause suppression of the sinus node and the conduction system.[70] Therefore, caution must be exercised in prescribing these drugs to patients who have sinus dysfunction or atrioventricular or intraventricular conduction disturbances.

Third, as nifedipine is a strong arteriolar vasodilator, it will potentiate the intraventricular pressure gradient in patients with hypertrophic obstructive cardiomyopathy. It might also cause a severe hot flushing sensation in young patients, and edema of the lower extremities in elderly patients without evidence of congestive heart failure. These symptoms may limit its clinical use in some patients.

OTHER POSSIBLE THERAPEUTIC AGENTS

As discussed above, β-blockers and calcium antagonists are the only drugs investigated that might improve impaired diastolic properties in HCM. There are two other categories of agents that might be effective, but have not yet been investigated. One is a group of drugs that might prevent hypertrophy or cause regression of hypertrophy. Angiotensin-converting enzyme inhibitors and α-adrenergic blocking agents are considered to belong to this category, and it seems worthwhile to investigate their effects in this disease. The other group is the so-called coronary vasodilators. Dipyridamole and nitrates such as isosorbide dinitrate and nicorandyl might prevent myocardial ischemia by preventing coronary spasm or dilating small vessels. It is worthwhile to conduct trials to evaluate the effects of these drugs.

REFERENCES

1. Braunwald, E., Morrow, A.G., Cornell, W.P., Aygen, M.M., and Hilbish, T.F. Idiopathic hypertrophic subaortic stenosis. Clinical hemodynamic and angiographic manifestations. *Am. J. Med.* **29**: 924–945, 1960.
2. Stewart, S., Mason, D.T., and Braunwald, E. Impaired rate of left ventricular filling in idiopathic hypertrophic subaortic stenosis and valvular aortic stenosis. *Circulation* **37**: 8–14, 1968.
3. Gaasch, W.H. and Zile, M.R. Evaluation of myocardial function in cardiomyopathic states. *Prog. Cardivasc. Dis.* **27**: 115–132, 1984.
4. Goodwin, J.F. Congestive and hypertrophic cardiomyopathies. A decade of study. *Lancet* **ii**: 731–739, 1970.
5. Toshima, H., Ueda, T., Aoyagi, M., Koga, Y., Miki, N., and Kimura, N. Peak negative dP/dt as an index of left ventricular relaxation. *Jpn. J. Med.* **15**: 322–327, 1976.
6. Sanderson, J.E., Traill, T.A., St. John Sutton, M.G., Brown, D.J., Gibson, D.G., and Goodwin, J.F. Left ventricular filling in hypertrophic cardiomyopathy. An echocardiographic study. *Br. Heart J.* **40**: 596–601, 1978.
7. Sanderson, J.E., Gibson, D.G., Brown, D.J., and Goodwin, J.F. Left ventricular filling in hypertrophic cardiomyopathy. An angiographic study. *Br. Heart J.* **39**: 661–670, 1977.
8. Hirota, Y. A clinical study of left ventricular relaxation. *Circulation* **62**: 756–763, 1980.
9. Hanrath, P., Mathey, D.G., Siegert, R., and Bleifeld, W. Left ventricular relaxation and filling pattern in different forms of left ventricular hypertrophy: an echocardiographic study. *Am. J. Cardiol.* **45**: 15–23, 1980.
10. Gidding, S.S., Snider, A.R., Rocchini, A.P., Peters, J., andarn Fsworth, R. Left ventricular diastolic filling in children with hypertrophic cardiomyopathy: assessment with pulsed doppler echocardiography. *J. Am. Coll. Cardiol.* **8**: 310–316, 1986.
11. Bryg, R.J., Pearson, A.C., Williams, G.A., and Labovitz, A.J. Left ventricular systolic and diastolic flow abnormalities determined by Doppler echocardiography in obstructive hypertrophic cardiomyopathy. *Am. J. Cardiol.* **59**: 925–931, 1987.
12. Peason, A.C., Labovitz, A.J., Mrosek, D., Williams, G.A., and Kennedy, H.L. Assessment of diastolic function in normal and hypertrophied hearts: comparison of Doppler echocardiography and M-mode echocardiography. *Am. Heart J.* **113**: 1417–1425, 1987.
13. Bonow, R.O., Ostrow, H.G., Rosing, D.R., Cannon, R.O. III, Lipson, L.C., Maron, B.J., Kent, K.M., Bacharach, S.L., and Green, M.V. Effects of verapamil on left ventricular systolic and diastolic function in patients with hypertrophic cardiomyopathy: pressure-volume analysis with a nonimaging scintillation probe. *Circulation* **68**: 1062–1073, 1983.
14. Bonow, R.O., Dilsizian, V., Rosing, D.R., Maron, B.J., Bacharach, S.L., and Green, M.V. Verapamil-induced improvement in left ventricular diastolic filling and increased exercise tolerance in patients with hypertrophic cardiomyopathy: short- and long-term effects. *Circulation* **72**: 853–864, 1985.
15. Chen, Y.T., Chang, K.C., Hu, W.S., Wang, S.J., and Chiang, B.N. Left ventricular diastolic function in hypertrophic cardiomyopathy: assessment by radionuclide angiography. *Int. J. Cardiol.* **15**: 185–193, 1987.
16. Lorell, B.H., Paulus, W.J., Grossman, W., Wynne, J., and Cohn, P.F. Modification of abnormal left ventricular diastolic properties by nifedipine in patients with hypertrophic cardiomyopathy. *Circulation* **65**: 499–507, 1982.
17. Takenaka, T., Dabestani, A., Gardin, J.M., Russell, D., Clark, S., Allfie, A., and Henry, W.L. Left ventricular filling in hypertrophic cardiomyopathy: a pulsed Doppler echocardiographic study. *J. Am. Coll. Cardiol.* **7**: 1263–1271, 1986.

18. Maron, B.J., Spirito, P., Green K.J., Wesley, Y.E., Bonow, R.O., and Arce, J. Noninvasive assessment of left ventricular diastolic function by pulsed Doppler echocardiography in patients with hypertrophic cardiomyopathy. *J. Am. Coll. Cardiol.* **10**: 733–742, 1987.
19. Ishida, Y., Meisner, J.S., Tsujioka, K., Gallo, J.I., Yoran, C., Frater, R.W.M., and Yellin, E.L. Left ventricular filling dynamics: influence of left ventricular relaxation and left atrial pressure. *Circulation* **74**: 187–196, 1986.
20. Choong, C.Y., Herrmann, H.C., Weyman, A.E., and Fifer, M.A. Preload dependence of Doppler-derived indexes of left ventricular diastolic function in humans. *J. Am. Coll. Cardiol.* **10**: 800–808, 1987.
21. Brutsaert, D.L., Rademakers, F.E., and Sys, S.U. Triple control of relaxation: implications in cardiac disatole. *Circulation* **69**: 190–196, 1984.
22. Hood, W.P. Jr., Rackley, C.E., and Rolett, E.L. Wall stress in the normal and hypertrophied human left ventricle. *Am. J. Cardiol.* **22**: 550–558, 1968.
23. Gaasch, W.H., Battle, W.E., Oboler, A.A., Banas, J.S. Jr., and Levine, H.J. Left ventricular stress and compliance in man. With special reference to normalized ventricular function curve. *Circulation* **45**: 746–762, 1972.
24. Hirota, Y., Furubayashi, K., Kaku, K., Shimizu, G., Kino, M., Kawamura, K., and Takatsu, T. Hypertrophic nonobstructive cardiomyopathy: a precise assessment of hemodynamic characteristics and clinical implications. *Am. J. Cardiol.* **50**: 990–997, 1982.
25. Henry, P.H., Shuchleib, R., Davis, J., Weiss, E.S., and Sobel, B.E. Myocardial contracture and accumulation of mitchondrial calcium in ischemic rabbit heart. *Am. J. Physiol.* **233**: H 677–H 684, 1977.
26. Shimizu, G., Zile, M.R., Blaustein, A.S., and Gaasch, W.H. Left ventricular chamber filling and midwall fiber lengthening in patients with left ventricular hypertrophy: Overestimation of fiber velocities by conventional midwall measurements. *Circulation* **71**: 266–272, 1985.
27. Spirito, P., Maron, B.J., Chiarella, F., Bellotti, P., Tramarin, R., Pozzoli, M., and Vecchio, C. Diastolic abnormalities in patients with hypertrophic cardiomyopathy: relation to magnitude of left ventricular hypertrophy. *Circulation* **72**: 310–316, 1985.
28. Kumada, T., Karliner, J.S., Pouleur, H., Gallagher, K.P., Shirato, K., and Ross, J. Jr. Effects of coronary occlusion on early ventricular diastolic events in conscious dogs. *Am. J. Physiol.* **237**: H542–H549, 1979.
29. Maseri, A., Severi, S., De Nes, M., L'Abbate, A., Chierchia, S., Marzilli, M., Ballestra, A.M., Parodi, O., Biagini, A., and Distante, A. "Variant" angina: one aspect of a continuous spectrum of vasospastic myocardial ischemia. Pathogenetic mechanisms, estimated incidence and clinical and coronary arteriographic findings in 138 patients. *Am. J. Cardiol.* **42**: 1019–1035, 1978.
30. McLaurin, L.P., Rolett, E.L., and Grossman, W. Impaired left ventricular relaxation during pacing-induced ischemia. *Am. J. Cardiol.* **32**: 751–757, 1973.
31. Mann, T., Goldberg, S., Mudge, G.H. Jr., and Grossman, W. Factors contributing to altered left ventricular diastolic properties during angina pectoris. *Circulation* **59**: 14–20, 1979.
32. Woods, J.D. Relative ischemia in the hypertrophied heart. *Lancet* **i**: 696–698, 1961.
33. Anderson, K.R., St. John Sutton, M.G., and Lie, J.T. Histopathological types of cardiac fibrosis in myocardial disease. *J. Pathol.* **128**: 79–85, 1979.
34. Malik, A.B., Abe, T., O'Kane, H., and Geha, A.S. Cardiac function, coronary flow, and oxygen consumption in stable left ventricular hypertrophy. *Am. J. Physiol.* **225**: 186–191, 1973.
35. Weiss, M.B., Ellis, K., Sciacca, R.R., Johnson, L.L., Schmidt, D.H., and Cannon, P.J. Myocardial blood flow in congestive and hypertrophic cardiomyopathy. Relationship to peak wall stress and mean velocity of circumferential fiber shortening. *Circulation* **54**: 484–494, 1976.
36. Yonekura, Y., Brill, A.B., Som, P., Yamamoto, K., Srivastava, S.C., Iwai, J., Elmaleh,

D.R., Livni, E., Strauss, H.W., Goodman, M.M., and Knapp, F.F. Jr. Regional myocardial substrate uptake in hypertensive rats: a quantitative autoradiographic measurement. *Science* **227**: 1494–1496, 1985.

37. Kostis, J.B., Moreyra, A.E., Natarajan, N., Hosler, M., Kou, P.T., and Conn, H.L. Jr. The pathophysiology and diverse etiology of septal perforator compression. *Circulation* **59**: 913–919, 1979.
38. Kitazume, H., Kramer, J.R., Krauthamer, D., El Tobgi, S., Proudfit, W.L., and Sones, F.M. Myocardial bridges in obstructive hypertrophic cardiomyopathy. *Am. Heart J.* **106**: 131–135, 1983.
39. Nishimura, K., Nosaka, H., Saito, T., and Nobuyoshi, M. Another possible mechanism of angina in hypertrophic cardiomyopathy. *Circulation* **68**: Suppl. 3; 162, 1983 (abstr).
40. Tanaka, H., Adachi, K., Yamashita, Y., Ogata, M., Terasawa, M., Ota, K., Toshima, H., Takahashi, N., Umezu, T., and Morimatsu, M. An autopsy case of diffuse myocardial fibrosis with wall hypertrophy of intramural coronary arteries in the family of hypertrophic cardiomyopathy. *Kokyu to Junkan* **33**: 1369–1374, 1985 (in Japanese).
41. Maron, B.J., Wolfson, J.K., Epstein, S.E., and Roberts, W.C. Intramural ("small vessel") coronary artery disease in hypertrophic cardiomyopathy. *J. Am. Coll. Cardiol.* **8**: 545–557, 1986.
42. Tanaka, M., Fujiwara, H., Onodera, T., Wu, D.J., Matsuda, M., Hamashima, Y., and Kawai, C. Quantitative analysis of narrowings of intramyocardial small arteries in normal hearts, hypertensive hearts, and hearts with hypertrophic cardiomyopathy. *Circulation* **75**: 1130–1139, 1987.
43. Mirsky, I., Cohn, P.F., Levine, J.A., Gorlin, R., Herman, M.V., Kreulen, T.H., and Sonnenblick, E.H. Assessment of left ventricular stiffness in primary myocardial disease and coronary artery disease. *Circulation* **50**: 128–136, 1974.
44. Grantz, S.A. and Parmley, W.W. Factors which affect the diastolic pressure volume curve. *Circ. Res.* **42**: 171–180, 1978.
45. Apstein, C.S. and Grossman, W. Opposite initial effects of supply and demand ischemia on left ventricular compliance: the ischemia-diastolic paradox. *J. Mol. Cell. Cardiol.* **19**: 119–128, 1987.
46. Lorell, B.H. and Grossman, W. Cardiac hypertrophy: the consequences for diastole. *J. Am. Coll. Cardiol.* **9**: 1189–1193, 1987.
47. Teare, D. Asymmetric hypertrophy of the heart in young adults. *Br. Heart J.* **20**: 1–8, 1958.
48. ten Cate, F.J. and Roelandt, J. Progression to left ventricular dilatation in patients with hypertrophic cardiomyopathy. *Am. Heart J.* **97**: 762–765, 1979.
49. Fujiwara, H., Onodera, T., Tanaka, M., Shirane, H., Kato, H., Yoshikawa, J., Osakada, G., Sasayama, S., and Kawai, C. Progression from hypertrophic obstructive cadiomyopathy to typical dilated cardiomyopathy-like features in the end-stage. *Jpn. Circ. J.* **48**: 1210–1214, 1984.
50. Yutani, C., Imakita, M., Ishibashi-Ueda, H., Hatanaka, K., Nagata, S., Sakakibara, H., and Nimura, Y. Three autopsy cases of progression to left ventricular dilatation in patients with hypertrophic cardiomyopathy. *Am. Heart J.* **109**: 545–553, 1985.
51. Frank, S. and Braunwald, E. Idiopathic hypertrophic subaortic stenosis. Clinical analysis of 126 patients with emphasis on the natural history. *Circulation* **37**: 759–788, 1968.
52. Wigle, E.D. Hypertrophic cardiomyopathy 1988. *Mod. Con. Cardiovasc. Dis.* **57**: 1–6, 1988.
53. Fouad-Taraji, F.M. and Liebson, P.R. Echocardiographic studies of regression of left ventricular hypertrophy in hypertension. *Hypertension* **9** (suppl. 2): 65–68, 1987.
54. Webb-Peploe, M.M., Croxson, R.S., Oakley, C.M., and Goodwin, J.F. Cardioselective beta-adrenergic blockade in hypertrophic obstructive cardiomyopathy. *Postgrad. Med. J.* **47**: 93–97, 1971.
55. Hubner, P.J.B., Ziady, G.M., Lane, G.K., Harderson, T., Scales, B., Oakley, C.M., and Goodwin, J.F. Double-blind trial of propranolol and practolol in hypertrophic cardiomyopathy. *Br. Heart J.* **35**: 1116–1123, 1973.

56. Saenz de la Calzada, S., Ziady, G.M., Harderson, T., Curiel, R., and Goodwin, J.F. Effect of acute administration of propranolol on ventricular function in hypertrophic obstructive cardiomyopathy measured by non-invasive techniques. *Br. Heart J.* **38**: 798–803, 1976.
57. Frank, M.J., Abdulla, A.M., Canedo, M.I., and Saylors, R.E. Long-term medical management of hypertrophic obstructive cardiomyopathy. *Am. J. Cardiol.* **42**: 993–1001, 1978.
58. Katz, A.M. Cyclic adenosine monophosphate effects on the myocardium: A man who blows hot and cold with one breath. *J. Am. Coll. Cardiol.* **2**: 143–149, 1983.
59. Katz, A.M. Influence of altered inotropy and lusitropy on ventricular pressure-volume loops. *J. Am. Coll. Cardiol.* **11**: 438–445, 1988.
60. Hess, O.M., Grimm, J., and Krayenbuehl, H.P. Diastolic function in hypertrophic cardiomyopathy: effects of propanolol and verapamil on diastolic stiffness. *Eur. Heart J.* (suppl. F) **4**: 47–56, 1983.
61. Suwa, M., Hirota, Y., and Kawamura, K. Improvement in left ventricular diastolic function during intravenous and oral diltiazem therapy in patients with hypertrophic cardiomyopathy: An echocardiographic study. *Am. J. Cardiol.* **54**: 1047–1053, 1984.
62. Kaltenbach, M., Hopf, R., and Keller, M. Calciumantagonistsche therapie bei hypertrophihobstruktiver Kardiomyopathie. *Dtsch. Med. Wschr.* **101**: 1284–1287, 1976.
63. Rosing, D.R., Kent, K.M., Borer, J.S., Seides, S.F., Maron, B.J., and Epstein, S.E. Verapamil therapy: a new approach to the pharmacologic treatment of hypertrophic cardiomyopathy. I. Hemodynamic effects. *Circulation* **60**: 1201–1207, 1979.
64. Bonow, R.O. Effects of calcium-channel blocking agents on left ventricular diastolic function in hypertrophic cardiomyopathy and coronary artery disease. *Am. J. Cardiol.* **55**: 172–178, 1985.
65. Anderson, D.M., Raff, G.L., Ports, T.A., Brundage, B.H., Parmley, W.W., and Chatterjee, K. Hypertrophic obstructive cardiomyoapthy. Effects of acute and chronic verapamil treatment on left ventricular systolic and diastolic function. *Br. Heart J.* **51**: 523–529, 1984.
66. Bonow, R.O., Dilsizian, V., Rosing, D.R., Maron, B.J., Bacharach, S.L., and Green, M.V. Verapamil-induced improvement in left ventricular diastolic filling and increased exercise tolerance in patients with hypertrophic cardiomyopathy: short- and long-term effects. *Circulation* **72**: 853–864, 1985.
67. Suwa, M., Hirota, Y., and Kawamura, K. Effects of nifedipine on left ventricular systolic and diastolic function in hypertrophic nonobstructive cardiomyopathy. *J. Cardiovasc. Ultrasonog.* **2**: 9–17, 1983.
68. Tyberg, J.V. Ventricular interaction and the pericardium. In: The Ventricle. Basic and Clinical Aspects, Levine, H.J. and Gaasch, W.H. (eds.), Martinus Nijhoff Publishing, Boston, 1985, pp. 171–217.
69. Toshima, H., Koga, Y., Nagata, H., Toyomasu, K., Itaya, K., and Matoba, T. Comparable effects of oral diltiazem and verapamil in the treatment of hypertrophic cardiomyopathy. Double-blind crossover study. *Jpn. Heart J.* **27**: 701–715, 1986.
70. Kawai, C., Konishi, T., Matsuyama, E., and Okazaki, H. Comparative effects of three calcium antagonists, diltiazem, verapamil and nifedipine, on the sinoatrial and atrioventricular nodes. Experimental and clinical study. *Circulation* **63**: 1035–1042, 1981.
71. Betocchi, S., Bonow, R.O., Cannon, R.O. III, Lesko, L.J., Ostrow, H.G., Watsom, R.M., and Rosing, D.R. Relation between serum nifedipine concentration and hemodynamic effects in nonobstructive hypertrophic cardiomyopathy. *Am. J. Cardiol.* **61**: 830–835, 1888.
72. Epstein, S.E. and Rosing, D.R. Verapamil: its potential for causing serious complications in patients with hypertrophic cardiomyopathy. *Circulation* **64**: 437–441, 1981.
73. Kawamura, K., Suwa, M., and Hirota, Y. Problems of beta blockades and calcium antagonists treatments in patients with hypertrophic cardiomyopathy. In the Report of the Study Group of Idiopathic Cardiomyopathy to the Department of Wellfare and Public Health of the Japanese Government 1985, pp. 411–416, 1986 (in Japanese).

Medical Management of Supraventricular and Ventricular Arrhythmias in Patients with Hypertrophic Cardiomyopathy

William J. McKenna and Michael P. Frenneaux

Cardiological Sciences, St George's Hospital Medical School, London, U.K.

ABSTRACT

Arrhythmias are common in hypertrophic cardiomyopathy. Approximately 45% of patients have paroxysmal or established supraventricular arrhythmias, while 25–30% have asymptomatic episodes of nonsustained ventricular tachycardia. Supraventricular arrhythmias are associated with thromboembolic complications, while nonsustained ventricular tachycardia is significantly more common in patients who die suddenly and is the best single marker for the identification of the high-risk patient. Treatment of high-risk patients with low-dose amiodarone is associated with improved survival.

INTRODUCTION

The natural history of patients with hypertrophic cardiomyopathy is characterized by a slow progression of symptoms, with death most often being sudden and unexpected.[1,2] A major problem in the management of patients is the prevention of complications, particularly sudden death. In adults, supraventricular arrhythmias are common and important, as they predispose to complications, while ventricular arrhythmias are a useful marker of patients who are at increased risk of sudden death.[3–6] In children and adolescents, arrhythmias are uncommon during ECG monitoring.[7] In these younger patients, electrical stability as determined by the extent of myocardial disarray is likely to be an important determinant of sudden death.

CLINICAL SIGNIFICANCE OF ARRHYTHMIAS

Incidence and Characteristics

In adults with hypertrophic cardiomyopathy arrhythmias are common.[3,5] Established atrial fibrillation is present at the time of diagnosis in 7% and can be expected to develop during five-year follow-up in another 5% of patients. Episodes of paroxysmal atrial fibrillation or supraventricular tachycardia are detected during 48-hr ECG monitoring in an additional 30%, while episodes of nonsustained ventricular tachycardia are found in 25–30% of consecutive adult patient populations (Table 1). The charac-

Adapted from: McKenna, W.J., Alfonso, F. Arrhythmias in the cardiomyopathies and mitral valve prolapse. In: Zipes, D.P. and Rowlands, D.J. (eds.), *Progress in Cardiology*, Philadelphia: Lea and Febiger, 1988: 59–77 and McKenna, W.J. Sudden death in hypertrophic cardiomyopathy: identification of the "high risk" patient. In: Brugada, P., Wellens, H.J.J., (eds.), *Cardiac Arrhythmias: Where to Go from Here?* New York: Futura Publishing Company Inc., 1987, pp. 353–365.

TABLE 1. Arrhythmias during 48–72-hr ECG Monitoring in 100 Consecutive Adults and 53 Consecutive Infants, Children, and Adolescents with Hypertrophic Cardiomyopathy

	Children and adolescents		Adults
	No.	%	No.
Established atrial fibrillation	0	0	14
Supraventricular tachycardia/ paroxysmal atrial fibrillation	4	8	27
Ventricular extrasystoles peak > 30/hr	0	0	24
Nonsustained ventricular tachycardia	4	8	29

(Data are taken from references 5–7)

teristics of the episodes of ventricular tachycardia are remarkably similar between patients. The ventricular tachycardia is slow (median rate 140 beats/min) and episodes occur during periods of relative vagal tone; the mean heart rate during the preceding minute is 70 beats/min, while 40% of episodes occur between midnight and 6:00 a.m.[6)] Arrhythmias in younger patients with hypertrophic cardiomyopathy, however, are much less common.[7)] Of 53 consecutive infants, children, and adolescents who underwent 48-hr ECG monitoring, all were in sinus rhythm and only four had episodes of supraventricular tachycardia and four of nonsustained ventricular tachycardia (Table 1). Repeated ECG monitoring at annual intervals in these younger patients revealed the development of both supraventricular and nonsustained ventricular arrhythmias in those aged 18 to 25 years.[7)]

Which adults with hypertrophic cardiomyopathy are prone to arrhythmias? The development of supraventricular arrhythmias, particularly established atrial fibrillation, is seen in patients who have more severe dyspnea on exercise, greater left and right ventricular hypertrophy, and increased echocardiographic left atrial dimension, while ventricular arrhythmias are particularly associated with older age, longer duration of symptoms, impaired systolic function with reduced ejection fraction and peak ejection rate, and increased left ventricular end-diastolic pressure.[3–9)] The presence of resting or provocable left ventricular gradients is not more common in patients with either supraventricular or ventricular arrhythmia, while the relation of abnormalities of diastolic function and arrhythmias has not been systematically assessed.

Hemodynamic Effects

The acute onset of atrial fibrillation is associated with the loss of atrial systolic contribution to filling volume as well as a rapid and irregular rhythm that reduces the time for diastolic filling of the ventricles. This may have disastrous effects with immediate hemodynamic collapse or the development of ischemia and lethal ventricular arrhythmias, even without accessory pathway conduction or excessively rapid ventricular rates.[10)] Occasionally, however, relatively rapid atrial fibrillation is well tolerated. Similarly the hemodynamic effect of established or paroxysmal atrial fibrillation with controlled ventricular response is variable. The likely response of the individual patient to the development of atrial fibrillation can often be determined from analysis of Doppler filling patterns or the diastolic portion of the left ventricular volume-time curve.[11,12)] Patients with slow filling who are dependent on atrial systole for 20% or more of filling volume experience significant worsening of their exercise capacity. In contrast, patients with rapid and early filling and small atrial contribution may be unaware of rhythm changes from sinus to atrial fibrillation providing the ventricular response is controlled. Although arrhythmias are common during ECG monitoring, most are not associated with either palpitation or symptoms of hemodynamic deterioration.[3,5,6] In particular, clinical episodes of ventricular tachycardia are invariably asymptomatic, and in our experience of more than 400 such episodes in 52 patients, none have degenerated or been associated with syncope or impaired consciousness. We are aware of a patient with ventricular tachycardia leading to sudden death, however, the arrythemia was preceded by ischemia and autonomic disturbance which have been documented in patients with nonsustained ventricular tachycardia.[12]

Relation to Prognosis

Although the development of atrial fibrillation has been considered to be a bad omen,[13] in our series of 52 patients who developed atrial fibrillation, overall survival, during a median follow-up of six years, was similar to that in those who remained in sinus rhythm.[14] The prognostic significance of atrial fibrillation, like the hemodynamic consequences, varies among patients. Although hemodynamic collapse and ventricular fibrillation have been documented following the development of atrial fibrillation with rapid ventricular response, neither established atrial fibrillation nor episodes of supraventricular tachycardia during ECG monitoring are associated with or are predictive of sudden cardiac death.[3,5,6] The development of atrial fibrillation carries a risk of thromboembolism, and therefore anticoagulation is important and should be considered in those with frequent or prolonged episodes of paroxysmal supraventricular arrhythmias. The precise risk is unknown but it is probably less than in dilated cardiomyopathy, where in one large series 20% of patients who were not anticoagulated developed thromboembolic complications during six years.[15]

In adults there is an annual mortality from sudden death of 2–3%.[1] Routine clinical, echocardiographic, and hemodynamic evaluation does not identify the majority of

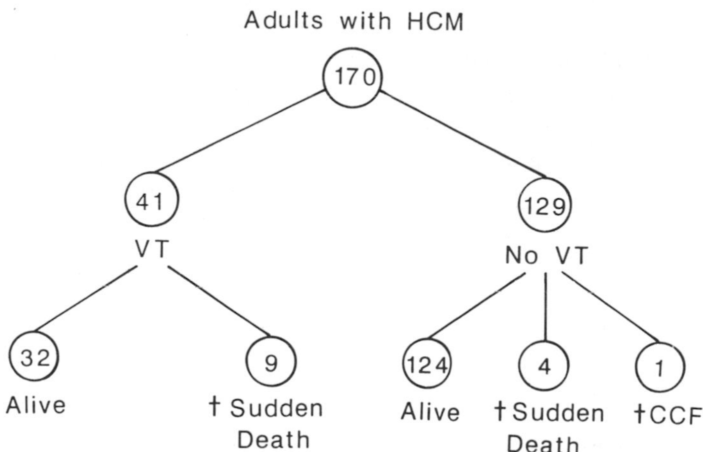

Fig. 1. Flow diagram showing clinical outcome in the 170 unoperated patients undergoing 24–72 hr of electrocardiographic monitoring. Eighty-four patients are from the series reported by Maron *et al.*[4]; 86 are from McKenna *et al.*[5] HCM = hypertrophic cardiomyopathy; VT = ventricular tachycardia; CCF = congestive cardiac failure.

during ECG monitoring is the most useful single feature in the prediction of sudden death, with a sensitivity of 69% and a specificity 80%. Figure 1 presents the results of ECG monitoring in unoperated patients from two independent studies at the NIH (Bethesda, Maryland)[4)] and the Hammersmith Hospital (London, U.K.).[5)] Thirteen of the 170 consecutive unoperated patients from the NIH and the Hammersmith Hospital died suddenly during three years; nine of these 13 had nonsustained ventricular tachycardia. In both studies, arrhythmia was significantly more common in those who died suddenly. This does not indicate a causal relationship but does establish that ventricular tachycardia is a marker of the adult who is at particular risk of sudden death. Indeed, in the adult with hypertrophic cardiomyopathy, episodes of nonsustained ventricular tachycardia during electrocardiographic monitoring are the best single feature in the prediction of sudden death, with a sensitivity of 69% and a specificity of 80% (Table 2). The reduced sensitivity, in part, reflects the inclusion of an 11-year-old girl (patient 1, Table 1, Maron *et al.*[4)]) who was recognized to be at high risk because of recurrent syncopal episodes but who did not have ventricular arrhythmias during ECG monitoring. It is now recognized that spontaneous arrhythmias are rare in children and adolescents and that other clinical features are of greater predictive value.[7)] In addition, all four of the patients who did not have ventricular tachycardia but died suddenly (two from NIH and two from Hammersmith) had only 24 hr of electrocardiographic monitoring; thus a sampling error is possible, particularly as ventricular arrhythmias in hypertrophic cardiomyopathy are known to exhibit marked biological variability.[7)] The finding of nonsustained ventricular tachycardia during electrocardiographic monitoring identifies adults at high risk with a sensitivity that is probably greater than 69%.

The fact that 32 of 41 patients with ventricular tachycardia survived is reflected in the low positive predictive accuracy (22%) of ventricular tachycardia for sudden death, and it raises the possibility that aggressive treatment of patients with nonsustained ventricular tachycardia would include a group who are not at increased risk. Although the number of patients in the subset with ventricular tachycardia in each study was small, there did not appear to be features that distinguished patients with ventricular tachycardia who survived from those who died suddenly. In the NIH study, patients with ventricular tachycardia and sudden cardiac catastrophe did not differ from survivors with regard to age or sex, ventricular septal thickness, or occurrence of an abnormal electrocardiogram.[4)] In the Hammersmith study, the symptomatic status, the proportion with a left ventricular gradient, and the incidence of supraventricular arrhythmias were similar in the survivors and patients who died suddenly.[5)] In addition, more detailed characterization of the episodes of nonsustained ventricular tachycardia from our study

TABLE 2.

	Sudden death	
	+	−
VT+	9	32
VT−	4	124
Sensitivity	69%	
Specificity	80%	
Prevalence	7.6%	
Positive predictive value	22%	
Negative predictive value	97%	

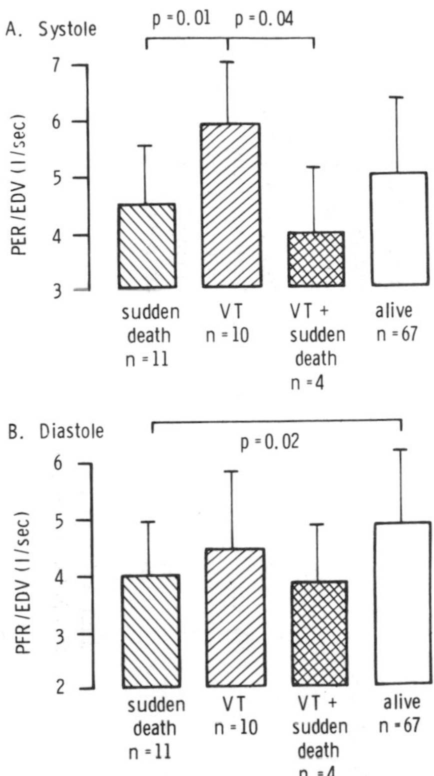

Fig. 2. Normalized indices of ventricular ejection and filling in 10 patients with ventricular tachycardia (VT) who survived and four who died suddenly, compared with all 11 patients who died suddenly and with 67 survivors. A: Peak ejection rates normalized by end-diastolic volume (PER/EDV) were higher in patients with ventricular tachycardia who survived than in those who died suddenly. B: Peak filling rates normalized by end-diastolic volume (PFR/EDV) were higher in the survivors than in patients who died suddenly. (Reproduced with permission from Newman *et al.*,[8] *JACC* **5**: 1064–1074, 1985.)

patients who will die suddenly.[1,16] The finding of nonsustained ventricular tachycardia did not identify subsets at increased risk, however, the data were insufficient to be conclusive. In another study of the relation of left ventricular function and prognosis in a subset of 14 patients with ventricular tachycardia, digitized angiographic analysis revealed that peak left ventricular ejection rate was significantly reduced in patients with ventricular tachycardia who died suddenly compared with those who survived (Fig. 2).[8] Impaired left ventricular function may be an important predictor of which patients with ventricular tachycardia are at increased risk, and further risk stratification of patients with nonsustained ventricular tachycardia would be useful.

What is the role of electrophysiologic testing in the identification of the high-risk patient with hypertrophic cardiomyopathy? Several groups have done electrophysiological studies in adults, many of whom were at "high risk" because of previous syncopal episodes or cardiac arrest (Table 3).[18–27] Anderson *et al.* performed right ventricular programmed electrical stimulation in the operating room in 17 patients with left ventricular outflow tract gradients who were undergoing myotomy/myectomy and in

TABLE 3. Programmed Electrophysiological Studies in Patients with Hypertrophic Cardiomyopathy

	Pts	Age (years) mean (range)	History	Holter	PES: PVS 2 ES	PES: PVS 3 ES	PES: PAS	FU (months)	Comments
Schiavone[18] 1986	26	51 (18–77)	S:14	NSVT:7 SVA:7	26 VF:1	5 VF:0	26 SVA:17	0	Syncope best predicted by hypotension induced during SVA
Anderson[19] 1983	17	46 (15–74)	S:5 CA:1	—	17 3-SPVT/VF–11	14	—	0	PVS performed preoperatively under anaesthesia
Kowey[20] 1984	7	54 (25–75)	CA:4 (3VF, 1VT) PS:2 Seizure:1	NSVT:3 T de P:1	4 VT:3	1 VF:1	SVA:2	6 to 30 (mean 17)	PES useful in identification of cause of symptoms; no events during FU on anti-arrhythmic Rx
Ingham[21] 1978	13	51 (25–74)	S, PS or P in all	SVA:7 NSVT:3	—	—	dual AV node 7/12 (no inducible SVA)	0	
Geibel[22] 1986	18	—	S:2 VF:3 SMVT:2	—	18 SMVT:2 SPVT:3		12 SMVT:1 SPVT:7	0	SMVT induced in 2/2 pts who had D-SMVT
Borgreffe[23] 1986	31	—	S:21 VT/VF:5 P:5	NSVT:9	31 SMVT:3 SPVT/VF:5	—	31 Acc P:2 AVNT:1 AFib:8 1:1 > 200 bpm:8	0	EPS identified a possible cause of Sx in 52% of pts

Kunze[24] 1986	26	45 (—)	S:4 VF:2	—	26 VF:3	23 VF:7	—	32±5	No events during FU, pts with S or VF Rx with amoidarone
Watson[25] 1987	18	36 (14–64)	S:4 NSVT:9 CA:3 MFH:2	NSVT:9	18 VF:5	13 VF:3	VF:1	0	Inducible arrhythmias common in high-risk pts
Kuck[26] 1988	54	48 (—)	S:8 CA:3	—	54 SMVT:3 SPVT:2 VF:3	—	54 VF:1	0	Inducible arrhythmia not specific to symptomatic pts

Legend: Numbers refer to patients unless otherwise stated in the column headings. S=syncope; CA=cardiac arrest; VT=ventricular tachycardia; NSVT=nonsustained ventricular tachycardia; SVA=supraventricular arrhythmia; T de P=torsdae de pointes; PVS=programmed ventricular stimulation; PES=programmed electrophysiologic stimulation; PAS=programmed atrial stimulation; SPVT=sustained polymorphic ventricular tachycardia; SMVT=sustained monomorphic ventricular tachycardia; VF=ventricular fibrillation; AV=atrioventricular; Acc P=accessory pathway; AVNT=atrioventricular nodal tachycardia; AFib=atrial fibrillation; FU=follow-up; Rx=treatment; D-SMVT=documented sustained monomorphic ventricular tachycardia; Sx=symptoms; MFH=malignant family history. Updated from McKenna, W.J., Ref. 27.

five control patients who were undergoing coronary artery bypass grafting.[19] In their protocol, which included three premature ventricular stimuli, 14 of 17 patients had inducible sustained ventricular tachycardia ($n=9$) or ventricular fibrillation ($n=5$), something not seen in the five control patients. Their findings indicate that with an aggressive stimulation protocol, inducible life-threatening arrhythmias are more common in patients with hypertrophic cardiomyopathy than in those without a primary heart muscle disorder. Watson *et al.* performed right ventricular programmed electrical stimulation in 18 "high-risk" patients with hypertrophic cardiomyopathy who had experienced cardiac arrest ($n=3$) or syncope ($n=4$), had a malignant family history ($n=2$), or had nonsustained ventricular tachycardia during electrocardiographic monitoring ($n=9$).[25] Ventricular fibrillation was induced in eight patients (47%) with up to three premature stimuli during programmed ventricular stimulation and in an additional patient during atrial stimulation. Other centers have also shown that programmed electrical stimulation can initiate sustained ventricular tachycardia or fibrillation in a significant proportion of patients (28 of 150, 19% using two premature ventricular stimuli; 16 of 41, 39% using three premature ventricular stimuli or incremental atrial pacing) (Table 3). The high rate of inducible ventricular tachycardia and fibrillation in low risk as well as apparently high-risk patients supports the contention that patients with hypertrophic cardiomyopathy may be unusually vulnerable to spontaneous ventricular tachyarrhythmias, particularly in the presence of ischemia or hemodynamic collapse.[25–27] The prognostic significance of these findings, however, will be uncertain until the clinical outcome has been determined in more patients.

What is the potential for programmed electrical stimulation to improve upon the sensitivity ($\geq 69\%$) of ECG monitoring for the identification of the high-risk adult with hypertrophic cardiomyopathy? As ECG monitoring identifies most of the adults who are at high risk, electrophysiological studies may be more profitably performed in selected "high-risk" patient populations. As discussed above, the predictive accuracy of ventricular tachycardia is low (22%). Programmed stimulation as well as assessment

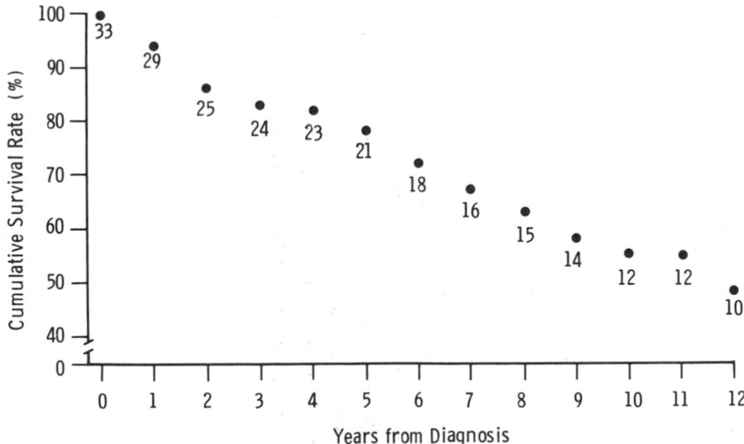

Fig. 3. Cumulative survival curve from the year of diagnosis for 33 medically treated patients. Their obability of death equals the total number of deaths for the year divided by the adjusted number at risk minus the number of deaths due to other causes. (Reproduced with permission from McKenna and Deanfield,[28] *Arch. Dis. Childhood* **59**: 971–975, 1984.)

of left and right ventricular function may provide measurements that will improve the predictive accuracy and identify those patients with episodes of nonsustained ventricular tachycardia during ECG monitoring who are at greatest risk and warrant more vigorous treatment.

Thus far we have reviewed the identification of the adult who is at high risk. Children and adolescents with hypertrophic cardiomyopathy, however, have a much higher annual mortality from sudden death, approximately 6%.[1,28] Patients with a family history of multiple sudden deaths are recognized to be at particular risk.[1,29] However, children and adolescents without such a "malignant" family history still have an annual mortality from sudden death of over 4% (Fig. 2).[28] Apart from syncopal episodes, which are associated with sudden death, other clinical features and electrocardiographic and hemodynamic measurements are similar in those who die suddenly and survive and do not help identify the young who are at particularly high risk. The majority of children and adolescents who die suddenly do not have significant limitation of exercise tolerance nor have they experienced syncope; when syncope does occur, however, this is ominous, and in our retrospective analysis of 37 young patients, it was 86% specific for subsequent sudden death.[28] In addition, arrhythmias during ECG monitoring are uncommon in children and adolescents and are not of prognostic value.[7] Thus, in patients with hypertrophic cardiomyopathy who are at greatest risk, many of whom are not only young but also asymptomatic, current clinical and hemodynamic evaluation is of limited value in the identification of most of those who will die suddenly.

Mechanism of Sudden Death

Patients with hypertrophic cardiomyopathy are often unable to maintain stroke volume and increase cardiac output appropriately during exercise, presumably because of the shortened time for filling of a poorly relaxing and noncompliant left ventricle.[30,31] It is well recognized that tachycardia may be associated with hypotension, ischemia, and symptoms of angina or impaired consciousness. A recent case report by Stafford *et al.* is of interest in this regard.[10] A 15-year-old youth who presented with cardiac arrest and documented ventricular fibrillation was found to have hypertrophic cardiomyopathy without a gradient but with diffuse left ventricular hypertrophy. At electrophysiological study there was no evidence of an accessory pathway, and no ventricular arrhythmias were inducible during programmed ventricular stimulation. Atrial stimulation, however, initiated sustained atrial fibrillation with a ventricular response of 180 to 190 beats/min. This rhythm, associated with hypotension and evidence of myocardial ischemia, degenerated into ventricular fibrillation.

The cause of sudden death in hypertrophic cardiomyopathy is rarely ascertained. The low incidence of spontaneous arrhythmias in the young suggests that, in this subgroup of patients, a primary arrhythmia is less likely. We speculate that in some adults, but particularly in the young, the precipitating event is most often hemodynamic, with a decrease in stroke volume and hypotension in relation to emotion- or exercise-related tachycardia; a primary supraventricular tachyarrhythmia as the cause of the tachycardia is also possible.[23,25,26,32] The outcome, survival sudden death, is then determined by the vulnerability of the myocardium to spontaneous life-threatening arrhythmias (Fig. 4). In the adult, nonsustained ventricular tachycardia during ECG monitoring may be a marker of this, while in children and adolescents, no such marker has been identified to date. The extent and severity of myocardial disarray must be an important determinant of the electrical stability of the myocardium. Myocardial disarray is greater in young patients who die suddenly than in adults who die suddenly or from other causes,

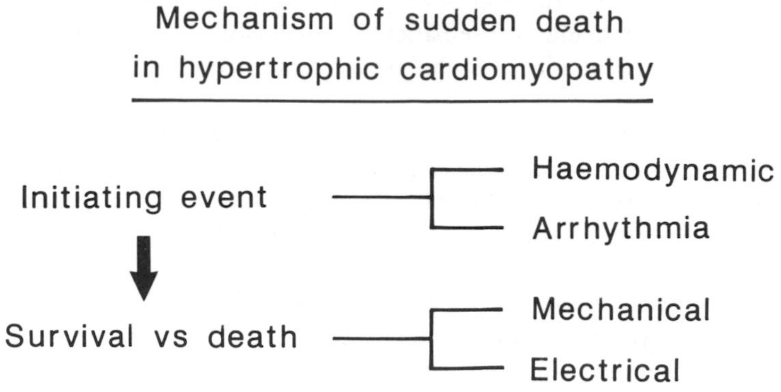

Fig. 4. See description in text.

but the severity and distribution of disarray is not closely related to the severity and distribution of hypertrophy and at present can only be reliably assessed at postmortem examination.[33,34]

MANAGEMENT

Supraventricular Arrhythmias

Established atrial fibrillation should be treated with conventional antiarrhythmic agents, digoxin, and when required, a β-blocker or verapamil for improved control of the ventricular response. Digoxin is contraindicated in patients with hyperdynamic systolic function and a significant gradient, but atrial fibrillation is unusual in such patients and more often occurs in those with normal or impaired indices of systolic performance. In our experience with amiodarone, restoration and maintenance of sinus rhythm is possible in approximately 35% of patients with chronic atrial fibrillation who have been refractory to cardioversion with or without a class 1 agent.[35] Restoration of sinus rhythm in patients who have been in atrial fibrillation for many years, however, is rarely associated with significant improvement in exercise capacity. Indeed the theoretical benefits of maintaining sinus rhythm overstate the situation. In most patients, the classical progression from a loud fourth heart sound to a palpable atrial beat without an audible fourth heart sound and the subsequent development of atrial fibrillation is usually associated with a progressive loss of atrial systolic contribution to stroke volume. As long as the ventricular response is controlled and is not excessively variable, patients may be unaware of changes from atrial fibrillation to sinus rhythm. When the recent onset of atrial fibrillation is associated with significant symptomatic deterioration, however, restoration of sinus rhythm is important and may be facilitated by treatment with amiodarone for four to six weeks prior to cardioversion.[35] We also use low-dose amiodarone (1,000 to 1,400 mg/week) for patients with refractory paroxysmal supraventricular arrhythmias with episodes which are frequent, prolonged, or symptomatic. Whether such therapy attenuates the development of atrial fibrillation or the risk of thromboembolism is unproven. Anticoagulation is necessary in patients with frequent or sustained supraventricular arrhythmias.

Many consider the use of amiodarone inappropriate in patients who have arrhythmias which are symptomatic but not life threatening. The well-known side effects profile of amiodarone, however, has been developed in patient populations that required plasma amiodarone concentrations of 1.5 to 2.5 mg/l, two to three times the levels necessary for successful management of supraventricular arrhythmias in hypertrophic cardiomyopathy.[35–38] In such patients with hypertrophic cardiomyopathy, the interaction of amiodarone with digoxin and particularly warfarin is an important unwanted effect of the drug.[35] Amiodarone increases the plasma concentration of digoxin and potentiates the effect of anticoagulants by mechanisms which are not clearly defined. A reduction of digoxin and warfarin dosages by approximately 50% and careful monitoring during the first two to three weeks is important to avoid complications.[38]

Ventricular Arrhythmias

Symptomatic or sustained ventricular arrhythmias in hypertrophic cardiomyopathy are rare. In our series, ventricular tachycardia was sustained (>30 sec) in only two of 52 patients with documented episodes, and both patients also had the uncommon finding of a left ventricular apical aneurysm with normal coronary arteries.[39] Reports from arrhythmia referral centers include eight patients with hypertrophic cardiomyopathy and documented clinical ventricular tachycardia or fibrillation[20,22,23]; such patients, even in tertiary referral centers, are uncommon. Although one study suggested that programmed electrical stimulation would define an arrhythmic cause of syncope or cardiac arrest,[20] larger series reveal that with conventional protocols arrhythmias are induced in an equal proportion of patients (approximately 20%) with and without such events.[23,26] The observed endpoint of sustained ventricular tachycardia or cardiac arrest may relate to a primary supraventricular or ventricular arrhythmia or be a consequence of structural and/or hemodynamic abnormalities. Such patients present a challenging management problem and require careful assessment to define the likely initiating mechanism in order to target therapy. This will be important in selecting appropriate patients for implanatation of automatic defibrillators.

Identification and Treatment of High-Risk Patients

In the evaluation of adults and particularly children and adolescents with hypertrophic cardiomyopathy, future studies should characterize patients in relation to likely mechanisms of sudden death. This should include an assessment of both the propensity for hemodynamic collapse as well as the vulnerability of the myocardium to life-threatening arrhythmias. The optimal method of acquiring this information has not been determined and may differ in patient subgroups, particularly in relation to age and perhaps in relation to the severity of both left ventricular hypertrophy and functional impairment. Noninvasive tests which simulate or record events during normal daily life, such as stress testing, response to physiological maneuvers, and ECG monitoring, can be broadly applied, while invasive investigations, particularly electrophysiological studies, are more appropriate in selected subgroups. It is important that patients with hypertrophic cardiomyopathy are better characterized in relation to likely mechanisms of sudden death, as the pharmacological and surgical treatments may significantly improve prognosis if they are applied appropriately.

The role of surgery in the prevention of sudden death remains to be defined. At present, surgery is usually reserved for patients with refractory symptoms who have features of left ventricular outflow tract "obstruction." Whether myotomy/myectomy will prevent hemodynamic collapse and improve prognosis requires evaluation. Although there is no convincing evidence to suggest that symptomatic therapy with β-blockers[1,16] or calcium antagonists improves prognosis, the use of low-dose amiodarone (initially 300 mg, more recently 200 mg daily) in patients with nonsustained ventricular tachycardia during ECG

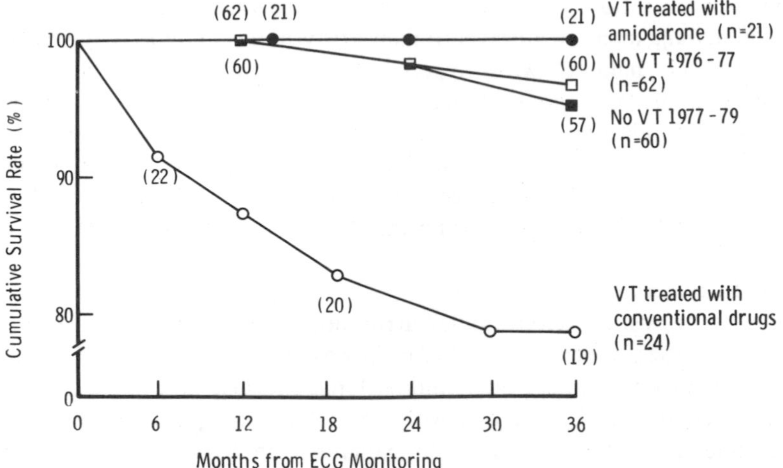

Fig. 5. Cumulative survival rate for 24 patients with ventricular tachycardia treated with conventional antiarrhythmic agents (○), 21 with ventricular tachycardia treated with amiodarone (●), and 122 without ventricular tachycardia (□). The probability of cardiac death is equal to the total number of deaths for the year divided by the adjusted number at risk minus the number of deaths due to other causes. (Adapted from McKenna *et al.*[40])

monitoring is associated with improved survival (Fig. 5).[40] There have been no deaths in 21 adults who received amiodarone and who have now been followed for at least five years, compared with 7% annual mortality over a three-year period in an earlier consecutive control group that received conventional class 1 agents. The two groups with nonsustained ventricular tachycardia were well matched for age and sex, clinical, prognostic, echocardiographic, and hemodynamic features, and arrhythmia characteristics.[40] In addition, all patients were evaluated during a period when referral sources, diagnostic criteria and methods, and symptomatic treatment did not change at our institution. Plasma amiodarone and desethylamiodarone concentrations of 1.4 ± 0.7 were necessary for suppression of episodes of nonsustained ventricular tachycardia.[35] Serious side effects were rare; however, troublesome unwanted effects, particularly photosensitivity and sleep disturbance, were common.[35]

The finding of nonsustained ventricular tachycardia during ECG monitoring is associated with subsequent sudden death, but it is now apparent that these arrhythmias are unlikely to be pathogenetic, i.e., directly or indirectly initiate ventricular fibrillation. The mechanism of the beneficial effect of amiodarone is uncertain. The drug has many actions, and suppression of supraventricular arrhythmias, control of the ventricular response, increased ventricular fibrillation thresholds, and sympathetic antagonism may all be relevant. It is of interest that the protective action of amiodarone has been maintained despite lower doses and recurrence of the "marker" arrhythmias and that there have been no sudden deaths after three years in 15 high-risk adolescents who also received very low-dose amiodarone (500–1,000 mg/week, with plasma concentrations of 0.5 mg/l).[7] The effect of low-dose amiodarone on mortality needs to be assessed in a prospective randomized trial in young patients with hypertrophic cardiomyopathy once a risk factor characterization has identified those who are particularly vulnerable to hemodynamic and/or electrical collapse.

REFERENCES

1. McKenna, W.J., Deanfield, J., Faruqui, A., England, D., Oakley, C.M., and Goodwin, J.F. Prognosis in hypertrophic cardiomyopathy: Role of age and clinical, electrocardiographic and hemodynamic features. *Am. J. Cardiol.* **47**: 532–538, 1981.
2. Maron, B.J., Bonow, R.O., Cannon, R.O. III, Leon, M.B., and Epstein, S.E. Hypertrophic cardiomyopathy. Interrelations of clinical manifestations, pathophysiology, and therapy. *N. Engl. J. Med.* **316**: 780–789, 1987.
3. Savage, D.D., Seides, S.F., Maron, B.J., Myers, D.M., and Epstein, S.E. Prevalence of arrhythmia during 24 hour electrocardiographic monitoring and exercise testing in patients with obstructive and nonobstructive hypertrophic cardiomyopathy. *Circulation* **59**: 866–875, 1979.
4. Maron, B.J., Savage, D.D., Wolfson, J.K., and Epstein, S.E. Prognostic significance of 24 hour ambulatory electrocardiographic monitoring in patients with hypertrophic cardiomyopathy. A prospective study. *Am. J. Cardiol.* **48**: 252–257, 1981.
5. McKenna, W.J., England, D., Doi, Y.L., Deanfield, J.E., Oakley, C.M., and Goodwin, J.F. Arrhythmia in hypertrophic cardiomyopathy: I. Influence on prognosis. *Br. Heart J.* **46**: 168–172, 1981.
6. McKenna, W.J., Krikler, D.M., and Goodwin, J.F. Arrhythmias in dilated and hypertrophic cardiomyopathy. *Med. Clin. N. Am.* **68**: 983–1000, 1984.
7. McKenna, W.J., Franklin, R.C.G., Nihoyannopoulos, P., Robinson, K.R., and Deanfield, J.E. Arrhythmia and prognosis in infants, children and adolescents with hypertrophic cardiomyopathy. *J. Am. Coll. Cardiol.* **11**: 147–153, 1988.
8. Newman, H., Sugrue, D.D., Oakley, C.M., Goodwin, J.F., and McKenna, W.J. Relation of left ventricular function and prognosis in hypertrophic cardiomyopathy: An angiographic study. *J. Am. Coll. Cardiol.* **5**: 1064–1074, 1985.
9. Spirito, P., Watson, R.M., and Maron, B.J. Relation between extent of left ventricular hypertrophy and occurrence of ventricular tachycardia in hypertrophic cardiomyopathy. *Am. J. Cardiol.* **60**: 1137–1142, 1987.
10. Stafford, W.J., Trohman, R.G., Bilsker, M., Zaman, L., Castellanos, A., and Myerburg, R.J. Cardiac arrest in an adolescent with atrial fibrillation and hypertrophic cardiomyopathy. *J. Am. Coll. Cardiol.* **7**: 701, 1986.
11. Maron, B.J., Spirito, P., Green, K.J., Wesley, Y.E., Bonow, R.O., and Arce, J. Noninvasive assessment of left ventricular diastolic function by pulsed Doppler echocardiography in patients with hypertrophic cardiomyopathy. *J. Am. Coll. Cardiol.* **10**: 733–742, 1987.
12. Bonow, R.O., Frederick, T.M., Bacharach, S.L., Green, M.V., Goose, P.W., Maron, B.J., and Rosing, D.R. Atrial systole and left ventricular filling in patients with hypertrophic cardiomyopathy. *Am. J. Cardiol.* **51**: 1386–1391, 1983.

12a. Nicod, P., Polikar, R., and Peterson, K.L. Hypertrophic cardiomyopathy and sudden death. *N. Engl. J. Med.* **318**: 1255–1257, 1988.

13. Glancy, D.L., O'Brien, K.P., Gold, H.K., and Epstein, S.E. Atrial fibrillation in patients with idiopathic hypertrophic subaortic stenosis. *Br. Heart J.* **32**: 652–659, 1970.
14. Robinson, K.R., Stockins, B., Dickie, S., and McKenna, W.J. Management of atrial fibrillation in hypertrophic cardiomyopathy (abstr.). *J. Am. Coll. Cardiol.* **9** (suppl. A): 117A, 1987.
15. Fuster, V., Gersh, B.J., Giuliani, E.R., *et al.* The natural history of idiopathic dilated cardiomyopathy. *Am. J. Cardiol.* **47**: 525–531, 1981.
16. Maron, B.J., Roberts, W.C., and Epstein, S.E. Sudden death in hypertrophic cardiomyopathy: A profile of 78 patients. *Circulation* **65**: 1388–1394, 1982.
17. Mulrow, J.P., Healy, M.J.R., and McKenna, W.J. Variability of ventricular arrhythmias in hypertrophic cardiomyopathy and implications for treatment. *Am. J. Cardiol.* **58**: 615–618, 1986.
18. Schiavone, W.A., Maloney, J.D., Lever, H.M., Castle, L.W., Sterba, R., and Morant, V.

Electrophysiologic studies of patients with hypertrophic cardiomyopathy presenting with syncope of undetermined etiology. *Pace.* **9**: 476–481, 1986.

19. Anderson, K.P., Stinson, E.B., Derby, G.C., Oyer, P.E., and Mason, J.W. Vulnerability of patients with hypertrophic obstructive cardiomyopathy to ventricular arrhythmia induction in the operating room. *Am. J. Cardiol.* **51**: 811–816, 1983.
20. Kowey, P.R., Eisenberg, R., and Engel, T.R. Sustained arrhythmias in hypertrophic obstructive cardiomyopathy. *N. Engl. J. Med.* **310**: 1566, 1984.
21. Ingham, R.E., Mason, J.W., Rossen, R.M., Goodman, D.J., and Harrison, D.C. Electrophysiologic findings in patients with idiopathic hypertrophic subaortic stenosis. *Am. J. Cardiol.* **41**: 811–816, 1978.
22. Geibel, A., Brugada, P., Zehender, M., Kersschot, I., and Wellens, H.J.J. Results of a standardized ventricular stimulation protocol in patients with hypertrophic cardiomyopathy (abstr.). *J. Am. Coll. Cardiol.* **7**: 195A, 1986.
23. Borggrefe, M., Podczeck, A., and Breithardt, G. Electrophysiologic studies in hypertrophic cardiomyopathy (abstr). *Circulation* **74** (suppl. II): II–1922, 1986.
24. Kunze, K.-P., Kuck, K.-H., Geiger, M., and Bleifeld, W. Programmed electrical stimulation in hypertrophic cardiomyopathy—specificity and sensitivity of different stimulation protocols (abstr.). *J. Am. Coll. Cardiol.* **7**: 195A, 1986.
25. Watson, R.M., Liberati Schwartz, J., Maron, B.J., Tucker, E., Rosing, D.R., and Josephson, M.E. Inducible polymorphic ventricular tachycardia and ventricular fibrillation in a subgroup of patients with hypertrophic cardiomyopathy at high risk for sudden death. *J. Am. Coll. Cardiol.* **10**: 761–774, 1987.
26. Kuck, K.-H., Kunze, K.-P., Schluter, M., Nienaber, C.A., and Costard, A. Programmed electrical stimulation in hypertrophic cardiomyopathy. Results in patients with and without cardiac arrest or syncope. *Eur. Heart J.* **9**: 177–185, 1988.
27. McKenna, W.J. Sudden death in hypertrophic cardiomyopathy: Identification of the high risk patient. In: Cardiac Arrhythmias: Where to Go from Here? Brugada, P., and Wellens, H.J.J. (eds.), Mount Kisco, New York, Futura Publishing Co., 1987, pp. 353–365.
28. McKenna, W.J. and Deanfield, J.E. Hypertrophic cardiomyopathy: an important cause of sudden death. *Arch. Dis. Child.* **59**: 971–975, 1984.
29. Maron, B.J., Lipson, L.C., Roberts, W.C., Savage, D.D., and Epstein, S.E. "Malignant" hypertrophic cardiomyopathy: identification of a subgroup of families with unusually frequent premature death. *Am. J. Cardiol.* **41**: 1133–40, 1978.
30. Goodwin, J.F. and Oakley, C.M. The cardiomyopathies. *Br. Heart J.* **34**: 545–552, 1972.
31. Edwards, R.H.T., Kristinsson, A., Warrel, D.A., and Goodwin, J.F. Effects of propranolol on response to exercise in hypertrophic cardiomyopathy. *Br. Heart J.* **32**: 219–225, 1970.
32. Krikler, D.M., Davies, M.J., Rowland, E., *et al.* Sudden death in hypertrophic cardiomyopathy: Associated accessory atrioventricular pathways. *Br. Heart J.* **43**: 245–251, 1980.
33. Maron, B.J. and Roberts, W.C. Quantitative analysis of cardiac muscle cell disorganisation in the ventricular septum of patients with hypertrophic cardiomyopathy. *Circulation* **59**: 689–706, 1979.
34. Maron, B.J., Anan, T.J., and Roberts, W.C. Quantitative analysis of cardiac muscle cell disorganisation in the ventricular wall of patients with hypertrophic cardiomyopathy. *Circulation* **63**: 882–894, 1979.
35. McKenna, W.J., Harris, L., Rowland, E., Kleinebenne, A., Krikler, D.M., Oakley, C.M., and Goodwin, J.F. Amiodarone for long-term management of hypertrophic cardiomyopathy. *Am. J. Cardiol.* **54**: 802–810, 1984.
36. Greene, H.L., Graham, E.L., Werner, J.A., *et al.* Toxic and therapeutic effects of amiodarone in the treatment of cardiac arrhythmias. *J. Am. Coll. Cardiol.* **2**: 1114–1128, 1983.
37. Haffajee, C.I., Love, J.C., Canada, A.T., Lesko, L.J., Asdourian, G., and Alpert, J.S. Clinical pharmacokinetics and efficacy of amiodarone for refractory tachyarrhythmias. *Circulation* **67**: 1347–1355, 1983.
38. Mason, J. Amiodarone. *N. Engl. J. Med.* **316**: 455–466, 1987.

39. Alfonso, F., Frenneaux, M.P., Cripps, T.R., Rowland, E., and McKenna, W.J. Clinical sustained monomorphic ventricular tachycardia in hypertrophic cardiomyopathy: Association with left ventricular apical aneurysm. *Br. Heart J.* 1988 (submitted).
40. McKenna, W.J., Oakley, C.M., Krikler, D.M., and Goodwin, J.F. Improved survival with amiodarone in patients with hypertrophic cardiomyopathy and ventricular tachycardia. *Br. Heart J.* **53**: 412–416, 1985.

Keyword Index

The numbers refer to the first pages of papers on these subjects.

adenylate cyclase, 113
adrenergic receptor, 141; α -,73; β -,73, 113
amiodarone, 335, 343, 373
angina, 335
apical hypertrophic cardiomyopathy, 293
apical hypertrophy, 203, 293
asymmetric hypertrophy of interventricular septum, 15
atrial fibrillation, 373
autosomal dominant trait, 171

biopsy of HCM, 59
BMHD (bizarre myocardial hypertrophy with disorganization), 59
β-blocking agents, 335, 348; *see also* propranolol

cAMP content, 113
calcium blocking agents, 335, 343; *see also* verapamil
cardiac output, 251
cardiac transit times, 251
case-control study, 203
cavity obliteration, 327
cell culture, 73
congestive heart failure, 129
contractile proteins, 73
color Doppler imaging, 271
coronary artery disease, occlusive, 335
coronary flow, 219; *see also* myocardial blood flow

definition of HCM, 3
diagnosis of HCM, 59
diastolic dysfunction, 171
diastolic filling, 219
disarray, 47; myocyte, 27
diurnal change, 155
dyspnea, 335

echocardiography, 283
electrophysiological study, 373
elederly HCM, 203
endomyocardial biopsy, 59
environmental factors, 193
epinephrine, 141
exercise tests, 251

familial cardiomyopathy, 187
familial occurrence, 203; *see also* genetics; inheritance
fatty acid metabolism, 237
fibrosis, 47; myocardial, 27

Gauer-Henry phenomenon, 327
gene regulation, 73
genetic counselling, 171
genetic factors, 193
genetics, 187; *see also* familial occurrence; inheritance
giant negative T wave, 155, 293
glucose utilization, 237

heart rate, 251
hemodynamics, 343
HLA, 187
hypertrophy;
cellular, 113; histological, 15; heart and myocyte, 47;myocardial, 15, 73; myocyte, 27,59; pathologic, 73, 113; physiologic, 113 ; *see also* left ventricular hypertrophy ; right ventricular hypertrophy
hypertension, 203, 293; heart with, 47
hypertrophic cardiomyopathy associated with systemic disorders, 27; in animals, 27; in elderly, 203
hypertrophic heart disease, 59

idiopathic hypertrophic subaortic stenosis, 311; *see also* muscular subaortic stenosis; obstructive hypertrophic cardiomyopathy
inheritance, 203, 293; *see also* genetics; familial occurrence
interstitial cleft, 15
intramyocardial vessel disease, 15; *see also* small vessel disease
isoproterenol, 155
isozymic heavy chain cDNA, 97

left ventricular hypertrophy, 59; pattern of, 171; progression of, 171; within pedigree, 171; *see also* hypertrophy

magnetic resonance imaging, 283
mid-ventricular obstruction, 271
mitral regurgitation, 271
mitral-septal contact, 327
monoclonal antibody, 97
muscular subaortic stenosis, 311; *see also* idiopathic hypertrophic subaortic stenosis; obstructive hypertrophic cardiomyopathy
myocardial blood flow, 237; *see also* coronary flow
myocardial ischemia, 219
myosin isozyme, 97

neural elements in hypertrophic cardiomyopathy, 27
nomenclature, 3
norepinephrine, 113, 129, 141
Northern blot hybridization, 97

obstructive hypertrophic cardiomyopathy, 271, 311; *see also* idiopathic hypertrophic subaortic stenosis; muscular subaortic stenosis
oncogene, cellular, 97
outflow obstruction, 15, 327

parasympathetic function, 155
phosphoinositides, 73
positron emission tomography (PET), 237
prognosis, 343
propranolol, 155, 251
protein kinase C, 73
pulmonary artery pressure, 251

quantitative analysis, 47

right ventricular hypertrophy, 59; *see also* hypertrophy

small coronary artery, stenosis of, 47
small vessel disease, 219
spade-shaped configuration, 293
sporadic occurrence, 171
stroke volume, 251
subvalvular myectomy, 251
sudden death, 373
sympathetic activity, 141

thallium scintigraphy, 219
thickening of anterior mitral leaflet, 27
thickening of endocardium of the left ventricular outflow tract, 27

vascular abnormalities, 27
ventricular arrhythmias, 251
ventricular emptying, 327
ventricular tachycardia, 373
verapamil, 251